Saunders
Nursing Survival Guide
Pathophysiology

Second Edition

Kathleen Jo Gutierrez, PhD, RN, ANP-BC, CNS-BC
Independent Practice, Littleton, Colorado
Associate Professor, School of Nursing
University of Colorado at Denver Health Sciences Center
Denver, Colorado

Phyllis Gayden Peterson, RN, MN, APRN
Assistant Professor, Division of Nursing
Our Lady of Holy Cross College
New Orleans, Louisiana

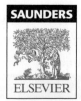

SAUNDERS

ELSEVIER

SAUNDERS
ELSEVIER

11830 Westline Industrial Drive
St. Louis, Missouri 63146

SAUNDERS NURSING SURVIVAL GUIDE: PATHOPHYSIOLOGY

ISBN-13: 978-1-4160-3048-5
ISBN-10: 1-4160-3048-4

Notice

Knowledge and best practice in this field are constantly changing. As new research and experience broaden our knowledge, changes in practice, treatment and drug therapy may become necessary or appropriate. Readers are advised to check the most current information provided (i) on procedures featured or (ii) by the manufacturer of each product to be administered, to verify the recommended dose or formula, the method and duration of administration, and contraindications. It is the responsibility of the practitioner, relying on their own experience and knowledge of the patient, to make diagnoses, to determine dosages and the best treatment for each individual patient, and to take all appropriate safety precautions. To the fullest extent of the law, neither the Publisher nor the Authors assumes any liability for any injury and/or damage to persons or property arising out or related to any use of the material contained in this book.

The Publisher

ISBN-13: 978-1-4160-3048-5
ISBN-10: 1-4160-3048-4

Acquisitions Editor: Catherine Jackson
Developmental Editor: Amanda Sunderman Politte
Editorial Assistant: Heather Bays
Publishing Services Manager: John Rogers
Project Manager: Kathleen L. Teal
Design Direction: Jyotika Shroff
Cover Art: Chris Sharp, GraphCom Corporation
Cover Designer: Jyotika Shroff

Printed in the United States of America

Last digit is the print number: 9   8   7   6   5   4   3   2   1

How to Use This Saunders Nursing Survival Guide

This book presents need-to-know information on pathophysiology in a complete, easy-to-learn format to help you master one of the most difficult subjects in nursing.

These headings walk you through each chapter:

What You WILL LEARN An introductory list of checkpoints to outline what is covered in each chapter.

What It IS A "short and sweet" section devoted to the definition and description of the topic.

What You NEED TO KNOW The essential information and skills to be mastered, with a discussion of why they are important.

What You DO Nursing interventions that apply everything you learned in the What You NEED TO KNOW section.

Do You UNDERSTAND? Various activities and exercises (with answers) so you may review and make sure you understand each topic.

Technical terms (and common hospital terms) are given with easy-to-understand explanations, and if you're likely to hear something referred to in a certain way in the hospital setting, we've highlighted the term in color.

These icons punctuate the text:

 Highlights the most important points to study or use in the clinical atmosphere.

 Alerts you to urgent information about dangerous conditions and how to avoid them.

 Points out age-related variations in signs and symptoms, nursing interventions, and patient teaching.

 Clues you in to possible variations related to a patient's cultural background.

 Instructs you to head to the Internet for additional resources.

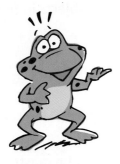

Tell Us What YOU Think

The *Saunders Nursing Survival Guide Series* has been created with the help of student feedback to serve your nursing review needs. In order to continue this tradition we invite you to voice your opinion. A website has been created to allow you the opportunity to Tell Us What YOU Think. Please, go to the website SNSGSurvey.elsevier.com, and help us continue to provide you with student focused and friendly review activities. Your ideas will be used to create new and fun ways for students like you to learn and review the difficult topics they face throughout their nursing education.

Go to: SNSGSurvey.elsevier.com and Tell Us What YOU Think. YOU Think.

About the Authors

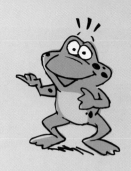

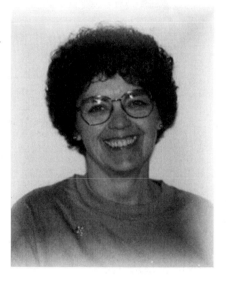

Dr. Kathleen Jo Gutierrez completed an associate degree in nursing from the Community College of Denver, a Bachelor of Science degree in nursing from Metropolitan State College of Denver, and a Master of Science degree from the University of Colorado at Denver Health Sciences Center. She also completed a post-master's program as an adult nurse practitioner through Beth El College in Colorado Springs. Her interest in education and professional development led her to a doctoral degree in education from the University of Denver.

Dr. Gutierrez is a primary health care provider in the Denver area. In the 20 years before entering private practice, she was an associate professor of nursing at Regis University in Denver and is presently an associate professor with the University of Colorado at Denver Health Sciences Center.

In addition to her work on *Saunders Nursing Survival Guide: Pathophysiology,* Dr. Gutierrez is the author and editor of *Pharmacotherapeutics: Clinical Reasoning in Practice, Pharmacotherapeutics: Clinical Decision-Making in Nursing, Pharmacology for Nursing Practice,* and co-author of *Saunders Nursing Survival Guide: Pharmacology.*

Dr. Gutierrez is named in "Who's Who in American Nursing", "Who's Who in American Education," "Who's Who in Medicine and Health Care", and most recently "Who's Who in American Women." She is board certified as both an adult nurse practitioner and medical-surgical clinical nurse specialist. She is a member of the American Nurses Association, the National Organization of Nurse Practitioner Faculties, the American Academy of Nurse Practitioners, the American Association of Diabetic Educators, and Sigma Theta Tau, the International Honor Society of Nursing.

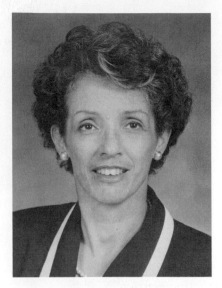

Phyllis Gayden Peterson has been a nurse for 25 years. Most of her nursing practice has been in adult medical oncology, with a special emphasis on the care of patients receiving chemotherapy and those undergoing bon e marrow transplantation. She has extensive experience as a staff nurse and in nursing administration. She holds a bachelor of arts degree in French and Spanish from Michigan State University. She earned a diploma in nursing from Charity Hospital School of Nursing in New Orleans in 1980 and a bachelor of science degree in nursing from Loyola University of the South in 1985. She completed her master's degree in adult health nursing at Louisiana State University Medical Center in 1990. She has been a member of the nursing faculty of Our Lady of Holy Cross College in New Orleans, Louisiana, since 1991. She is a clinical nurse specialist and a chemotherapy trainer for the Oncology Nursing Society, and has been a featured guest speaker at international oncology conferences. Her professional interests are biomedical ethics, symptom management, and geriatric oncology.

Contributors to the First Edition

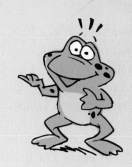

Tracey D. Allen, BSN, BS
Certified Gerontological Nurse
Nurse Consultant
New Orleans, Louisiana

Leslie S. Arceneaux, FNP, MAFN
Family Nurse Practitioner, Board Certified
Endocrinology
Ochsner Foundation Clinic
New Orleans, Louisiana

Sheila A. Arrington, MSN, RN, GNP,
   CS, OCN
Nurse Practitioner
Hematology/Oncology Department
Wake Forest University Baptist Medical Center
Winston-Salem, North Carolina

Joanne M. Bullard, BSN, MN, APRN
Assistant Professor of Nursing
Our Lady of Holy Cross College
New Orleans, Louisiana

Karen L. Beard-Byrd, MSN, RN, GNP, OCN
Nurse Practitioner
Hematology/Oncology Department
Wake Forest University Baptist Medical Center
Winston-Salem, North Carolina

Charlotte M. Cline-Taylor, MSN, RN,
   CNS, C-FNP
Nurse Practitioner Associates, Inc.
Franklin, Louisiana

Kathleen Jo Gutierrez, PhD, RN, ANP, CNS
Independent Practice, Internal Medicine
Littleton, Colorado
Affiliate Faculty
Regis University
Denver, Colorado

Linda Eilee Schmidt McCuistion, PhD, RN
Associate Professor, Division of Nursing
Our Lady of Holy Cross College
New Orleans, Louisiana

Margaret M. Mulhall, MSN, RN
Assistant Professor of Nursing
Regis University
Denver, Colorado

Mary Ann Nemcek, DNS, RN
Assistant Professor of Nursing
Loyola University
New Orleans, Louisiana
Continuing Education Coordinator
Home Care Services
Egan Health Care Services
Metairie, Louisiana

Phyllis Gayden Peterson, RN, MN, APRN
Assistant Professor
Division of Nursing
Our Lady of Holy Cross College
New Orleans, Louisiana

Karen L. Rice, MSN, APRN
Adult Nurse Practitioner and Geriatric
    Resource Nurse
Division of Nursing
Alton Ochsner Foundation Hospital
New Orleans, Louisiana

Susan M. Sciacca, RN, BSN
Staff Nurse
Craig Hospital
Englewood, Colorado

Gwen Pfeffer Skaggs, RN, BSN
Staff Nurse/Registered Nurse
Pediatric Emergency Room, Medicine Clinic
University Hospital, Medical Center of Louisiana
New Orleans, Louisiana

Eileen H. Stoll, MSN, CCRN
Assistant Professor
Division of Nursing
Our Lady of Holy Cross College
New Orleans, Louisiana

Lynn C. Wimett, EdD, MSN, RN, BSN, ANT
Assistant Professor of Nursing
Regis University
Denver, Colorado

Contributors

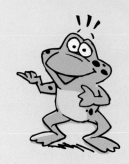

Elizabeth Wise Kissell, RN, MS
LaCasa-Quigg Newton Family Health Center
    Denver, Colorado

Linda Eilee Schmidt McCuistion, PhD, RN
Professor
Division of Nursing
Our Lady of Holy Cross College
New Orleans, Louisiana

Susan M. Sciacca, RN, BSN
Affiliate Faculty
Regis University
Denver, Colorado

Eileen Hellwig Stoll, MSN, RN, CCRN
Assistant Professor
Division of Nursing
Our Lady of Holy Cross College
New Orleans, Louisiana

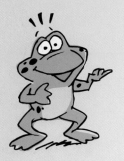

Reviewers

Nancy Burruss, RN, MSN, CCRN, APRN, BC
Assistant Professor
Bellin College of Nursing
Green Bay, Wisconsin

Therese Morgan
Parkwest Hospital
Knoxville, Tennessee

Preface

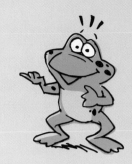

Nursing is an art, as well as a science. To assess, plan, and successfully implement a plan of care, nurses must possess a basic understanding of pathophysiology. Knowledge of pathophysiology helps you to anticipate and prevent, or at least to minimize, complications of disease processes. This book is intended to serve as a resource, offering easy-to-read information on common diseases and helping you to understand the role of nursing interventions in your patients' plans of care.

As with the first edition, we have included many features in the margins to help you focus on the most important information you will need to succeed in the classroom and in the clinical setting. TAKE HOME POINTS are composed of both study tips and "pearls of wisdom" to assist you in caring for patients. Both study tips and pearls are drawn from our many years of combined academic and clinical experience. Content marked with an alert icon ▼ is vital and usually involves considerations that may have life-threatening consequences or those that may significantly affect patient outcomes. The lifespan icon and the culture icon ☯ highlight points that are necessary for specific age or ethnic groups. A weblinks icon directs you to sites on the Internet that will give more detailed information on specific topics. Each of these icons specifically helps you focus on patient care and positive patient outcomes. Captions have now been paired with illustrations in the margin to help highlight concepts and information.

We have also continued the use of consistent headings that emphasize specific nursing actions. **What You WILL LEARN** provides a list of concepts to be learned in that chapter. **What It IS** provides a brief definition of the disease or disorder, along with a summary of the physical changes that take place as a result of a disease process. When applicable, At-Risk Populations are also specified. **What You NEED TO KNOW** summarizes the clinical manifestations, as well as prognoses and treatment regimens. **What You DO** includes bulleted lists of nursing interventions and responsibilities. As professionals, we are responsible for providing comprehensive care for our patients, including patient teaching. Finally, **Do You UNDERSTAND?** provides questions and exercises that are both entertaining and useful to reinforce the topic's concepts. This five-step approach provides information and helps you learn how to apply it in the clinical setting.

We hope this book continues to make a sometimes difficult topic easier and provide you with new insights and understanding of the affects of illness and disease. Please share the knowledge you gain with others; most of all, use this information to make a positive difference in the lives of your patients.

Kathleen Jo Gutierrez
PhD, RN, ANP-BC, CNS-BC
Phyllis Gayden Peterson
RN, MN, APRN

My heartfelt appreciation, gratitude, and thanks to
my husband and soulmate, Pat,
and to our children, Mike, Pam, and Brad,
for their undying support and understanding.

Blessed are those who have learned to admire without envy,
to follow without mimicking, to praise without flattery,
and to lead without manipulation.
Kathleen Jo Gutierrez

This book is dedicated to all those students and faculty who endured hurricane
Katrina and continue to pursue their dreams.
"When I get a little money I buy books and if any is left
I buy food and clothes."   *Erasmus*
Phyllis Gayden Peterson

Acknowledgments

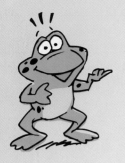

Special thanks are due to many people who participated in the preparation of the second edition of this book. Comments and suggestions from students in the original focus group provided the initial concept for this series and valuable insights from the perspective of the students of nursing education. Student nurse reviewers from Our Lady of Holy Cross College and Charity Delgado School of Nursing generously gave their time to scrutinize and critique the chapters while still in draft form and helped make the text more "student friendly."

The content in this book was provided by many different nurse experts from across the country. Without the help of our contributors, this book would not have been possible. We also extend our appreciation to Heather Bays, Amanda Politte, and Catherine Albright Jackson, editors in the nursing division of W.B. Saunders, for their patience and persistent guidance in all aspects of the publishing process.

Kathleen Jo Gutierrez
Phyllis Gayden Peterson

Contents

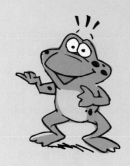

Alterations in Immune and Inflammatory Response

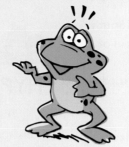

What You WILL LEARN

After reading this chapter, you will know how to do the following:

- ✔ Explain cellular defense mechanisms.
- ✔ Compare and contrast the various types of hypersensitivity reactions.
- ✔ Discuss the role of abnormal immunologic responses in the development of autoimmune diseases.
- ✔ Explain how the human immunodeficiency virus (HIV) causes immunodeficiency.
- ✔ Identify appropriate nursing interventions for the various types of hypersensitivity reactions.
- ✔ Describe nursing interventions for patients with autoimmune disorders.
- ✔ Discuss nursing interventions for patients with HIV disease.

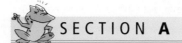

SECTION **A**

HYPERSENSITIVITY REACTIONS

This section provides information on the body's immune system, and conditions and disorders that may adversely affect this protective mechanism.

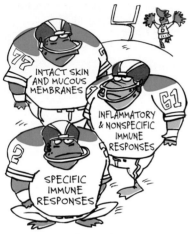

Defensive line.

Review of the Physiologic Aspects of Cellular Defense Mechanisms

The body has three main lines of defense against injury and disease. These defenses include anatomic barriers such as intact skin and mucous membranes, the inflammatory and nonspecific immune responses, and specific immune responses by antigens and activated cells. If pathogenic or disease-causing organisms penetrate the physiologic barriers, the inflammatory response will be activated.

When properly functioning, immunity is both specific and nonspecific. The immune system must recognize an invading organism as a threat and mount an appropriate response. In addition, the immune system must distinguish between foreign substances and those of our own bodies, otherwise autoimmune disorders can result.

Inflammation is a mechanism that allows cells to be repaired when subjected to stress or damage. The body has a two-pronged response to injury that is both vascular and cellular in nature. During the vascular phase, there is an increase in blood flow and capillary permeability in the damaged area. After a brief period of vasoconstriction, vasodilation occurs, increasing blood flow to the damaged area. Subsequent increased pressure in capillaries increases the movement of plasma and blood cells into the tissues, which then causes the redness and swelling that is characteristic of inflammation.

Certain agents secreted by the body are responsible for regulating the inflammatory response (mediators). Examples of these mediators include histamine, leukotrienes, prostaglandins, and platelet-activating factors. These mediators cause dilation of blood vessels, fever, and narrowing of the airways in the lungs. Further, these mediators affect the activity and effectiveness of a wide variety of white blood cells in the event of tissue damage.

Inflammatory Mediators

Mediator Type	Function
Histamine	Temporary constriction of large vessels, increased vascular permeability
Leukotrienes	Contraction of smooth muscle, greater permeability of vessels, increased motility of neutrophils and eosinophils (chemotaxis)
Prostaglandins	Increased smooth muscle contraction, vascular permeability; may modulate inflammation by suppressing the release of histamine
Platelet-activating factor	Increased vascular permeability; helps to facilitate the movement of white cells out of the vessels to damaged tissue; activates platelets

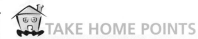 **TAKE HOME POINTS**

Drugs such as nonsteroidal antiinflammatory drugs (NSAIDs) and cyclooxygenase-2 (COX-2) inhibitors are useful in the control of pain and inflammation because they block the release of prostaglandins.

During the cellular response phase, granulocytes, (specialized white blood cells) move out of the circulatory system and into the tissues, where they clean up debris and deactivate potentially dangerous foreign organisms such as bacteria and viruses. If a similar attack occurs in the future, these specialized white cells "remember" invading organisms, a process that helps them launch a response that is significantly more rapid and aggressive.

Immune Cell Review

Cell Type	Function
Macrophages	Engulf cellular debris, present foreign proteins or antigens to lymphocytes. Phagocytic cells can be found throughout the body. Provides long-term defense and can stimulate the growth of granulocytes within the bone marrow.
Neutrophils	Move to areas of tissue damage. Important defenders against bacterial colonization and infection. Engulf and destroy cellular debris and bacteria within damaged tissue.
Eosinophils	Important in preventing parasitic infections. Active in adaptive immunity.
Basophils	Protect mucosal surfaces. Release cell mediators that promote the inflammatory response.
Mast cells	Secrete cellular mediators that support and maintain the immune response.
B lymphocytes	Produce antibodies. Provide specific immunity for antigens found outside of the host cells. Most humoral immunity requires interaction with T lymphocytes.
Antibodies (immunoglobulins [IGs])	Bind to specific antigens and promote inflammation by attracting phagocytic cells. IgG: Most common antibody to respond to infection. IgA: Prevents germs from entering through external openings. IgM: Active in primary responses; mediates cytotoxic responses. IgE: Mediates type I hypersensitivity reactions. IgD: Function unknown.
T lymphocytes	Have three main functions: helper, killer, and suppressor. Able to destroy antigens and regulate the activity of other immune cells.

Chronic or recurrent infections frequently trouble patients who have defects in cellular immunity. Genetic disorders, disease processes, malnutrition, and abuse of alcohol and certain drugs (e.g., steroids) can adversely affect white cell function.

What IS a Type I Hypersensitivity Reaction?

Hypersensitivity reactions are the result of an extreme response of the immune system to an antigen and are characterized by the destruction of healthy tissue. An antigen is a foreign protein that stimulates an immune response in a susceptible individual. Type I reactions are noted for their rapid and occasionally dramatic onset of symptoms. Symptoms of type I reactions range from the sniffling and runny nose commonly present with hay fever to the respiratory distress, generalized edema, and cardiopulmonary arrest commonly observed with anaphylaxis. Atopic symptoms affect the skin, respiratory, and gastrointestinal systems because these tissues contain a large number of mast cells.

Pathogenesis

Type I reactions are the result of an excessive or inappropriate production of immunoglobulin (Ig) E antibodies after exposure to an environmental antigen. With initial exposure to the allergen, IgE forms, attaches to mast cells, and forms a complex. The complex is a large molecule and is more likely to stimulate an allergic response. With subsequent exposure to the allergen, tiny sacs in the mast cells break open and release a vasoactive substance known as histamine, which then triggers the inflammatory response.

At-Risk Populations

Allergies tend to be hereditary. The children of allergic mothers are likely to have allergies. When both parents have allergies, the likelihood that their offspring will be allergic is at least 80%.

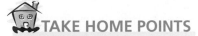

TAKE HOME POINTS

The vascular phase results in three cardinal signs of inflammation—redness, warmth, and swelling in an area of tissue damage. A normal inflammatory response promotes healing from injury due to trauma, burns, or pathogens. In some cases, an exaggerated, prolonged, or inappropriate inflammatory response damages the host, resulting in chronic inflammatory diseases and even life-threatening complications, such as septic shock.

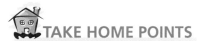

TAKE HOME POINTS

Type I reactions result from exposure to an environmental allergen. Common environmental allergens include animal dander, dust, dust mites, bee stings, certain drugs (particularly penicillin), molds, fungi, pollen, feathers, wheat, eggs, peanuts, chocolate, shellfish, and dairy products. Typically, the patient must be exposed repeatedly to the allergen to cause sufficient production of IgE to sensitize and produce an allergic response.

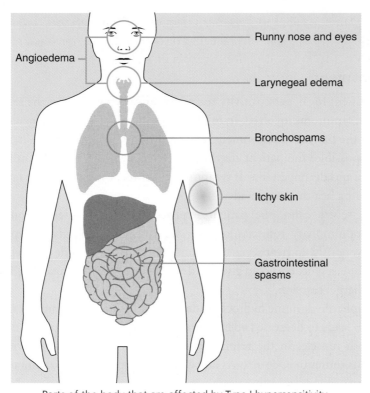

Parts of the body that are affected by Type I hypersensitivity.

- Runny nose and eyes
- Angioedema
- Larynegeal edema
- Bronchospams
- Itchy skin
- Gastrointestinal spasms

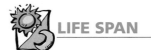

LIFE SPAN

Native Americans and African Americans are more likely to be allergic to foods containing lactose than are those of Middle European ancestry.

What You NEED TO KNOW

Clinical Manifestations

Type I hypersensitivity reactions have a sudden onset. The signs and symptoms may include watery, reddened eyes, runny nose, sneezing, wheezing, itching, shortness of breath, rashes, swelling of the face, tongue, and hands, diarrhea, and abdominal pain.

Prognosis

In most cases, type I hypersensitivity reactions can be reversed with prompt treatment and removal of the offending antigen.

What You DO

Treatment

Treatment for hypersensitivity reactions varies depending on the severity of the symptoms involved. In mild cases, removing the offending allergen from the patient's environment may be the only requirement. When this is impossible, the patient may benefit from over-the-counter antihistamines and decongestants. If symptoms continue, the patient may need to consult a health care provider.

In severe cases, the patient requires emergency intervention and cardiopulmonary resuscitation. Various drugs may be given, typically intravenously, to treat severe reactions. These drugs include methylprednisolone, a glucocorticoid given to decrease inflammation associated with the allergic reaction.

Diphenhydramine hydrochloride is given for its antihistaminic effect, which leads to decreased edema formation and decreased constriction of smooth muscles in the respiratory tract. Epinephrine can be given via various routes to open airways and constrict blood vessels to maintain the patient's blood pressure.

Nursing Responsibilities

Many patients believe they are allergic to a drug when, in reality, they are experiencing a side effect or adverse reaction caused by the drug. The patient should also know the difference between allergic and adverse reactions.

The nurse should do the following:

- Ask all patients about allergic reactions as part of the initial assessment and before administering medications. Remember to inquire about food and environmental allergies as well.
- Tell the patient to report any allergic reaction to the appropriate health care provider immediately. Document the allergy in the patient's medical record.
- Be alert to your patient's complaints. Take special note of complaints of rashes, watery eyes, runny noses, or itching, particularly in the absence of fever.
- Reevaluate the patient's initial assessment information, looking for possible explanation for the allergic reaction such as new drugs, a change in diet, or the environment. Obtain orders, as appropriate, to treat the allergic symptoms.

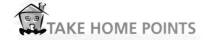

TAKE HOME POINTS

The most common drugs producing a type I hypersensivity reaction in the hospital setting, are penicillin and cephalosporin antibiotics. Patients who have an allergy to a drug in one class may also react to another drug in the same class.

- Educate your patients as to the potential for reactions from the environment, and assist them in changing their lifestyle to avoid exposure to the allergen.
- Recognizing the signs and symptoms of hypersensitivity reaction is important. For some individuals, initial hypersensitivity symptoms rapidly progress to acute respiratory distress and, ultimately, cardiopulmonary arrest.
- Teach patients with severe allergic responded to wear Medic-Alert identification at all times.

Patients with severe respiratory failure who fail to respond to drug therapy may require supportive measures, including endotracheal intubation or a tracheostomy, to maintain their airway. Respiratory support with a mechanical ventilator may also be required to help these patients breathe, in addition to further drug therapy to support their heart and vascular system.

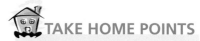
TAKE HOME POINTS

- Make certain that the patient understands ways to avoid allergen exposure in the future. Repeated exposure to an allergen puts a patient at risk for anaphylaxis, a potentially life-threatening reaction.
- Suspect an allergic reaction when itching and rash are present. Remember that cross-sensitivities can occur between related categories of drugs.
- Be prepared to initiate emergency measures for severe reactions and monitor the patient for potentially life-threatening progression of symptoms. Be certain that emergency resuscitation equipment and rescue drugs such as diphenhydramine hydrochloride, methylprednisolone, and epinephrine are readily available.

Do You UNDERSTAND?

DIRECTIONS: **Choose the option that most accurately completes the sentence.**

_____ 1. An antigen is
   a. A foreign protein capable of stimulating an immune response in anyone with a healthy immune system.
   b. A foreign protein capable of stimulating an immune response in a susceptible individual.
   c. A protein that binds with an antibody.
   d. A protein that is released by the immune system.

_____ 2. An anaphylactic reaction is an example of
   a. Type I hypersensitivity.
   b. Type II hypersensitivity.
   c. Type III hypersensitivity.
   d. Type IV hypersensitivity.

_____ 3. Histamine is released by
   a. T lymphocytes.
   b. B lymphocytes.
   c. Monocytes.
   d. Mast cells

_____ 4. Signs and symptoms of a type I reaction usually appear
   a. After chronic exposure to the allergen.
   b. 12 to 24 hours after exposure to the allergen.
   c. After only one exposure to the allergen.
   d. Soon after exposure to the allergen.

What IS a Type II Hypersensitivity Reaction?

In a type II hypersensitivity reaction, antibodies react with an antigen on the surface of a cell. In most cases, the antibodies are IgG and IgM types. The antigen can be found on the membranes of red blood cells received during a transfusion, resulting in a transfusion reaction, or from a drug adhering to the surface of the patient's own cells. Antibodies produced by the patient's own cells may cause autoimmune hemolytic anemia.

Pathogenesis

Type II reactions involve the activation of complement by antibodies, which in turn results in destruction of cells. Complement is a series of proteins that control the immune response. In the healthy individual, complement distinguishes the individual's own cells from foreign substances **(self-tolerance or self-recognition).** When this ability is lost, the individual is susceptible to autoimmune diseases.

Type II hypersensitivity reactions result primarily from blood transfusions and mismatches between the blood of a mother and her fetus. This is a tissue-specific reaction that can damage or destroy cells. After receiving a transfusion, antibodies are produced to the recipient's own blood cells that then triggers the process of hemolysis.

In some cases, disease can cause hemolytic anemia. Patients with chronic lymphocytic leukemia tend to have small, ineffective lymphocyte cells. When these cells produce antibodies, they attach to the patient's red blood cells. Hemolytic anemia has also been associated with systemic infection. Type II reactions are also thought to cause autoimmune thrombocytopenia, a platelet disorder.

TAKE HOME POINTS

- Type II hypersensitivity reactions result from the interaction of an antigen with an antibody.
- Type II reactions are observed primarily as the result of blood transfusions or mismatches between the blood of a mother and her fetus.
- Drugs occasionally cause type II reactions that result in hemolysis and anemia.

Answers: 1. b; 2. a; 3. d; 4. d.

At-Risk Populations

Anyone receiving a transfusion or drug therapy is at risk for a type II hypersensitivity reaction. Banking the patient's own blood before surgery and using donated blood only when absolutely necessary reduces the risk for a hypersensitivity reaction.

What You NEED TO KNOW

Clinical Manifestations

Signs and symptoms of type II reactions vary depending on the overall physical status of the patient and the nature of the precipitating factors. In the case of transfusion-associated hemolytic anemia, symptoms can range from mild to life-threatening. Mild symptoms include chills, fever, backache, and headache. Other symptoms include apprehension, chest pain, flank pain, elevated heart and respiratory rates, hypertension, and hemoglobinuria. Severe cases may progress to disseminated intravascular coagulation, renal failure, and circulatory collapse.

A 10% mortality rate is common when large amounts of incompatible blood are transfused.

When a pregnant woman who is Rh$^-$ becomes sensitized to the red blood cells of her Rh$^+$ fetus, *erythroblastosis fetalis* occurs in subsequent pregnancies. Ultimately, the mother's antibodies cross the placenta to attack the red cells of the fetus. Infants of mothers with toxemia, mothers who have undergone manual removal of the placenta, or mothers who have had caesarean deliveries are at additional risk for developing hemolytic anemia because these events tend to mix fetal and maternal blood. Jaundice usually appears in the neonate within 24 hours after birth. An enlarged spleen and liver can be detected in the neonate through a clinical examination. Varying degrees of anemia, ranging from mild to severe, may be present.

Autoimmune hemolytic anemia associated with disease in the adult has a wide range of symptoms depending on the severity of the anemia. In mild cases, the patient will be pale and complain of fatigue and weakness. In severe cases, the patient may be hypoxic and breathless and have symptoms of heart failure.

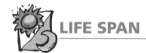

LIFE SPAN

A condition called erythroblastosis fetalis (hemolytic disease of the newborn) occurs when there is an Rh or ABO incompatibility between the blood of the mother and her fetus. As a result of the hemolytic process, the red blood cells of the fetus are destroyed.

Prognosis

The prognosis for the patient with a type II allergic reaction is highly individual and depends on the patient's underlying state of health and the severity of the reaction. Vulnerable or otherwise compromised patients are much less likely to survive an acute event.

What You DO

Treatment

In most cases, patients who are experiencing a mild type II hypersensitivity reaction may require only monitoring and supportive care. Transfusion-associated hemolytic transfusion reactions are treated with acetaminophen, antiinflammatory drugs, and intravenous fluids. Whenever a transfusion reaction is suspected, the infusion of blood should be stopped immediately and the health care practitioner notified. Do not remove the IV line. It may be needed for IV drugs used to treat the reaction. Patients with severe reactions may require aggressive measures, supportive care, and hemodialysis to survive.

Hemolytic anemia associated with disease or infection usually is refractory to treatment until the underlying cause of the problem is corrected. These patients will require supportive care, including transfusions, until they can complete appropriate treatment for their disease or illness. Hemolytic anemia is an indication for discontinuing drug therapy. In most cases, when the drug is discontinued, the hemolytic process resolves without further intervention.

Nursing Responsibilities

Transfusion-associated reactions can be prevented with meticulous cross-matching between the blood product and the proposed recipient by blood bank personnel and the nurse. In the instance of transfusion-associated hypersensitivity reactions, the nurse's most important function is preventive. Nurses must also adhere to institutional protocols and safety measures in order to ensure that all patients receive the correct blood product. When blood is drawn for a type and crossmatch for the transfusion, the nurse must be *absolutely certain* that the blood is drawn from the correct patient and labeled appropriately.

Patients who have been heavily transfused or those who have certain forms of cancers are at risk for hypersensitivity reactions and may require

⚠ • Patients with severe reactions can have damage to the renal tubules because hemoglobin prescipitates in the urine. As a result of the decreased blood flow to the kidneys, circulatory shock associated with a severe reaction can also contribute to renal failure.
• Many potentially fatal complications can result from hemolytic disease: infants who are severely affected can have hypoxia, brain damage, heart failure, and abnormal accumulations of fluid (effusions) in the heart, lungs, and abdomen.

premedication with acetaminophen and diphenhydramine before the transfusion. When blood products arrive from the blood bank, nurses must take special precautions to ensure that the correct blood product is given to the patient for whom it is intended.

When a transfusion is ordered, the nurse should do the following:
- Obtain baseline blood pressure, pulse, and temperature prior to starting the transfusion.
- Check the patient's identification band against the blood product, and the transfusion order with a second nurse.
- Take vital signs every 15 to 30 minutes during the transfusion. A decrease in blood pressure and an increase in heart rate or body temperature may indicate an early transfusion reaction.
- Observe for the presence of early symptoms such as fever and chills. These mild symptoms may indicate a need to discontinue the transfusion.
- Carefully monitor patients for evidence of a transfusion-associated hypersensitivity reaction.
- Report signs and symptoms of an hypersensitivity reaction to the health care provider in a timely fashion.

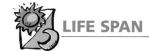

LIFE SPAN

- Treatment for erythroblastosis fetalis may include intrauterine transfusions and phototherapy following birth to decrease jaundice. Phototherapy involves exposing the infant to fluorescent light to promote the excretion of bilirubin. When phototherapy fails, a series of exchange transfusions can be performed to replace the infant's blood with compatible blood.
- *Erythroblastosis fetalis* can be prevented with appropriate obstetric care. Shortly after their first delivery, women who do not have the Rh antigen in their blood should receive the drug RhoGAM to prevent sensitization of the mother to the Rh factor.

Do You UNDERSTAND?

DIRECTIONS: **Choose the option that most accurately completes the sentence.**

_____ 1. Type II reactions can be the result of
   a. Drug therapy.
   b. Blood transfusions.
   c. Disease.
   d. All of the above.

_____ 2. While monitoring a patient receiving a blood transfusion, the nurse notes that the patient's blood pressure has fallen from 140/90 to 116/70, and the heart rate has increased from 84 to 110 beats per minute. The nurse's most immediate action should be to
   a. Decrease the rate of the transfusion.
   b. Increase the rate of the transfusion.
   c. Stop the transfusion but maintain a patent IV line.
   d. Call the health care provider

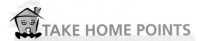

TAKE HOME POINTS

Most type II reactions can be prevented with appropriate nursing and medical care.

_____ 3. To prevent a hemolytic transfusion reaction, it would *not* be helpful to give _____ and _____.
   a. Morphine
   b. Meperidine
   c. Diphenhydramine
   d. Acetaminophen

_____ 4. Erythroblastosis fetalis is the result of
   a. ABO incompatibility between the blood of the fetus and the blood of the mother.
   b. Rh incompatibility between the blood of the fetus and the blood of the mother.
   c. Drug therapy given during pregnancy.
   d. Sensitization to foreign antibodies.
   e. Both b and d.

_____ 5. RhoGAM is given after childbirth to
   a. Treat jaundice in the neonate.
   b. Decrease hemolysis of the red blood cells in the neonate.
   c. Recent hyperbilirubinemia in the mother.
   d. Prevent sensitization of the mother to the Rh factor.

What IS a Type III Hypersensitivity Reaction?

Type III hypersensitivity reactions are the result of the body's failure to rid itself of antigen-antibody immune complexes. Immune complexes are large molecules that form when antibodies attach to antigens. The size of the complexes influence whether they remain in plasma or lodge in tissues, where they set up an inappropriate immune response that eventually results in tissue damage. Type III reactions can produce local manifestations or be systemic.

Pathogenesis

Persistent immune complexes in the circulation set up a cascade of abnormal immune responses. While in the circulation, the immune complexes may cause damage to the walls of veins, arteries, and capillaries. Eventually, these complexes deposit in areas of the body with increased vascular permeability, increasing the likelihood of disruptions in blood flow that result from increased pressure and turbulence within the vascular system. As a result, complement is released. Complement attracts macrophages and neutrophils to the area, and these release cytokines and activate the inflammatory response. This inappropriate inflammatory response can damage and destroy healthy tissue. Tissue destruction then leads to further activation of the immune response, and a vicious cycle begins. Histamine is released from mast cells, which results in increased capillary permeability and vasodilation. Increased capillary wall permeability causes edema, which then permits greater activity of inflammatory components.

The exact mechanism that causes this damaging reaction is not fully understood. Two possible causes include the formation of the antigen from a foreign protein, such as a virus or bacteria, or the formation of antibodies against self-components **(endogenous antigens).** Because autoimmune disorders tend to occur in families, a genetic link may exist for many of these disorders. Three common illnesses thought to be the result of type III reactions are glomerulonephritis, lupus, and rheumatoid arthritis.

At-Risk Populations

Patients with a family history of hypersensitivity reactions should be monitored carefully for the development of these disorders. In addition, patients with persistent infections from bacterial, viral, fungal, or protozoan organisms or people receiving treatment with allergenic drugs should be evaluated carefully for the development of hypersensitivity reactions. Prompt detection and treatment can minimize complications from tissue damage.

TAKE HOME POINTS

- Type III reactions are the result of persistent antigen-antibody complexes that set up an inappropriate immune response. This faulty immune response leads to destruction of normal healthy tissue.
- Causes of type III reactions include low-grade infections, inhalation of antigens in the environment, and the formation of autoantibodies.

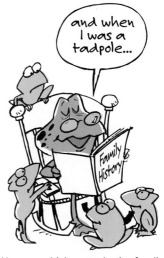

Hypersensitivity runs in the family.

TAKE HOME POINTS

- Untreated, glomerulonephritis may eventually lead to chronic renal failure, necessitating dialysis.
- Systemic lupus erythematosus (SLE) can affect any organ in the body and can cause arthritis, anemia, coagulopathies, and disturbances in central nervous system function, among other sequelae. Approximately 15% of people with SLE die within the first 5 years after diagnosis.
- Because of damage to the cartilage and joints by immune complexes, rheumatoid arthritis causes chronic, severe pain and disability. This disease also affects arteries, which may then lead to damage to major organs, including the heart, lungs, skin, and eyes.

What You NEED TO KNOW

Clinical Manifestations

Symptoms of type III hypersensitivity reactions vary depending on the organ affected by the abnormal accumulation of immune complexes. Because many symptoms are vague and nonspecific, an individual with an autoimmune disorder may be ill for quite some time before a diagnosis is established.

Prognosis

The outcome of type III hypersensitivity reactions is highly variable and is a function of the nature of the reaction and whether major organs are damaged. Other factors affecting the outcome include the ability of the individual to seek and comply with medical care, as well as the existence of other diseases and conditions that may adversely affect health.

What You DO

Treatment

Treatment involves the use of antiinflammatory drugs, antihistamines, and glucocorticoids to suppress the inflammatory response, thereby protecting healthy tissues from damage and preserving normal function. Severe cases may require the use of immunosuppressants, which can leave the individual prone to infections. The following drugs are commonly used in the treatment of hypersensitivity reactions.

- aspirin
- salsalate
- ibuprofen
- azathioprine
- cyclophosphamide
- hydroxychloroquine
- hydrocortisone sodium succinate

- methylprednisolone
- dexamethasone
- montelukast
- prednisolone
- tacrolimus

Nursing Responsibilities

Nursing care begins with a careful assessment and evaluation of the needs of the individual. Special attention should be paid to the individual with a medical history or family history of allergies. Whenever possible, ask the individual to discuss in detail the nature of the reaction. What many consider as an allergic reaction, particularly when dealing with drugs, may actually be an adverse reaction (e.g., nausea and vomiting) that is commonly observed with oral antibiotic therapy. The nurse should do the following:

- Educate patients with autoimmune diseases on the ways to cope with their disease. Include the causes of the disease, factors that may lead to an exacerbation of the symptoms, treatment regimens, and lifestyle adjustments that will help the patient minimize distressing symptoms and associated problems. Patients with autoimmune disease often require lifelong immunosuppressive therapy in order to minimize tissue damage and complications associated with these disorders.
- Teach patients the importance of adhering to a medication regimen to avoid more severe consequences, up to and including organ damage and death. Many medications prescribed for hypersensitivity reactions and associated autoimmune disorders have side effects and toxicities.
- Teach patients about symptoms that indicate a need to seek immediate medical intervention to prevent the advent of severe illness.

Do You UNDERSTAND?

DIRECTIONS: Fill in the blanks to complete the sentences using the words listed below. Words are used only once, and not all words are used.

1. Histamine is released by _____.
2. Histamine release results in _____ vascular permeability and _____.
3. _____ probably does not represent a hypersensitivity reaction.
4. Corticosteroids are helpful in the treatment of hypersensitivity reactions because they _____.

decrease	itching	vasoconstriction
increase	mast cells	vasodilation
inflammation	nausea	

What IS a Type IV Hypersensitivity Reaction?

Type IV hypersensitivity reactions differ from other hypersensitivity responses in that they are mediated by sensitized T cells. This reaction is delayed, typically occurring 24 to 72 hours after exposure to the offending antigen.

Pathogenesis

Type IV hypersensitivity is regulated by T lymphocytes that are damaging to cells **(cytotoxic)**. T lymphocytes secrete lymphokines that release inflammatory cytokines, which, in turn, attract monocytes, neutrophils, and basophils. Cytokines also activate macrophages. These cells and substances augment the inflammatory response, which serves to inactivate and destroy foreign substances. This type of reaction is a protective form of defense against certain pathogens, including mycobacteria, fungi, and parasites. However, in some circumstances this protective mechanism can backfire and result in disease, particularly when exposure to the offending antigen is over a prolonged period.

Delayed hypersensitivity reactions tend to occur in response to exposure to large antigens that are poorly soluble and difficult for the body to attack and destroy. Type IV reactions are initiated when a sensitized individual is exposed to this type of antigen. Various conditions and disorders can result from type IV reactions, including contact dermatitis due to exposure to metals or poison ivy, positive reactions to tuberculin tests, and transplant rejection.

At-Risk Populations

Even normal, healthy individuals can experience a type IV reaction if they have been previously sensitized to an antigen. Tuberculin skin testing is an example of how this reaction can be used for diagnostic purposes. Contact dermatitis is another example of a common type IV hypersensitivity reaction.

Certain chronic diseases and autoimmune conditions can also be the result of cell-mediated hypersensitivity reactions. Allergic alveolitis occurs in response to inhaled organic dusts or antigens that may be found in the home or work environment. When exposure to the antigenic substance is prolonged, chronic irreversible lung disease can result. Other disorders thought to result from type IV hypersensitivity reactions include type 1 diabetes mellitus and multiple sclerosis. In both cases, T cells react with normal host antigens to launch an inflammatory response that results in destruction of normal tissue.

Organ transplantation is also associated with type IV reactions. T lymphocytes of the organ recipient recognize foreign antigens on the cells of the donated organ. CD_8 cells mature into cytotoxic T lymphocytes and initiate the release of cytokines that mediate the inflammatory response. CD_4 cells release cytokines that lead to increased vessel permeability and promote the local accumulation of lymphocytes and macrophages, all of which begins the process of breaking down the foreign grafted tissue. When uncontrolled, the tissue damage will lead to eventual rejection of the grafted or transplanted organ.

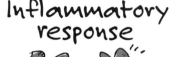

TAKE HOME POINTS

- Type IV hypersensitivity reactions are delayed reactions mediated by T lymphocytes.
- Common causes of type IV hypersensitivity reactions include chemicals, aerosolized cleaning compounds, cosmetics, plant toxins, drugs, and dyes.

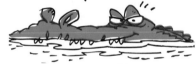

Inflammatory response

What You NEED TO KNOW

Clinical Manifestations

Symptoms of a type IV hypersensitivity reaction are highly variable depending on the body system affected and the nature of the exposure. Because this reaction is delayed, identifying the triggering factor can be difficult.

Sensitizing agents that are inhaled by susceptible individuals can cause respiratory and upper airway symptoms, such as wheezing, coughing, and shortness of breath. Repeated, prolonged exposures can lead to chronic respiratory symptoms and permanent respiratory impairment.

Prognosis

The prognosis for recovery from a type IV hypersensitivity reaction depends on the nature of the exposure and the severity and duration of the damage imposed to organs by the reaction. Contact dermatitis, one example of this type of reaction, is usually readily treated through the removal or avoidance of the causative agent.

Hypersensitivity involving the respiratory system is more problematic. Particularly after prolonged exposure, patients can develop chronic, disabling lung disease that leaves them unable to work, dependent on others for care, and with a shortened life expectancy because of eventual respiratory failure.

What You DO

Treatment

Treatment modalities for type IV hypersensitivity reactions are directed toward identifying and removing the causative agent or agents and using pharmacologic measures when necessary to speed the patient's recovery. Antihistamines such as diphenhydramine and topical and systemic corticosteroid therapy may be indicated.

Nursing Responsibilities

When caring for a patient who is experiencing a delayed hypersensitivity reaction, the nurse should do the following:

- Obtain an accurate, detailed history to help identify the source of the problem.
- Implement treatment modalities such as soothing baths, lotions, and ointments for skin involvement, as well as the administration and management of pharmacologic therapy, such as corticosteroids.
- Educate the patient regarding the nature of the allergic reaction. Help the patient develop strategies to avoid the allergic triggers and understand the ways to treat reactions if they occur in the future.

Do You UNDERSTAND?

DIRECTIONS: Unscramble the letters to form the names of diseases or situations related to type IV hypersensitivity reactions.

1. _____

   (ontcatc istredamti)

2. _____

   (brecluntui etts)

3. _____

   (jircteneo splartnat)

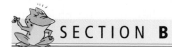

SECTION B

IMMUNODEFICIENCY DISORDERS

This section provides an overview of immunodeficiency diseases, specifically human immunodeficiency virus (HIV) disease, acquired immunodeficiency syndrome (AIDS), and B- and T-cell disorders. Since the identification of the virus that causes HIV, medical research has made significant strides in understanding of the immune system and its role in maintaining health and normal function.

Answers: 1. contact dermatitis; 2. tuberculin test; 3. transplant rejection.

What IS HIV Disease?

AIDS is the result of infection by one of two retroviruses: HIV type 1 or HIV type 2. The HIV-2 virus is more common in Africa and on the Asian continent, and also causes an AIDS type of illness. Different subtypes of both the HIV-1 and the HIV-2 virus exist, making it possible for a person to be infected with more than one type of virus.

These viruses selectively attack and destroy cells within the immune system. In the HIV retrovirus, genetic information is carried on RNA rather than DNA. A person infected with either of these viruses is said to be "HIV-positive," meaning that he or she has contracted the virus. HIV disease is a chronic illness that can be asymptomatic or manifest itself with a wide variety of symptoms. Characteristics of this disease include profound immunosuppression, opportunistic infections, cancers, and neurologic dysfunction. Patients infected with HIV experience the gradual destruction of their immune system. New drug therapies have delayed the progression of the disease and offer hope of an eventual cure.

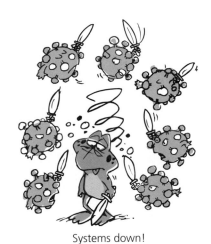

Systems down!

Pathogenesis

HIV tends to gravitate to certain types of cells within the body, including a type of lymphocyte called CD_4 cells and macrophages **(helper-inducer cells or T4 lymphocytes).** In normal states of health, lymphocyte cells play a vital role in maintaining immune function. In a healthy individual, these cells are responsible for initiating the immune response. After these helper-inducer cells recognize foreign antigens and infected cells, they stimulate B lymphocytes to produce antibodies, mobilize phagocytic cells, and influence cell-mediated immunity.

HIV is attracted to protein molecules on the surface of CD_4 cells and is also capable of infecting macrophages, monocytes, and dendritic cells. HIV is covered with a protein called gp120. This protein envelope binds to the CD_4 receptor. The virus then enters the host's cells and uses an enzyme to copy its own RNA into the host cell's DNA. Depending on the type of cell infected, the infected cell may then enter a dormant phase or release the virus into the bloodstream, where it infects other cells. Early in the disease process, HIV colonizes lymphoid tissue, particularly the spleen and lymph nodes. These areas are reservoirs for infected cells. The virus may then continue to replicate, killing the CD_4 cells and thereby promoting the spread of the infection.

Patients with HIV also suffer from abnormal B-cell function and are unable to mount an antibody response to a new antigen. Impairments in humoral immunity cause people with HIV to be at risk for infections caused by *Cytomegalovirus*, *Streptococcus pneumoniae*, and *Haemophilus influenzae*, to name but a few. Overall, patients with HIV are susceptible to a wide variety of infections, many of which cause no significant mortality or morbidity in patients with normal immune systems. Because these infections rarely occur in the healthy population, but are relatively common in patients with HIV, many of these infections are considered to be diagnostic indicators.

Because HIV generates billions of viral particles on a daily basis, the virus ultimately wins the battle against the host's immune defenses. In most cases, the CD_4 count gradually declines and the viral load in the host's blood gradually increases. As the CD_4 count decreases and virus count rises, patients experience more symptoms associated with AIDS.

In nearly all cases, the progression of HIV infection is a reflection of the host's immunologic status. Most individuals infected with HIV experience phases of the infection, as summarized in the following table.

Phases of HIV Infection

Phase	Symptoms	Physiologic Events	CD_4 Count
Incubation	None		No detectable change
Early	Fever, sore throat, mucosal ulcers, myalgias, fatigue, weight loss, enlargement of cervical lymph nodes, transient faint pink maculopapular rash. Neurologic symptoms include headache, photophobia, muscle pain, and neuropathy	Increased levels of viral production, viremia, seeding of lymphoid tissues. CD_4 lymphocytes may be depleted and the CD_4:CD_8 ratio may be reversed.	Normal
Middle or latent period	May be asymptomatic or have minor trouble—some opportunistic infections May also develop persistent generalized lymphadenopathy with symmetrical, firm, mobile and nontender nodes	Immune system intact, especially when virus is clinically latent	Normal
Crisis	Persistent fever, fatigue, weight loss, and diarrhea. Previously acquired infections such as herpesvirus may be reactivated Onset of opportunistic infections, cancers, and neurologic disorders	Failure of host defenses against virus	<500

Some individuals with HIV disease appear to have a nonprogressive form and remain asymptomatic for 10 years or more with stable CD_4 counts. Untreated, HIV infection progresses to AIDS in most individuals within 7 to 10 years.

At-Risk Populations

Transmission of HIV has been clearly proven to be via the exchange of body fluids.

High-risk behaviors include the following:

* Unprotected sexual intercourse with multiple partners, or with one partner who has engaged in high-risk behavior such as sharing needles for intravenous drug use or unprotected sexual intercourse with others. Studies indicate that rectal intercourse conveys a greater risk of transmission to the receptive partner, likely because of the increased probability of damage to the rectal mucosa. In heterosexual intercourse, male-to-female transmission of the virus is more common than is female-to-male transmissions

* Transfusions of blood and blood products before 1985, before the advent of routine screening for the AIDS virus in blood donors

* Accidental exposure to contaminated blood or body fluids in the health care setting

Because a small number of health care workers have contracted the AIDS virus through occupational exposure, the Centers for Disease Control and Prevention (CDC) recommends that universal blood and body fluid precautions be used for all patients within the health care setting.

The Occupational Safety and Health Administration (OSHA) has also mandated that personal protective gear, including latex gloves, face masks, eye shields, and waterproof gowns, must be made available to all health care workers when necessary.

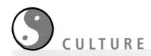

CULTURE

Risk of contracting HIV is not limited to any specific socioeconomic group or ethnic population, but is rather influenced by high-risk behaviors and situations.

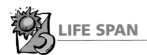

LIFE SPAN

Perinatal transmission occurs from an infected mother to her fetus. Transmission is thought to occur either in utero, during labor and delivery, or by breast-feeding after birth.

What You NEED TO KNOW

Clinical Manifestations

AIDS is not a single isolated disease process; rather, it is a syndrome with a wide variety of symptoms. During the period of initial infection, some patients experience flulike symptoms from 2 to 8 weeks after the initial exposure. These symptoms include fever, chills, headache, arthralgia, vomiting, diarrhea, sore throat, and rash. During this period, an accelerated rate of viral replication occurs, which may temporarily lower the CD_4 count. Within several weeks, the body's immune system is able to suppress viral replication.

This initial infection begins a period of latency that may last 7 to 10 years before other symptoms occur. In some cases, patients experience persistent generalized swelling of the lymph nodes (**lymphadenopathy**). Two or more sets of lymph nodes in different locations in the body may remain chronically swollen and painful for 3 months or more. During the period of latency, the CD_4 cells gradually decrease. Eventually, the individual becomes susceptible to opportunistic infections and malignancies, most of which are rare in the healthy individual.

With progressive impairment in the immune system, the typical adult patient is seen with malnutrition, weight loss, diarrhea, and gastroenteritis. Infections that attack the mucosal lining of the gastrointestinal system impair the functioning, causing profuse, watery diarrhea that can lead to a fluid loss of several liters per day. The herpes simplex virus and cytomegalovirus can cause ulcerations beginning in the mouth and extending all the way to the anus. These viral infections cause severe pain and interfere with normal digestive processes. *Candida* infections of the mouth and esophagus can cause difficulty eating and swallowing, leading to further weight loss and malnutrition. Opportunistic organisms may infect almost any organ of the immunocompromised HIV patient.

Other symptoms involve the respiratory tract. Early complaints include a persistent dry cough and progressive shortness of breath during exertion. *Pneumocystis carinii* is a common organism found both in soil and in living spaces that does not cause illness in people with a normal immune system. In people with suppressed immune systems, this organism multiplies rapidly and causes pneumonia.

Central nervous system (CNS) abnormalities are present in many AIDS patients. These symptoms can be the consequence of secondary infections from organisms such as *Toxoplasma gondii*, or may be a result of the effects of the retrovirus on the CNS. Progressive multifocal leukoencephalopathy causes a loss of the myelin covering of the nerves in the CNS. Lesions in the brain lead to dementia, blindness, and paralysis. Few people with this condition survive more than 1 year.

AIDS dementia complex has been identified as a neurologic syndrome associated with HIV. Symptoms of this disorder include a gradual decrease in cognitive function, changes in behavior, impaired concentration and

TAKE HOME POINTS

- Overall, people with coexisting sexually transmitted diseases (STDs) are at an increased risk for transmitting HIV, particularly when the STD causes genital ulceration.
- Tears and saliva have not been proven to transmit the virus.

All patients must be thought of as potential carriers of HIV.

TAKE HOME POINTS

- The person with immunocompromise from AIDS is susceptible to unusual diseases and infections including toxoplasmosis, systemic histoplasmosis, rare malignancies, and neurologic deterioration.
- AIDS is a terminal disease transmitted by the exchange of body fluids.
- With appropriate, early treatment, the average life expectancy of the person with AIDS is 10 to 15 years.

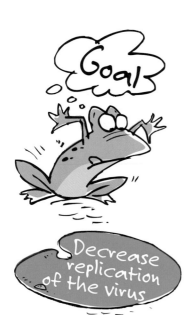

Goal

Decrease replication of the virus

memory, psychomotor slowing, and social withdrawal. Some patients experience depression and psychosis.

Various forms of neuropathy affect patients with AIDS, causing severe pain in the legs and feet, postural hypotension, and intractable diarrhea.

Because of damage to the immune system imposed by the virus, people with AIDS tend to have a higher incidence of certain malignant tumors, some of which are considered indicator diseases for the diagnosis of AIDS. Malignancies frequently present in the AIDS population include Kaposi's sarcoma, rapidly progressive cervical carcinoma, non-Hodgkin's lymphoma, and primary CNS lymphoma.

Prognosis

Although a small percentage of individuals who are HIV-positive have been identified as having nonprogressive forms of the disease, AIDS is nonetheless considered a terminal disease. Recent advances in the field of antiretroviral therapy have allowed many people with AIDS to experience a complete regression of symptoms and live normal lives, although they continue to harbor the virus and can transmit it to others. With the advent of highly active antiretroviral treatment (HAART), the immune function of patients with HIV is preserved with subsequent dramatic improvements in life expectancies.

What You DO

Treatment

Currently, the goal of therapy for HIV disease is to decrease replication of the virus. Combinations of several different antiretroviral drugs can prolong life and delay the development of full-blown AIDS. Properly taken, these drugs can suppress the virus to clinically undetectable levels. The therapy itself can pose many problems for HIV patients. In order to accomplish the greatest therapeutic benefit, the drugs must be taken on time, at precise intervals, and in such a manner that maximum absorption of the drugs is achieved.

Combination drug therapy can be extremely costly and is frequently difficult for patients to obtain. Paying the cost of medical care is a significant concern for AIDS patients, since they are often too sick to work because of their illness and, consequently, may have no health insurance benefits. Additionally, combination drug therapy has many side effects that may cause patients to be noncompliant with their medication regimen. The other goal of treatment is to provide prompt aggressive therapy for secondary diseases and complications associated with HIV.

Nursing Responsibilities

The nurse's role in caring for the patient with HIV is multifactorial. The nurse must do the following:

- Help patients with HIV achieve and maintain an optimal level of health for as long as possible.
- Prevent the spread of HIV to uninfected people. In view of the pandemic proportions of HIV infection, the general public must be educated in detail about measures to prevent the spread of the virus, but without inspiring fear to the extent that HIV-positive individuals are shunned, stigmatized, or isolated from the rest of society.
- Design and implement a series of interventions tailored to meet the specific needs of the individual throughout the course of the illness. Extensive education forms a core component of care for the patient with HIV. Most patients experience a state of shock and despair after being diagnosed with HIV. These individuals will require extensive emotional support, guidance, and counseling from the entire health care team.
- Provide information about the implications of the illness when the patient indicates they are ready to receive it. Even then, the nurse must be prepared to reinforce information with repetition and written literature. Severe emotional distress impairs the patient's ability to recall and use vital information.
- Teach the patient and family about measures to prevent spreading the disease:
  - Avoid sharing needles.
  - Use barrier precautions to prevent the exchange of body secretions during intercourse.
  - Refrain from donating blood in the presence of high-risk behaviors or possible exposure to HIV.
- Provide detailed information about treatment regimens and how to appropriately self-administer antiretroviral and other required medications. Failure to take these medications correctly may lead to a decreased therapeutic effect and drug-resistant strains of the virus.
- Teach patients how to manage side effects associated with treatments and medications.

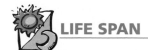

LIFE SPAN

Without treatment, the chances are 35% that the child of a mother infected with HIV disease will develop AIDS by age 5. Children with HIV disease respond well to highly active antiretroviral therapy and may have a better response to therapy than adults. Complications associated with pediatric HIV include cognitive dysfunction, impaired growth, and cardiac abnormalities.

- Antiretroviral drugs must be taken correctly and on a tightly fixed schedule to obtain maximal therapeutic benefit.
- Immunocompromise renders patients with AIDS extremely vulnerable, and they experience a high rate of mortality, particularly when timely treatment for complications of AIDS is not implemented.

HIV/AIDS Treatment Information Service (ATIS)

Provides information in English and Spanish about federally approved treatment guidelines for HIV and AIDS

http://www.hivatis.org

AIDSmeds.com

Contains complete and easy-to-read information on the treatment of HIV and AIDS

http://www.aidsmeds.com

National AIDS Treatment Advocacy Project

Dedicated to informing the HIV-positive population about the latest HIV treatment and advocating on the treatment and policy issues for people with HIV

http://www.natap.org/

HIV Insite Knowledge Base

http://hivinsite.ucsf.edu/InSite?page=all

- Teach the patient and family measures that help to reduce factors contributing to immune compromise such as:
  - Protein-calorie malnutrition
  - Pregnancy
  - Stress
  - Alcohol excess
  - Intravenous and recreational drug use
- Teach self-care measures to minimize disease-related symptoms, such as wasting and malnutrition.
- Teach strategies that help prevent opportunistic infection:
  - Avoid contact with contagious individuals and organisms found in soil, water, and human and animal feces.
  - Adhere to food safety precautions.
  - Encourage careful washing of produce.
  - Avoid raw or undercooked eggs.
  - Avoid nonpasteurized dairy products.
  - Avoid raw meats or seafood.
  - Teach hand-washing precautions.
  - Provide chemoprophylaxis against *P. carinii,* cytomegalovirus, and *T. gondii.* Teach patients how to take drugs appropriately.
- Provide skills to cope with body image changes.
- Provide information regarding where to obtain counseling, legal advice, and psychosocial support. Enlist the aid of a social worker to obtain financial assistance for the patient when necessary.
- Teach signs and symptoms that indicate the need to seek medical intervention, such as fever greater than 100.5° F, cough, and shortness of breath, intractable diarrhea, and significant weight loss.

Careful monitoring and evaluation for AIDS-associated complications must be carried out with each patient contact. Fever, cough, shortness of breath, weight loss, and changes in mental status are all potential indications of secondary diseases that must be addressed promptly to maximize the patient's chances for survival.

Nurses caring for patients with HIV and AIDS must also be prepared to cope with the emotional and social implications. For many people, this disease carries a great deal of shame and stigma. Patients may have been rejected by friends and family because of their sexual orientation, or they may have hidden their sexual orientation and now suffer severe depression and isolation because they are separated from a partner during their illness. Extensive and compassionate emotional support must be provided for this population.

Do You UNDERSTAND?

DIRECTIONS: **Choose the correct answer to each of the following questions and write the corresponding letter in the spaces provided.**

_____ 1. Which one of the following is stimulated by CD_4 cells to produce antibodies?

a. Monocyte

b. Neutrophil

c. T lymphocyte

d. B lymphocyte

_____ 2. Which one of the following is a sign and symptom of AIDS dementia?

a. Cognitive impairment

b. Loss of short-term memory only

c. Hyperactivity

d. Gait disturbances

_____ 3. A patient with AIDS has shown sudden changes in his physical status and behavior, including declining ability to perform simple tasks such as cooking a meal or caring for personal hygiene and grooming. Other symptoms include poor coordination and lethargy. Which one of the following is a possible cause of these changes?

a. CNS infection

b. CNS lymphoma

c. Multifocal leukoencephalopathy

d. All of the above

_____ 4. The AIDS virus is more likely to be transmitted in the presence of which of the following?

a. Dry, chapped skin

b. Genital ulcerations

c. Preexisting illness

d. Other infections

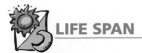

LIFE SPAN

Primary deficiencies may be either present at birth (congenital) or acquired and are not related to other causes.

_____ 5. The period of latency for HIV infection usually ends within which time frame?
a. 2 to 5 years
b. 5 to 7 years
c. 7 to 10 years
d. None of the above

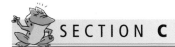

SECTION C

AUTOIMMUNE DISORDERS

Disturbances in the immune system can result in a variety of complications, including the development of autoimmune diseases. Generally, a disease is considered to be autoimmune when the body creates autoantibodies and there is T-cell activity against the host tissue. This section provides an overview of systemic lupus erythematosus (SLE), one of the more commonly occurring autoimmune diseases, and myasthenia gravis (MG). Two other diseases are also discussed: scleroderma and Sjögren's syndrome. These conditions can occur in conjunction with lupus or appear separately.

What IS Lupus?

SLE (**lupus**) is a chronic, progressive inflammatory disease characterized by periods of exacerbation and remission of symptoms. There are two forms of this disease. Discoid lupus erythematosus tends to involve only the skin and generally does not affect the internal organs. SLE eventually affects not only the skin, but also internal organs, including the kidneys, joints, lungs, heart, CNS, and gastrointestinal tract.

Pathogenesis
Lupus develops because the body forms antibodies (**autoantibodies**) to its own normal healthy tissue, including erythrocytes, coagulation

proteins, lymphocytes, and platelets. These antibodies react with the patient's tissues and lead to the formation of immune complexes. Immune complexes are accumulations of antigens and their corresponding antibodies. These immune complexes leave the circulation and may be deposited in capillaries, joints, skin, and internal organs, in which they initiate an immune response. The severity of the disease is thought to be a reflection of the degree of immune response initiated by the immune complexes. Lupus is characterized by faulty regulation of the immune response by T-cells and abnormal production of cytokines, especially interleukins 1 and 2.

The cause of this disease is unknown. Research suggests that the development of autoantibodies may be a result of many different factors, including genetic traits, hormonal influences, and immunologic and environmental factors. Environmental influences include exposure to chemicals, ultraviolet light, certain foods, and infectious agents. The disease may be exacerbated by hormone replacement therapy, oral contraceptives, and viral exposure.

The tendency of certain drugs to invoke a lupus-like reaction in susceptible individuals is well documented. Drug-induced lupus is most commonly observed with procainamide, isoniazid, hydralazine, and D-penicillamine. Contrary to the primary form of the disease, drug-induced lupus usually goes into complete remission when the causative agents are eliminated.

At-Risk Populations

SLE occurs most commonly in women between the ages of 20 and 40, although it has been diagnosed in both young children and elderly individuals.

> **!** African-American women have 3 times the incidence of lupus than Caucasian women. In this population, the disease tends to develop at a younger age and have a higher rate of serious complications and mortality than other ethnic groups.

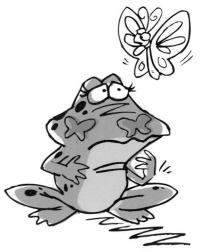

Butterfly-shaped rash=lupus.

What You NEED TO KNOW

Clinical Manifestations

Lupus has been called "the great pretender" because of the way it mimics many other diseases, which frequently causes it to be misdiagnosed. One of the few "classic" symptoms of lupus is a red, butterfly-shaped rash that covers the nose and cheeks. SLE causes a diffuse vasculitis that affects capillaries, venules, and arterioles. In mild cases the presenting symptoms may be only arthralgias and fatigue.

Less commonly observed symptoms involving the skin include mottled redness on the sides of the palms and the fingers, redness and swelling around the fingernails, and bruises (purpura). Approximately 40% of patients with lupus are sensitive to the sun.

The majority of lupus patients experience joint pain and arthritis-like symptoms at some time over the course of the disease. The arthritis associated with lupus rarely causes joint destruction, but complications such as osteonecrosis, local heat and swelling, stiffness, joint pain, and ulnar deviation of the fingers are frequently present.

Other symptoms include persistent fevers and malaise (in the absence of proven infections), vascular headaches, seizures, and psychoses. Symptoms involving connective tissue can include arthritis-like joint pain that is occasionally present for years before other evidence of the disease appears. Renal compromise can appear at any time over the course of the disease, even when other symptoms of lupus are absent.

Over one half of patients with lupus experience skin changes that may potentially cause pain, itching, and scarring. The facial butterfly rash characteristic of lupus can range from faint redness to severe eruptions and scaling. Ulcerations may also develop in the mucosa, and scalp hair loss occurs in up to one half of lupus patients. Severe itching can occur with lupus skin lesions.

Pericarditis, myocarditis, and vasculitis are frequently part of the disease process. Vascular abnormalities cause the patient to have an increased risk of venous and arterial blood clots (arterial thromboses) in the extremities. Complaints of chest pain that worsens with deep inspirations (pleuritic chest pain) are believed to be a result of inflammation of the pleural lining. These abnormalities can result in decreased cardiac function, impaired gas exchange, and poor tissue perfusion.

Most patients with lupus have asymptomatic renal damage as a consequence of their disease. Fewer than one half of patients with lupus have clinically detectable renal disease. Potential warning signs include nausea and vomiting, pruritus, anorexia, facial swelling, weight gain, edema of the lower extremities, breathlessness, cough, proteinuria, nocturia, and urinary frequency.

Neurologic changes secondary to lupus are common and can vary in severity. Cerebrovascular accidents occur in approximately 15% of patients, and up to 20% of patients develop seizure disorders. Cranial and peripheral neuropathies limit self-care ability and have a significant effect on quality of life. Cognitive impairment can also occur. Patients may develop epilepsy and migraines.

⚠ Cardiac abnormalities are among the most significant factors causing mortality and morbidity in patients with lupus. Myocardial infarctions secondary to atherosclerosis have been observed in patients under 35 years of age.

Prognosis

The outcome of lupus is highly variable and depends on the severity of the disease, the degree of organ damage, and the presence of drug-induced complications. Patients who require long-term immunosuppressive drug therapy to control lupus are at increased risk for malignancies and complications associated with infection. Chronic long-term use of corticosteroids can lead to coronary artery disease, diabetes, osteoporosis, and aseptic necrosis of the bones. When the initial acute phase of the disease is adequately controlled and the patient has access to health care, the long-term prognosis is usually good, with more than 95% of patients surviving 10 years after diagnosis.

What You DO

Treatment

Care is directed toward preventing tissue and organ damage from the disease and complications of treatment. Mild or sporadic flares of lupus require little or no treatment. Body aches can be controlled with NSAIDs, and judicious use of aspirin can be helpful. Antimalarial drugs such as hydroxychloroquine can be given to decrease the inflammatory response.

Corticosteroid therapy is indicated for severe disease to preserve organ function. Generally, combinations of prednisone and immunosuppressive therapy such as azathioprine and cyclophosphamide are used. For patients with coagulopathies, heparin and maintenance therapy with warfarin may be required.

Because of complications associated with long-term corticosteroid and immunosuppressive therapy, medical management is directed toward using the minimal possible dosages of either type of drug required to control symptoms of the disease. After control of symptoms is achieved, corticosteroid doses are gradually decreased, the goal being to eliminate steroids completely.

Nursing Responsibilities

Nursing management of the patient with lupus is directed toward controlling adverse symptoms, optimizing overall health, and promoting the patient's ability to cope with the disease. Because the disease has such a

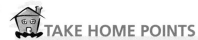
TAKE HOME POINTS

- Lupus is a chronic autoimmune disease that affects connective tissue and is characterized by periods of exacerbation and remission.
- Lupus is thought to develop as a consequence of antibodies the body creates against its own healthy tissue.
- The development of lupus has been linked to genetic influences, estrogen, environmental factors, and exposure to drugs.
- Lupus can affect the skin, serous membranes, lungs, heart, joints, muscles, kidneys, and blood-forming system.

wide spectrum of symptoms that change over time, and because the disease often has periods of exacerbation and remission, the nurse must frequently reassess the patient's status and adjust nursing care and interventions accordingly. For the patient with lupus, the nurse should do the following:

- Conduct and document a baseline neurologic assessment at the time of diagnosis.
- Regularly monitor the patient throughout the course of the disease for evidence of neurologic changes, including abnormalities of the cranial nerves, changes in mental status, depression, and cognitive decline. Symptoms of cognitive decline include confusion, difficulty in understanding abstract concepts, organizing, and solving problems.
- Because pharmacologic therapy for this disease is often complex, teach patients how to correctly self-administer medications, as well as how to monitor for treatment-associated side effects.

Nursing Management of Skin Manifestations

- Conduct a baseline assessment of the skin to evaluate the appearance, severity, and duration of skin lesions.
- Educate the patient regarding skin care measures and avoidance of exposure to ultraviolet (UV) rays from the sun, as well as fluorescent and halogen lights. Warn the patient that glass does not provide complete protection from UV rays. Teach the patient to use a sunscreen with a sun-protection factor (SPF) of at least 15 or higher every time he or she is exposed to the sun, and advise the patient to wear protective clothing such as broad-brimmed hats, long-sleeved shirts, and pants made of fabric capable of blocking UV rays. Hair dyes and over-the-counter creams and lotions can increase photosensitivity, as do certain drugs.

Nursing Management of Musculoskeletal Manifestations
Nursing management is directed toward helping the patient maintain joint function and increasing muscle strength.

- Inform the patient that an inflamed or swollen joint should not bear weight; however, gentle range of motion exercises can be helpful to maintain flexibility. A regular exercise plan should be maintained during periods of remission to promote muscle tone and overall fitness.
- Treat pain cautiously with analgesics but only under direct medical supervision.

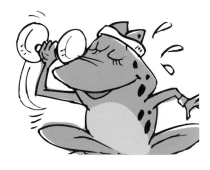

One...
and
Two...

- Remind the patient not to self-medicate with over-the-counter drugs without obtaining the health care provider's approval.

Nursing Management Associated with Cardiac Involvement

- Conduct a careful physical assessment.
- Monitor for evidence of cardiovascular complications and thrombus formation.
- Teach patients the measures to maintain cardiovascular health, including frequent monitoring of blood pressure, regular aerobic exercise (when not otherwise contraindicated), and avoidance of smoking, and the importance of following a diet low in fat and sodium.
- Teach the patient signs and symptoms of cardiac and pulmonary compromise that warrant medical intervention.

Nursing Management Associated with Renal Involvement

- Regularly assess renal function.
- Monitor diagnostic laboratory studies.
- Conduct a periodic evaluation for signs and symptoms of renal compromise.
- Decrease fluid retention and edema.
- Maintain electrolyte balance.
- Institute measures to decrease the risk of infection.
- Instruct the patient with dietary and fluid restrictions on the importance of daily weighing for evidence of fluid retention and on the correct way to measure blood pressure.
- Teach the patient about the signs and symptoms of fluid overload and the point at which to seek assistance of the health care provider.

National Institutes of Health Lupus: A Patient Care Guide for Nurses and Other Health Professionals
http://www.niams.nih.gov/hi/topics/lupus/lupusguide/chp1.htm
Systemic Lupus Erythematosus
http://www.medicinenet.com/systemic_lupus/article.htm

TAKE HOME POINTS

- Warm baths or heating pads after arising can help to loosen stiff joints and improve comfort.
- Corticosteroid and immunosuppressive therapy places the patient at risk for infections. Teach the patient about the signs and symptoms of urinary tract infection, including frequent urination, urgency, burning, cloudy urine, and incomplete emptying of the bladder. Advise the patient to avoid contact with people having contagious illnesses such as upper respiratory infections and influenza. Patients may need intensive psychologic and emotional support in order to cope effectively with this disease.

Do You UNDERSTAND?

DIRECTIONS: **Choose the correct answer to each of the following questions and write the corresponding letter in the spaces provided.**

_____   1. When is a disease considered to be autoimmune?

    a. B-cell activity against host tissue is present.

    b. T-cell activity against host tissue is present.

    c. Persistent inflammatory response is present.

    d. Macrophage activity is accelerated.

_____ 2. When deposited in tissue, immune complexes tend to do what to an immune response?
   a. Initiate
   b. Delay
   c. Suppress
   d. Maintain

_____ 3. The most important aspect of skin care for the patient with lupus involves which of the following?
   a. Keeping the skin moist and lubricated with a protective cream
   b. Using mild soaps
   c. Avoiding over-the-counter skin care preparations
   d. Avoiding exposure to ultraviolet rays

_____ 4. Patients whose lupus is currently in remission should be advised to do which of the following?
   a. Maintain a regular exercise program to improve muscle strength.
   b. Avoid contact with people with contagious illnesses.
   c. Gradually taper doses of corticosteroids.
   d. Avoid stress.

_____ 5. A patient with previously well-controlled lupus notes facial and pedal edema, along with dyspnea on exertion, over the last few days. The patient should do which of the following?
   a. Decrease salt and fluid intake.
   b. Elevate the feet.
   c. Take a diuretic.
   d. Notify the physician.

What IS Systemic Sclerosis?

Systemic sclerosis is a term used to describe a disorder that can affect not only the skin, but also most of the internal organs. This disease causes changes in connective tissue that can affect the synovium, skin, blood vessels and internal organs. Thickening and tightening of the skin is a

Answers: 1. b; 2. a; 3. d; 4. a; 5. d.

hallmark of the disease. Previously called *scleroderma*, this term is now most commonly used when the disorder affects only the skin. Systemic sclerosis is a relatively rare chronic autoimmune condition that is characterized by large deposits of collagen that lead to thickening and fibrosis of the skin, particularly on the hands and face. In some patients, the disease is limited to the skin, but the more severe form can also adversely affect vascular, organ, and immunologic function.

Pathogenesis

Currently, the cause of the abnormal autoimmune process leading to systemic sclerosis is unknown. The exact mechanisms of this disease are also poorly understood. The current consensus is that systemic sclerosis is the consequence of abnormal inflammatory mechanisms, similar in nature to those that cause lupus. Autoantibodies and abnormal accumulations of T cells cause damage to arterioles. The damaged vessels then leak plasma into the surrounding tissues. Chemical factors are released that lead to the excess production of collagen, a tissue protein. This collagen accumulates leading to hardening and tightening of the skin. Similar to lupus, this disorder has many different manifestations. Inflammation, fibrosis, and sclerosing of not only the skin but also the vital organs are all characteristics of progressive systemic sclerosis.

At-Risk Populations

No genetic link has been identified, although connective tissue disorders tend to occur more commonly in some families. Some studies suggest that scleroderma may be linked to exposure to chemicals, coal, silica dust, and plastics.

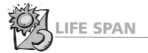 **LIFE SPAN**

Systemic sclerosis is most prevalent in women between the ages of 35 and 54.

What You NEED TO KNOW

Clinical Manifestations

Presenting symptoms vary from patient to patient and also depend on the stage and type of sclerosis encountered. Typically, patients will have painless edema both in the hands and the fingers, which can extend to the upper and lower extremities and the face. The skin is taut and shiny and lacks elasticity. As the disease progresses, the edematous areas become tight, hard, and thickened. Because of decreased elasticity, patients can

Involvement of internal organs can lead to severe hypertension, heart failure, and respiratory and renal failure.

lose range of motion in joints and develop contractures, occasionally to the extent that they are unable to perform activities of daily living (ADLs) independently. Calcium deposits in the subcutaneous tissue cause small, white lumps under the skin that may leak and drain.

When the sclerosis is progressive, this process of hardening and fibrosis can adversely affect internal organs and structures. Disruption of the gastrointestinal tract is common and is manifested by complaints of persistent indigestion, reflux, bloating, and early satiety with meals. Fibrotic changes in the esophagus lead to dysmotility, along with dysphagia and reflux disease. Peristalsis is decreased, which can cause symptoms similar to a small bowel obstruction.

Fibrotic changes in the myocardium may lead to electrocardiogram changes, abnormal heartbeats, chest pain, and heart failure. Most patients experience some degree of compromise in arterial circulation to the hands and feet, causing severe pain and even loss of fingers and toes. When exposed to emotional stress or cold, arterioles in the fingers and toes constrict, causing the digits to become blue, cold, and painful. In severe cases, the tips of the fingers and toes become necrotic. Renal involvement can lead to malignant hypertension and death. Changes in blood pressure may be the first indication of renal compromise.

Symptoms of pulmonary involvement include shortness of breath and a nonproductive cough. Fibrosis of the lung tissue is present in nearly all patients with progressive disease, although many individuals are asymptomatic.

Prognosis

The prognosis for systemic sclerosis is variable, depending on the type of disease and the presence of other comorbid factors. Most patients with involvement limited to their skin have a good prognosis. However, approximately 10% will gradually develop severe respiratory compromise over a period of approximately 10 to 20 years. Patients with rapidly progressing skin involvement or organ involvement tend to have a poorer prognosis. Currently, slightly more than one half of these patients survive for 10 years or longer.

What You DO

Treatment

Unfortunately, no effective therapy for systemic sclerosis is available. Medical care is directed toward control of symptoms and support of organ function. Some alleviation of symptoms has been obtained with drug therapy, specifically immunosuppressive drugs, antiinflammatory drugs, and some drugs with vasodilation effects. Gastrointestinal drugs such as lansoprazole, omeprazole, or famotidine can be used to support and maintain gastrointestinal function.

During the early stages of the disease, patients benefit from occupational and physical therapy to prevent contractures of the fingers and arms. Rapidly progressive tightening of the skin can cause pressure, pain, and inflammation of underlying muscles and tendons, leading to a painful inflammation of the muscles (myositis). This condition may be improved by the administration of low-dose oral steroids.

Nursing Responsibilities

For the patient with systemic sclerosis, the nurse should do the following:
- Assess all skin surfaces carefully for evidence of circulatory compromise or vasculitic lesions. Treat ulcers and breaks in skin integrity promptly, because poor peripheral circulation will make healing problematic.
- Teach the patient how to protect the skin in areas with poor circulation. Mild soap, lubricating lotions, and protective gloves and socks should be worn if the patient is able to tolerate the contact against the skin. For cases of severe skin involvement, a bed cradle and/or footboard can be helpful in removing bed linens from sensitive areas.
- Instruct the patient to avoid cold temperatures whenever possible because of the increased risk of vasospasm.
- Advise the patient to avoid tobacco and caffeine because of their vasoconstrictive effects.
- Offer the patient with esophageal dysfunction small and frequent meals that are soft and bland.
- Advise patients to avoid spicy and foods high in fat and alcohol because these ingredients stimulate the production of gastric acid.

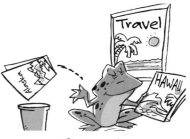

Stay warm!

- Teach the patient to keep the head elevated for at least 2 hours after eating. Histamine2 antagonists can be beneficial for some patients to decrease production of gastric acid.
- Monitor the patient on an ongoing basis for signs and symptoms of organ involvement. Changes in blood pressure, cardiovascular, pulmonary, and renal status should be reported to the health care provider immediately.
- Because of the toxic effects of many drugs used to treat systemic sclerosis, careful medical monitoring and frequent diagnostic testing is indicated to detect adverse effects before damage is severe or irreversible.

Do You UNDERSTAND?

DIRECTIONS: Fill in the blanks by unscrambling the letters.

1. The most common symptom of systemic sclerosis is _____ _____ of the skin. *(chengtinik)*
2. Systemic sclerosis is thought to be the result of damage to _____ _____. *(triolesare)*
3. A patient with systemic sclerosis complains of difficulties with dysphagia, bloating, and indigestion after eating. This patient is most likely experiencing _____ involvement. *(tarestalingsotin)*
4. Precautions to maintain _____ is one of the most important education topics for patients with systemic sclerosis. *(inks triginety)*

TAKE HOME POINTS

- Sjögren's syndrome is a progressive, chronic autoimmune disorder that is characterized by dry eyes and dry mouth.
- This disease results from abnormal infiltration of exocrine glands by T lymphocytes.
- Complications of Sjögren's syndrome include damage to the eyes, periodontal disease, and oral infections.

What IS Sjögren's Syndrome?

Sjögren's syndrome (SS) is a progressive, incurable autoimmune disorder characterized by dry eyes and dry mouth (**keratoconjunctivitis sicca [KCS] and xerostomia**). SS can occur as an isolated disorder, or it can be present in association with other autoimmune diseases such as

Answers: 1. thickening; 2. arterioles; 3. gastrointestinal; 4. skin integrity.

rheumatoid arthritis or lupus. This disease affects primarily the tear glands and salivary glands, although it may occasionally affect other exocrine glands, including those lining the vagina or the respiratory and gastrointestinal tract. SS is the result of abnormal infiltration of the lacrimal and salivary glands by T lymphocytes. The exact cause of this disease is unknown. Some research indicates that the syndrome may be triggered by viruses or bacteria that cause inappropriate stimulation of the immune system. Various genes have also been correlated with the development of this syndrome.

Pathogenesis

During the early stages of SS, molecules that attract lymphocytes are released from the venules. T lymphocytes adhere to the venules and migrate into the gland, where they are activated and release interleukin-2 and tumor necrosis factors. Activated B cells in the gland produce antibodies. With progressive infiltration and inflammation of the glandular tissue, glandular function decreases and the patient experiences the characteristic dryness of the mouth, the eyes, and the vagina.

At-Risk Populations

Approximately 90% of people with this disease are women. Most women are diagnosed after menopause, although this disorder can appear in younger women. Approximately 50% of cases occur in conjunction with another autoimmune or connective tissue disorder.

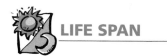

LIFE SPAN

Children of women with this disease have an increased risk of serious cardiac defects.

What You NEED TO KNOW

Clinical Manifestations

Patients with SS usually complain of painful, burning, dry eyes. Many people will complain of a foreign body sensation when they blink. These symptoms are a result of a decreased volume of flow of tears. For some patients, the corneal dryness is so severe that they have corneal ulcerations.

An additional symptom is a severely dry mouth. The patient may require water to swallow food and may be forced to carry water at all times. The patient may experience changes in taste perception and difficulty in swallowing. Diminished production of saliva can lead to a sore,

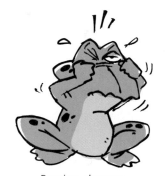

Burning, dry eyes.

inflamed tongue; painful, irritated oral mucosa; oral *Candida albicans* infections; and severe dental caries.

This disease can adversely affect any organ in the body. Signs and symptoms of musculoskeletal involvement include arthralgias and myalgias. Other potential sites of organ involvement include the lungs, the liver, kidneys, and the hematopoietic system. Diagnoses commonly observed with organ involvement include inflammation of the lungs (**pneumonitis**), biliary cirrhosis, interstitial nephritis, leukopenia, thrombocytopenia, and anemia.

Fatigue is common and can be severe and debilitating. In the presence of active immune disease, the fatigue is thought to be a result of the action of cytokines such as interleukin 1 or tumor necrosis factor on the CNS.

Prognosis

In the absence of other diseases or organ involvement, the rate of long-term survival for patients with SS is good. Importantly, however, these patients may suffer multiple complications such as dental and ophthalmic diseases, as well as poor quality of life and persistent prolonged discomfort.

What You DO

Treatment

Management of SS is directed primarily toward palliation of distressing symptoms and prevention of complications. Oral dryness may be alleviated with saliva substitutes and oral moisturizers. A variety of solutions is available and has been used with varying degrees of success in different patients. Sialogogues (drugs that stimulate the production of saliva) can also offer some benefit to patients who have some remaining functional salivary glands. Pilocarpine hydrochloride has been shown to be safe and effective for long-term use and has been approved by the U.S. Food and Drug Administration for this purpose. Patients with dry eyes will require frequent instillations of artificial tears and ophthalmic lubricants.

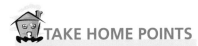

TAKE HOME POINTS

Treatment for Sjögren's syndrome includes the use of oral and ophthalmic lubricants.

Nursing Responsibilities

The nurse should do the following:

- Advise patients suffering from dry mouth to drink liquids throughout their waking hours, but to avoid caffeinated beverages such as tea and coffee. Sugarless candy and gum can help stimulate the flow of saliva.
- Warn patients to avoid alcohol and tobacco because these substances damage delicate oral mucosa.
- Teach the patient to maintain meticulous oral hygiene, avoid acidic foods, and see a dentist at frequent intervals to avoid the high risk of cavities and periodontal disease.
- Recommend using artificial tears to help the treatment of dry eyes. Because of the decreased volume of natural tears, some drugs with preservatives can cause increased pain and irritation. Preservative-free liquid tears are available in single-dose units, which decreases the risk of pathogens growing in the solution. Ocular lubricants can also be helpful at night, but are usually unsuitable for use during waking hours because of their tendency to cloud the vision. A minor surgical procedure that occludes tear drainage, which then allows tears to accumulate and moisten the eyes, can help relieve severe dryness of the eye.

> ⚠ Patients with persistent swelling of the parotid or submandibular glands should be carefully evaluated for malignancies. Patients with Sjögren's syndrome have a greatly increased risk of developing non-Hodgkin's lymphoma, particularly in the lymph nodes of the neck.

Do You UNDERSTAND?

DIRECTIONS: **Choose the correct answer to each of the following questions and write the corresponding letter in the spaces provided.**

_____   1. Sjögren's syndrome is characterized by which one of the following?
   a. Dry mucous membranes
   b. Weight loss
   c. Fluid retention
   d. Anorexia

_____ 2. Preventive screening measures for all patients with Sjögren's syndrome include which one of the following?
   a. Testing of stool for occult blood
   b. Evaluation of pulmonary function
   c. Annual colonoscopy
   d. Frequent evaluation for head and neck cancers

_____ 3. A patient with Sjögren's syndrome has persistent swelling in the left parotid gland. The nurse should do which one of the following?
   a. Apply an ice pack to the area.
   b. Apply a heating pad to the area.
   c. Suggest that the patient take over-the-counter NSAIDs.
   d. Inform the patient's health care provider.

_____ 4. Which nursing intervention would not be appropriate for a patient with Sjögren's syndrome?
   a. Offer the patient saliva substitutes and oral moisturizers.
   b. Advise the patient to use an alcohol-based mouthwash to maintain oral hygiene.
   c. Suggest the patient use gum and hard, sugarless candy to stimulate flow of saliva.
   d. Instruct the patient to use liquid tears in single-dose units.

_____ 5. Which foods or beverages should be avoided?
   a. Coffee
   b. Red meats
   c. Milk
   d. Caffeine-free sodas

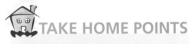

TAKE HOME POINTS

Myasthenia gravis is a disease that causes severe muscle weakness and impairs a person's ability to breathe or swallow.

What IS Myasthenia Gravis?

Myasthenia gravis (MG) is a disease that causes disturbances in the transmission of impulses between motor neurons and innervated muscle cells. It is characterized by fatigue and diminished muscle strength, particularly after repetitive or prolonged muscle activity.

Answers: 1. a; 2. d; 3. d; 4. b; 5. a.

Pathogenesis

MG occurs as a result of an abnormal immune process that causes antibodies to form against acetylcholine receptors in the neuromuscular junction. Approximately 80% of patients lose receptors, which ultimately results in fatigability and weakness of muscles. Although 10% to 20% of MG patients do not have serologically detectable antibodies, research indicates that this is an antibody-mediated autoimmune disease.

T cells can bind to the acetylcholine receptor site and can promote the production of B-cell antibodies. In addition, most patients with myasthenia gravis have abnormal thymus glands, which probably stimulates the abnormal immune responses associated with this disease.

Genetic factors are also thought to contribute to the development of myasthenia gravis. Certain human lymphocyte antigen (HLA) types are associated with this disease, including DRw3, DQw2, and HLA-B.

At-Risk Populations

MG is more common in women in their 20s and 30s and in men over the age of 60.

What You NEED TO KNOW

Clinical Manifestations

MG typically first presents with ocular muscle weakness, which causes drooping eyelids (ptosis) and double vision (diplopia). When the disease progresses, generalized muscle weakness will result, causing problems with respiratory muscles, chewing, swallowing, and moving. Often weakness is more pronounced in the proximal muscles of limbs, which causes difficulty climbing stairs and lifting objects. In most cases, symptoms worsen as the day progresses, with partial recovery with medication and rest. As the disease progresses, facial muscles are impaired, causing problems with speech.

Prognosis

With appropriate medical care, most patients with MG will have a normal life expectancy.

What You DO

Treatment

Therapy for this disease involves suppressing the abnormal immunologic process that appears to trigger this disorder. Various pharmacologic agents are used, including immunosuppressive medications, corticosteroids, and anticholinesterase agents. Plasmapheresis (an exchange of the patient's own plasma for donated plasma) may be used to remove antibodies, and thymectomy (removal of the thymus gland) is a treatment option for patients who do not respond satisfactorily to other therapies.

Nursing Responsibilities

Patients who are hospitalized should have their muscle strength tested every 4 hours or less, depending upon their status. Report deterioration in muscle strength to the health care provider. Patients with MG need extensive information on how to manage their disease, as well as when to seek help.

Instruct patients on the following:
- Self-administration of medications
- Lifestyle adjustments
- Myasthenic crisis—characterized by severe muscle weakness and difficulty breathing and swallowing
- Cholinergic crisis—caused by excessive anticholinesterase drugs; symptoms include muscle weakness, nausea, vomiting, gastrointestinal distress, diarrhea, pallor, excessive salivation, and miosis

A myasthenic crisis may be precipitated by stress, electrolyte imbalances, infection, and the administration of certain drugs that may increase weakness in myasthenic patients. These drugs include aminoglycoside antibiotics, beta blockers, procainamide, quinine, quinidine, and phenytoin. Patients with severe respiratory insufficiency will require intubation and ventilatory support.

Patients who are having difficulty swallowing or must support their chin on their hand in able to speak are at risk for respiratory failure and must be observed accordingly.

Do You UNDERSTAND?

DIRECTIONS: **Choose the correct answer to each of the following questions and write the corresponding letter in the spaces provided.**

_____ 1. _____ is an early symptom of MG.
  a. Exopthalmos
  b. Diaphoresis
  c. Blepharospasm
  d. Ptosis

_____ 2. Which drug may increase muscle weakness in the MG patient?
  a. diazepam
  b. phenytoin
  c. furosemide
  d. albuterol

_____ 3. A patient with MG is nauseated and also complains of diarrhea and gastrointestinal upset. The nurse notes that the patient's hand grasps are weaker than previously. This patient may be experiencing a
  a. Myasthenic crisis.
  b. Cholinergic crisis.
  c. Adverse drug reaction.
  d. Allergic reaction to a drug.

_____ 4. A patient with MG comments "It's my muscles that aren't working. Why do they want to take a CAT scan of my chest?" Which of the following would be the nurse's best answer?
  a. "To evaluate the status of your heart"
  b. "To evaluate the status of your lungs"
  c. "To see if you have any problems with your ribs that will hinder your breathing"
  d. "To see if your thymus gland is normal"

_____ 5. The most severe complication associated with MG is
  a. Impaired vision.
  b. Cardiac compromise.
  c. Respiratory failure.
  d. Renal insufficiency.

Answers: 1. d; 2. b; 3. b; 4. d; 5. c.

References

AIDS Knowledge Base: *Classification, staging and surveillance of HIV disease*, 1999, URL http://hivinsite.ucsf.edu/akb/current/01class index.html.

AIDS Knowledge Base: *Epidemiology of HIV/AIDS in the United States*, 1999, URL http://hivinsite.ucsf.edu/akb/current/01epius/index.html.

Bullock BA, Henze RL: *Focus on pathophysiology*, Philadelphia, 2000, Lippincott Williams & Wilkins.

Burns MV: *Pathophysiology: a self-instructional program*, Stamford, CT, 1998, Appleton & Lange.

Copstead LC, Banasid JL: *Pathophysiology: biological and behavioral perspective*, ed 4, Philadelphia, 2000, WB Saunders.

Corey L, Handsfield HH: Genital herpes and public health: addressing a global problem, *JAMA* 283:791, 2000.

Cotran RS, Kumar V, Collins T: *Pathologic basis of disease*, ed 6, Philadelphia, 1999, WB Saunders.

Crowley L: *An introduction to human disease: pathology and pathophysiology correlations*, ed 5, Sudbury, Mass, 2001, Jones and Bartlett.

Cunha M, Bullock BL: Altered immunity. In Bullock BA, Henze RL, editors: *Focus on pathophysiology*, Philadelphia, 2000, Lippincott.

Ellis P, Johnson DP: Dermatologic complications in HIV, *Nurse Pract Forum* 10(2):87, 1999.

Fox RL: Sjögren syndrome: new approaches to treatment, Medscape, 2000, URL http://www.medscape.com/Medscape/heumatology/TreatmentUpdate/2000/tu01/pnt–tu01.html.

Gamponia MJ, Graber MA: AIDS (acquired immunodeficiency syndrome). In *University of Iowa family practice handbook*, ed 3, 2000, URL http://www.vh.org/Providers/ClinRef/FPHandbook/Chapter16/ 01-16.html.

Guyton AC, Hall JE: *Human physiology and mechanisms of disease*, ed 6, Philadelphia, 1997, WB Saunders.

Guyton AC, Hall JE: *Textbook of medical physiology*, ed 9, Philadelphia, 1996, WB Saunders.

Halperin DT: Heterosexual anal intercourse: prevalence, cultural factors, and HIV infection and other health risks, Part I, *AIDS Patient Care STDS* 13(12):717, 1999.

Porth CM: *Pathophysiology: concepts of altered health states*, ed 5, Philadelphia, 1998, Lippincott-Raven.

Rhodus NL: Sjögren's syndrome, *Quintessence Int* 30(10):689, 1999.

Rote NS, Huether SE, McCance KL: Hypersensitivities, infections, and immunodeficiences. In Huether SE, McCance KL: *Understanding pathophysiology*, ed 2, St Louis, 2000, Mosby.

US Public Health Service and Infectious Diseases Society of America: Guidelines for the prevention of opportunistic infections in persons infected with human immunodeficiency virus: a summary, *MMWR* 44(RR-8), 1999, URL http://www.ams–assn.org/special/hiv/ treatmnt/ guide/rr4810/rr4810/ref.htm.

NCLEX® Review

Section A

1. If a patient has an inadequate inflammatory response, which would be the most likely consequence?
   1 Accelerated healing of damaged tissue
   2 Decreased risk for infection
   3 Impaired tissue healing and repair
   4 Increased pain in the presence of tissue damage

2. While monitoring a patient receiving a blood transfusion, the nurse notes that his blood pressure has fallen from 140/90 to 100/50, and his heart rate has increased from 84 to 118 beats per minute. He is also complaining of chills and low back pain. What should the nurse do first?
   1 Decrease the rate of the transfusion
   2 Increase the rate of the transfusion
   3 Stop the transfusion
   4 Notify the health care provider

3. While receiving an intravenous antibiotic for the first time, a patient complains of an itchy, runny nose and swollen lips. What should the nurse do?
   1 Continue the infusion.
   2 Decrease the rate of the infusion.
   3 Continue the infusion and notify the patient's health care provider.
   4 Stop the infusion and notify the health care provider immediately.

4. Which symptom indicates a possible allergic reaction?
   1 Fever
   2 Diaphoresis
   3 Rash
   4 Chills

5. Which drug would be most useful in treating a severe allergic reaction?
   1 Hydromorphone
   2 Cortisone
   3 Methylprednisolone
   4 Furosemide

6. When treating hypersensitivity reactions, epinephrine can be given to
   1 Decrease smooth muscle constriction.
   2 Decrease the heart rate.
   3 Control HTN.
   4 Maintain the inflammatory response.

7. A patient is highly allergic to cats. The nurse is aware that this is probably a _____ hypersensitivity reaction.
   1 Type I
   2 Type 2
   3 Type 3
   4 Type 4

8. A patient complaining of allergies to house dust is asking for advice regarding over-the-counter drugs that will help to control his or her symptoms. Which advice is most appropriate in this situation?
   1 Seek a physician's order for a prescription medication.
   2 Purchase a HEPA filter for home use.
   3 Look for a decongestant or antihistamine medication.
   4 Try to have someone else do housecleaning.
   5 3 and 4 only

9. RhoGAM is given after childbirth to
   1 Treat jaundice in the neonate.
   2 Decrease hemolysis of red blood cells in the neonate.
   3 Treat hyperbilirubinemia in the mother.
   4 Prevent sensitization of the mother to Rh factor.

10. Bronchospasm associated with hypersensitivity reactions is the result of
    1 Histamine release.
    2 Pulmonary vasodilation.
    3 Dilation of the alveoli.
    4 Inadequate antibody production.

11. Allergic reactions and allergies should be documented in multiple places including the _____, _____, and _____.

12. Antibodies do *not* participate in type _____ hypersensitivity reactions.
    1 I
    2 II
    3 III
    4 IV

Section B

13. A patient who is HIV-positive now has a CD_4 count of 380 and has asked the nurse to explain the implications of this result. The best response would be
    1 "Your immune system is still intact, but you are somewhat susceptible to infection."
    2 "This is a result that we routinely see with all patients who are HIV-positive."
    3 "This value indicates that the medication you are taking is working well."
    4 "Your immune system has been severely damaged, and you are highly susceptible to infection."

14. A patient with AIDS complains of sudden severe breathlessness and a persistent cough. The nurse should suspect possible
    1 Disseminated herpetic infection.
    2 Candidiasis of the esophagus.
    3 *Pneumocystis carinii* pneumonia.
    4 *Toxoplasmosis gondii* infection.

15. Failure to take antiretroviral drugs correctly may result in
    1 Adverse drug reactions.
    2 Development of a drug-resistant strain of the AIDS virus.
    3 Increased side effects.
    4 Decreased effectiveness.
    5 2 and 4

Section C

16. People with lupus are most at risk for which of the following disorders?
    1 Cardiac abnormalities
    2 Liver failure
    3 Decreased coagulation
    4 Psychiatric problems

17. Myasthenia gravis is the result of
    1 Decreased antibody formation.
    2 Excess numbers of acetylcholine receptors.
    3 Abnormal antibody formation against acetylcholine receptors.
    4 A hypoactive immune response.

18. One of the first symptoms of myasthenia gravis is often
    1 Ptosis.
    2 Weight loss.
    3 Anorexia.
    4 Muscle weakness upon arising.

19. A hospitalized patient with myasthenia gravis is having sudden difficulty swallowing and severe profound muscle weakness. Rank the interventions listed below in priority order by selecting the sequence of interventions that is most appropriate.
    1 Notify the health care provider.
    2 Position the patient to optimize respiratory expansion.
    3 Bring an ambu bag to the patient's bedside.
    4 Anticipate the possible need for endotracheal intubation.

20. Which group is most likely to develop systemic lupus erythematosus?
    1 Teenage girls of any race
    2 Caucasian men
    3 Caucasian women
    4 African American women

21. Signs and symptoms associated with systemic sclerosis (scleroderma) include which of the following?
    1 Taut, shiny skin
    2 Small, white lumps under the skin
    3 Hyperactive bowel sounds
    4 Large wheals on the skin

22. Patients with Sjögren's syndrome should have life-long monitoring for
    1 Cardiac disease.
    2 Renal compromise.
    3 Ophthalmic disease.
    4 Vascular insufficiency.

NCLEX® Review Answers

Section A

1. **3** A normal inflammatory process must be present in order for tissue healing and repair to take place. Excessive inflammatory processes may lead to local pain, and prolonged exaggerated immune responses that ultimately will cause tissue damage.

2. **3** The symptoms cited reflect a possible hemolytic reaction to the transfusion. The transfusion must be stopped immediately and the health care provider notified so appropriate treatment can be provided. Continuing the transfusion, no matter the rate, places the patient at risk for renal failure and even death. The IV line should remain in place for emergency drugs.

3. **4** Itching and swelling are signs of an allergic reaction. The infusion must be stopped and the health care provider notified. If the infusion continues, then the patient's airway may begin to swell, placing the individual at risk for respiratory arrest.

4. **3** Rash may be present with hypersensitive allergic reactions. Fever, diaphoresis (sweating), and chills are symptoms of infection.

5. **3** Methylprednisolone, a corticosteroid, has a stronger, more immediate effect than cortisone and prevents tissue response to inflammatory mediators and lysosomal enzyme release. Hydromorphone is an opioid analgesic, cortisone is a corticosteroid used in treatment of inflammatory disorders, and furosemide is a loop diuretic.

6. **1** Epinephrine results in the stimulation of beta$_1$ receptors, which leads to an increased heart rate and relaxation of smooth muscles. Epinephrine causes vasoconstriction, which leads to elevated, not decreased, blood pressure. Epinephrine does not affect the inflammatory response.

7. **1** A protein found in cat saliva is the antigen that stimulates the allergic reaction typically seen in susceptible individuals. Type I reactions are typically dramatic, sudden in onset, and are characterized by a runny nose, sniffling, and itching. In extremely sensitive individuals the reaction may progress to anaphylaxis.

8. **5** Prescription allergy medications should only be used if over-the-counter drugs provide inadequate relief. HEPA filters are generally costly and require special maintenance. Help the patient identify ways to avoid exposure to the offending allergen (house dust), and if possible find over-the-counter medications such as decongestants and antihistamines that safely suppress symptoms.

9. **4** RhoGAM is given as a preventive agent. It is an immune serum given to prevent an Rh$^-$ mother from becoming sensitized to the blood cells of her Rh$^+$ fetus. RhoGAM will not treat or decrease jaundice in the neonate, but it might prevent it from occurring if given to the mother appropriately during pregnancy.

10. **1** Histamine constricts smooth muscle, resulting in bronchiolar constriction, and causes increased permeability of the vessels, resulting in vascular congestion and edema. Histamine has no direct action on the alveoli and antibody production but is responsible for mediating the immune response.

11. **4** Patient's record; current chart; on the patient's (armband)

12. **4** Type IV hypersensitivity reactions are the result of sensitized T lymphocytes. Also called delayed reactions, type IV reactions tend to occur 24 to 72 hours after exposure to an antigen. Types I, II, and III reactions involve antibody formation.

Section B

13. **4** The CD_4 count of 380 indicates that the patient has AIDS and is severely immunocompromised. Not all patients who are HIV-positive are immunodeficient. A very low CD_4 count such as this indicates either the need to begin antiretroviral therapy or that the current treatment is ineffective.

14. **3** Severe breathlessness and a dry persistent cough of acute onset are typical symptoms of *P. carinii* pneumonia in the patient with AIDS. A disseminated herpes infection would be more likely to cause systemic symptoms such as fever, myalgia, and skin lesions. *Candida* in the esophagus would not cause respiratory findings. *T. gondii* infection usually affects the gastrointestinal tract.

15. **5** Failure to take antiretroviral drugs consistently and on time may result in the development of drug-resistant strains of the AIDS virus and may cause increased side effects due to drug-drug interactions.

Section C

16. **3** Most patients with lupus die of cardiovascular complications. Vascular abnormalities can also lead to renal and liver damage and/or renal or liver failure. These patients tend to experience hypercoagulable states and are at increased risk for venous and arterial thromboses. The stress of a serious chronic illness can lead to psychiatric problems, but lupus does not, in and of itself, cause psychiatric problems.

17. **1** Abnormal antibodies attack and damage acetylcholine receptors at the neuromuscular junction, which interferes with the transmission of muscle impulses.

18. **1** Drooping eyelids, particularly when the patient is asked to sustain a prolonged upward gaze, are a frequent finding in the early stages of myasthenia gravis. In the early stages, the disease does not affect body weight or appetite. Muscle weakness typically occurs after repeated muscle activity.

19. **3** Difficulty swallowing, and drooling, are warnings of impending respiratory failure in the patient with myasthenia gravis. Affected individuals should be positioned in such as way that respiratory expansion and risk of aspiration is minimized. In the event of respiratory arrest, an ambu bag can be used to maintain ventilation of the patient while the appropriate health care provider is notified. Patients with myasthenia gravis who have respiratory failure may require intubation and respiratory support with a ventilator until their condition has stabilized.

20. **4** African American women have 3 times the incidence of lupus as Caucasian women. However, this disease can develop in any race and at any age, although it is more common between the ages of 20 and 40.

21. **4** Excess collagen accumulates in the tissues and causes taut, shiny skin that eventually becomes thick and hard. Abnormal calcium deposits in the skin form small lumps that can leak and drain. Patients with sclerosis tend to experience decreased peristalsis, which can cause symptoms similar to a bowel obstruction.

22. **3** Although Sjögren's syndrome can affect almost any organ, one of its most common complications is eye disease.

Notes

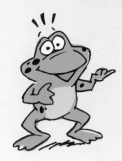

Chapter 2

Alterations in Neurologic Function

What You WILL LEARN

After reading this chapter, you will know how to do the following:

- ✔ Differentiate between a cerebrovascular accident and a transient ischemic event.
- ✔ Describe the various types of cerebrovascular accidents.
- ✔ Recognize the signs and symptoms of a cerebrovascular attack.
- ✔ Discuss the care of a patient who has had a cerebrovascular attack.
- ✔ Describe the pathogenesis of meningitis.
- ✔ Explain the physiologic changes associated with head injuries.
- ✔ Discuss nursing interventions for the patient with a head injury.
- ✔ Explain the pathogenesis of movement disorders.
- ✔ Compare and contrast the various types of seizure disorders.
- ✔ List nursing interventions suitable for a patient with a degenerative neurologic disorder.

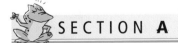

SECTION A

ACUTE CEREBRAL DISORDERS

Head injury is a common problem and is one of the most frequently observed diagnoses in children and adults seeking emergency care. Approximately 500,000 people each year need hospitalization for treatment of head trauma. Individuals who survive a head injury can be left with severe neurologic deficits. This section addresses various types of injury, including concussions, coup and contrecoup, hematomas, and skull fractures.

What IS a Head Injury?

Head injury involves physical damage to brain tissue that is caused by external physical force. Depending on the severity of the insult and the location of the brain injury, the changes in brain tissue and function can be temporary or permanent. Head injuries are categorized according to the type of damage that occurs or the nature of the mechanism that caused the injury.

Pathogenesis

Closed Head Injury. A closed head injury means that after a blow, the skull is left intact and no obvious external damage has occurred. This type of injury is usually the result of sudden acceleration-deceleration accidents. Because the brain is suspended in a hard container (the skull) and is surrounded by a layer of cerebrospinal fluid (CSF), the process of rapid acceleration-deceleration can result in injury at the site of impact. After the initial blow, the brain "bounces" back in the other direction within its container, striking the hard, rough inner surface of the skull. Another name for this type of injury is "coup, contrecoup."

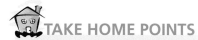

TAKE HOME POINTS

Head injuries are categorized according to the type of damage that occurs. A closed head injury means that the skull is left intact. An open head injury means that the skull, the scalp, the meninges, or the brain has been penetrated.

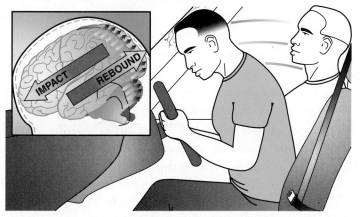

Mechanism of coup-contrecoup head injury.

Open Head Injury. An open head injury occurs when penetration of the scalp, the skull, the meninges, or the brain has occurred. Open head injuries are typically associated with skull fractures and carry a high risk of infection. Depressed or broken fragments of the skull may penetrate brain tissue, causing further damage.

After a blow to the head, both primary and secondary injuries can occur. Primary injuries are those that occur as a direct consequence of the physical trauma and are further categorized as focal or diffuse. Examples of focal primary injuries include contusion, laceration, and hemorrhage. Diffuse injuries include concussion, contusion, diffuse axonal injury, and hypoxic brain injury. Diffuse axonal injuries are commonly associated with strong acceleration-deceleration forces that cause damage to axons and neuronal pathways. Severe diffuse axonal injury can cause coma and autonomic dysfunction. The damage results in microscopic hemorrhages throughout the brain.

Concussions. Concussions are the least severe form of axonal injury. Sudden movement of the brain within the cranial vault that leads to diffuse but reversible injury is characteristic of concussions.

Skull Fractures. Fractures of the skull, a relatively common head injury, do not, in and of themselves, cause neurologic damage. An open skull fracture means that the dura mater is torn. This type of injury requires surgery. With closed skull fracture, the dura mater is intact. Blows to the face and nose can fracture the bones of the floor of the skull, creating an abnormal opening between the sinuses and the brain through which infectious organisms can enter the central nervous system (CNS).

Secondary brain injury occurs as a consequence of the original insult. The initial injury generates an inflammatory response that becomes maladaptive because the reaction is taking place within the tight confines of the skull. The inflammatory response leads to cerebral edema and increased intracranial pressure (ICP). Because increased pressure damages cells, the inflammatory response worsens. Cerebral edema compromises blood flow to cerebral tissue. Subsequent hypoxia causes anaerobic glycolysis and failure of the sodium and potassium pump, leading to an excess accumulation of sodium in the cell. Water moves into the cell, causing further swelling and a decrease in cerebral perfusion. Scarring and fibrosis of brain tissue occurs as a consequence of this process.

Hematomas. Hematomas are an indirect consequence of head trauma. A hematoma is an accumulation or a collection of blood that escapes from a damaged vessel. Ordinarily, a hematoma would be no great cause for concern, because the body eventually resorbs the blood.

However, cerebral perfusion may be jeopardized if blood accumulates within the confines of the cranial vault. The patient experiences increased ICP, tissue damage, and activation of the inflammatory response.

Hematomas are described based on the location where they occur. *Epidural hematomas* are usually the result of arterial bleeding from a skull fracture. Because arteries are under high pressure, a rapid accumulation of blood in the epidural space usually occurs. This rapid accumulation of blood in a confined space tends to cause sudden, dramatic symptoms in the affected person.

Subdural hematomas have a wide range of symptoms and can be acute, subacute, or chronic in nature. These hematomas are typically associated with torn cerebral veins but can occasionally occur from arterial sources. Acute subdural hematomas tend to appear rapidly and are characterized by a sudden decline in neurologic status. This type of intracranial bleeding is an emergency that requires immediate surgical intervention.

Subacute subdural hematomas are of venous origin; blood tends to accumulate more slowly. Symptoms appear anywhere from 4 to 21 days after the injury and typically involve neurologic deficits, changes in mental status, and complaints of severe headache.

Chronic subdural hematoma does not typically develop until several weeks after the initial injury. This type of injury can result from seemingly insignificant head trauma. Symptoms are vague, nonspecific, and are often mistakenly diagnosed as dementia or stroke.

Subarachnoid hemorrhage occurs as a result of head trauma that damages vascular structures in the subarachnoid space or a rupture of cerebral aneurysms within intracerebral arteries. This type of injury can cause vasospasm of cerebral blood vessels, which leads to hypoxia and ischemia of brain tissue, leaving the patient at risk for further brain damage.

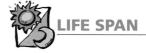

LIFE SPAN

Chronic subdural hematoma is commonly observed in older patients or in younger adults with a history of alcohol abuse.

At-Risk Populations

Head injuries can happen to anyone in the course of normal daily activities. One half of all brain injuries occur as a result of motor vehicle, pedestrian, bicycle, or pedestrian-vehicle accidents. Males are more than twice as likely as females to sustain a brain injury. Alcohol is thought to be a factor in one half of all traumatic head injuries. However, changes in speed limits and highway design have helped to decrease the incidence of head trauma. A second, less drastic peak in prevalence occurs in children age 5 and under.

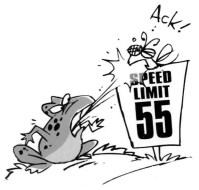

Slow down!

What You NEED TO KNOW

Clinical Manifestations

Signs and symptoms of head injury vary according to the location and extent of the damage to cerebral tissue.

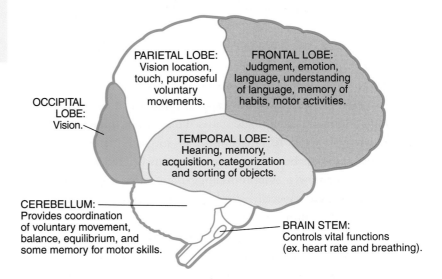

PARIETAL LOBE: Vision location, touch, purposeful voluntary movements.

FRONTAL LOBE: Judgment, emotion, language, understanding of language, memory of habits, motor activities.

OCCIPITAL LOBE: Vision.

TEMPORAL LOBE: Hearing, memory, acquisition, categorization and sorting of objects.

CEREBELLUM: Provides coordination of voluntary movement, balance, equilibrium, and some memory for motor skills.

BRAIN STEM: Controls vital functions (ex. heart rate and breathing).

After the initial trauma, patients may experience a brief or prolonged loss of consciousness, decreased level of consciousness (LOC), somnolence, confusion, and disorientation, as well as psychologic, cognitive, and motor deficits. A decline in level of consciousness is frequently the first sign of increasing ICP. Other signs and symptoms include headache, nausea, restlessness, increasing systolic blood pressure, decreasing pulse rate, and changes in pupillary reaction.

A localized injury can cause specific symptoms, whereas a more diffuse injury involving shifting of cerebral tissue results in a different pattern of injury, including changes in level of consciousness, contralateral muscle weakness, and coma. Injury scan also produce changes in physical, cognitive, mental, and emotional functioning. Patients with a severe diffuse axonal injury may be deeply comatose, with decerebrate or decorticate posturing and disruption of vital organ function and temperature regulation.

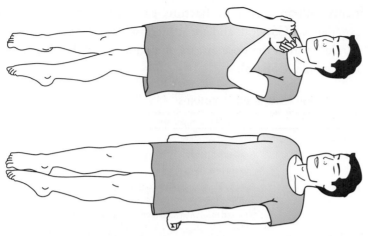

Decorticate posturing (*top figure*). Decerebrate posturing (*bottom figure*).

A brief loss of consciousness is characteristic of a concussion. Most patients recover fully without any neurologic deficit, although research suggests that a postconcussion syndrome involving headache, irritability, insomnia, and poor concentration may occur. These symptoms can persist for several months after the initial injury.

Even after the individual is recovered and medically stable, a variety of neurologic and psychomotor deficits can exist. Although they may appear physically normal, many survivors of traumatic brain injury have many functional problems that make it difficult for them to fulfill their previous role. These problems include difficulties in attention, concentration, language use, and visual perception. Learning ability may be altered, and previously acquired complex knowledge and skills may be lost. Behavioral alterations include verbal and physical aggression, agitation, impulsivity, and social disinhibition. Changes in personality, labile emotions, depression, and anxiety are also common findings.

Depending on the degree and location of damage, brain injury can impair motor function and cause hemiparesis or hemiplegia. Although some patients may retain voluntary control over movement, they may have problems with spasticity and abnormal posturing. Decorticate posturing is present in the patient with lesions in the corticospinal pathways. Decerebrate posturing is typically observed in patients with damage in the brainstem.

Depending on the extent, location, and severity of injury, deficits can be permanent, show partial improvement, or resolve completely. However, even patients with mild traumatic brain injury can experience permanent damage.

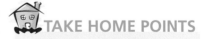

TAKE HOME POINTS

Internal rotation and flexion of the patient's arms, wrists, and fingers and plantar flexion of the legs are characteristic of *decorticate posturing*. *Decerebrate posturing* involves extension of the patient's arms and legs, pronation of the arms, arching of the back, and hyperextension of the head.

Patients with an open skull fracture, particularly of the basilar area, may experience a CSF leak and are at increased risk for CNS infections. Clear drainage from the nose or ears of a patient with head trauma is a warning sign of a CSF leak.

Brain Injuries and Associated Symptoms

Location of Injury	Associated Symptoms
Right hemisphere	Left-sided paralysis
Left hemisphere	Right-sided paralysis
Broca's area	Expressive aphasia
Wernicke's area	Poor auditory comprehension; fluent speech but with phrasing error and/or meaningless jargon
Cerebellum	Impaired movement and balance; loss of fine motor function
Frontal lobe	Impairments in fine motor movements, speech, and the ability to use and manipulate tools
Temporal lobe	Hearing disturbances; long-term memory loss
Occipital lobe	Decreased ability to interpret the meaning of visual images

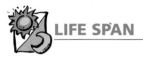

LIFE SPAN

The highest incidence for traumatic brain injury is for people aged 15 to 24 years and those 75 and older. Falls among elderly adults and young children are the second most frequent cause of brain trauma.

Prognosis

The chances of recovery from brain injury depend on the location and severity of the injury and the extent of damage. Even minor injuries such as a concussion can leave a patient with residual neurologic deficits such as memory loss.

Patients with more severe injuries have improved outcomes when appropriate medical treatment is initiated within the first hour after the injury. Patients with severe injuries have mortality rates of 35% or more. Survivors of this type of injury frequently experience profound personality changes, as well as neurologic and psychologic deficits.

Patients with elevated ICP that does not respond adequately to therapy tend to have a poor outcome. After the acute phase of injury is resolved, rehabilitative care significantly influences the degree of recovery of neurologic function. Individuals with damage so severe that they are unable to benefit from rehabilitative care usually require placement in a long-term care facility.

What You DO

Treatment

For optimal outcomes, treatment must begin as soon as possible after the injury. Initial interventions involve radiologic assessment of the brain for lesions, such as a hematoma or a depressed skull fracture, that require surgical intervention.

Generally, the goal of medical care is to restore and maintain normal ICP, oxygen and CO_2 levels, and blood supply to cerebral tissue. Because of the high risk for CNS infections, patients with open head injuries are typically treated with prophylactic antibiotics. ICP monitoring may be required to evaluate the status of the patient and facilitate prompt treatment of elevations in pressure. Patients requiring invasive monitoring will need placement in an intensive care unit.

A variety of pharmacologic approaches may be needed to decrease ICP. Restlessness and agitation, frequently present with head injury, can increase ICP and can be successfully treated with narcotics and benzodiazepines. When no benefit is obtained from sedation and the patient has rising ICP, has increased muscle tone, or is resisting the ventilator, paralyzing agents such as pancuronium or vecuronium may be used. Mannitol may be given to decrease ICP by osmotic diuresis. High-dose glucocorticoids are given to decrease cerebral edema. As a last step to control rising ICP, large doses of barbiturates may be used to induce coma. Patients with expanding brain injury, such as from a growing intracerebral hematoma, may require surgical intervention to remove the hematoma and preserve the integrity of cerebral tissue.

Nursing Responsibilities

Nurses must be actively involved in educating the public about measures that help decrease the incidence of head injury. Appropriate assessment of safety and the risk of falls can lead to interventions that will decrease the risk of injury. These interventions may include the use of assistive devices such as walkers and handrails and early screening and treatment of osteoporosis.

The goals of nursing care for the patient with a head injury are to decrease ICP, promote the delivery of oxygen and nutrients to the brain, and minimize complications and adverse effects associated with the brain injury. Immediately after the injury, patients with major head trauma

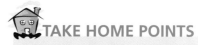

TAKE HOME POINTS

Safety precautions such as the use of safety belts, helmets, air bags, and child and infant seats can help prevent head injuries.

🏠 TAKE HOME POINTS

- Medical care for the patient with a head injury is directed toward restoring and maintaining normal ICP, oxygen and CO_2 levels, and blood supply to cerebral tissue.
- A lumbar puncture is contraindicated in the presence of known or suspected head injury.
- Patients with head injury are likely to have a cervical spine injury as well. Radiologic evaluation as a part of the initial diagnostic evaluation after the injury should rule out this possibility.

require supportive measures in an intensive care setting to maintain all vital functions.

Begin with a comprehensive assessment to establish a baseline, and document findings in the patient's record.

- Assess the patient carefully for evidence of seizure activity. In many cases, seizure activity is limited to one part of the body, such as an eyelid, corner of the mouth, or fingers, hand, or arm (i.e., focal seizures). Any focal seizure can progress to generalized seizures. Seizures are cause for concern because they can lead to cerebral hypoxia.

- After the initial baseline has been established, comprehensive examinations may be required as often as every hour. Temperature regulation can be a problem for patients with head injury, particularly when they have suffered damage to the hypothalamus. A correlation frequently exists between elevated temperature and poor outcomes in this population. Moderate hypothermia causes a reduction in cerebral blood flow and thus decreases ICP.

- Pay special attention to oxygenation levels and blood pressure. Hypotension has been shown to reduce cerebral perfusion pressure and oxygenation. A blood pressure that is too low compromises cerebral blood flow and increases damage to cerebral tissue. Uncontrolled hypotension has been associated with twice the mortality rates in head injury patients. Autoregulation of vital signs is often adversely affected by brain injury. Blood pressure must be carefully controlled. Elevated blood pressure can increase cerebral blood volume and indirectly cause more cerebral ischemia. Mechanical ventilation may be required to maintain adequate control of oxygen and CO_2. Keeping CO_2 levels within normal ranges is important. Excess levels of CO_2 causes increased cerebral blood flow and ICP, ultimately leading to cerebral ischemia. Decreased levels of CO_2 can cause constriction of cerebral arteries.

- Report findings suggestive of a skull fracture, including blood behind the eardrum, "raccoon's eyes" **(periorbital ecchymosis)**, or bruising over the mastoid bone **(Battle's sign)** to the health care provider immediately. Clear, thin fluid coming from the nose or ears is suggestive of a CSF leak. When the drainage is CSF, it will test positive for glucose and form a halo when applied to tissue paper. Patients with a CSF leak may also complain of a persistent salty or sweet taste. For patients with a confirmed CSF leak, avoid placing anything in the patient's nose or ears because of the increased risk for CNS infection.

- Teach the patient with a skull fracture to avoid blowing the nose and apply a "mustache" dressing over the upper lip to absorb drainage.
- Elevate the head of the patient's bed 15 to 30 degrees, unless contraindicated.
- Avoid flexing the patient's neck or knees or turning the patient's head to either side. Abnormal muscle tone, spasticity, posturing, and disrupted motor reflexes make positioning a brain-injured patient in normal anatomic alignment difficult. Special care must be taken in positioning to compensate for abnormal reflexes and muscle tone. These patients may require supportive devices such as pillows, foam wedges, and rolls to maintain good body alignment. Unless other medical contraindications exist, such as increased ICP, these patients should have routine passive and active range of motion exercises within the levels of their ability and should also be inspected daily for evidence of skin breakdown. Keep in mind that abnormal movement and spasticity can cause skin breakdown in unusual locations.
- Minimize extraneous stimulation such as loud noise, conversations, and lights, all of which have been shown to increase ICP. Suctioning, painful procedures, baths, and emotionally charged conversations within the patient's hearing can also increase ICP.

Sedatives and analgesics may be required to decrease fear, anxiety, and pain. These drugs can also help decrease combativeness and agitation and facilitate mechanical ventilation. Because these drugs can make evaluating mental and neurologic status difficult, they may have to be withheld periodically to obtain an accurate assessment. Sedation can mask symptoms of neurologic deterioration and should not be used without ICP monitoring.

After the patient is medically stable, a referral should be made to a brain injury rehabilitation team. Recovery from head injury is frequently prolonged and difficult not only for the patient, but also for the patient's significant others.

- Increasing ICP is an emergency and must be treated. Without prompt intervention, the patient may suffer permanent brain damage or death.
- Any suspected seizure activity must be reported immediately so that antiepileptic drug therapy can be initiated.
- Subtle changes such as drowsiness may be indicative of further intracranial bleeding. Any subsequent deterioration in baseline neurologic examination must be reported immediately.
- In contrast to other types of head injuries, the patient with a basilar skull fracture should be placed nearly flat to prevent pressure on the brainstem, unless other contraindications exist.

Do You UNDERSTAND?

DIRECTIONS: **Provide answers for the following questions.**

1. What type of head injury carries the greatest risk for infection?

   _____

2. A patient with a recent head injury complains of a persistent sweet taste. This is likely a result of what?

   _____

3. What position is safest for the patient with a basilar skull fracture? Why?

   _____

4. Why should hypotension be avoided when treating a patient with a head injury?

   _____

What ARE Headaches?

Headaches may cause varying types of pain and neurologic symptoms, depending upon the causative factors. Headaches are usually classified according to their etiology or cause. The three most common types, tension, migraine and cluster headaches, will be discussed in this section. The different types of headaches probably have physiologic factors in common.

What IS a Tension Headache?

Tension headaches may be episodic or chronic in nature. Episodic tension headaches usually occur in association with stressful events. Chronic tension headaches may occur daily and are associated with contracted muscles of the scalp and neck.

Answers: 1. open; 2. CSF leak; 3. flat, prevents pressure on the brain stem; 4. hypotension leads to decreased cerebral perfusion pressure and oxygenation.

Pathogenesis

Tension headaches are thought to have both physical and psychologic components. A variety of factors may precipitate a tension headache including emotional conflicts, depression, anger, repressed hostility, and fatigue. These factors lead to abnormal, sustained contractions of the muscles in the face, scalp, neck, and shoulders, which ultimately cause pain because of muscular irritation, inflammation, and decreased blood flow.

At-Risk Populations

Usually, people who are prone to tension headaches begin to experience them in early adulthood. Women are more likely to have tension headaches than men.

Clinical Manifestations

In contrast to other types of headaches, symptoms of a tension headache include a throbbing pain that gradually increases. Patients tend to complain of a feeling of pressure or tightness. The pain is often located either in the frontal or occipital lobes and may be bilateral. These headaches are frequently present upon arising from sleep and may persist for as little as 30 minutes or as long as 7 days. Usually, tension headache pain does not change with activity levels.

Prognosis

Unless caused by other underlying disease processes, nearly all tension headaches can be successfully treated. Successful resolution of headaches may require lifestyle changes and elimination of stressors.

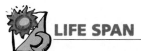

In young children and patients over the age of 50, new onset of headache is uncommon. It may signal underlying pathology such as tumors or cerebral disease and injury and should always be thoroughly investigated.

LIFE SPAN

In the older individual headaches may be a symptom of glaucoma, sinusitis, hemorrhagic stroke, subarachnoid hemorrhage, subdural hematoma, temporal arteritis, and temporomandibular joint syndrome.

What You DO

Treatment

Initial therapy of all headaches is directed toward providing prompt relief of symptoms; pharmacologic agents are usually effective, particularly if used before the headache becomes severe. Nonsteroidal antiinflammatory drugs (NSAIDs) can be helpful because they reduce serotonin release and block the synthesis of prostaglandin, as well as decrease platelet aggregation. These actions help to decrease inflammation and improve cerebral blood flow.

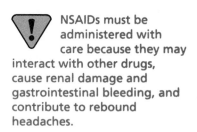

NSAIDs must be administered with care because they may interact with other drugs, cause renal damage and gastrointestinal bleeding, and contribute to rebound headaches.

Opioid analgesics may cause drug dependence.

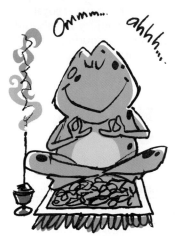

Meditate to relieve headaches.

For patients with infrequent headaches, barbiturates in combination with acetaminophen can be used to induce relaxation and relieve pain. Examples of other drug combinations that can be helpful include butalbital, aspirin and caffeine; acetaminophen and codeine; and acetaminophen and oxycodone.

Nonpharmacologic measures that are also helpful include physical therapy, exercise programs, and counseling regarding lifestyle modification to eliminate or reduce stressors.

Nursing Responsibilities

Using a holistic approach to headache treatment helps patients cope with and resolve headache pain. The nurse should do the following:

- Teach the patient how to safely self-administer prescribed analgesics when a headache occurs.
- Help the patient identify coping measures that reduce stress such as meditation, exercise, and progressive muscle relaxation.
- Give assistance and support to patients who smoke regarding smoking cessation. Nicotine constricts blood vessels, with subsequent reduction in cerebral blood flow and oxygenation of cerebral tissues.

Do You UNDERSTAND?

DIRECTIONS: **Indicate which statements are *true* (T) and which are *false* (F). If false, correct the statement in the margin space to make it true.**

_____ 1. Tension headaches are caused by abnormal dilation of cranial blood vessels.

_____ 2. Relaxation exercises can be helpful in the control of tension headaches.

_____ 3. Men are more likely to get tension headaches than women.

_____ 4. Most tension headaches occur in individuals over the age of 50.

_____ 5. Tension headaches usually require treatment with opioid analgesics.

Answers: 1. F: Sustained contractions of the muscles in the face, scalp, neck, and shoulders, ultimately cause pain; 2. T; 3. F: Women are more likely than men to have tension headaches; 4. F: People prone to tension headaches begin to experience them in early adulthood; 5. F: Nonsteroidal antiinflammatory drugs and non-drug therapies pharmacologic agents are also helpful. In most cases it is inappropriate to use an opioid analgesic for tension headaches.

What IS a Migraine Headache?

Migraines are the second most common type of headaches and are estimated to affect up to 20% of the U.S. population. There are two main types of migraine headaches: the classic migraine and a common migraine. About 75% of migraines are the common type. Another type of headache, related to migraine, is the cluster headache.

Pathogenesis

Migraine headaches are thought to be due to changes in cerebral vessel tone and neurotransmitter levels. Falls in serotonin levels cause the brain to become more sensitive to triggers of migraines such as hormonal changes, stress, chemicals, ingestion of tyramine-containing foods, and sleep deprivation. Blood vessels in the brain become abnormally dilated and stretch the nerves surrounding the vessels. This causes the release of inflammatory cytokines, with subsequent transmission of pain impulses to the hypothalamus via the trigeminal nerve.

Cluster headaches are migraine-like headaches marked by attacks of unilateral intense pain over the eyes and forehead. The attacks last up to 3 hours and occur in clusters. The cause of cluster headaches is not clearly understood. Possible etiologies include changes in neurovascular tone, initiation of abnormal firing of neurons by the trigeminal nerve, and hypothalamic activity. In some individuals cluster headaches may be precipitated by small amounts of histamines. Other possible causes include stress, allergens, nitroglycerin, and alcohol. Of patients with this condition 80% are heavy smokers, and half have a history of heavy alcohol use.

At-Risk Populations

Women are 3 times more likely than men to have migraines. About two thirds of patients who have migraines experience a dramatic decrease in migraines after menopause. However, there are many other migraine triggers: these range from eating certain foods—such as wine, chocolate, caffeine, and aged cheeses, among others—to stress. People who suffer from migraines often have a distinctive personality type that is characterized by a meticulous, neat, compulsive, and somewhat rigid personality. When migraines occur in childhood, they are more commonly seen in boys.

Cluster headaches are 6 times more common in men than women. In men, these headaches begin in the 30s; they have a somewhat later onset in women. Possible precipitating factors of cluster headaches include inadequate rest, excessive physical activity, strong emotions, and smoking or the odor of tobacco smoke.

What You NEED TO KNOW

Clinical Manifestations

Classic migraine headaches start with a warning sign, called an *aura*. Auras are painless, sensory disturbances that occur in 20% to 25% of patients before the migraine attack. Auras last 15 to 30 minutes and are thought to be related to ischemia in certain regions of the brain. Auras may manifest as sudden blind spots (scotomas), disruptions of the visual fields, alterations in smell or hearing, and rarely in neurologic dysfunction. Auras may occur before or after the head pain; sometimes the pain and aura overlap; or the pain might never occur.

Classic migraine headache pain is usually of more sudden onset than tension headache, and is usually unilateral in nature. The pain tends to be of a pounding quality. It is severe in intensity and usually occurs either around or behind the eyes. Migraines may be accompanied by systemic symptoms such as sonophobia and photophobia and changes in appetite, mood, and libido. Most, if not all patients, will experience some degree of nausea, vomiting, and light-headedness.

Common migraines don't start with an aura. Common migraines usually start more slowly than classic migraines, last longer, and interfere more with daily activities. The pain of common migraines may be on only one side of the head.

Cluster headaches, also called histamine headaches, are an uncommon, severe type of headache. They are characterized by pain that is lancinating (stabbing), severe in quality, and located on one side of the face; or, it can be felt along the first and second divisions of the trigeminal nerve. There is a sensation that the eye is being pushed out of the socket. The onset is sudden, with a peak in 15 minutes or less, and the headaches may last from 10 minutes to 3 hours. These headaches may occur at the same time every day for several weeks until the "cluster period" is finished. Cluster periods may occur every few months and can be frightening and disabling.

⚠ Pain associated with cluster headaches is excruciating. Suicides have been reported in people who have frequent and severe cluster headaches.

Physical examination of patients who are having cluster headaches may reveal injection of the conjunctiva, ptosis on the same side that the pain is felt, and lack of sweating on that side of the face. Some patients experience bradycardia and facial flushing. Other symptoms associated with cluster headaches are nasal congestion, lacrimation (excess production of tears), nausea, sweating, restlessness, and agitation.

In both cluster and migraine headaches, blood vessels dilate, but the blood vessels behind the eyes pulsate only in cluster headaches. What causes these events and how they relate to cluster headaches are still unclear.

Prognosis

The frequency and severity of common and classic migraine headaches can be reduced with appropriate medical management. Currently there is no cure for cluster headaches. With the right therapy, most people can learn how to manage their symptoms and have fewer, better-controlled headache episodes.

Patients with migraine require prompt evaluation to verify that the headache is not due to underlying pathology such as cerebral aneurysms, meningitis, stroke, or intracranial bleeding.

What You DO

Treatment

Treatment of migraine and cluster headaches is directed toward obtaining prompt relief of pain, as well as using drugs to decrease the frequency and severity of headaches. Drug therapy is the mainstay of therapy for common and classic migraine headaches. Nonpharmacologic measures that are often helpful include bedrest in a quiet, dark environment, and cold compresses applied directly to painful areas.

Patients in the throes of a severe migraine may require intravenous opioids and antiemetics to relieve the pain and nausea that typically accompanies a migraine headache. Other drugs are given to reduce the frequency and severity of the attacks. These drugs include 5-HT1 (serotonin) receptor agonists such as sumatriptan. Eletriptan is a selective serotonin agonist that acts on receptors in cranial blood vessels and sensory nerve endings to relieve pain. Other helpful adjuncts include ergot alkaloids and derivatives, which act by constricting smooth muscles of cranial blood vessels. In some cases, antiepileptic drugs such as topiramate or carbamazepine, muscle relaxants such as cyclobenzaprine, and antidepressant drugs may help. If used early, administration of 100% oxygen may help relieve a cluster headache.

When applied to the nasal mucosa, capsaicin cream may lower the number and severity of cluster headaches. Corticosteroids and NSAIDs may also help to decrease the inflammatory component of these headaches, but may take up to 12 hours to offer the patient relief.

For severe cases that do not respond to pharmacologic interventions, nerves may be injected with alcohol to interrupt the transmission of pain impulses along the nerve fibers. Chronic refractory cases may require resection of the nerves in order to offer relief. Surgery is used only when all other therapies have failed.

Nursing Responsibilities

As soon as the patient's pain is controlled, obtain a baseline history. Ask how long the patient has been experiencing migraines, what the patient has done in the past to deal with attacks, and whether or not he or she is aware of any precipitating factors. Do a physical examination to detect any neurologic deficits. In addition, the nurse should do the following:

- Help the patient identify headache triggers and learn how to avoid them.
- Report any neurologic deficits or changes immediately to the patient's health care provider.
- Promptly administer drug therapy to control migraine symptoms and help the patient learn how to prevent and control triggering factors.
- Inform the patient about alternative measures which may help control symptoms including meditation, tai chi, and yoga.
- Teach the patient and a family member how to administer drug therapy at home in the event of an attack, especially since some drugs must be given via an injection or as a nasal inhalation.
- Advise patients that use of opioids for pain control may cause intermittent cluster headaches to transform into chronic cluster headaches and become more frequent.
- Instruct patients who have cluster headaches to avoid high altitudes, which may precipitate an attack, or using capsaicin intranasally for headache treatment without first checking with their health care provider.

Do You UNDERSTAND?

DIRECTIONS: Fill in the blanks to complete the following statements.

1. Migraines are typically _____ or _____ in onset.
2. Migraine pain is most often _____.
3. _____ and _____ are the two of the common symptoms associated with migraine headache.

Circle the best answer.

4. Which food or beverage should be eliminated from the diet of a patient with frequent tension headaches?
   a. Red meat
   b. Acidic fruits
   c. Coffee
   d. Cola type soft drinks
   e. c and d only
5. Oxygen may be helpful in the treatment of
   a. Tension headaches
   b. Migraine headaches
   c. Cluster headaches
   d. None of the above

What IS Vertigo?

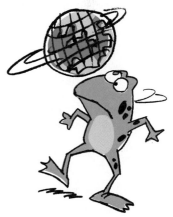

Vertigo is the perception that either one's self or the environment is moving. For some people the perception of movement may be exaggerated. Patients with objective vertigo perceive that their environment is moving while they are standing still. Subjective vertigo patients have the perception that their body is moving while their surroundings are not. A patient with benign paroxysmal positional vertigo (BPPV) has a short-lasting but severe vertigo that can be immobilizing because the individual is often too dizzy to walk.

The world isn't spinning... it's vertigo.

Answers: 1. sudden or acute; 2. unilateral; 3. nausea, vomiting; 4. c and d; 5. c.

Pathogenesis

Vertigo is not in and of itself a disease, but rather a manifestation of an underlying problem. Dysfunction of the inner ear or labyrinth, the medulla or cerebellum of the brain, or systemic and metabolic disturbances can cause vertigo. Neurologic and medical conditions that may contribute to vertigo include stroke, multiple sclerosis, Parkinson's disease, infection, hypoglycemia, and alcohol abuse.

BPPV is often related to the dislodging of calcium crystals that are normally deposited on the small hair-like structures within the ear. The calcium crystals weight the hairs and help modulate the response when the head is turned. When those crystals are dislodged, the hair response when the head is moved becomes hypersensitive and much more rapid. In approximately a quarter of cases of vertigo, no cause is ever found.

At-Risk Populations

People with a history of inner ear problems are more likely to develop this symptom. It may also be seen after head trauma or a severe cold. Women are twice as likely to be affected as men.

What You NEED TO KNOW

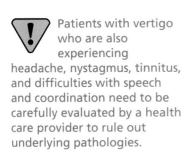 Patients with vertigo who are also experiencing headache, nystagmus, tinnitus, and difficulties with speech and coordination need to be carefully evaluated by a health care provider to rule out underlying pathologies.

Clinical Manifestations

Patients with vertigo typically describe a subjective sensation of dizziness or spinning when objectively they know that no movement is present. Other symptoms may include an unsteady gait, confusion, nausea, and feeling faint.

BPPV is exacerbated by movement. Actions such as rolling over in bed or turning the head can give rise to intense periods of dizziness. Symptoms of BPPV are usually worse in the morning upon arising.

Prognosis

Vertigo can often be resolved, particularly if the underlying cause can be successfully treated.

What You DO

Treatment

Therapy for vertigo varies depending upon the underlying cause of the condition. Antihistamines, antiemetics, and benzodiazepines can be helpful in controlling symptoms of nausea and vomiting. Scopolamine may help to reduce dizziness.

Patients with BPPV may gain relief from vertigo by performing an Epley or Hall-Pike maneuver, a series of movements of the patient's head that will move displaced calcium crystals out of the posterior semicircular canal into the part of the inner ear where they belong. Symptoms are thus relieved. Even without therapy, most cases of BPPV are self-limited and will subside spontaneously over a period of several weeks.

Nursing Responsibilities

Nursing care is directed toward controlling symptoms and preventing patient injury. Help the patient who is dizzy to stand up and change positions slowly. Teach patients how to safely administer their own drug therapy. Advise patients to use caution when driving and to avoid alcohol until the effects of the drugs are known. Dizzy and confused patients may need to have direct visual supervision at all times to protect them from injury.

Do You UNDERSTAND?

DIRECTIONS: Circle the correct answer.

1. A patient with a history of diabetes walks into the emergency room and complains that he feels very weak and dizzy. The nurse should first
   a. Do a baseline physical examination.
   b. Ensure the patient's safety.
   c. Do a capillary glucose level.
   d. Report the patient's presence to the emergency room physician.
2. Vertigo is often due to
   a. Middle ear disorders.
   b. Metabolic disorders.
   c. Cardiovascular disease.
   d. Any of the above.

Answers: 1. b; 2. d.

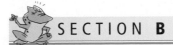

SECTION **B**

ISCHEMIC DISEASE AND STROKE

The nervous system allows humans to interact with and respond to the world around them. Regardless of the cause, dysfunctions in the nervous system can adversely affect the ability to think, reason, predict, or carry out simple activities of daily living.

The CNS may be considered the master control system of the body; it allows us to interpret, use, and act on the input from our senses, and it helps protect and maintain the integrity and normal function of the body. The nervous system has central and peripheral components. The brain and spinal cord are the major components of the CNS.

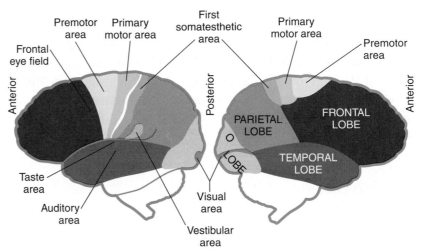

Major components of the CNS.

The autonomic nervous system (ANS) is responsible for maintaining and regulating the function of glands and smooth muscles within the body and promoting the coordinated functioning of the visceral organs. The ANS has two subdivisions: the sympathetic and the parasympathetic systems. The sympathetic nervous system is responsible for initiating the protective "fight-or-flight" response when the body is exposed to stress.

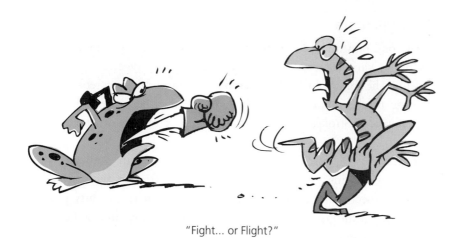

"Fight... or Flight?"

The parasympathetic system transmits impulses to the visceral organs and is responsible for "vegetative" functions of the body that are not under conscious control.

Nerve cells have a limited ability to recover from damage, which is an important consideration when considering the effect of disease and trauma to the CNS. The brain is a delicate organ and requires a constant supply of glucose and oxygen. At any given time, the brain receives 15% of cardiac output (blood ejected by the heart) and consumes 20% of the body's total oxygen requirements. Any event or process that decreases the brain's supply of oxygen and nutrients is a serious threat to the normal integrity and function of the brain and CNS.

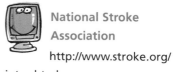

National Stroke Association
http://www.stroke.org/intro.html
National Institute of Neurologic Disorders and Stroke
http://www.ninds.nih.gov/

What IS a Cerebrovascular Accident?

Cerebrovascular accidents (CVA) are also called strokes or brain attacks. A stroke occurs when a sudden interruption of blood flow to a part of the brain occurs. A stroke should not be confused with a transient ischemic attack (TIA). A stroke is defined as a neurologic deficit lasting over 24 hours that occurs as a result of interrupted arterial blood flow to a part of the brain. With a stroke, the interruption of oxygen and nutrients to brain cells can cause permanent brain damage and impaired functioning. A TIA is a neurologic deficit that lasts for less than 24 hours. Most TIAs resolve within a few hours, and the patient regains full neurologic functioning.

Pathogenesis

CVAs or brain attacks are the result of disturbance in blood flow of the brain. Various factors can deprive the brain of oxygen and nutrients, causing the brain tissue to become ischemic. Most cerebrovascular damage to the brain is the indirect result of either atherosclerosis or hypertension. Strokes are generally occlusive, embolic, or hemorrhagic in origin.

Occlusive. Atherosclerosis of the vessels in the brain can lead to the gradual narrowing or stenosis of the cerebral arteries, with complete blockage (occlusion) as the ultimate result. Alternatively, fatty plaques can break off into the circulation and form a thrombus in distal cerebral vessels, ultimately causing a blockage.

Hemorrhagic. Hypertension can lead to damage to cerebral vessels and subsequent intracerebral hemorrhage. Bleeding can occur into the ventricular, subdural, or subarachnoid spaces. Other vascular conditions leading to cerebral hemorrhage include ruptured cerebral aneurysms and arteriovenous malformations (AVM). An aneurysm is an abnormally dilated area or blister on the arterial wall. When subjected to increased pressure from hypertension, the arterial wall becomes progressively thinner and more fragile and eventually ruptures, allowing blood to leak into the cerebral tissues.

An AVM is a tangle of twisted, abnormally shaped blood vessels that are frequently described as resembling a "nest of worms." These vessels can become abnormally dilated and fragile and frequently leak blood, which can cause a stroke.

Embolic. Cardiovascular conditions such as atrial arrhythmias and recent myocardial infarction can cause clots (emboli) to be released into the systemic circulation, where they may lodge in a cerebral vessel obstructing blood flow. Certain blood disorders and hyperviscosity syndromes increase an individual's risk for stroke. The abnormal hemoglobin associated with sickle cell disease causes abnormally shaped, rigid red blood cells to form, resulting in increased viscosity and microvascular sludging. Myeloproliferative disorders such as polycythemia vera can cause increased blood viscosity and impaired blood flow to vital organs.

Whatever the cause, the result of impaired arterial blood flow to the brain is ischemia and hypoxia of cerebral tissues. The brain's oxygen supply is exhausted within 10 seconds after cessation of blood flow. Irreversible tissue damage occurs within 2 to 4 minutes after the stroke unless the blood supply is reestablished. These tissues then undergo anaerobic glycolysis. Lactic acid accumulates, and ionic gradients are altered, allowing sodium, calcium, chloride, and water to enter the cells. Excess intracellular calcium leads to further damage of the cells, causing prostaglandins, cytokines, and leukotrienes to be released, resulting in further cell damage. Synaptic transmission is decreased as a result of inadequate adenosine triphosphate (ATP). When blood flow is restored promptly, the damage may be reversed. Otherwise, intracellular homeostasis is permanently disrupted, with subsequent cellular swelling and the death of neurons.

In the case of hemorrhagic strokes, damage to delicate brain tissue is compounded by the presence of blood within the tissue, which tends to cause increased intracranial pressure and subsequent extension of brain damage.

At-Risk Populations

Any individual with disease that compromises normal blood flow is at risk for a stroke. Such diseases include prolonged uncontrolled hypertension, diabetes mellitus, heart disease, atherosclerosis, and blood disorders such as sickle cell anemia and polycythemia vera. Regardless of race or ethnicity, strokes are increasingly likely to occur in people over the age of 60.

To some extent, the tendency toward cardiovascular disease appears to be an inherited trait. Patients with a strong family history of cardiovascular disease including myocardial infarction or hypertension, particularly in people under the age of 50, are at risk. Behaviors strongly correlated with an increased risk for stroke include the use of alcohol, tobacco, and cocaine.

Age, gender, and race are nonmodifiable risk factors, that is, not under patient control. Modifiable risk factors involve individual decisions, and are frequently, but not always, subject to the patient's control. Lifestyle modification and elimination of high-risk behaviors, such as smoking, and consuming a diet low in fat and sodium can accomplish a great deal in decreasing the risk of stroke and cardiovascular disease.

African American men have a higher incidence of stroke than Caucasian men, and they appear to experience increased mortality and morbidity from stroke. One possible cause for this phenomenon is an increased incidence of hypertension at an early age. Other contributing factors include inadequate access to preventive health care and financial constraints that limit their ability to adhere to a prescribed medical regimen.

Women over the age of 35 who take oral contraceptives have an increased risk of stroke. The risk is even higher when the individual smokes.

Preventive measures should include careful management and, when possible, elimination of risk factors. People who are physically active, maintain ideal body weight, consume a diet low in animal and saturated fats, and abstain from smoking have a significantly decreased risk for coronary and vascular disease. Patients who have problems with hypertension or hyperlipidemia, or those with a family history of stroke or cardiovascular disease, require careful monitoring and care by the health care provider.

What You NEED TO KNOW

Clinical Manifestations

Signs and symptoms of a stroke vary according to the area of the brain that has been affected. Symptoms can be gradual in onset or sudden and acute. Strokes from cerebral thrombosis exhibit fluctuating symptoms characterized by periods of regression and improvement. Progression of the blockage can be seen as a pattern of increasing neurologic deficits. This process is referred to as a "stroke in evolution." Early symptoms of a thrombotic stroke include confusion, aphasia, vertigo, and headache. Patients who have a TIA recover baseline function within 24 hours, but have a significantly increased risk of stroke in the future.

Hemorrhagic strokes tend to occur during activity. Of the three main types of strokes, hemorrhagic strokes tend to have the highest mortality rate. Intracerebral bleeding occurs abruptly, and the symptoms evolve quickly. Early warning signs of a cerebral hemorrhage include severe headache and nausea.

Embolic stroke tends to cause symptoms that are sudden and acute in onset. In contrast to hemorrhagic strokes, embolic strokes tend to occur during sleep. Symptoms of embolic stroke include weakness or numbness on one side of the body, visual changes or blindness, paralysis, and difficulty speaking or understanding speech. Speech difficulties experienced by the patient with a stroke can be particularly distressing because they deprive the patient of the ability to communicate. Strokes can also cause cognitive impairment and decreased self-care ability.

Strokes involving the right portion of the brain tend to adversely affect visual and spatial awareness and orientation, but leave the patient unaware of any deficits. These patients tend to be impulsive in their behaviors and exhibit poor judgment. In contrast, the left hemisphere of the brain is, for most people, the center for language, math, and analytic skills. A stroke in this area can result in varying degrees of aphasia. Sensory deficits can cause significant impairment, leaving the patient unable to read, write, or carry out purposeful activities, such as shaving or grooming. Patients with this type of injury tend to be slower and more cautious in their behavior, are often anxious and depressed, and tend to have labile emotions.

Neglect syndrome is a result of this sensory deficit, rendering the patient unaware of the paralyzed side. This problem tends to be more severe in patients with a right hemispheric stroke. Patients with this syndrome may leave the affected leg dragging underneath a wheelchair or neglect to comb one side of their hair, shave one side of their face, or eat off of one side of a plate.

Motor deficits associated with CVAs tend to affect the opposite side of the body from the cerebral hemisphere in which the stroke occurred. However, if the brainstem is involved, symptoms may be seen on both sides of the body. Depending on the nature and extent of the injury, muscle tone can be flaccid or spastic. Neurologic damage can also result in a spastic bladder and problems with bowel function.

Prognosis

The chance for recovery from a stroke is highly variable and depends on the extent and severity of cerebral tissue damage. Hemorrhagic stroke has a mortality rate of up to 70% and is particularly high when intracerebral bleeding is extensive. Overall, approximately 10% to 15% of patients with an ischemic stroke do not survive. Approximately 20% of individuals who manage to survive require long-term institutionalization, and up to one half of those remaining experience varying degrees of disability.

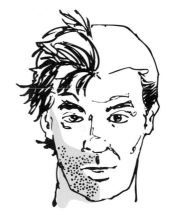

Neglect syndrome.

What You DO

Treatment

To determine a course of treatment, the exact cause of the stroke must be identified as soon as possible. Computerized tomography (CT) or magnetic resonance imaging (MRI) is used to evaluate the brain and identify the presence of a hemorrhage or aneurysm. Cerebral angiograms or magnetic resonance angiography (MRA) may be used to evaluate the brain vasculature and to detect clots and areas of vasospasm or rupture.

Depending on the extent of the damage involved, most patients who have had a stroke are kept in a fasting state immediately after the attack. Many of these patients have difficulty with the mechanics of speech and swallowing and are consequently at risk for aspiration. Indications of potential problems with eating include slurred speech and an absent or diminished gag reflex.

Medical management of a patient with a stroke is directed toward minimizing damage resulting from the stroke, maintaining adequate cerebral perfusion, and decreasing the risk of extension of the stroke and a subsequent recurrence. Tissue plasminogen activator (tPA) may reverse the effects of the stroke if given within 3 hours of the onset of symptoms. Patients with an embolic or thrombotic stroke usually receive heparin for anticoagulation and will likely require long-term anticoagulant therapy after leaving the hospital. Alternative management involves the administration of platelet aggregation inhibiters that are given to decrease the risk of clot formation.

Coexisting medical conditions that may have contributed to the stroke, such as diabetes mellitus or hypertension, are also evaluated and treated in an attempt to decrease the patient's future risk of another stroke. As soon as the patient is medically stable and does not appear at risk for extension of the stroke, rehabilitation therapy can begin to help minimize the effect of neurologic deficits.

During the acute phase, care is focused on timely implementation of therapeutic measures and on careful monitoring for evidence of extension of the stroke. Optimal care of the patient with a stroke involves collaboration among many different disciplines. The nurse is frequently responsible for ensuring that care is coordinated among the various disciplines and that the care is implemented in an effective, timely manner.

After a hemorrhagic stroke has been ruled out with diagnostic studies, patients with an ischemic or thrombotic stroke can benefit from the administration of thrombolytic therapy, particularly when treated within 3 hours of the initial occurrence of symptoms. The patient, who has had a previous stroke in the last 2 months, has active internal bleeding, or who has a history of aneurysms is not a candidate for thrombolytic therapy.

Nursing Responsibilities

Because of their potentially devastating, even lethal outcomes, strokes should be prevented whenever possible. Nurses have a duty to educate the public on cardiovascular health, including the role of exercise,

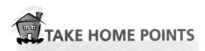

TAKE HOME POINTS

The rehabilitative phase of stroke care is directed toward helping the patient regain lost function or learn new ways of carrying out activities of daily living.

weight management, abstinence from smoking, and prompt aggressive control of hypertension and diabetes. Meticulous nursing care and collaboration with other health care disciplines, including dietitians, physical therapists, occupational therapists, and social workers, help minimize the damage associated with stroke and facilitate the patient's recovery.

Care of the patient with a stroke is directed toward maintaining adequate cerebral tissue perfusion and decreasing the risk for increased intracranial pressure with careful positioning. A precise history of symptoms help identify the area of the brain affected and can also help identify possible causes of the stroke. The nurse should do the following:

- Gather information on the nature of the symptoms, the length of time that they have been present, and whether the symptoms have resolved, are improving, or appear to be worsening.
- Obtain the patient's medical history, particularly of risk factors such as diabetes, cardiovascular disease, and hyperlipidemia.
- Assess neurologic function: level of consciousness; motor and sensory deficits; cognitive, memory, or intellectual impairments; and difficulties with speech, hearing, or vision. Because of the possibility of cognitive and memory deficits, obtain a description of baseline status before the stroke from a friend or family member.
- Evaluate the patient for evidence of further neurologic deterioration or increased intracranial pressure throughout the hospital stay. A comprehensive neurologic assessment should be performed at least every 2 to 4 hours. Complete vital signs must be obtained at least every 4 hours.
- Elevate the head of the bed to 30 degrees; the head and neck should be in a neutral position. Extreme hip and neck flexion should be avoided. Procedures that increase intracranial pressure, such as bathing or suctioning, should be widely spaced to allow rest periods.
- Evaluate oxygen saturation levels frequently, keeping oxygen levels above 95% when possible. Elevated carbon dioxide (CO_2) levels tend to increase intracranial pressure.
- Place patients who have hemiplegia or hemiparesis in proper body alignment at all times, and begin passive and active range of motion exercises when feasible. Supportive devices such as hand and wrist splints, slings, and footboards may be needed to keep the patient in normal anatomic alignment and prevent contractures.
- Reposition immobile patients every 2 hours and assess every 8 hours for skin breakdown, particularly over bony prominences.

- Plan care to accommodate for possible sensory deficits. Communication can be difficult, particularly when the patient has aphasia. Avoid the temptation to finish patient sentences, and be prepared to devise alternate methods of communication. For example, a patient with expressive aphasia may have difficulty saying, "I'm thirsty," but may be able to point to a picture of a glass of water.
- Approach the patient from the unaffected side, and place frequently used items within the patient's visual field.
- Touch the affected side frequently when the patient has neglect syndrome, and protect these areas from injury.
- Collaborate with physical and occupational therapy to put together a treatment plan that will either help the patient regain function or compensate for deficits. Helping a patient relearn old skills or relearn new ways of doing old tasks takes a great deal of time, repetition, and patience.
- Make the patient's family and caregivers a part of the rehabilitation process while keeping them informed about the goals of care, so they can promote and encourage independence whenever possible.
- Protect the patient from falls and potential sources of injury
- Answer the patient's calls for assistance promptly and offer the chance for toileting every 2 hours while awake to decrease episodes of incontinence.
- Place patients who have poor impulse control directly across from the nurses' station and use passive restraints (as needed) to keep them safely seated in a wheelchair. Electronic alarms may also be used to alert staff to a patient who is attempting to get out of bed or out of a chair unsupervised. These alarms are also safer than a restraint device.

Emotional and personality changes and intellectual deficits are frequently the most devastating of all the complications experienced by a stroke patient. Because of cognitive changes, break complex instructions into short, simple, concrete steps, and be prepared to repeat instructions frequently. Distractions in the environment must be minimized, and expectations must be realistic and achievable.

The patient who is emotionally labile requires a safe, supportive, predictable environment with routine and structure. Nurses and caregivers must learn to disregard emotional outbreaks and be respectful of the patient's dignity at all times. Family and friends must be advised that behavior and personality changes are a consequence of the illness and may be irreversible.

TAKE HOME POINTS

- Any deterioration in neurologic status must be reported to the health care provider immediately.
- Do not offer food to patients who have had a stroke without a health care provider's order or without the evaluation of his or her swallowing ability by a speech pathologist.
- Be careful to support joints and extremities when performing passive range of motion activities. Patients with flaccid muscle tone are at risk for dislocations and joint damage.

Do You UNDERSTAND?

DIRECTIONS: **Fill in the blanks to complete the following statements.**

1. The _____ lobe of the brain is responsible for vision.

2. The _____ lobe of the brain is responsible for judgment.

3. A stroke patient tends to be impulsive and falls frequently. This patient's stroke likely occurred in the _____ side of the brain.

4. The _____ type of stroke is usually treated with heparin.

DIRECTIONS: **Circle the correct answer.**

5. Which diseases and disorders increase a patient's risk for stroke?

diabetes mellitus   asthma   sickle cell anemia

hypertension   hemolytic anemia

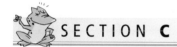

SECTION C

SPINAL CORD AND PERIPHERAL NERVE DISORDERS

What IS Multiple Sclerosis?

Pathogenesis

Multiple sclerosis (MS) is a disease of the CNS that is characterized by recurrent scattered areas of inflammation of neural tissue. MS is also characterized by the random formation of plaque in the CNS, along with destruction of the myelin sheath. Damage to the myelin sheath disrupts transmission of nerve impulses. Although this process can occur at any location within the CNS, commonly affected areas include the optic

Answers: 1. occipital; 2. frontal; 3. right; 4. thrombotic or embolic; 5. diabetes mellitus, hypertension, and sickle cell anemia.

nerves, cervical spinal cord, and the region between the thoracic and lumbar spine. In the initial stages, this disease is characterized by periods of exacerbation and remission of symptoms.

The origin of the abnormal inflammatory process has yet to be identified. Research is ongoing regarding the possible role of viral and bacterial infections, trauma, autoimmunity, and heredity.

At-Risk Populations

MS is most common along the 40th parallel and in cold climates. Because MS is more likely to occur in people who have a first-degree relative with the disorder, a genetic component to the development of this disease may exist. Epidemiologic studies indicate that there are both environmental and genetic factors that contribute to the development of MS. This disease is most frequently observed in people ages 15 to 50 and is more frequent in women than it is in men.

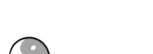

CULTURE

People of European origin are more likely to develop MS than are those of Asian, African, or Native American descent.

What You NEED TO KNOW

Clinical Manifestations

The signs and symptoms of MS depend on the area of the CNS affected. Common presenting symptoms include blurred vision, double vision, weakness in the arms and legs, a history of falls, and difficulty walking. Early symptoms can be transient, and the patient may experience a period of remission before symptoms occur again. Older individuals often present with muscle weakness, leg spasticity, difficulty walking, and bladder dysfunction. Other symptoms include sensory loss, especially sensation and vision, problems with coordination, dexterity, depression, emotional lability, and cognitive impairment.

As the disease advances, periods of remission no longer occur. Nerve cells are destroyed, and new symptoms appear, leading to gradually increasing disability. Late symptoms of the disease typically include involuntary movement of the eyes (nystagmus), intention tremors, difficulty speaking, paraplegia, and emotional lability.

Prognosis

MS is a chronic, incurable disease with a variable clinical course. Many people with MS are able to walk and maintain gainful employment for decades after their diagnosis. Most MS patients live nearly as long as people without the disease. Patients who demonstrate progressively worsening symptoms from the onset, or those who radiologically demonstrate abnormal findings with the beginning of symptoms, tend to experience greater disability and have a worse overall prognosis. Some research indicates that infections of any type will increase the risk for exacerbation of the disease, probably because of activation of the immune system.

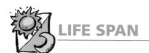

LIFE SPAN

Women and people under 40 years of age at the time of diagnosis appear to have a more favorable prognosis.

What You DO

Treatment

Treatment of multiple sclerosis is directed toward control of symptoms, prevention of complications, and maintenance and promotion of normal function. Patients with early relapsing and remitting disease have been shown to benefit from periodic doses of intravenous methylprednisolone, which has been shown to slow disease progression. Immunomodulating drugs shown to be helpful include interferon β-1b and interferon β-1a, glucocorticosteroids, and immunosuppressant drugs, such as azathioprine and methotrexate.

Spasticity may be helped by a combination of physical therapy and pharmacologic agents such as baclofen and diazepam. Dystonic spasms (repeated, painful posturing of one or more extremities) may be helped by carbamazepine or phenytoin. Fatigue associated with MS, when not a consequence of depression, may be treated with amantadine or modafanil. Because these two drugs decrease serum antibodies, therapeutic plasma exchanges have been shown helpful in some cases as well.

Nursing Responsibilities

Successful management of MS requires a multidisciplinary approach involving the efforts of many disciplines including the primary care provider, physical therapy, occupational therapy, and psychologic counseling. Coordinating the various levels of care is frequently the responsibility of the nurse and includes the following:

- Teach the patient about the proper ways to administer medications safely and to follow and adhere to an exercise regimen, as well as the need for adequate rest, stress reduction, skin care, and prevention of infection.

- Teach patients to avoid people with contagious respiratory illnesses and to avoid prolonged inactivity whenever possible. Remind the patient to receive the vaccination for pneumococcal pneumonia and a yearly influenza vaccination. Some patients experience an exacerbation of symptoms when febrile or in an excessively heated environment, which may be helped by the use of fans, air conditioning, and cool showers.
- Provide for, and teach the patient and family active and passive range of motion exercises; inspect the patient's skin daily for evidence of breakdown, paying special attention to pressure points this helps minimize complications, including decubitus ulcers and contracted extremities.
- Placing grab bars and handrails in strategic places in the patient's home to help decrease the risk of injury from falls. Assistive devices such as walkers, canes, and wheelchairs can help the patient maintain independence and mobility.

TAKE HOME POINTS

- Infection is a major complication of MS, usually occurring in the lungs or urinary tract. Infection can also trigger an exacerbation of the disease.
- Patients with MS are at increased risk for falls. Monitor ambulatory patients and provide assistive devices whenever possible.

Do You UNDERSTAND?

DIRECTIONS: **Indicate which statements are *true* (T) and which are *false* (F). If false, correct the statement in the margin space to make it true.**

_____ 1. MS is more likely to affect men than women.

_____ 2. MS typically occurs in women over the age of 60.

_____ 3. Symptoms associated with MS are the result of the disruption of the transmission of nerve impulses.

_____ 4. Biologic response–modifying drugs can be helpful in slowing the progression of the disease.

Answers: 1. F; 2. F—MS typically occurs in women ages 15 to 50; 3. T; 4. T.

What IS Amyotrophic Lateral Sclerosis?

Pathogenesis

Amyotrophic lateral sclerosis (ALS), also known as Lou Gehrig's disease, is a neurologic disease affecting motor neurons with a slow degeneration of the anterior horn cells and corticospinal tracts. Eventually complete paralysis will occur, including paralysis of respiratory muscles. At this time, no single cause of ALS has been identified.

At-Risk Populations

ALS occurs more often in men than in women, and tends to strike between the ages of 40 and 60. As of this time, no other risk factors have been identified, but up to 10% of patients have a family history of ALS, which suggests an autosomal dominant mode of transmission. Autoimmunity, enzyme mutations, and mitochondrial dysfunction have also been suggested as possible causes for this disease.

What You NEED TO KNOW

Clinical Manifestations

Muscle weakness usually begins in the upper part of the body and involves the upper arms, the shoulders, and then muscles of the neck and throat. As the disease progresses, the trunk and legs are affected. Neurologic findings vary depending upon the part of the body affected. Upper motor neuron involvement causes spasticity and hyperactive reflexes. Lower motor neuron damage results in weakness, atrophy of muscles, cramps, and fasciculations. Dysphagia and slurred speech are from involvement of the corticobulbar tract. As the diaphragm and intercostals muscles become affected, the patient's respirations become shallow and weak. Eventually the ability to muster an effective cough is lost. Over the course of the disease, patients remain cognitively intact, with control of bowel and bladder function even though they may be otherwise totally debilitated by the illness.

Prognosis

ALS is a progressive terminal illness. Most patients die 2 to 5 years after their diagnosis, usually because of pneumonia or respiratory failure.

What You DO

Treatment

Currently there is no cure for this disease. Riluzole has been shown to prolong the lives of patients with ALS by a few months, but its mechanism of action is unknown. Treatment is otherwise supportive and directed toward prevention of complications.

Nursing Responsibilities

The nurse should do the following:
- Help the patient with ALS to maintain independent function as long as possible by offering suggestions for modifications in lifestyle, activity levels, and diet. Plan care activities so as to conserve patient energy levels. Leg braces, canes, and walkers may help the patient retain the ability to walk for a longer period of time.
- Take measures to prevent aspiration of food as the patient's activity tolerance and motor function decreases. Position the patient upright with his or her head flexed slightly forward to aid in swallowing.
- Provide small, high-calorie nutrient-dense feedings. Have suction equipment readily available at the patient's bedside in case of aspiration.
- Encourage patients to use an alternative means of communication if speech becomes slurred or unintelligible. Writing may be used, and some patients may benefit from other devices such as an alphabet board.
- Encourage patients who smoke to stop because of safety issues, as well as to improve their respiratory status.
- Teach patients and their family members to avoid contact with individuals who have contagious respiratory illnesses.
- Offer the patient and family emotional support. Give them the opportunity to speak about the losses, fears, and feelings.
- Encourage the patient and family, when appropriate, to consider whether or not they wish to have life-prolonging measures such as mechanical ventilation.

Do You UNDERSTAND?

DIRECTIONS: **Circle the correct answer.**

1. Which drug is prescribed to delay the progression of ALS?
   a. anastrazole
   b. clotrimazole
   c. riluzole
   d. avetek
2. ALS patients typically die from
   a. Heart failure
   b. Respiratory failure
   c. Liver failure
   d. Kidney failure

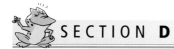

SECTION D

CNS INFLAMMATION AND INFECTION

Despite the physical and innate protection the body affords to the brain and CNS, infectious and inflammatory agents can disrupt normal functioning of the CNS. This section describes and discusses infectious and inflammatory processes affecting the CNS.

What IS Meningitis?

Infections and inflammatory processes of the CNS are identified based on the portion or portions of the CNS affected. The term meningitis is used to describe the infectious process that is limited to the subarachnoid space and meninges. Meningitis tends to spread rapidly because the infection is readily disseminated throughout the CNS by cerebrospinal fluid (CSF).

Answers: 1.c, 2.b.

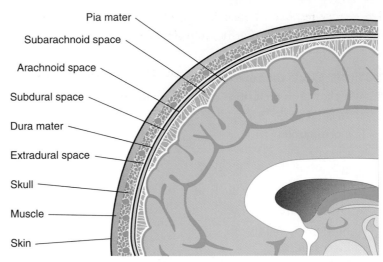

Pia mater
Subarachnoid space
Arachnoid space
Subdural space
Dura mater
Extradural space
Skull
Muscle
Skin

Cross section of the skull and meninges.

Pathogenesis

In most cases, either bacteria or enteroviruses cause meningitis. Common bacteria include *Haemophilus influenzae, Neisseria meningitidis, Streptococcus pneumoniae,* and *Escherichia coli.* Bacterial meningitis can occur when an infection elsewhere in the body spreads into the CNS via the bloodstream. Enteroviruses grow and replicate in the intestinal tract, from which they are ultimately transmitted to the brain and nervous system. Fungal organisms can also infect the CNS, particularly when the patient is immunocompromised.

Many different types of viruses, including the Epstein-Barr, mumps, Coxsackie, and human immunodeficiency viruses can cause viral meningitis. Viruses enter the body through many different routes, including the nose and mouth, animal or mosquito bites, and by passing across the placenta to the fetus.

Common sources of infectious organisms include the respiratory tract, the sinuses, the mastoid sinuses, and middle ear. Infectious organisms enter the CNS by one of three routes: the blood, either via the arterial route or through connections between facial veins and the cerebral circulation; traumatic insertion of an organism, such as during a medical procedure; or by local extension from an established infection.

Problems associated with a CNS infection are the result of organisms or bacterial toxins that cause either direct or indirect damage to tissue. The presence of endotoxins and cell wall fragments is thought to activate the immune response, with subsequent tissue damage resulting from the inflammatory response. Research suggests that inflammatory mediators disrupt the blood-brain barrier, allowing pathogens, neutrophils, and protein into the CSF.

Occasionally, patients who have cancer develop meningitis because of infiltration of the meninges by tumor cells. The result is increased intra-cranial pressure, fibrosis, and further inflammation of brain tissue.

At-Risk Populations

Risk factors for meningitis include living in cramped, crowded quarters such as military barracks or college dormitories, or the presence of a basilar skull fracture, otitis media, sinusitis or mastoiditis, neurosurgery, dermal sinus tracts, certain types of immunocompromise, and systemic sepsis.

By no means are all CNS infections preventable, although prudent health care measures can help decrease the incidence and severity of infection. With the availability of effective oral antibiotics, the incidence of serious otitis media has decreased significantly in the last few decades, thereby decreasing what was once a major risk factor for meningitis. Early detection and prompt treatment of infection, particularly when involv-ing the head, the neck, and the respiratory system, can also decrease the risk for meningitis and encephalitis. Careful hand washing with bacterio-cidal agents can also help decrease the transmission of disease-causing organisms.

Vaccination against childhood illnesses, particularly mumps, measles, rubella, and varicella, conveys a high degree of protection against these diseases and is also an important measure to decrease the risk for meningitis. Vaccination is available against certain organisms such as *N. meningitidis* and *S. pneumoniae* and should be offered to high-risk groups.

What You NEED TO KNOW

Clinical Manifestations

Symptoms associated with meningitis vary depending on the causative organism, as well as the extent and location of the infection. A headache, fever, myalgia, malaise, photophobia, pain in the eyes and neck, stiffness in the neck and back, and a positive Kernig's sign are all characteristic of meningitis.

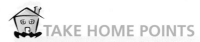

TAKE HOME POINTS

- Risk factors for meningitis include cramped, crowded living quarters, basilar skull fractures, otitis media, sinusitis or mastoiditis, and systemic sepsis.
- Bacteria, fungi or enteroviruses can cause meningitis.
- Common sources and reservoirs for infection include the respiratory tract, the sinuses, the mastoid sinuses, and the middle ear.

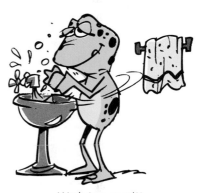

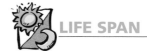

Wash 'em good!'

LIFE SPAN

Bacterial meningitis is common in children under 5 years of age. The extremely young and the extremely old as a group tend to experience the highest rates of mortality from meningitis. Pneumococcal meningitis is a major threat for the extremely young and the extremely old, particularly when these individuals are compromised by coexisting illnesses.

Meningococcal meningitis usually causes a petechial rash, in addition to the previously mentioned symptoms. Patients may develop tremors and convulsions. A decreased level of consciousness is usually present, with progressive confusion and drowsiness that will eventually progress to a coma and death if prompt, aggressive treatment is not initiated.

Microscopic examination and cultures of the CSF are important in differentiating between bacterial and viral meningitis. In bacterial meningitis the CSF is cloudy, with elevated neutrophil and protein levels and a low glucose level. In contrast, with viral meningitis, examination of the CSF typically reveals an elevated leukocyte count, a mild to moderate elevation in protein, and a normal glucose level.

Prognosis

Most patients with viral meningitis completely recover within 10 to 14 days of the onset of symptoms, although some patients complain of persistent fatigue and weakness for months afterward. In a patient who is otherwise healthy, viral meningitis is usually self-limiting, and the patient responds well to symptomatic and supportive care.

What You DO

Treatment

Infections of the CNS are emergencies and require immediate medical intervention. Because the signs and symptoms of viral and bacterial meningitis can be similar, obtaining a thorough health history and diagnostic evaluation is important to aid in determining the possible cause and source of infection, particularly in the absence of a positive culture.

Medical treatment for bacterial meningitis emphasizes prompt initiation of antibiotic therapy because of the high risk for mortality. Meningococcal meningitis is usually susceptible to penicillin, which represents first-line therapy. Alternate drugs include ceftriaxone and cefotaxime.

Because meningococcal infections are contagious, people who have had close contact with patients with meningococcal meningitis should be given prophylactic antibiotic therapy to decrease their risk for developing the infection. Chemoprophylaxis can be accomplished with rifampin, ciprofloxacin, or a single dose of ceftriaxone. In cases caused by other bacteria such as *H. influenzae*, corticosteroids can be helpful as adjunct

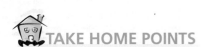

TAKE HOME POINTS

To test for Kernig's sign, instruct the patient to lie on the back with one leg bent at the knee. Raise the knee toward the chest and flex the patient's head. Pain with this maneuver is considered to be a positive Kernig's sign, the result of meningeal irritation.

therapy to reduce the incidence of disease-related complications (e.g., hearing loss) and to decrease the chance of other neurologic deficits.

Medical treatment of acute viral infections of the CNS is directed toward supportive care, prevention and treatment of complications, and alleviation of distressing symptoms. Even patients with severe cases involving coma and seizures are likely to make a full recovery but may require management in an intensive care unit in which respiratory and nutritional support can be provided.

Nursing Responsibilities

The nurse should do the following:

- Perform a comprehensive physical and neurologic assessment at least every 4 hours during the acute phases of the infection.
- Report changes in vital signs and deterioration in neurologic status promptly to the health care provider.
- Carefully and accurately administer scheduled antibiotics and anti-infectives on time.
- Monitor serologic studies routinely, particularly electrolyte, renal, and liver function tests, to detect potential drug-induced toxicities.
- Assess the patient for evidence of drug-induced adverse reactions, such as gastrointestinal distress, rashes, and allergic reactions.
- Leave low-grade fevers untreated unless they are causing the patient discomfort. Low-grade fevers are thought to enhance the body's natural immune defenses. Temperatures of 40° C (104° F) or higher usually require vigorous treatment with antipyretics and possibly a cooling blanket.
- Routinely assess all four extremities for normal pulses and adequate perfusion. Severe bacterial infections carry an increased risk of septic emboli, with subsequent obstruction of microcirculation in the hands and feet.
- Assess carefully for evidence of abnormal bleeding, such as unexplained bruises and resumption of bleeding from old venipuncture sites. Septic emboli can also trigger the clotting cascade and cause disseminated intravascular coagulation (DIC).
- Establish seizure precautions for all patients. Keep the side rails up at all times, and have a portable suction device plugged in and ready for immediate use at the bedside in the event of aspiration. An oral airway is kept at the seizure-prone patient's bedside.

Bacterial meningitis tends to have high rates of mortality and morbidity and is likely to be fatal if prompt treatment is not initiated. One third of survivors have neurologic sequelae including deafness, hydrocephalus, and mental retardation.

- Monitor intake and output and collaborate with the health care provider to make certain that adequate fluids and nutrition are provided, particularly in patients with decreased LOC.
- Elevate the head of the bed 30 to 45 degrees at all times to decrease ICP, (unless otherwise contraindicated). Activities that increase ICP, such as deep endotracheal suction, should be carried out only when necessary and with extreme caution.
- Carry out routine nursing measures for the immobilized, obtunded, or comatose patient so as to prevent the complications associated with immobility (e.g., decubitus ulcers and renal calculi).
- Discharge planning should include the need for possible physical therapy and rehabilitation to help the patient regain prior levels of functioning.

Do You UNDERSTAND?

DIRECTIONS: **Fill in the blanks to complete the following statements.**

1. The covering of the brain closest to the skull is called the _____.

2. At least three measures help prevent the development of CNS infection including _____, _____, and _____.

3. Meningococcal meningitis usually causes a _____, in addition to other neurologic symptoms.

4. _____ meningitis tends to have a high rate of mortality and morbidity.

What IS Encephalitis?

The term encephalitis refers to an inflammation of the brain, which is usually due to a viral infection. Arboviruses transmitted by mosquitos and ticks are the most common cause of encephalitis. Mosquitos are the vectors for western equine encephalomyelitis and West Nile viruses, and herpes simplex encephalitis occurs sporadically as a result of the spread of a herpes infection to the CNS. Viral encephalitis in the United States is most commonly associated with western equine encephalomyelitis, West Nile virus, and the herpes simplex virus. Other infectious organisms that may cause encephalitis include the following:

- Varicella-zoster virus
- Epstein-Barr virus
- Lyme disease
- Toxoplasmosis
- Rubeola ("hard measles")
- Mumps
- Rubella ("German measles")

Pathogenesis

Mosquitos and ticks inoculate the host with the arbovirus. The virus replicates outside the CNS and disseminates either through the bloodstream or neural pathways. After crossing the blood-brain barrier the virus causes perivascular congestion and inflammation, which diffusely affects gray matter of the brain. Herpes-related encephalitis is thought to be due to the reactivation of the virus lying dormant in the spinal ganglia. Immunocompromise and physiologic stress present an opportunity for the virus to grow and replicate, causing active disease in the host.

At-Risk Populations

People who are ill, debilitated or immunocompromised are more likely to develop encephalitis. Otherwise, anyone who lives or works in areas where mosquito-borne viruses are common is at risk, particularly if they engage in many outdoor activities. In general, mosquito-borne infections are more prevalent during warm months, which are the prime mating and breeding times for birds, mosquitos, and ticks.

What You NEED TO KNOW

Clinical Manifestations

Mild cases of encephalitis may be totally asymptomatic and resolve without treatment. Other individuals may complain of headache, irritability or lethargy. Severe encephalitis may cause drowsiness, confusion, changes in level of consciousness, seizures, sudden high fevers, severe headaches, photophobia, stiff neck, and bulging of the fontanels of infants.

Prognosis

Even in otherwise healthy people, severe cases of viral encephalitis may be fatal. Those who do recover may have permanent cognitive impairment, including loss of memory, problems with speech, muscle coordination, hearing and vision. Without treatment, herpes simplex encephalitis has a mortality rate of 50% to 75%, and nearly 100% of survivors have permanent mental deficits. Other strains of arbovirus encephalitis have a more benign course, with mortality rates ranging from 2% to 25%. Regardless of age or gender, people who are very young or elderly are at highest risk for mortality and morbidity from viral encephalitis.

What You DO

Treatment

Unfortunately no therapy is available for many arbovirus infections. Treatment is mainly supportive and emphasizes maintaining vital functions, treating pain, and suppressing inflammation, particularly if there is evidence of ICP.

Nursing Responsibilities

Accurate diagnosis and treatment should be undertaken as soon as possible. Accordingly, the nurse should do the following:

- Obtain a baseline history and physical assessment, with special attention to the possibility of mosquito, tick, or animal bites.
- Obtain a platelet count and coagulation studies before invasive procedures are carried out to rule out the possibility of DIC. Testing is particularly important for patients who have bruising or bleeding abnormalities.
- Anticipate the need for a lumbar puncture to obtain cerebrospinal fluid for testing and culture. Blood will be drawn for viral serology studies to determine the cause of the illness.
- Instruct the patient and family that an emergency CT scan of the head (with and without contrast) may be needed to determine the presence of elevated ICP or obstructive hydrocephalus, both of which can be a complication of the disease.

- Protect patients who have an altered mental status from injury and should be protected accordingly. Initiate seizure precautions and take steps to protect the patient's airway.
- Monitor vital signs closely, inserting a large-bore intravenous (IV) line so as to infuse crystalloids as ordered for patients with severe infection who are at risk for hypotension and septic shock.
- Administer analgesics and antipyretics as ordered to decrease pain and fever. If the encephalitis is due to the herpes virus or varicella-zoster, begin acyclovir administration immediately as prescribed by the health care provider. Foscarnet may also be used to treat cytomegalovirus (CMV) and herpetic infections.
- Administer a corticosteroid such as decadron as ordered to help decrease inflammation and increased ICP.
- Monitor the patient routinely for evidence of changes in mental status and decline in neurologic function, and report changes promptly. Patients who have recovered but are left with cognitive or neurologic deficits may benefit from rehabilitative therapy.
- Educate the public about ways to prevent encephalitis. Encourage people to wear protective clothing and use mosquito repellant in areas where insect vectors are present. Repair holes in screens and cracks under doors to keep insects out of the home. Eliminate sources of standing water, such as drains and flowerpots, empty birdbaths, and unused containers. Report sick or dying birds to the local health department.

Do You UNDERSTAND?

DIRECTIONS: **Circle the correct answer.**

1. Encephalitis may be caused by
   a. Viruses.
   b. Fungi.
   c. Bacteria.
   d. All of the above.
2. One of the most lethal forms of encephalitis is caused by the ___.
   a. Cytomegalovirus.
   b. Epstein-Barr virus.
   c. Herpes simplex virus.
   d. Varicella-zoster virus.

Answers: 1. d; 2. c.

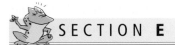

SECTION E

CHRONIC DISORDERS OF NEUROLOGIC FUNCTION

This section provides an overview of neurologic diseases that alter motor and sensory function, also known as movement disorders. Neurologic diseases frequently deprive the individual of independence. The nature of the disease reflects a process of loss, which may be both cognitive and physical. The functional rate of decline will vary depending on the particular disease process and the individual patient. In addition, adjustments and ability to cope will depend on the patient's perception of the loss of function. This section provides information on commonly observed neurodegenerative diseases. An understanding of these disorders will assist the nurse in developing strategies that will help patients cope with loss and set realistic goals.

What IS a Seizure Disorder?

Pathogenesis

A seizure is an abnormal discharge of electrical impulses within the brain. Abnormal impulses result in changes in awareness, sensory alterations, and involuntary muscle movement. Seizures can be a symptom of an underlying condition or illness and may resolve spontaneously when the problem is treated. Three or more recurring seizures are usually a result of a disease called *epilepsy*. Epilepsy is characterized by changes in subjective awareness, altered awareness, and involuntary movements.

Isolated seizures occur from a variety of conditions and disorders, including electrolyte imbalance, renal and liver failure, hypertensive encephalopathy, and acute head trauma. In patients with epilepsy, a lesion or injury to the brain may be identified. In many cases, the structural lesion causing the disease is never identified. Approximately 40% of epilepsy in adults and children is inherited.

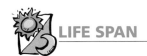

LIFE SPAN

Epilepsy frequently causes depression and a sense of social isolation, particularly in children and adolescents. Children with undiagnosed absence seizures are frequently accused of inattentiveness and inappropriate behavior, particularly in the classroom setting. Any child with a sudden change in behavior requires physical evaluation by a qualified health care provider.

At-Risk Populations

Patients with seizure disorders have more than one risk factor in their medical history. Patients who have had a single, isolated seizure have a 25% risk of developing epilepsy.

Seizures can occur in infants and young children because of birth injury, hypoxia, or high fever. In the older adult, seizures can occur after a stroke. Newborns with birth trauma or hypoxia, or those with a family history of seizures or neurologic diseases are at risk for seizures.

What You NEED TO KNOW

Clinical Manifestations

Seizures are classified according to their clinical symptoms. Seizure activity varies, depending on the area of the brain involved. Simple partial seizures do not involve loss of consciousness and can begin with involuntary twitching of an extremity, loss of ability to speak, or strange vocalizations. The patient may also express fear or a sense of impending doom.

Complex partial seizures involve impaired levels of consciousness, with automatic repetitive movements noted such as chewing, swallowing, or picking at clothes. Partial seizures can evolve into tonic-clonic seizures (previously known as grand mal seizures).

Absence seizures are characterized by loss of awareness and loss of muscle tone, typically lasting from 10 to 15 seconds. Patients with uncontrolled absence seizures can have one hundred or more episodes per day.

Myoclonic seizures are characterized by jerking of one or more muscle groups, with a tendency to occur early in the morning. Tonic-clonic seizures begin on both sides of the body. During the initial tonic phase the muscles are rigid, and the patient may stop breathing for a brief period. The clonic phase involves a rhythmic jerking of muscles, with deep breathing at the end of the seizure. The patient may bite the tongue and become incontinent of urine and feces. After returning to consciousness, the patient may be confused, complain of headache, and be sleepy. Some patients with epilepsy experience an aura—an abnormal sensation or sensory perception that is a warning of an impending seizure.

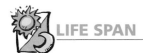

• Patients with epilepsy are at increased risk of death resulting from accidents, especially drowning and motor vehicle accidents. Patients with severe chronic epilepsy are at risk for death resulting from cardiac arrhythmia, pulmonary edema, and myocardial infarction.
• Status epilepticus, a condition involving persistent, prolonged tonic-clonic seizures is life-threatening and requires immediate emergency medical intervention.

Individuals with recurrent seizures must begin drug therapy immediately to avoid further damage to brain tissue. They must be instructed to avoid discontinuing antiepileptic drugs without medical assistance and supervision because of the danger of recurrent seizures, including status epilepticus.

LIFE SPAN

Pregnancy lowers the seizure threshold. Patients of childbearing age should be cautioned about possible adverse effects of antiseizure medications on a developing fetus.

Prognosis

Approximately 80% of patients with epilepsy respond to drug therapy, have good quality of life, and live a normal life span. Most other cases can be cured by surgery. A few patients who are unable to or unwilling to comply with drug therapy can succumb to complications of status epilepticus, usually a stroke or heart failure.

What You DO

Treatment

Patients who have a single seizure, have no risk factors for epilepsy, and have a normal electroencephalogram (EEG) and neurologic examination require no antiepileptic treatment. However, they should be screened for an underlying cause of the seizure episode.

After ruling out underlying causes of seizures, such as metabolic disorders or structural defects within the brain, patients may be started on antiepileptic medication. Therapy is directed toward suppressing seizures, avoiding drug-related adverse effects, and maintaining the patient's normal quality of life. Approximately 40% to 60% of patients obtain complete control of seizure activity with drugs such as phenytoin, carbamazepine, or primidone. The remainder of patients may require more than one drug to control their seizures satisfactorily.

A small percentage of patients have refractory seizures that fail to respond to drug therapy. These patients may be helped by neurosurgery that involves destroying or ablating the epileptic focus within the brain or sectioning the corpus callosum between the hemispheres to decrease the transmission of abnormal impulses.

Nursing Responsibilities

Care of the patient with a seizure disorder is complex and involves intensive education and emotional support. The nurse should do the following:
• Help the patient to manage drug therapy and appropriately cope with unavoidable drug-induced adverse effects.
• Teach the patient to avoid precipitating factors including stress, excessive heat, alcohol, sleep deprivation, and certain drugs.
• Teach the patient's family safety measures that are to be implemented when a seizure occurs, the importance of adherence to drug therapy, and the ways to manage adverse effects.

- Advise patients who have a history of poorly controlled or recurrent seizures to avoid driving a car or engaging in activities in which they can be at risk for injury. Children or adults may require helmets or other protective devices to decrease the risk for injury.
- Encourage patients with epilepsy to express their concerns and referring them to a support group available in their area.

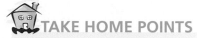

TAKE HOME POINTS

When caring for a patient having a seizure, the primary consideration is to protect and maintain the patient's airway. Do not attempt to move patients except to roll them on their side to prevent aspiration. Remove any potential sources of injury such as furniture from the immediate environment. Never try to pry open the clenched jaws of a patient who is having a seizure or put your fingers in their mouth! Both you and the patient can be seriously injured.

Do You UNDERSTAND?

DIRECTIONS: **Indicate which statements are *true* (T) and which are *false* (F). If false, correct the statement in the margin space to make it true.**

_____ 1. Seizure disorders can be inherited.

_____ 2. Adults can experience febrile seizures.

_____ 3. To be diagnosed with epilepsy, a person must have three or more seizures.

_____ 4. Pregnancy can lower the seizure threshold.

What IS Multiinfarct Dementia?

Multiinfarct dementia (MID) (vascular dementia) is a nondegenerative type of dementia.

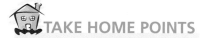

TAKE HOME POINTS

MID is a nondegenerative type of dementia occurring as a result of cerebral infarction. Mental slowing, dysphagia, shuffling gait, and urinary incontinence are classic symptoms of MID.

Pathogenesis

Multiple cortical embolic infarcts are responsible for neurologic symptoms. In individuals with subcortical white matter or lacunar infarctions, progressive deterioration in cognition without focal deficits may be present. Carotid and cardiac emboli, cerebral arterial and venous thrombosis, and vasculitis all contribute to MID. Infarcts seen on CT or MRI scans are necessary to establish a diagnosis. Many patients diagnosed with MID are found to have a mixture of MID and Alzheimer's disease (AD) on autopsy.

Answers: **1. T; 2. F—children most often experience febrile seizures; 3. T; 4. T.**

At-Risk Populations

Hypertension, heart disease, positive family history, hypercholesterolemia, cocaine abuse, and smoking place patients at an increased risk for MID.

What You NEED TO KNOW

Clinical Manifestations

The hallmark findings of MID include mental slowing, dysphagia, shuffling gait, urinary incontinence, and bilateral motor abnormalities. There are fewer behavioral problems associated with MID compared with other types of dementia. When other symptoms commonly associated with AD are present, such as wandering, mixed dementia should be included in the differential diagnosis.

Prognosis

Because MID is a nondegenerative disease, prevention of additional cerebral infarcts preserves cognitive function and positively affects the prognosis of the disorder.

What You DO

Treatment for MID

The goal of treatment for the patient with MID is to optimize the patient's functional level of independence. Treatment strategies include the following:

- Encouraging physical and cognitive activities that promote the highest level of functional ability
- Therapies directed at correcting underlying medical conditions
- Drug therapies such as aspirin or antiplatelet agents (ticlopidine or clopidogrel) to minimize the risk of recurrent stroke
- Minimizing environmental stressors
- Avoiding concurrent use of drugs that have CNS effects
- Managing behavioral problems

Treatment for AD

Currently, no cure for AD is available. Treatment is limited to palliation. Behavioral and drug therapies focus on improving both cognitive and physical levels of function. Newer drugs that increase acetylcholine levels, called cholinesterase inhibitors (e.g., donepezil and rivastigmine), can improve cognitive function when initiated in the early stages of AD. Antipsychotic drugs are frequently used to manage hallucinations and delusions. In high doses, vitamin E may slow disease progression. Psychotropic drugs such as risperidone, olanzapine, and trazadone may be helpful in managing psychiatric symptoms such as delusions and agitation that are associated with the disease.

Nursing Responsibilities for MID and AD

Nursing responsibilities for both MID and AD focus on optimizing the patient's level of cognitive and physical function. When a diagnosis is established early, patients are usually mentally competent and capable of making decisions regarding end-of-life care. In these situations, the health care provider is in a strategic position to facilitate dialogue among the patient, family, and health care providers regarding later issues of tube feeding, nursing home placement, and resuscitative efforts.

Consistency, stability, and active participation are essential in enhancing cognitive function. The following programs have been identified as helpful adjuncts:

- **Social skills therapy:** Reinforcing behaviors used when interacting with others positively
- **Communication therapy:** Improving speech patterns; minimize sensory deprivation
- **Memory retaining therapy:** Providing reality orientation
- **Reminiscence therapy:** Using story telling and memory recall of past experiences
- **Stress management:** Identifying factors that minimize stress and methods of effective management
- **Behavioral therapy:** Maintaining consistency and structure to identify behavioral expectations; using written directions and schedules to assist with activities; provide day care programs
- **Pharmacologic therapy:** Using drug therapy to improve cognitive function and manage behaviors

TAKE HOME POINTS

- Consistent, stable routines help to maximize the function and coping ability of patients with AD. Treatment of AD is limited to palliation.
- Stress the importance of compliance with treatment of the underlying cause of MID as an essential element in preserving cerebral function.
- Cholinesterase inhibitors and antipsychotic drugs are frequently used to improve cognitive function and manage psychotic behavior in AD and MID.

- For the patient with MID or AD, the nurse should do the following:
  - Administer cholinesterase inhibitors (e.g., donepezil and rivastigmine) as ordered. These drugs can improve cognitive function when initiated in the early stages.
  - Administer antipsychotic drugs as ordered. Antipsychotics are frequently required to manage behavioral problems.
  - Minimize stressors to optimize cognitive function as a result of associated decreases in acetylcholine levels from catecholamine surges.
  - Regularly assess patient drug therapy for other health problems, paying particular attention to effects on baseline mental status. For instance, drugs that have anticholinergic properties also negatively affect acetylcholine levels and can significantly affect cognitive function.
  - Educate caregivers about the nutritional and physical needs of the patient. Caregiver stress tends to increase with progressive decline in independence, particularly in patients who exhibit wandering behaviors. Ongoing assessment of caregiver burden and referral to support groups becomes important because of the effect on the patient's care.

Do You UNDERSTAND?

DIRECTIONS: **Indicate which statements are *true* (T) and which are *false* (F). If false, correct the statement in the margin space to make it true.**

_____ 1. MID is not preventable.

_____ 2. Day care programs are not as effective in patients with MID as they are in patients with AD.

_____ 3. Platelet aggregation inhibitors play an essential role in treatment of MID.

_____ 4. Patients with MID are at an increased risk for falls.

What IS Alzheimer's Disease?

Alzheimer's disease (AD) is a chronic, progressive, degenerative disorder involving the brain. The disease is characterized by profound impairment of cognitive function.

Pathogenesis

The cognitive impairment commonly observed in AD is thought to be a result of abnormalities in cholinergic neurotransmitters, which cause a decrease in acetylcholine synthesis. Confirmation of the diagnosis can be made only at autopsy, during which cerebral atrophy and cellular degeneration are documented. The cellular degenerative changes occur primarily in the temporoparietal and anterior frontal areas and include neurofibrillary tangles and amyloidal plaque deposits.

The exact cause of AD is unknown. However, deficits in the neurotransmitter acetylcholine, which is necessary for memory, are thought to be responsible for symptoms. Approximately 10% of cases have been linked to a gene located on chromosome 21. This gene is closely linked to the genes for apo-protein and for beta amyloid, which are present in increased concentrations in patients with AD.

At-Risk Populations

A positive family history of AD and the presence of Down syndrome appear to be the only two risk factors. Other proposed risk factors include previous head trauma, a family history of Down syndrome, thyroid disease, hearing loss, maternal age, and exposure to aluminum. However, the evidence is conflicting and insufficient.

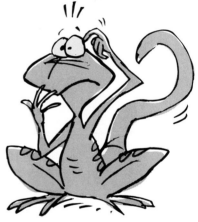

Memory Loss.

TAKE HOME POINTS

- AD involves a predictable progressive decline in cognitive and physical function.
- Continuous activity places client at risk for safety, agitated delirium, and dehydration.
- In the final stage, families are faced with making end-of-life decisions regarding initiation of tube feeding, nursing home placement, and hospice.

What You NEED TO KNOW

Clinical Manifestations

Progressive deterioration of short- and long-term memory is responsible for the clinical manifestations of AD. In many instances, depression is one of the first symptoms. Although the stages vary between patients, characteristic behaviors have been identified.

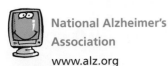

National Alzheimer's Association
www.alz.org
National Institute of Health Alzheimer's disease Page
www.ninds.nih.gov

Stage 1: Early (2 to 4 Years After Diagnosis)

- Exhibits forgetfulness; usually subtle
- May attempt to cover up using lists and notes
- Demonstrates declining interest in environment, people, and affairs
- Demonstrates uncertainty and hesitancy in initiating tasks
- Performs poorly at work, may be terminated from job

Stage 2: Middle (2 to 12 Years After Diagnosis)

- Exhibits progressive memory loss
- Hesitates when questioned; shows signs of aphasia
- Displays difficulty following simple instructions or completing simple calculations
- Exhibits bouts of irritability
- Becomes anxious, evasive, and physically active
- Wanders at night rather than sleeping

Stage 3: End-stage

- Becomes apraxic for basic activities
- Loses important papers
- Loses way in familiar surroundings or inside own home
- Forgets to pay bills; neglects household chores; becomes noncompliant with drug therapy
- Loses possessions, then claims someone stole them; exhibits paranoid delusions
- Neglects personal hygiene
- Loses social graces; embarrasses family and friends
- Exhibits dysphagia; refuses to eat and drink fluids in adequate amounts
- Is unable to communicate verbally or in writing
- Fails to recognize family
- Is incontinent of urine and feces
- Is predisposed to major seizures
- Loses ability to stand and walk
- Death usually results from sepsis (i.e., aspiration pneumonia)

Prognosis

Progressive decline generally reaches the final stage in 10 to 12 years. Death generally occurs within 6 to 9 months after reaching the final stage.

Do You UNDERSTAND?

DIRECTIONS: **Indicate in the spaces provided whether the listed activity is likely to *increase* (I) or *decrease* (D) the functional level of independence for the patient with AD.**

_____ 1. Being home alone
_____ 2. Watching old movies
_____ 3. Taking a 25-mg phenergan suppository
_____ 4. 1500-calorie diet in the middle-stage patient
_____ 5. Day care program
_____ 6. Diphenhydramine 25 mg by mouth for sleep
_____ 7. Trips to the zoo
_____ 8. Scheduled toileting every 3 hours while awake

What IS Parkinson's Disease?

Pathogenesis

Parkinson's disease is a progressive neurologic disorder resulting from degeneration of dopaminergic neurons of the substantia nigra in the midbrain. The loss of neurons causes a decline in the amount of the neurotransmitter dopamine. Dopamine is responsible for controlling movement. Damage to this area causes the rigidity, abnormal movement, and muscle tone that are characteristic of this disorder. Impairment of other neurotransmitters is thought to contribute to the autonomic symptoms and depression that may be seen in conjunction with this disease.

Parkinson's disease is classified as either primary (of unknown cause) or secondary. This disorder is slightly more common in men than it is in women. Some research suggests a genetic component to primary Parkinson's disease. Secondary Parkinson's is the result of conditions that interfere with the activity of dopamine. These conditions include the ingestion of certain drugs such as haloperidol and reserpine, as well as hydrocephalus, cerebrovascular disease, and lesions in the midbrain. Other causes of Parkinson's include the ingestion of toxins such as mercury or ethanol, or postencephalitic conditions.

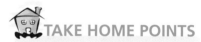

TAKE HOME POINTS

Parkinson's disease is a degenerative neurologic disorder characterized by resting tremors, cogwheel rigidity, a festinating gait, and bradykinesia. Approximately one third of all patients with this disease will experience dementia, which is thought to be a consequence of degeneration of the cholinergic nucleus basalis.

Answers: 1. D; 2. I; 3. D; 4. D; 5. I; 6. D; 7. I; 8. I.

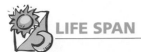

LIFE SPAN

The primary form of Parkinson's is most common in men over the age of 60. Older women are more likely to develop drug-induced Parkinson's than are men. On rare occasions, Parkinson's disease develops in children and adolescents.

At-Risk Populations

In rare cases, Parkinson's disease is an autosomal dominant condition. People with cerebrovascular disease or those who take certain drugs are also at risk for secondary Parkinson's. In patients with a drug-induced version of the disease, the symptoms may or may not resolve after the drugs are discontinued.

What You NEED TO KNOW

Clinical Manifestations

Parkinson's disease (also referred to as parkinsonism) is a clinical syndrome characterized by four important signs: resting tremors, bradykinesia (slow movements), rigidity, and difficulty maintaining a balanced posture. One subtype of the disorder has tremor as the most noticeable feature; the other type tends to cause more problems with postural instability and walking.

In the early stages, patients may notice a decrease in the speed of their movement and their ability to carry out certain tasks. Generalized stiffness and poorly localized muscle pain may also be present. Friends and family members may remark that the patient has a masklike facial expression (**masked facies**) and that the voice is softer and more monotonous in tone.

Tremors typically occur when the patient is at rest or when the arms are raised. The tremor is frequently described as a "pill-rolling" because the hands move from supination to pronation as the fingers are flexing and extending. The tremor usually decreases with voluntary movement. In many patients, the legs are also affected, causing a shuffling gait and problems with posture and balance. As the disease progresses, the patient's automatic movements gradually decrease. Patients frequently have difficulty rising from a sitting position and may have problems with balance, resulting in falls. Eye blinking, smiling, crossing the legs, and swinging the arms while walking are typically affected.

The term *bradykinesia* is used to describe the slowing of voluntary and involuntary movement. The length of the patient's stride becomes progressively smaller, causing the patient to take small, shuffling steps (**festinating gait**). Patients with this disease tend to have stiff muscle tone (**cogwheel rigidity**). The stiff muscle tone produces a ratchet-like

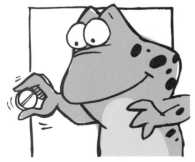

Pill-rolling.

resistance when performing range of motion activities. Other problems encountered by these patients include problems with swallowing, which results in a tendency to drool, *micrographia* (small handwriting), and freezing of motion. Affected individuals may be unable to pick up their feet to take a step, or roll over in bed.

Prognosis

The prognosis for Parkinson's disease varies, depending on the severity of symptoms, the presence of dementia at the time of diagnosis, and the patient's responsiveness to medical therapy. In the later stages of the disease, patients may require 24-hour care. Many patients die of complications of the illness such as aspiration pneumonia and falls. Patients with milder forms of the disease may continue to work for as long as 10 years after diagnosis. Individuals with more severe, rapidly progressive forms of the illness may survive only 5 to 7 years after diagnosis.

What You DO

Treatment

Drugs are the mainstay of therapy for Parkinson's disease. Selegine is a neuroprotective drug that is often used in the early stages of the disease, and may be used in combination with other anticholinergic drugs. When symptoms are no longer satisfactorily controlled by these drugs, dopamine agonists such as pergolide or ropinirole may be used. When these drugs fail to satisfactorily suppress symptoms, levodopa combined with carbidopa is initiated and gradually increased depending upon the therapeutic response and the patient's ability to tolerate the drugs. These drugs must be given at frequent intervals because of their short duration of action. Other drugs shown to be beneficial include dopamine agonists, monoamine oxidase (MAO) inhibitors, and catechol O-methyltransferase (COMT) inhibitors.

Because some patients ultimately become resistant to drug therapy, neurosurgical interventions can be helpful in some cases. Thalamotomy, thalamic stimulation, and pallidotomy have been shown to decrease and, in some cases, eliminate tremors. Some research indicates that the implantation of fetal substantial nigra cells into the striatum may be beneficial. The use of fetal tissue as a therapy poses an ethical dilemma that is beyond the scope of this book.

Nursing Responsibilities

Nursing care is directed toward helping the patient maintain the activities of daily living while minimizing symptoms and complications and includes the following:

- Teaching the patient and family about drugs the patient is taking, including adverse effects and drug-drug interactions.
- Focusing on minimizing complications of the disease itself and maximizing existing system functioning. Physical therapy and regular exercise can help patients improve gait, postural stability, joint flexibility, and range of motion.
- Seeing to it that the patient is upright when eating or drinking to prevent aspiration. A suction device should be placed at the bedside. Loss of spontaneous automatic movements such as swallowing can decrease a patient's food intake and place him or her at risk for aspiration. Patients who have a problem with drooling (sialorrhea) may require evaluation by a speech pathologist to determine if they are able to swallow food safely.
- Encouraging the use of dietary supplements as needed to supplement nutritional intake. The texture and consistency of the patient's diet may require modification according to the patient's swallowing ability.
- In the hospital as well as the home setting, place the call bell within the patient's reach at all times. Encourage the use of safety devices such as hand rails, walkers, canes, and elevated toilet seats. Because of impaired gait and postural instability, patients are at significant risk for falls.
- Allow the patient sufficient time to communicate because speech is frequently difficult in later stages of the disease. Do not finish patients' thoughts for them.

Do You UNDERSTAND?

DIRECTIONS: **Fill in the blanks to complete the following statements.**

1. Parkinson's disease is caused by the loss of _____, a neurotransmitter.

2. The most disabling symptom of Parkinson's disease is problems with initiation of _____.

3. The most common causes of secondary Parkinson's include _____ and _____.

What IS a Cerebellar Disorder?

The cerebellum is a part of the brain that looks like a cauliflower and is located below the occipital lobes at the base of the skull, just above the brainstem. The cerebellum acts in the regulation of muscle tone and coordination of fine movement.

The three main anatomic subdivisions of the cerebellum are the archicerebellum, the paleocerebellum, and the neocerebellum. The archicerebellum helps coordinate movements of the eyes, head, and neck, and helps to maintain balance. Movements of the trunk and legs are coordinated by the paleocerebellum. Fine movements of the arms are coordinated by the neocerebellum. Damage to the cerebellum can cause problems with gait, disruption in fine motor control, tremors and underreaching or overreaching of targets (dysmetria). There is recent evidence that the cerebellum can also affect thought processes (cognition) and emotion.

Pathogenesis

Cerebellar dysfunction or disease may be due to various causes including intracranial bleeding, infarcts, tumors, alcoholism, exposure to toxins such as carbon monoxide and heavy metals, high fevers, and repeated head trauma. In rare cases, cerebellar dysfunction is the presenting symptom of occult malignancies, particularly of the female reproductive organs. Some cerebellar disorders are hereditary; others occur sporadically.

Answers: 1. dopamine; 2. movement; 3. cerebrovascular disease, drugs.

Ataxia-telangectasia (A-T) and Friedreich's ataxia (FA) are two examples of inherited forms of cerebellar disease. Both diseases have autosomal recessive modes of transmission, which means that two copies of the abnormal chromosome must be inherited, one from each parent, for the disease to manifest.

FA causes nerve cells to deteriorate over time. Symptoms of the disease tend to develop during adolescence and cause changes in the spinal cord, the heart, and the pancreas, and in speech and vision. Almost everyone with this disease will ultimately be confined to a wheelchair.

A-T is characterized by progressive neurologic dysfunction, varying degrees of immunocompromise, increased sensitivity to x-rays, the formation of ocular and cutaneous telangiectasia (permanently dilated and enlarged blood vessels), and increased risk of cancer. The disease causes spinocerebellar degeneration, with spinal muscular atrophy and neuropathy of the peripheral nerves. Both forms of ataxia are characterized by a progressive decline in neurologic function.

At-Risk Populations

People exposed to neurologic toxins, as well as those with a family history of cerebellar disorders, are at risk for the development of cerebellar disease. Nearly all individuals with FA are of European, North African, or Middle Eastern ancestry.

What You NEED TO KNOW

Clinical Manifestations

Signs and symptoms depend upon the part of the cerebellum affected and the degree of damage to cerebellar and neural tissue. Midline cerebellar syndromes tend to cause imbalance; patients have difficulty standing steadily upright with eyes open or closed, and are unable to walk heel-to-toe. Many patients have a characteristic staggering, broad-based gait. Patients may have difficulty sitting upright unsupported. Eye movements may be abnormal, with nystagmus, ocular dysmetria, and difficulty focusing on a single object.

Syndromes affecting the cerebellar hemispheres cause poor coordination of the limbs, dysmetria, and difficulty performing rapid alternating movements (dysdiadochokinesis). Both kinetic and intention tremors may be present.

Patients with FA will experience progressive difficulties with gait between the ages of 5 and 15, followed by cognitive decline, loss of reflexes, and cardiomyopathy. They may also develop talipes (club foot) and other bony deformities of the foot, and scoliosis.

Symptoms of A-T become apparent in infancy, usually when the child begins to walk. Ataxia is associated with abnormal movements of the head, as well as choreoathetoid (twisting, worm-like) movements. Ocular and cutaneous telangectasia are uniformly present; they tend to appear after the age of 6 and sometimes not until adolescence. Deep tendon reflexes become diminished or absent by the age of 7 to 8 years. Typically, affected children will be wheelchair-bound by 10 or 11 years of age. Most patients have a dull, sad facial expression and tend to be stooped, with the head held forward and tilted to one side. Thirty percent of patients have mild mental retardation.

> ! Patients with A-T have a 100-fold greater incidence of cancer than the normal population, and should be monitored accordingly.

Prognosis

Currently there is no cure for cerebellar disease. With appropriate supportive care, patients with FA may survive 35 years or more after their diagnosis. Patients with A-T tend to die prematurely of pulmonary and malignant diseases.

What You DO

In patients who have no family history of cerebellar disorders, a careful search should be made for a causative agent, that is, a neurologic toxin. In some cases, when the offending agent is removed the individual may regain normal neurologic function.

All patients who have a family history of A-T or FA should receive genetic counseling. Patients with FA should be followed by an endocrinologist and a cardiologist because of the risk for diabetes and cardiac disease. Patients with A-T should be aggressively screened for the development of malignancies.

Distressing symptoms can be improved with drug therapy. Haloperidol and the phenothiazines may alleviate chorea and tic syndromes; reserpine may be helpful for tardive dyskinesia. Klonopin may help to decrease myoclonus and spasticity.

Medical management is directed toward prevention of complications and maintaining muscle function for as long as possible. Patients with

A-T who have immunocompromise may be helped by regular injections of immunoglobulin. These individuals also require frequent screening for ophthalmic disease. Educational and physical rehabilitation measures are important. These patients require multidisciplinary care from a variety of professionals including physical, occupational, and speech therapists. Parents of affected children may require psychologic and emotional support from counselors, social workers, or psychotherapists to help them cope with the stress of raising a child with a serious medical illness.

Nursing Responsibilities

For the patient with cerebellar dysfunction, the nurse should do the following:

- Do a careful baseline history and physical examination to rule out the possibility of underlying causes of cerebellar dysfunction.
- Collaborate with other members of the health care team to develop a plan of care that preserves muscle function and independence to the maximum extent possible.
- Obtain equipment and adaptive devices that maintain independence such as walkers, commode chairs, and adaptive utensils to use when eating.
- Educate the affected individual and family or caregivers regarding the importance of exercise regimens that help to maintain muscle strength and coordination. Helpful fitness programs include swimming, horseback riding (with special assistance), the use of specially adapted bicycles, and a graduated program of weight lifting.

Do You UNDERSTAND?

DIRECTIONS: **Fill in the blanks to complete the following statements.**

1. A wide-based, staggering gait is characteristic of _____.
2. Dysmetria means that someone _____.
3. Freidreich's ataxia is an autosomal _____ disease.
4. One of the most important aspect of nursing care of the patient with cerebellar disease is to _____.

Answers: 1. cerebellar disease 2. overreaches their target 3. recessive; 4. help the patient maintain muscle function.

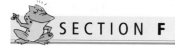

SECTION **F**

GENETIC AND DEVELOPMENTAL DISORDERS

What IS Huntington's Disease?

Huntington's disease (HD) is an autosomal dominant degenerative brain disease characterized by dementia and involuntary movements (**chorea**).

Pathogenesis

HD results from genetically programmed degeneration of neurons in certain areas of the brain. The genetic defect responsible for HD is a small sequence of DNA on chromosome 4 that contains an unstable nucleotide. Neurons of the basal ganglia are specifically affected, causing uncoordinated movement. Within the basal ganglia, HD targets the striatum, particularly neurons in the caudate nuclei and pallidum. The cerebral cortex is also affected, and this is responsible for symptoms associated with psychiatric disorders and dementia.

A small number of cases are sporadic in that they occur despite the absence of family history. A new genetic mutation is thought to be the cause of these cases; it occurs during sperm development and brings the number of amino acid (CAG) repeats into the range that causes HD.

At-Risk Populations

HD is a result of an inherited autosomal dominant disorder. This means that children of an affected parent have a 50% chance of developing the disease. A person who inherits the HD gene and survives long enough will eventually develop the disease.

Genetics of Huntington Disease
http://www.ninds.nih.gov/disorders/huntington/huntington.htm
National Institute of Stroke and Neurologic Diseases
www.ninds.nih.gov; http://www.ninds.nih.gov/disorders/huntington/huntington.htm

What You NEED TO KNOW

Clinical Manifestations

Early manifestations of the disease vary. Adult-onset HD with its disabling chorea frequently begins in middle age. However, other variations of HD are distinguished not simply by age at onset, but rather by the clinical picture.

Initially symptoms may be overlooked as mood swings or uncharacteristic irritability that progresses to depression, hostile outbursts, and dementia. In some patients, symptoms begin with mild clumsiness, balance problems, or continuous uncontrollable movement in the fingers, the feet, the face, or the trunk. Their gait may be dance-like and unsteady. These movements frequently intensify with anxiety. Because chorea causes problems with walking, increased falls result. As neurodegeneration progresses, speech becomes slurred and associated functions, such as swallowing, eating, and speaking, continue to decline. Cognitive changes include short-term memory loss and impaired judgment.

Prognosis

The duration of the illness ranges from 10 to 30 years. Generally, the earlier the symptoms appear, the more rapidly the disease progresses. The most common causes of death are sepsis and injuries related to a fall.

What You DO

Treatment

At this time there is no cure for HD. Muscle dystonia may be helped with supportive therapy, including relaxation training, muscle relaxants, and injections of botulinum toxin. Benzodiazepines, antipsychotic drugs, and muscle relaxants may help alleviate choreic movements, as well as control hallucinations, delusions, and violent outbursts. Antidepressants can be helpful during the early stages of HD. Antipsychotic drugs such as haloperidol or fluphenazine may also be used to control psychiatric manifestations and dementia.

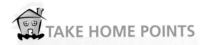

TAKE HOME POINTS

Continuous involuntary movements and dementia are characteristic of HD.

Nursing Responsibilities

Nursing responsibilities focus on optimizing the patient's level of cognitive and physical function. Because of the genetic predisposition for HD, patients may receive explicit directions regarding the aggressive nature of their care and end-of-life issues. Nursing management of the patient with Huntington's chorea includes doing the following:

- Explain the indications and adverse effects of all prescribed drugs to patients, their families, and their caregivers.
- Instruct caregivers on preventing skin problems and preventing aspirations. Choreic movements frequently cause limited mobility and difficulties with swallowing.
- Educate families regarding the importance of genetic counseling.

Do You UNDERSTAND?

DIRECTIONS: **Indicate which statements are *true* (T) and which are *false* (F). If false, correct the statement in the margin space to make it true.**

_____ 1. Lorazepam is frequently used to treat the choreic movements associated with HD.

_____ 2. Aspiration is an uncommon occurrence in the patient with HD.

_____ 3. Patients with HD frequently die from complications associated with fractures.

_____ 4. Families with a positive history for HD should be referred for genetic counseling.

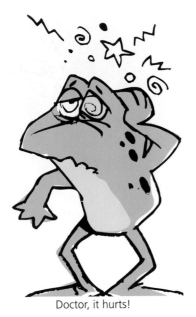

Doctor, it hurts!

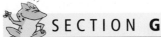 SECTION **G**

PAIN SYNDROMES

Pain is the symptom that most commonly prompts a person to seek professional help; it is a complex phenomenon that is subjective and a personal experience. According to the International Association for the Study of Pain, "pain is an unpleasant sensory and emotional experience associated with actual or potential tissue damage, or described in terms of such damage." Failure to recognize and manage pain not only causes unnecessary suffering, but can delay recovery and prolong hospitalization. Pain can serve as a protective mechanism; for example, touching a very hot object causes us to remove our hand quickly, thereby preventing further injury.

Pain can also be a source of suffering, causing prolonged recovery from illness and extended hospital stays. Suffering occurs when pain is poorly controlled, the source of the pain is undetermined, the meaning of the pain is perceived as dire by the patient, and when the pain is chronic in nature. To provide comprehensive care to patients, health care providers need to understand the physiology of pain and basic principles of pain management so that pain can be controlled and managed, and needless suffering avoided.

Pathogenesis

The physiologic process involved in the transmission of pain signals within the CNS is called **nociception.** Nociceptors are simply free nerve endings found under the epidermis, within deep tissues, muscles, tendons, and subcutaneous tissue. Nociceptors aren't evenly distributed throughout the body, which accounts for variations in relative sensitivity to pain. Nociception has four distinct stages: transduction, transmission, perception, and modulation.

Transduction involves the stimulation of nerve fibers that react to thermal, chemical, and mechanical stimuli. Once activated, the nerve fibers transmit the information to the spinal cord and then the brain. Many different substances are active in transduction including potassium, hydrogen, histamine, serotonin, and prostaglandins.

Transmission occurs when activated nociceptors send impulses to the CNS by way of specialized nerve fibers. Aδ fibers are larger and myelinated, which allows them to transmit pain impulses much more rapidly than the smaller, unmyelinated C fibers. Aδ fibers transmit sharp, stinging, cutting, and pinching sensations, whereas C fibers transmit dull, aching, and burning sensations. Rapid transmission along Aδ fibers allows a person to localize the pain quickly and withdraw from a potential source of injury. Pain signals transmitted by C fibers are of greater duration and poorly localized, and tend to cause more distress for the patient.

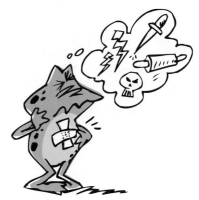

Perception is everything.

Pain *perception* takes place within the cerebral cortex, and is not always related to the degree of tissue damage. Pain may be altered or modulated at various points along the nerve pathways. Pain perception may be *modulated* by the administration of drugs, by initiating other stimuli (such as rubbing a painful area), or by the release of endogenous endorphins within the body.

Pain is classified and described according to the cause of the pain and the duration of symptoms. *Acute pain* is usually the result of direct tissue injury has an immediate onset and resolves when the damaged tissue heals, usually in 3 months or less. This type of pain often causes stimulation of the sympathetic nervous system, with changes in vital signs as well as nausea, sweating, and pallor. Patients with acute pain can usually pinpoint their pain within a single area and tend to use descriptors such as throbbing, stabbing, intense, gnawing, sharp, or aching when describing their pain. Acute unrelieved pain may increase cardiac workload and oxygen demands, with subsequent increased risk for myocardial infarction. Severe unrelieved pain may also cause splinting and inadequate respiratory expansion and be a predisposing factor for pneumonia, especially in postoperative patients. *Acute nociceptive pain* occurs with sprains and fractures, burns, tension headaches, and unstable angina, among other examples. Without intervention, acute nociceptive pain may progress to acute neuropathic pain or a chronic nociceptive pain.

Pain is considered *chronic* in nature when it persists for 6 months or more or beyond the expected healing time after the initial tissue injury. Chronic pain is not always accompanied by sympathetic nervous system activity because the nervous system becomes desensitized to the noxious pain stimulus. The pain may be continuous or recurrent. Chronic pain occurs with stable angina, gastritis, gout, tendonitis, and diverticulitis, among other conditions.

Somatic pain, a form of nociceptive pain, is due to activation of somatic primary afferent nerve fibers. *Visceral pain,* another type of somatic pain,

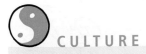

is caused by the stimulation of receptors located within the viscera of the body.

Neuropathic pain is caused by injury to nerves. The injury may be due to disease (such as diabetes, fibromyalgia), infection, trauma, surgery, injury from tumor growth, and antineoplastic and radiation therapy. Neuropathic pain is not completely understood and is thought to be due to changes in central nervous system processing of nociceptive input. Many patients have allodynia, which is pain in response to a stimulus that would not ordinarily be painful. Particularly when an extremity is affected, the painful area will be cold and eventually atrophy, with changes in the patterns of hair distribution and appearance of the skin.

Some patients may have *referred pain,* which is defined as pain that is present in an area or part of the body that is distant from its point of origin. This phenomenon occurs because nerve signals from different parts of the body often travel along the same pathways going to the spinal cord and brain.

Ischemic pain is caused by the loss of blood flow to tissues in a particular part of the body. Failure to perfuse the area causes tissue hypoxia and damage, which leads to the release of inflammatory cell mediators and chemicals that stimulate nociceptors. Angina is an example of pain that is due to ischemia.

Cancer-related pain can have many different causes. Tumors may compress or obstruct vital organs, resulting in visceral pain. Cancers may also infiltrate nerve fibers, causing neuropathic pain. Adverse effects of certain cancer therapies such as antineoplastic or radiation may indirectly cause pain. This type of pain may cause physical and emotional distress for the patient because of fear that it is a symptom of progressive disease.

At-Risk Populations

Pain is a common complaint. All persons are at risk for pain at sometime in their life.

What You NEED TO KNOW

Clinical Manifestations

Pain is a highly variable, subjective experience and is affected by the patient's physiologic, emotional, cultural, and sensory state. Perceptions of pain in the same individual may vary over the course of time depending upon all of these factors. Physiologic aspects that influence pain perception include the cause of the pain; the intensity, quality, frequency, and duration of the pain; the patient's emotional state; previous experience with pain; and level of anxiety.

The ability to tolerate pain is also highly individual. Factors that influence pain tolerance include family support, role expectations, spiritual beliefs, cultural beliefs, gender roles, personality, and coping ability.

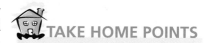

TAKE HOME POINTS

Vital signs used in isolation are unreliable indicators of the extent of the pain a patient has. Pain reporting is the single best measure of pain for the person who is able to communicate.

Types of Pain	Associated Descriptions
Somatic	Aching, squeezing, stabbing, throbbing, intense, unbearable, heavy, sharp, nagging, exhausting, tiring, shooting
Visceral	Cramping, gnawing
Ischemic	Burning, prickling, or aching in quality
Neuropathic	Constant, severe ache that is overlaid by bursts of burning, or shocklike stabbing pain

Agency for HealthCare Research and Quality. (Formerly the Agency for Health Care Policy and Research). Clinical Practice Guidelines.

http:www.ahrq.gov

Prognosis

Resolution of pain usually depends upon the cause and type of pain experienced by the patient. Ideally, the underlying cause of the pain should be treated and corrected, but this isn't always possible, particularly in the case of cancer-related pain. All types of pain can be alleviated with appropriate therapy, and in many cases pain can be completely eradicated.

What You DO

Treatment

Particularly when pain is severe, successful pain management requires that a therapeutic, trusting relationship be established between the patient and health care providers. Factors such as anxiety, fear, and the need for distraction must be addressed as well as investigating and correcting the underlying causes of pain when appropriate. Treatment for pain should include both pharmacologic and nonpharmacologic measures. Pain should always be prevented rather than treated after the fact, because pain is more difficult to eradicate than to prevent. Analgesics should be consistent with the nature and severity of the patient's pain.

The World Health Organization recommends a stepwise approach to analgesic therapy. Opioids such as morphine, hydromorphone, and

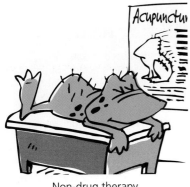

Non-drug therapy.

methadone should be used for acute moderate-to-severe nociceptive pain. Milder opioids such as codeine and oxycodone are suitable for mild to moderate pain. For mild pain, agents such as NSAIDs and acetaminophen are helpful. Adjunctive drug therapies include antidepressants, anticonvulsants, muscle relaxants, steroids, and anesthetics.

Non–drug treatment measures include physical therapy, cognitive and behavioral therapy, distraction measures, guided imagery, progressive muscle relaxation, dermal stimulation, transcutaneous electrical nerve stimulation (TENS), and applications of heat and cold. For patients who do not achieve satisfactory relief with pharmacologic and nonpharmacologic measures, acupuncture, percutaneous electrical nerve stimulation (PENS), nerve blocks, and neurosurgical interventions may offer relief.

Nursing Responsibilities

Thorough evaluation of a patient's pain must be done in order for it to be adequately managed. Remember that only the patient can describe or quantify the pain he or she is experiencing, and that not all patients will complain of or show symptoms of pain such as grimacing or groaning. The history of the patient's pain should contain the components listed in the accompanying box.

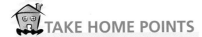

TAKE HOME POINTS

Pain is the fifth vital sign and should be assessed routinely with each patient contact.

Assessing Pain—The Fifth Vital Sign

- Intensity (e.g., "On a scale of 1-10, how would you rate your pain?")
- Location (e.g., "Where is the pain?")
- Onset and pattern (e.g., "When did it start? Was it sudden or develop over time? Is it continuous or intermittent?")
- Extension or radiation (e.g., "Does the pain move to other areas?")
- Duration (e.g., "How long does the pain last?")
- Character or quality (e.g., "Is it sharp? Dull? Shooting? An ache?")
- Precipitating, aggravating, and alleviating factors (e.g., "What starts the pain? What makes it worse? What makes it better?")
- Associated manifestations (e.g., "Do you suffer from anorexia? Nausea? Restlessness? Insomnia?")
- Effects on activities of daily living (e.g., "Has the pain affected things like your sleep, appetite, concentration, work, school, interpersonal relationships, marital relations, sex, home activities, driving, walking, leisure activities, or your emotional state?")

A numeric pain rating scale can be used to help the patient quantify the intensity of pain. There are many specific assessment tools available to assess pain in adults and children. For young children or adults who are cognitively impaired or unable to read, a color scale or a scale showing smiling or weeping faces may be used.

Establish a helping relationship with the patient, family members, and significant others. Present a calm, nonjudgmental manner when interviewing the patient. Many individuals who suffer chronic pain are mistakenly labeled as "drug-seeking" by health care providers, and have learned not to trust that their pain will be believed in or adequately relieved by health care providers. Ask patients what level of pain control will be satisfactory for them. Many people prefer to experience some pain rather than cope with the adverse effects of large doses of opioid and opioid-like analgesics, particularly if they have a chronic pain syndrome.

In collaboration with the patient, develop a plan of care tailored to the individual patient's needs. Administer prescribed analgesics on time, keeping in mind possible adverse effects such as respiratory depression, sedation, confusion, constipation, nausea, and pruritus. Most patients should receive around-the-clock dosing to prevent pain from occurring, along with supplemental drugs to treat break-through pain. Remember to evaluate the level of pain relief after interventions are performed, and make adjustments in the plan of care.

Be an educator and patient advocate for the patient and family. Teach the patient ways to minimize and control his or her own pain, including measures such as self-hypnosis, progressive muscle relaxation, guided imagery, and exercise when not otherwise contraindicated. Instruct the patient on how to self-administer the drugs, and to store them in a safe place, away from children in the home environment.

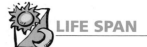

LIFE SPAN

Be aware of the physiologic changes of aging when using pain drugs in the very young and in older adult patients. Physiologic changes alter drug absorption, distribution, metabolism, and elimination. Careful observation of the elderly patient is vital to effective and safe pain management.

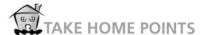

TAKE HOME POINTS

Remember: pain is a subjective and highly variable experience. Pain is defined differently by each patient based on values, beliefs, culture, and physiology. Pain can only be defined and expressed by the person experiencing it.

Do You UNDERSTAND?

DIRECTIONS: **Circle the correct answer.**

1. Acute pain is usually the result of
   a. Direct tissue injury.
   b. Indirect tissue injury.
   c. Abnormal transmission of pain signals.
   d. None of the above.
2. Changes in vital signs associated with severe acute pain are related to
   a. An abnormal autonomic response.
   b. Sympathetic nervous system activation.
   c. Parasympathetic stimulation.
   d. Stimulation of C fibers.

Using the examples below, identify whether the pain is typically acute, chronic, or both.

3. _____ Sensations felt the first few weeks after a mastectomy
4. _____ Migraine headache
5. _____ Persistent low back pain
6. _____ Chest pain due to myocardial infarction
7. _____ Osteoarthritis of the knee
8. _____ Diabetic peripheral neuropathy
9. _____ Postoperative incisional pain
10. _____ Tumor of the sacral nerve plexus

References

Acute Pain Management Guideline Panel: *Acute pain management: operative or medical procedures and trauma,* Clinical Practice Guideline, AHCPR Pub. No. 92-0032. Rockville, Md, 1992, U.S. Department of Health and Human Services.

Agency for HealthCare Research and Quality: Clinical practice guidelines, URL http:www.ahrq.gov.

Answers: **1. a; 2. b; 3. acute; 4. acute; 5. chronic; 6. acute; 7. chronic; 8. chronic; 9. acute; 10. acute and chronic.**

Blanda M: *Headache, tension*, 2004, URL www.emedicine.com/EMERG/topic231. htm.

Brookoff D: *Chronic pain. 2. The case for opioids*, 2005, URL www.hosppract.com/issues/2000/09/brook.htm.

Cacchione PZ: Cognitive and neurologic function. In Lueckenotte AG, editor: *Gerontologic nursing*, ed 2, St Louis, 2000, Mosby.

Chang AK: *Benign positional vertigo*, 2005, URL www.emedicine.com/emerg/topic57.htm.

Fahn S: Huntington disease. In Rowland LP, editor: *Merritt's neurology*, ed 10, Philadelphia, 2000, Lippincott–Williams & Wilkins.

Friedland R, Wilcock GK: Dementia. In Evans GJ et al: *Oxford textbook of geriatric medicine*, ed 2, Oxford, 2000, Oxford University Press.

Fulmer T et al: Providing care for elderly people who exhibit disturbing behavior. In Evans GJ et al, editors: *Oxford textbook of geriatric medicine*, ed 2, Oxford, 2000, Oxford University Press.

Ghajar J: Traumatic brain injury, *Lancet* 356(9233):923, 2000.

Gottschalk A, Smith, DS: New concepts in acute pain therapy: preemptive analgesia, *Am Fam Phys* 63(10):1979, 2001.

Henze RL: Traumatic and vascular injuries of the central nervous system. In Bullock BA, Henze RL, editors: *Focus on pathophysiology*, Philadelphia, 2000, Lippincott–Williams & Wilkins.

Jozwiak S: *Ataxia-telangiectasia*, 2005, URL www.emedicine.com/drem/topic691. htm.

Lazoff M: Encephalitis, 2005, URL www.emedicine.com/emerg/topic163.htm.

Lundgren CL: Chronic sorrow in long-term illness across the life span. In Miller JF, editor: *Coping with chronic illness*, ed 3, Philadelphia, 2000, FA Davis.

Mendizabal J: *Cluster headache*, 2005, URL www.emedicine.com/NEURO/topic70. htm.

Morris GF, Marshall LF: Injury of the head and spinal cord. In Goldman L, Bennett JC, editors: *Cecil textbook of medicine*, Philadelphia, 2000, WB Saunders.

National Guideline Clearinghouse: *Assessment and management of acute pain*, 2005, URL www.guideline.gov.

Nikhar NK: *Neuropathy of Friedreich Ataxia*, 2001, URL www.emedicine.com/neuro/topic265.htm.

Sargeant L: *Headache, cluster*, 2005, URL www.emedicine.com/EMERG/topic229. htm.

Small SA, Mayeux R: Alzheimer's disease and related dementias. In Rowland LP, editor: *Merritt's neurology*, ed 10, Philadelphia, 2000, Lippincott–Williams & Wilkins.

Waldren, SJ: *Atlas of Common Pain Syndromes*, Philadelphia, 2002, WB Saunders.

NCLEX® Review

Section A

1. A 79-year-old woman is admitted for evaluation of changes in mental status. The patient's daughter reports that the patient fell and struck her head 1 month ago and has been progressively more lethargic and confused over the past few days. A large, fading bruise is visible on her forehead. The patient may have a/an
   1 Epidural hematoma.
   2 Subdural hematoma.
   3 Arterial intracranial bleeding.
   4 Concussion.

2. A teenager is about to be discharged from the emergency room after receiving treatment for a concussion. Discharge teaching for the patient and family should include which type of statement?
   1 "You may have intermittent headaches for several months after this injury."
   2 "It is possible that you will have problems with gait and coordination until you recover."
   3 "You will probably need a lot more sleep during the next several months."
   4 "You shouldn't have any trouble keeping up with your studies."

3. Patients with an injury to their frontal lobe may experience
   1 Expressive aphasia.
   2 Problems with long-term memory.
   3 Impairments in fine motor movements.
   4 Hearing disturbances.

4. Moderate hypothermia may be beneficial for the patient with a head injury because it
   1 Increases cerebral blood flow.
   2 Decreases intracranial pressure.
   3 Increases oxygen levels.
   4 Increases oxygen requirements.

5. Which of the following is a potential complication of injury to the occipital lobe?
   1 Changes in personality
   2 Left-sided paralysis
   3 Loss of vision
   4 Aphasia

6. Epidural hematomas are usually the indirect result of a
   1 Venous leak.
   2 Skull fracture.
   3 Capillary leak.
   4 Coagulation defect.

7. Headache, irritability, and the decreased ability to concentrate are thought to be symptoms of
   1 Cerebral hypoxia.
   2 Postconcussion syndrome.
   3 Subdural hematoma.
   4 Autonomic dysfunction.

8. Which type of intracranial hematomas can occur several weeks after the injury?
   1 Acute subdural hematomas
   2 Epidural hematomas
   3 Chronic subdural hematomas
   4 Subarachnoid hematomas

9. Which of the following signs are suggestive of skull fracture?
   1 Clear, thin fluid coming from the nose and ears
   2 Bruising around the jaw
   3 Areas of local edema in the scalp
   4 Bloody drainage from the ears

10. A patient describes excruciating pain behind his left eye. His left eye is also watery and reddened and his left nostril is congested. This patient is experiencing a/an
    1 Attack of acute sinusitis.
    2 Tension headache.
    3 Migraine headache.
    4 Cluster headache.

11. Self-care measures for the patient with chronic headaches include
    1 Avoiding caffeine.
    2 Maintaining healthy sleep habits.
    3 Abstaining from all aerobic exercise.
    4 Drinking moderate amounts of alcohol.

12. A patient complains of severe dizziness that is made worse with movement and activity. The nurse is aware that this patient may have
    1 Benign paroxysmal positional vertigo.
    2 Acute vertigo.
    3 Chronic vertigo.
    4 None of the above.

Section B

13. A patient mentions that he experienced transient slurred speech and numbness in one arm that lasted for approximately 2 hours and then subsided spontaneously. What did this patient likely experience?
    1 Stroke
    2 Brain attack
    3 Transient ischemic attack
    4 Hypertensive episode

14. An arteriovenous malformation is best defined as a (an)
    1 Ballooning of the arterial wall.
    2 Nest of abnormally shaped, twisted vessels.
    3 Abnormally shaped vessel that forms because of atherosclerosis.
    4 Stroke.

15. The wife of a patient who has had a stroke reports that her husband woke up with slurred speech and was unable to get out of bed without assistance. Two days later, the patient is still experiencing neurologic deficits. What did this patient probably experience?
    1 Hemorrhagic stroke
    2 Thrombotic stroke
    3 Syncopal event
    4 Transient ischemic attack

16. Risk factors for thrombotic strokes include
    1 Atrial arrhythmias.
    2 Thyroid disease.
    3 Renal disease.
    4 All of the above.

17. Which of the following measures would be contraindicated for a patient with a recent stroke?
    1 Keeping the head of the bed elevated at all times
    2 Keeping the patient's hips flexed
    3 Grouping the patient's care together to facilitate undisturbed rest for the remainder of the day
    4 Widely spacing procedures that increase intracranial pressure, such as bathing

Section C

18. Which of the following signs and symptoms is uncharacteristic of multiple sclerosis?
    1 Blurred vision or diplopia
    2 Weakness in the extremities
    3 History of falls
    4 Muscle rigidity

19. Patients with multiple sclerosis with early disease may benefit from
    1 High doses of IgG.
    2 High-dose intravenous methylprednisolone.
    3 Routine doses of NSAIDs.
    4 All of the above.

20. Early symptoms of amyotrophic lateral sclerosis usually include
    1 Weakness in the arms and shoulders.
    2 Hypoactive reflexes.
    3 Swallowing difficulty.
    4 Confusion.

Section D

21. Meningitis means that infection is present in the
    1 Subarachnoid space.
    2 Epidural space.
    3 Pia mater.
    4 Cerebral cortex.

22. Viral meningitis can enter the body as a result of
    1 Mumps infection.
    2 Hand washing.
    3 Chicken pox infection.
    4 Eating undercooked meats.

23. Which of the following factors is *not* a typical symptom associated with meningitis?
    1 Decreased level of consciousness
    2 Headache
    3 Agitation
    4 Rash

24. Patients with which of the following disorders are likely to make a complete recovery within 10 to 14 days?
    1 Fungal encephalitis
    2 Bacterial meningitis
    3 Viral meningitis
    4 Bacterial encephalitis

25. The nurse notes that a patient with bacterial meningitis is oozing blood from old venipuncture sites. What should the nurse do first?
    1 Apply a pressure bandage
    2 Avoid invasive procedures whenever possible
    3 Evaluate the patient for other sources of infection
    4 Notify the primary care provider immediately

26. Which form of encephalitis may be prevented by avoiding exposure to mosquito bites?
    1 Cytomegalovirus
    2 West Nile
    3 Herpes simplex
    4 Varicella-zoster

27. A patient with a presumptive diagnosis of encephalitis arrives at the emergency department with altered mental status, temperature of 97.4° F, and a blood pressure of 80/40. The nurse should first
    1 Apply a warming blanket.
    2 Start a large-bore IV and begin fluids.
    3 Do a complete neurologic assessment.
    4 Offer the patient something for pain.

28. A patient with encephalitis has petechiae and several bruises. The nurse should be concerned that the patient may
    1 Have fallen.
    2 Have disseminated intravascular coagulation.
    3 Have bone marrow failure.
    4 Be experiencing an adverse drug reaction.

Section E

29. Which of the following is the cause of Parkinson's disease?
    1 Loss of acetylcholine
    2 Excess secretion of acetylcholine
    3 Loss of dopamine
    4 Excess secretion of dopamine

30. Which of the following is *not* a symptom associated with Parkinson's disease?
    1 Cogwheel rigidity
    2 Broad-based gait
    3 Tremors
    4 Bradykinesia

31. Which of the following interventions is most appropriate for a patient experiencing a seizure?
    1 Restrain the patient's arms and legs to ensure that the patient is not injured
    2 Use a gloved hand to clear the patient's airway.
    3 Roll the patient on his or her side.
    4 Move the patient to a hospital bed.

32. Symptoms associated with Alzheimer's disease are thought to be a result of
    1 Genetic defects.
    2 Deficits in neurotransmitters.
    3 Trauma.
    4 Excess acetylcholine.

33. Which class of medication can have a negative effect on the patient with Alzheimer's disease?
    1 Anticholinergics
    2 Calcium channel blockers
    3 Angiotensin converting enzyme (ACE) inhibitors
    4 Diuretics

34. Multiinfarct dementia is *not* commonly associated with
    1 Carotid emboli.
    2 Vasculitis.
    3 Arterial thrombosis.
    4 Head trauma.

35. Pharmacologic therapies to prevent multiinfarct dementia include which of the following?
    1 aspirin
    2 furosemide
    3 haloperidol
    4 ibuprofen

36. Identify the symptom of cerebellar dysfunction.
    1 Difficulty sitting unsupported
    2 Hemiparesis
    3 Hyperactivity
    4 Ptosis of the eyelids

37. Which preventive screening measures would not ordinarily be indicated for patients with ataxia-telangectasia?
    1 Yearly mammography
    2 MUGA scan
    3 Colonoscopy
    4 Assessment of skin

Section F

38. Huntington's disease is a hereditary autosomal dominant disorder. This means that children of a parent with this disease have a _____ chance of developing the disease.
    1 25%
    2 50%
    3 75%
    4 100%

Section G

39. Endorphins are found in the brainstem and
    1 Increase pain perception.
    2 Decrease pain sensations.
    3 May increase or decrease pain transmission.
    4 Has no effect on pain sensation.

40. Acute pain is most characterized by sympathetic nervous system responses such as
    1 Increased blood pressure and pulse.
    2 Pink skin and skeletal muscle tension.
    3 Constricted pupils and dry skin.
    4 Decreased or normal blood pressure and pulse.

41. Chronic pain is characterized by parasympathetic nervous system responses such as
    1 Increased blood pressure and pulse.
    2 Pallor and skeletal muscle tension.
    3 Dilated pupils and diaphoresis.
    4 Decreased or normal blood pressure and pulse.

42. Which of the following statements is true regarding pain?
    1 The majority of pain is caused by physical trauma.
    2 Pain is a subjective experience best defined by the patient.
    3 The individual most qualified to evaluate pain is the health care provider.
    4 Pain is an objective experience that can be measured quantitatively.

43. Name 5 factors influencing a patient's response to pain.

NCLEX® Review Answers

Section A

1. **2** Subdural hematomas involve venous circulation and are characterized by a slow accumulation of blood within the subdural space, which would cause a gradual onset of symptoms. Arterial bleeds within the brain and epidural hematomas have a more rapid accumulation of blood, which would cause sudden, dramatic onset of symptoms. Concussion would not cause gradual deterioration of neurologic status.

2. **1** Postconcussion syndromes are characterized by persistent headaches, insomnia, and difficulty concentrating for as long as several months after the injury. Problems with gait and coordination would be seen with a more severe injury than a concussion.

3. **3** Frontal lobe injury causes impairment in fine motor movements, speech, and the ability to use and manipulate tools. The temporal lobe controls long-term memory and hearing. Expressive aphasia may be a result of damage to Broca's area.

4. **2** Lower body temperatures decrease metabolic processes and reduce intracranial pressure in the head injury patient. Oxygen requirements are decreased rather than increased, and oxygen levels are unaffected by hypothermia.

5. **3** Injury to the occipital lobe may cause loss of the ability to interpret visual images and blindness.

6. **2** Epidural hematomas usually form as a consequence of arterial bleeding from a skull fracture. Coagulation defects may cause the hematoma to accumulate more rapidly, but do not in and of themselves cause the hematoma to occur. Venous and capillary leaks do not typically affect the epidural space.

7. **2** The sequelae of concussion cause persistent pain, inflammation, and problems with cognition in some individuals. Hematomas, hypoxia, and autonomic dysfunction would all cause a more severe array of symptoms.

8. **3** Chronic subdural hematomas may not become symptomatic until several weeks after the initial injury because of slow accumulation of blood in the subdural space.

9. **1** Always suspect a skull fracture if the patient has thin, clear fluid draining from the nose and ears. Cerebrospinal fluid will test positive for glucose. Bloody drainage from the ears is suggestive of a ruptured tympanic membrane. Edema in the scalp and bruising around the jaw indicate trauma to the head, but are not necessarily indicative of a skull fracture.

10. **4** Cluster headache pain is usually extreme, localized and around or behind one eye. Tension headaches are characterized by less severe pain which is more generalized. Migraine headaches tend to be more unilateral, and don't cause the symptoms of nasal congestion and ipsilateral lacrimation.

11. **2** Sleep deprivation may precipitate headaches in susceptible individuals. Caffeine can help to relieve headaches rather than worsening them, because it causes constriction of abnormally dilated cerebral vessels. Moderate exercise may help to relieve headache pain. Alcohol tends to precipitate headaches in susceptible individuals and should be avoided.

12. **1** Dizziness with movement is the hallmark symptom of BPPV.

Section B

13. **3** Transient ischemic attacks are typically brief in duration and leave no permanent deficit. A true stroke or brain attack is likely to leave permanent neurologic deficits. Hypertensive episodes are generally asymptomatic.

14. **2** An arteriovenous malformation is best defined as a nest of abnormally shaped, twisted blood vessels. A dilation (ballooning) of a vessel wall is more consistent with an aneurysm; however, these can form in any vessel, not in arteries alone. Atherosclerosis does not change the shape of a blood vessel. A stroke or brain attack is an interruption of blood flow to the brain.

15. **2** Thrombotic strokes tend to occur at night, during sleep. A hemorrhagic stroke is characterized by sudden onset of symptoms. A syncopal event, also known as fainting, does not result in neurologic deficits. A transient ischemic attack is a neurologic deficit lasting for less than 24 hours.

16. **2** Atrial arrhythmias tend to allow blood to pool within the atria, which provides an opportunity for clots to form. Those clots may then be ejected out into the systemic circulation and cause myocardial infarctions and stroke.

17. **2** Hip flexion is contraindicated because it may increase intracranial pressure in the patient who has had a recent stroke. All other measures cited will help to decrease intracranial pressure.

Section C

18. **2** Multiple sclerosis does not cause muscle rigidity. All other symptoms cited are characteristic of the disease.

19. **2** High-dose methylprednisolone may help to decrease the inflammatory component of MS, thereby obtaining a remission of symptoms. NSAIDs offer no particular benefit for patients with MS.

20. **1** Weakness in the arms and shoulders are one of the most common presenting symptoms of ALS. Loss of reflexes and swallowing difficulty appear with disease progression. The disease does not cause confusion or cognitive decline.

Section D

21. **1** The term *meningitis* refers to infection that is limited to the meninges in the subarachnoid space.

22. **1** Viral meningitis can be caused by the mumps virus. Frequent hand washing is a good precaution against the spread of viral meningitis. Chicken pox does not cause viral meningitis. Eating undercooked meats can lead to several conditions, including salmonella poisoning, *E. coli* infection, and tuberculosis.

23. **3** Agitation is not typically observed with a central nervous system infection. More commonly present are headache, rash, and altered levels of consciousness.

24. **3** Viral syndromes (e.g., viral meningitis) are typically self-limiting and resolve within 10 to 14 days. Bacterial and fungal central nervous system infections such as fungal encephalitis, bacterial meningitis, and bacterial encephalitis require intensive therapy in the acute-care setting.

25. **1** The nurse should first attempt to control bleeding with a pressure bandage and then notify the primary care provider immediately, because oozing from old puncture sites can be a symptom of disseminated intravascular coagulation, a potentially life-threatening complication. Avoidance of invasive procedures and evaluation of the patient for sources of infection occur later in care.

26. **2** The West Nile virus is the only one of these organisms that is transmitted via mosquito bites.

27. **2** The patient may be in septic shock. Therefore the most appropriate intervention would be to start an IV and begin aggressive volume replacement to maintain perfusion to vital organs. Next, a complete neurologic assessment should be done, followed by administration of analgesics if not otherwise contraindicated. A warming blanket would not be indicated in this scenario.

28. **2** Petechiae and ecchymoses are a possible indication of DIC, often seen as a sequela of sepsis. A fall might cause bruises but not petechaie. Bone marrow failure is not a complication of encephalitis. Drug reactions would more likely be allergic in nature.

Section E

29. **3** Parkinson's disease is the result of a loss of dopamine. A rise or fall in the acetylcholine level does not cause Parkinson's disease.

30. **4** Bradykinesia is not characteristic of Parkinson's disease. Cogwheel rigidity; small, shuffling steps; and tremors are associated with Parkinson's disease.

31. **3** Rolling the patient to his or her side decreases the patient's risk of aspiration. Restraining the patient's arms and legs may cause injury to the caregiver and fractures for the patient. Never insert hands or fingers in the patient's mouth during a seizure. Moving the patient to a hospital bed must wait until the seizure is finished.

32. **2** Symptoms associated with AD are thought to be the result of defects in neurotransmitters. Genetic defects may lead to development of the disease but are not responsible for the development of symptoms. Head trauma may cause neurologic damage but does not cause the progressive decline in neurologic function that is associated with this disease. Excessive acetylcholine does not cause neurologic damage.

33. **1** Medications with anticholinergic properties can adversely affect acetylcholine levels and may cause further decline in cognitive function. Calcium channel blockers, ACE inhibitors, and diuretics may be given to Alzheimer's disease patients when necessary to treat other medical conditions.

34. **4** Head trauma has not been shown to cause cerebral infarcts, although it may cause neurologic damage.

35. **1** Aspirin will inhibit platelet activity and thereby decrease the risk of embolic formations that cause multiinfarct dementia. The other drugs mentioned do not affect cerebral blood flow.

36. **1** Patients with midline damage to the cerebellum have difficulty sitting unsupported. Patients with cerebellar disease have limitations in muscle function, which inhibits activity. Ptosis of the eyelids is a symptom of myasthenia gravis.

37. **2** Patients with A-T have a risk for malignancies that is 100 times greater than the normal population and should be aggressively screened for malignancies.

Section F

38. **2** Presuming that only one parent has Huntington's disease, a child of the affected parent has a 50% chance of inheriting a defective copy of the gene.

Section G

39. **2** Endorphins reduce pain sensations rather than increase them. Endorphins are not related to transmission of painful impulses or their interpretation.

40. **1, 2, 3, 4** All are representative of parasympathetic nervous system activity.

41. **4** Options 1, 2, and 3 are sympathetic nervous system responses and are characteristic of an acute pain response.

42. **2** All pain is subjective. The best person to evaluate the pain is the patient, not the health care provider.

43. Previous experience with pain; family and occupational roles; spiritual belief system; physical influences such as sleep or stress; pain threshold; pain quality, location, duration, type; patient personality; communication skills

Notes

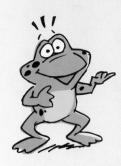

Alterations in Hemostasis and Coagulation

What You WILL LEARN

After reading this chapter, you will know how to do the following:

✔ Describe how the body controls bleeding.
✔ Differentiate between idiopathic thrombocytopenia purpura and thrombotic thrombocytopenia purpura.
✔ List nursing interventions for a patient with a bleeding disorder.
✔ Explain the pathogenesis of hemophilia.
✔ Identify treatment measures for hemophilia.
✔ List the various causes of anemia.
✔ Identify treatment measures and nursing interventions for anemia.
✔ Discuss complications of sickle cell disease.
✔ Develop a plan of care for the patient with sickle cell disease.

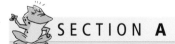

SECTION A

COAGULATION DISTURBANCES

In this section, diseases and disorders affecting coagulation of the blood are examined. Coagulation is an essential, protective mechanism. **Hemostasis,** or the cessation of blood flow, prevents blood loss when a vessel is damaged. **Coagulation** is the ability of blood to change from a fluid to a semisolid mass. This mechanism of clot initiation and formation involves a series of sequential cascadelike reactions that employ several factors in the blood and injured tissue. Control of bleeding is accomplished through the following sequence:

1. Immediately after the wall of a vessel is injured, contraction of the vessel decreases the flow of blood into and out of the vessel. This constriction is a protective mechanism because it helps limit blood loss.

2. Damage to the blood vessel causes platelet plugs to form. With disruption of the endothelial lining of the vessel, the underlying collagen is exposed. Platelets contain enzymes necessary for the synthesis of prostaglandins, an important part of hemostasis.

3. When platelets are exposed to collagen or other foreign substances such as antigen-antibody complexes, thrombin, proteolytic enzymes, endotoxins, or viruses, they undergo a change. The platelets begin to swell and form irregular shapes with processes protruding from their surfaces. Eventually, these platelets become sticky and adhere to the collagen and basement membrane of the vessel.

4. The platelets release adenosine diphosphate (ADP), which attracts other platelets and aids in platelet adhesion and aggregation. ADP is also released from disrupted red blood cells and damaged tissue.

5. Enzymes released from the platelet cause the formation of thromboxane A in the plasma.

6. Both ADP and thromboxane A activate platelets that adhere to the original platelets. The platelet plug results, causing the damaged endothelial vessel wall to adhere to the collagen fibers. When the tear is small, the plug stops further blood loss. The conversion of fibrinogen into fibrin creates a mesh that cements the platelets and other blood components in place.

Coagulation is achieved through three basic reactions, which constitute the sequential pathway for blood coagulation. The intrinsic or extrinsic pathway, activated in response to tissue or endothelial damage, causes prothrombin activator to form. Prothrombin activator catalyzes the conversion of prothrombin to thrombin. Thrombin catalyzes the conversion of soluble fibrinogen to solid fibrin polymer threads. These fibrin threads form the meshwork on which plasma, blood cells, and platelets aggregate to make the clot.

Clot formation must occur before coagulation can be achieved. Clotting factors are a series of plasma proteins that are generally inactive forms of proteolytic enzymes. The enzymatic proteolytic actions cause successive reactions of the clotting process in a cascade-like sequence. One factor is important for the activation of the next factor. Most of the

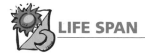

LIFE SPAN

Pregnancy and oral contraceptives can adversely affect the coagulation process.

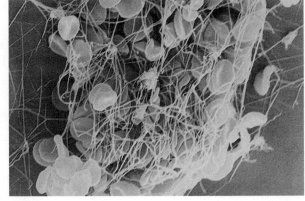

A blood clot or thrombus, showing blood cells trapped by fibrin strands. *(From Stevens ML: Fundamentals of clinical hematology, Philadephia, WB Saunders, 1997. With permission.)*

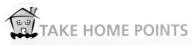

TAKE HOME POINTS

Fibrinogen, prothrombin, and factors VII, IX, and X are essential procoagulation factors that are synthesized in the liver according to the body's requirements.

factors that promote coagulation are proteins that are synthesized in the liver. In order for adequate synthesis to take place, the patient must have a healthy liver and adequate amounts of vitamin K and calcium.

What IS Idiopathic Thrombocytopenia Purpura?

Idiopathic thrombocytopenia purpura (ITP) is an autoimmune bleeding disorder characterized by the formation of platelet antibodies and a marked increase in platelet destruction, resulting in multiple bruises and hemorrhage into the tissue. The disorder may be either acute or chronic in nature.

Pathogenesis

Low platelet count (**thrombocytopenia**) results from immunologic platelet destruction. ITP resulting from autoantibodies directed against certain platelet antigens is the most common type of immune thrombocytopenia.

At-Risk Populations

Acute ITP is most commonly seen in children, usually after a viral infection. The reported prevalence of ITP in adults and children is 1 to 13 per 100,000 persons. In children, both sexes are affected; in adults, the disease predominates in women. Typically the chronic form is

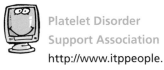

Platelet Disorder Support Association http://www.itppeople. com/

National Heart Lung and Blood Institute—What Is Idiopathic Thrombocytopenia Purpura? http://www.nhlbi.nih.gov/health/dci/Diseases/Itp/ITP_WhatIs.html

idiopathic (of unknown origin), but it may occur in association with other autoimmune disorders such as lupus and thyroid disease. Fewer than 40% of all patients with ITP are younger than 10 years of age. Pregnant women may also be affected with ITP.

What You NEED TO KNOW

Patients with ITP who are refractory to medical therapy may require splenectomy. For these individuals, immunization is important. They should receive haemophilus influenza type B conjugated vaccine, polyvalent pneumococcal vaccine, and quadrivalent meningococcal polysaccharide vaccine at least 2 weeks before elective splenectomy.

Clinical Manifestations

Results of the physical examination are usually normal except for purpura. A platelet count of less than 20,000/mm^3 and a prolonged bleeding time are indicative of ITP. Platelet size and appearance may be abnormal, and anemia may be present when extensive bleeding has occurred. Bone marrow studies reveal an abundance of megakaryocytes. Platelet survival time is decreased from 3 to 7 days to only several hours.

Prognosis

Spontaneous remission occurs in children 83% of the time compared with 2% in adults. Rare intracranial hemorrhage is the most common cause of death, affecting only 3% to 4% of patients.

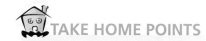

TAKE HOME POINTS

- Patients with the human immunodeficiency virus (HIV) may also have associated ITP.
- ITP has the same damaging secondary consequences associated with a chronic disease, for example, time lost from work or school.
- Weight gain and mood swings, observed with steroid treatment, are also a concern of some patients.

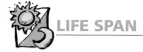

LIFE SPAN

Older patients have hemorrhagic complications more often than younger patients with the same platelet counts. Chronic acute idiopathic or autoimmune thrombocytopenia purpura (AITP) occurs most frequently in adults.

What You DO

Treatment

The main goal of therapy is to reduce the production of platelet autoantibodies and to remove antibody-coated platelets from the circulation. Treatment emphasizes the prevention of life-threatening complications such as intracranial hemorrhage. Medical management of ITP ranges from a simple steroid treatment to a splenectomy with long-term follow-up.

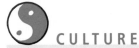

LIFE SPAN

Treatment of children with acute ITP continues to be debated. Usually, AITP resolves spontaneously within 6 months. Children are usually treated with a short course of tapering steroids. Unless an emergency exists, platelet transfusions are not administered.

CULTURE

The Jehovah's Witness population does not permit transfusion of blood products. Their religious beliefs may preclude the use of IVIG, primarily because it is derived from blood.

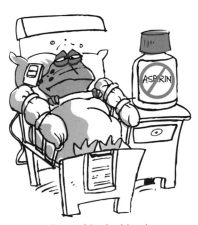

Don't thin the blood.

Avoid all aspirin in any form and other drugs that can impair coagulation.

ITP can be present for many years and is characterized by periodic flare-ups or exacerbations. Supportive care and the institution of bleeding precautions are advised.

Adults with ITP are given corticosteroids as the initial treatment to promote capillary integrity. Intravenous immunoglobulin (IVIG) may also be administered on a weekly basis. Other treatments include intravenous azathioprine, danazol, immunosuppressive therapy, plasmapheresis, and splenectomy. Splenectomy is not performed as initial therapy in patients who have bleeding symptoms or minor purpura.

Nursing Responsibilities

When caring for a hospitalized patient with clotting problems, the nurse should take every precaution against bleeding and should do the following:

- Protect the patient from trauma, keeping the side rails up and padded when possible.
- Promote the use of an electric razor and soft toothbrush.
- Avoid invasive procedures such as venipuncture or urinary catheterization when possible.
- Monitor platelets at least daily.
- Test for blood: in stool, in the urine, and in emesis.
- Watch for symptoms of bleeding such as petechiae, ecchymosis, surgical or gastrointestinal bleeding, and menorrhagia.
- Advise the patient to avoid constipation, straining during bowel movements, and coughing, which can lead to increased intracranial pressure. Before discharge, instruct the patient on appropriate safety measures to use at home, including avoidance of injury due to falls. Children with ITP may require protective gear such as helmets and elbow and knee pads.
- During periods of active bleeding, enforce strict bed rest.
- When administering platelet transfusions, remember that platelets are fragile; therefore infuse quickly with the proper administration set.

Do You UNDERSTAND?

DIRECTIONS: **Choose the correct answer to each of the following questions and write the corresponding letter in the spaces provided.**

_____ 1. A patient diagnosed with ITP will have which of the following?

    a. High platelet count and hemoglobin

    b. High platelet count and low hemoglobin

    c. Low platelet count

    d. High hemoglobin

_____ 2. Nursing management of the patient diagnosed with ITP should include what?

    a. Monitoring of bleeding

    b. Heme testing of stools and emesis

    c. Padding bed rails when bed rest is necessary

    d. Instructions for the patient to avoid taking over-the-counter medications, particularly aspirin products

    e. All of the above

    f. a, b, and d

What IS Thrombotic Thrombocytopenia Purpura?

Thrombotic thrombocytopenia purpura (TTP) is a syndrome characterized by intravascular thrombosis with extreme thrombocytopenia, extreme elevation of lactate dehydrogenase (LDH), neurologic symptoms, fever, and renal dysfunction.

Pathogenesis

TTP is a syndrome with diverse etiologic aspects and many possible precipitating causes. More than 90% of cases of TTP develop without an apparent cause or underlying disease process. Medications implicated in development of TTP include oral contraceptives, antineoplastic drugs, immunosuppressive drugs, antibiotics, iodine, and ticlopidine hydrochloride.

Infectious agents have also been associated with TTP. Disseminated thrombotic occlusions of the microcirculation and end-organ injury facilitate the symptoms. Evidence suggests that platelet or endothelial cell injury may be the initial pathologic event. A number of factors in the patient's plasma, including immunoglobulins, can mediate cellular injury.

At-Risk Populations

Patients with lymphoma, acute myelogenous leukemia, some adenocarcinomas, and bone marrow transplant patients are at risk. Patients who have *Escherichia coli* infection, Coxsackie B virus, mycoplasma pneumonia, HIV, or a nonspecific upper respiratory infection can develop the disease.

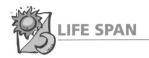

LIFE SPAN

Patients who are most at risk are young pregnant women because of hormonal effects that appear to trigger the onset of TTP.

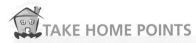

TAKE HOME POINTS

- TTP is a syndrome characterized by microvascular thrombosis with thrombocytopenia, neurologic symptoms, fever, and renal dysfunction.
- Plasma exchange or infusion is the single most important therapeutic intervention for TTP.

What You NEED TO KNOW

Clinical Manifestations

Profound thrombocytopenia, intravascular hemolysis with erythrocyte fragmentation (schistocytosis), extreme elevations in serum LDH, and mental status changes occur with TTP. The blood supply to the brain is compromised in approximately 50% to 75% of TTP episodes. Neurologic symptoms may be intermittent and fluctuate but are usually the most common presenting symptom. Headaches of unknown origin, confusion, stupor, coma, paresis, and cranial nerve palsies are common.

Hemorrhagic complications are the second most common presenting symptom. Approximately 40% of patients present with bleeding complications and 80% to 90% of patients develop bleeding complications. A patient may experience overwhelming hemorrhage as characterized by petechiae, purpura, and bruises (ecchymoses), and hemorrhage from the gastrointestinal or urinary tracts.

Fever is an uncommon presenting symptom but eventually occurs in 60% to 100% of patients and may be as high as 102° to 105° F. Usually, no source of infection is found. Fever may also be the result of tissue necrosis, release of the products of hemolysis, or the release of endogenous pyrogenic substances from leukocytes damaged by the antigen-antibody reaction.

Renal dysfunction is common. Approximately 80% to 90% of patients are seen with hematuria. Proteinuria is observed in 50% of patients.

Prognosis

Without treatment, 90% of patients will die of their disease, and 10% of patients die in spite of therapy.

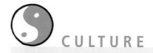

CULTURE

Patients who are unwilling to accept transfusion with blood products or plasma because of cultural issues or religious beliefs can die from uncontrolled hemorrhage.

What You DO

Treatment

Treatment includes steroid therapy, dipyridamole, daily aspirin, and fresh frozen plasma (FFP) at the rate of 1 unit per hour until plasmapheresis can be arranged. Plasma exchange or infusion is the single most important intervention for improved outcomes. Patients must receive plasma exchange daily or twice per day, depending on their LDH levels, platelet levels, and symptoms. Other treatments include immunosuppressive drugs such as cyclophosphamide, azathioprine, and intravenous gamma globulins.

Splenectomy has an 87% response rate when performed in conjunction with administration of steroids and dextran.

Nursing Responsibilities

Nurses should institute bleeding precautions, as previously discussed for ITP. Meticulous hand washing before contact with the patient and between patients to prevent spread of infection is important. Intravenous lines must be swabbed with alcohol before entry. Central venous catheters must have dressings changed per institutional guidelines and be monitored for infection. Renal function should improve with plasmapheresis. The nurse should do the following:

- Protect the patient from harm by padding side rails and having the patient use an electric razor.
- Test for blood in stool, urine, and in emesis.
- Instruct the patient to avoid all aspirin products.
- Administer stool softeners, when necessary, to help patients avoid straining with bowel movements.
- Advise the patient not to engage in sexual intercourse of any kind while platelet counts are below institutional guidelines.

- No intramuscular injections or suppositories should be used in patients with TTP.
- Monitoring for the symptoms of serious bleeding complications is imperative in patients with TTP.
- A patient with an unstable pulse and blood pressure and falling hemoglobin and hematocrit may be experiencing occult internal hemorrhage

Do You UNDERSTAND?

DIRECTIONS: Choose the correct answer to each of the following questions and write the corresponding letter in the spaces provided.

_____ 1. TTP is associated with which of the following?
   a. Renal dysfunction
   b. Neurologic manifestation
   c. Thrombocytopenia and bleeding
   d. All of the above

_____ 2. Plasmapheresis is which of the following?
   a. Blood transfusion
   b. Plasma exchange
   c. IVIG
   d. Platelet exchange

_____ 3. Patients diagnosed with TTP usually have which of the following?
   a. Elevated LDH, 5 to 10 times greater than the normal limit
   b. Elevated blood urea nitrogen (BUN) and creatinine levels
   c. High platelet counts
   d. Elevated bilirubin
   e. a, b, and d

What IS von Willebrand's Disease?

Characterized by a prolonged bleeding time, moderate deficiency of clotting factor VIII (antihemophilic factor), and impaired platelet function, von Willebrand's disease (VWD) is the most common hereditary bleeding disorder. This genetic disorder may be either autosomal dominant or recessively inherited. The von Willebrand factor gene is found on chromosome 12. The hallmark feature of this disorder is

Answers: 1. d; 2. b; 3. e.

impaired platelet plug formation and thrombus formation, both of which cause increased risk for bleeding problems.

Pathogenesis

A glycoprotein that is synthesized in the megakaryocytes and endothelial cells is the von Willebrand's factor (VWF). The primary hemostatic property is the binding of VWF to the subendothelium and platelet glycoproteins. This binding forms a bridge between platelets and subendothelium. VWF promotes platelet-to-platelet binding. VWF's additional hemostatic effect is its binding with factor VIII to form a stable complex and protect it from rapid removal from circulation.

At-Risk Populations

VWD occurs equally in men and women. Although determining the prevalence is difficult since mild cases often go undetected, the worldwide prevalence of the disorder is estimated to be as high as 1%.

What You NEED TO KNOW

Clinical Manifestations

VWD can be distinguished from classic hemophilia because (1) both sexes are equally affected because of the autosomal mode of inheritance, (2) the bleeding time is prolonged, and (3) mucosal bleeding manifestations are typical, although deep tissue hemorrhage is rare.

The clinical symptoms include bleeding episodes involving the skin and mucous membranes, nosebleed **(epistaxis),** easy bruising, gingival bleeding, and menorrhagia. Epistaxis is the most common manifestation and is frequently the first indication of the bleeding disorder. Severe forms of this disease can cause hemorrhage after laceration or surgery, menorrhagia, and gastrointestinal bleeding.

Also, the blood group O has been associated with low levels of VWF.

Typical laboratory test results include a prolonged bleeding time (more than 6 minutes), slightly prolonged partial thromboplastin time (more than 45 seconds), absent or reduced levels of factor VIII–related antigens, low factor VIII–activity level, defective in vitro platelet aggregation, and normal platelet count with normal clot retraction. The same patient will have varying levels of VWF at different episodes. No single laboratory test to define VWD is available.

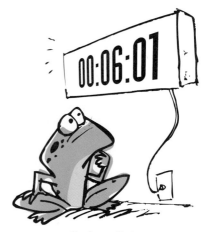

6-minute limit.

Prognosis

Patients with VWD usually respond well to treatment. Fatal hemorrhage is rare.

What You DO

Treatment

Therapy is aimed at shortening the bleeding time by local measures and replacement of factor VIII by infusion of cryoprecipitate or blood fractions that are rich in factor VIII. Before surgery, intravenous infusion of cryoprecipitate or FFP generally shortens bleeding time. Factor VIII should be 50% of normal before invasive procedures begin. Superficial bleeding can be managed with topical hemostatic drugs, pressure dressings, and sutures. Women treated with the exogenous administration of estrogen are reported to have increased levels of VWF and factor VIII. The administration of DDAVP (**desmopressin**) is widely used for mild cases of VWF to regain hemostasis in bleeding episodes. DDAVP may be given intravenously, subcutaneously, and intranasally.

Nursing Responsibilities

The nurse should do the following:

- Teach patients local measures to control bleeding during bleeding episodes: immediately elevate the injured part and apply cold compresses and gentle pressure to the site.
- Instruct patients on ways to prevent bleeding, unnecessary trauma, and complications.
- Warn patients to inform health care providers and other medical personnel that they have a bleeding disorder before undergoing invasive procedures.

Do You UNDERSTAND?

DIRECTIONS: Fill in the blanks to complete the following statements.

1. VWD is the most common _____
_____.

2. The treatment for VWD is _____
of _____.

3. von Willebrand's disease is _____ and
_____.

What IS Hemophilia?

Pathogenesis

Hemophilia is a group of inherited blood coagulation disorders. A deficiency exists of one of the factors necessary for blood coagulation, which leads to hemorrhage or excessive bleeding, even from minor injuries. The two most common forms are hemophilia A (classic) and hemophilia B **(Christmas disease).** Approximately 80% of persons with the disease have classic hemophilia, which is the result of a deficiency or absence of antihemophilic factor VIII. In hemophilia B, factor IX is missing, which causes a deficiency of plasma thromboplastin compound.

At-Risk Populations

Hemophilia is usually inherited in males as an X-linked recessive trait. If a female carrier of the hemophilia genetic trait has children, offspring of both sexes have a 50% chance of being a carrier of the trait. Hemophilia is estimated to occur in 25 per 100,000 males.

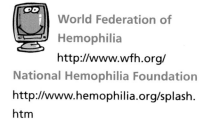

World Federation of Hemophilia
http://www.wfh.org/
National Hemophilia Foundation
http://www.hemophilia.org/splash.htm

Hemophilia is frequently first noted as a result of circumcision. During the toddler years, children may repeatedly develop blood within the joints **(hemarthroses),** which can lead to chronic synovitis or the destruction of bone and cartilage.

All patients with hemophilia develop excessive bleeding after dental extraction. Any surgery or trauma should be considered life-threatening.

What You NEED TO KNOW

Clinical Manifestations

The plasma levels of factors VIII or IX procoagulation activity affect the severity of the illness and bleeding manifestations. Patients with levels less than 1% have an increased chance of spontaneous and severe bleeding complications.

Hematuria, mucous membrane bleeding, and intracranial hemorrhage can also occur. Moderately affected patients (with factor VIII:C or factor IX:C levels below 5% or normal) bleed after trauma or surgery. These patients can also develop spontaneous bleeding. Hematuria and gastrointestinal bleeding are also common, especially when the patient has a local lesion (e.g., ulcer, polyp, inflammatory process).

Prognosis

With appropriate treatment and precautions, the life expectancy of the hemophiliac patient is comparable to that of the unaffected male population.

What You DO

Treatment

Treatment consists of replacement with factor VIII or factor IX concentrates. Factor VIII has a half-life of about 12 hours and must be given at least twice daily to maintain therapeutic benefit. This replacement may be administered to treat bleeding episodes or as a prophylactic in patients with severe disease. Replacement factors are also administered before surgery or dental extraction. DDAVP or antifibrinolytic drugs or both may be administered as a prophylactic measure. Social and psychologic support is especially important. Patients and their significant others should be encouraged to join a support group of specialized health care providers.

Nursing Responsibilities

The patient who is diagnosed with hemophilia can be faced with exposure to viral infection and HIV from replacement factors derived from human blood. The use of recombinant factors VIII and IX have made exposure less of an issue in recent times. This chronic disease places a stress on the family socially, psychologically, and financially. Guilt on the part of the mother, who may have not known she was a carrier, may also be present. The nurse should do the following:

- Counsel parents about the importance of avoiding injury in children with hemophilia.
- Encourage regular check-ups with the dentist.
- Teach parents of young children with hemophilia and adult patients about the administration of factors VIII and IX concentrates. The goal of therapy is to minimize the development of chronic synovitis or progressive arthropathy.
- Treatment of acute hemarthrosis must begin immediately, with intensive therapy and pain control, physical therapy, wedging casts, night splints, or traction in conjunction with regular infusions of factor concentrates. Prevention of repeated episodes of hemarthroses is important in order to avoid joint fibrosis, contractures, and permanent disability. Parents of children with hemophilia should be encouraged to seek genetic counseling.

 Patients and their families need to be educated early about complications and the need for immediate therapy.

TAKE HOME POINTS

- Therapy should begin promptly for the patient who is diagnosed with hemophilia to prevent further complications. If the bleeding cannot be controlled immediately, the patient should be advised as to the ways to contact their health care provider for possible plasmapheresis and further treatment.
- The patient and family should receive counseling and guidance at diagnosis. Many social and psychologic problems affect the patient and significant others.
- A high incidence of drug addictions is present with hemophiliac patients because of the frequent need for pain medication.

Do You UNDERSTAND?

DIRECTIONS: **Unscramble the italicized words to complete the statements.**

1. Hemophilia is inherited as an X-linked defect from the _____ _____. *(thremo)*

2. Hemophiliac patients develop excessive bleeding after _____ _____. *(nadtle tronixctea)*

Answers: 1. mother; 2. dental extraction.

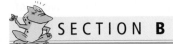

SECTION **B**

DISORDERS OF ERYTHROPOIESIS AND ERYTHROCYTE FUNCTION

This section discusses diseases and disorders affecting red blood cells (erythrocytes). The erythrocyte is a component of blood that the body uses to transport oxygen to the tissues. Under the microscope, these cells appear flat and concave. The red blood cell is sturdy and flexible, which allows it to travel through small capillaries and vessels without being trapped or destroyed. Hemoglobin is an important component of the red cell because of its ability to bind with oxygen and carbon dioxide. The hemoglobin contained in red blood cells releases oxygen to the tissues and organs through gas exchange in the capillaries.

The average life span of the red blood cell is approximately 4 months, after which time it is removed from the circulation by macrophages in the spleen and liver. Bone marrow must rapidly create new cells. The body must have adequate amounts of iron to create hemoglobin. Vitamin B_{12} and folic acid are required for the synthesis of the erythrocyte precursors needed for the formation of properly functioning cells.

What IS Anemia?

Anemia is a decrease in hemoglobin concentration, circulating red blood cells (RBCs), or hematocrit (packed RBC volume). Anemias are classified according to their cause and the appearance of the RBCs when viewed under a microscope. The size of the RBCs may be larger (macrocytic) or smaller (microcytic) than is normal, and the hemoglobin concentration will be pale (hypochromic) or more highly colored (hyperchromic) than is usual.

Pathogenesis

Three possible causes for anemia include blood loss, destruction or hemolysis of RBCs because of disease or drugs, and ineffective production of RBCs as a result of disease or nutritional deficits.

At-Risk Populations

Anemia can occur in nearly any age group and be the consequence of a wide variety of physical disorders. Any person with poor nutrition can develop anemia.

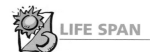

LIFE SPAN

Individuals who are particularly at risk include children, pregnant women, and older adults.

What You NEED TO KNOW

Clinical Manifestations

Because RBCs are responsible for carrying oxygen throughout the body, the symptoms of anemia are usually reflective of the degree of oxygen deficiency **(hypoxemia).** Some patients are asymptomatic if their anemia developed gradually. Blood tests during a routine examination can first detect the problem. Initially, some general fatigue and weakness may be present. Other symptoms include breathlessness, angina, leg pain, and palpitations. As hypoxemia progresses, patients experience headaches, tinnitus, roaring in the ears, light-headedness, and near syncope.

As the body tries to compensate for the decrease in available oxygen, patients may progress from dyspnea on exertion (DOE) to shortness of breath at rest with accompanying tachycardia or cardiac arrhythmia. Patients with cardiovascular disease are particularly at risk for anemia-related problems, including congestive heart failure and angina. Other symptoms are associated with specific causes of the anemia.

TAKE HOME POINTS

Caucasian patients with anemia may be pale or have pallor. In the dark-skinned individual, pallor may be noted in the conjunctiva, oral mucosa, the palms of the hands, and the plantar surfaces of the feet.

Prognosis

Most patients recover completely from anemia when the underlying cause is treated.

What You DO

Treatment

Treatment of anemia includes not only correcting the imbalance, but also finding and treating the underlying cause or causes of the condition. Supplementation with oral or parenteral iron, folic acid, and vitamin B_{12} may be indicated. Transfusions with packed red blood cells are indicated in severe anemias associated with acute blood loss or in patients with

Lab Tests On-Line / Information About Anemias

http://www.labtestsonline.org/ understanding/conditions/anemia. html

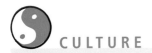

TAKE HOME POINTS

Oxygen therapy helps to decrease dyspnea and treat compensatory tachycardia.

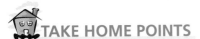

CULTURE

Jehovah's Witnesses may decline treatment with blood products because of their religious beliefs.

coexisting cardiopulmonary disease. Whole blood may be required for patients who are anemic and hypovolemic.

Nursing Responsibilities

Diagnostic evaluation of anemia is targeted toward identifying the source of the problem. The nurse should do the following:

- Help patients understand the cause of and treatment for their anemia.
- Counsel the patient to conserve energy during treatment. Nurses can help patients explore ways to avoid fatigue and overexertion.
- Conduct laboratory studies that include a complete blood count with hemoglobin, hematocrit, RBC count, white blood cell (WBC) count, indices, and differential. Additional blood tests may include a reticulocyte count, folate level, vitamin B_{12} level, serum iron level, total iron binding capacity (TIBC), and transferrin saturation. When hemolysis is suspected, the haptoglobin and direct and indirect Coombs' tests may be ordered.
- In some patients, diagnostic examinations of the upper and lower gastrointestinal tract for occult blood loss may be indicated.
- Assist with bone marrow biopsies when necessary to rule out potential problems with hematopoiesis.
- Administer transfusions, when ordered.
- Teach patients about the risks associated with transfusions.
- Monitor for transfusion reactions.

Do You UNDERSTAND?

DIRECTIONS: **Unscramble the italicized letters to form a term key to understanding anemia.**

1. Three _____: *(ussace)*
2. _____ loss *(odlob)*
3. _____ of RBCs *(trudetonics)*
4. Ineffective _____ of RBCs *(dropnutcoi)*

Answers: **1. causes; 2. blood; 3. destruction; 4. production.**

What IS Vitamin B$_{12}$ Deficiency Anemia?

Vitamin B$_{12}$ deficiency anemia (**pernicious anemia**) is a megaloblastic anemia in which the RBCs appear larger than normal on examination under the microscope. This condition is reflected in laboratory studies indicating an elevated mean corpuscular volume (MCV), which estimates the size of RBCs. The RBCs are large and immature and thus unable to function normally, which results in premature removal of the cells from circulation. Hypersegmented neutrophils can be noted on the blood smear during microscopic examination. The diagnosis is confirmed with a serum B$_{12}$ level and a Schilling test. The Schilling test involves the administration of radiolabeled cyanocobalamin (vitamin B$_{12}$) and a 24-hour urine collection to determine malabsorption of B$_{12}$.

Pathogenesis

Vitamin B$_{12}$ is needed for the formation of DNA, which is essential for the growth of mature, properly functioning RBCs. Vitamin B$_{12}$ deficiency anemia is nearly always the result of an inadequate absorption of this nutrient in the ileum from a lack of intrinsic factor. Intrinsic factor is normally secreted by the gastric mucosa to promote the absorption of vitamin B$_{12}$.

At-Risk Populations

Many patients at risk for vitamin B$_{12}$ deficiency anemia are those who have undergone gastrectomy, ileal resection, or those with inflammatory bowel syndromes. Individuals with poor dietary habits or alcoholism are also at risk for this disorder. All foods of animal origin contain vitamin B$_{12}$. Although uncommon, dietary deficiency of this vitamin may occur in strict vegetarians who avoid all meat, fish, and dairy products.

Patients with this disorder are usually older, and an autoimmune component to this anemia may be present.

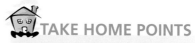

TAKE HOME POINTS

- Individuals at risk include older adults and those who have undergone gastrectomy or ileal resection, or those with an inflammatory bowel disease, poor dietary habits, or alcoholism.
- Treatment involves daily vitamin B$_{12}$ injections.

What You NEED TO KNOW

Clinical Manifestations

Vitamin B_{12} deficiency anemia usually develops slowly, over years, primarily because the body can have a 3-year store of vitamin B_{12}. The body compensates for the gradual loss of RBCs, and the symptoms of anemia as listed may not become apparent until late in the development of the anemia. Because vitamin B_{12} is also essential for myelin integrity in the nervous system, symptoms can include neurologic manifestations. Gradually worsening soreness and burning of the tongue can occur. Patients may complain of symmetric numbness or tingling in the extremities, and ataxia or a loss of vibratory sense may be noted. Affected individuals may exhibit changes in mental status, memory loss, dementia, and depression. Indigestion, constipation, or diarrhea can also be present.

Prognosis

Without treatment, pernicious anemia will result in irreversible neurologic damage and cause life-threatening complications, particularly for the weak or vulnerable patient who is already compromised from preexisting conditions or age.

What You DO

Treatment

Treatment can begin with daily vitamin B_{12} injections while the patient is hospitalized, after which the injections can then become monthly. People with this disorder will require lifelong therapy.

Nursing Responsibilities

The nurse should do the following:
- Help patients understand that treatment must continue for their life span, except in cases in which the underlying cause of the condition is reversible.
- Provide assistance with ambulation, and take appropriate safety precautions in patients with neurologic deficits from vitamin B_{12} deficiency, when needed.

- Teach the patient or caregiver the proper way to administer B_{12} injections at home.
- Neurologic deficits do not always resolve with treatment. Patients may need physical or occupational therapy directed toward helping them maintain independent activities of daily living.

Do You UNDERSTAND?

DIRECTIONS: **Fill in the numbers to complete each statement.**
1. The body can store vitamin B _____ for _____ years.
2. The Schilling test involves collecting urine for _____ hours.

What IS Folate Deficiency Anemia?

Folic acid is required for the synthesis of DNA and the development of red cells in the bone marrow. A deficiency of folic acid will cause a megaloblastic anemia with large RBCs and an elevated MCV. In addition, decreased folate levels in the serum are present. In contrast to vitamin B_{12} deficiency, folic acid deficiency does not produce neurologic symptoms.

Pathogenesis

Chronic alcohol abuse is the classic cause of folate deficiency anemia. People who abuse alcohol frequently have an inadequate diet and tend to have decreased absorption of nutrients in the gut. This deficiency can also be the result of malnutrition or an increased need for folate as in pregnancy, hemolysis, or malabsorption syndromes in the bowel. Common drugs that interfere with folate absorption are phenytoin, methotrexate, trimethoprim, and triamterene.

At-Risk Populations

Individuals with an inadequate diet as a result of either environmental factors or biologic factors are at risk for folate deficiency anemia. Groups that tend to have an inadequate diet are those from low socioeconomic

Answers: 1. 12, 3; 2. 24.

classes, persons who abuse drugs or alcohol, those with nutritional disorders (e.g., bulimia, anorexia), the elderly, and pregnant women.

During pregnancy, low folate levels in the mother can lead to an increased risk of neural tube defects in the newborn. For this reason, pregnant women or those who are attempting to conceive should have daily supplements of oral folic acid.

What You NEED TO KNOW

Clinical Manifestations

Because folate stores in the body only last for 3 months, symptoms can be more pronounced than those in vitamin B_{12} deficiency anemia. Signs and symptoms include weakness, fatigue, pallor, dyspnea, and tachycardia. Irregular, brown, patchy pigmentation of the skin may be present, particularly in the folds of the skin and nail beds. Some patients may have a sore, inflamed tongue. No neurologic symptoms occur.

Prognosis

Most patients recover completely after the nutritional deficiency is corrected.

What You DO

Treatment

Treatment consists of oral folate therapy until hemoglobin or hematocrit levels are adequate. Nurses should provide nutritional counseling for patients to insure adequate folate intake in the future. Foods high in folate include liver, leafy green vegetables, broccoli, legumes, and brewer's yeast. Cooking destroys 60% to 90% of the folic acid found in food. Patients who are seriously depleted may require oral supplementation with 5 mg daily for approximately 4 months to replace body stores. Any underlying cause of the deficiency such as malabsorption syndromes should also be treated, or the problem will recur. Refer patients for counseling or therapy when alcoholism is suspected or known.

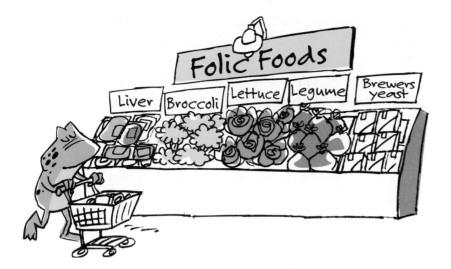

Nursing Responsibilities

The nurse should do the following:

- Educate the patient about folate therapy.
- Encourage regular use of folic acid, as ordered.
- Counsel the patient on prevention of folate deficiency anemia in the future.
- When alcoholism, drug abuse, or a nutritional disorder is suspected, refer the patient to the appropriate specialist.

TAKE HOME POINTS

- Folate reserves in the body last only 3 months.
- Pregnant women should take folic acid supplements to prevent neural tube defects in the fetus.

Do You UNDERSTAND?

DIRECTIONS: **Indicate which statements are *true* (T) and which are *false* (F). If false, correct the statement in the margin space to make it true.**

_____ 1. Chocolate is high in folate.

_____ 2. Women should avoid taking folic acid supplements when they are trying to conceive.

_____ 3. Alcoholics tend to have increased absorption of nutrients in the gut.

Answers: 1. F. Liver, green vegetables, broccoli, legumes, and brewer's yeast are high in folate acid; 2. F. Pregnant women should take folic acid supplements to prevent neural tube defects; 3. F. Alcoholics have a decreased absorption of nutrients in the gut.

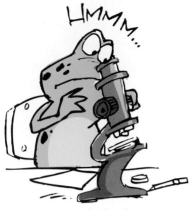

These look pale!

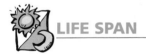

Heavy menstruation is a common cause of iron deficiency anemia in women.

What IS Iron Deficiency Anemia?

Iron deficiency anemia is a microcytic anemia. The RBCs are smaller than are normal RBCs (microcytic) on examination under a microscope, and the MCV is decreased. The RBCs are also deficient in hemoglobin (hypochromic), and the RBCs appear pale under the microscope. A low serum iron and an elevated TIBC confirm the diagnosis. Iron deficiency anemia is the most common type of anemia and may be a result of an inadequate intake of iron, excessive blood loss, or poor absorption of iron.

Pathogenesis

Inadequate amounts of iron inhibit the synthesis of hemoglobin. Decreased levels of hemoglobin in the blood cause a decrease in the amount of oxygen that can be transported to the tissues.

At-Risk Populations

Iron deficiency anemia is also associated with blood loss from the gastrointestinal tract. Poor iron intake among young children or vegetarians can lead to anemia. The excessive use of antacids or gastrectomy can also lead to an inadequate absorption of iron. Additionally, iron deficiency anemia can be observed in patients with chronic renal failure who require hemodialysis.

What You NEED TO KNOW

Clinical Manifestations

Pica is a classic symptom of iron deficiency anemia in which patients have a craving for nonfood substances such as ice, clay, or starch. Sore tongue and cracked lips (cheilitis) are common. The tongue may appear bright red and shiny as a result of the loss of papillae. The nails can become soft and curl, a phenomenon known as "spoon" nails. The hair may become brittle in texture. The body is initially able to compensate for the loss of iron, but weakness, fatigue, pallor, dyspnea, tachycardia, and other symptoms of anemia occur with worsening disease. Extensive medical evaluation with complete gastrointestinal examinations may be indicated to locate bleeding sites, particularly in older patients. Treatment with oral iron preparations is usually adequate after the cause of the iron deficiency anemia is diagnosed.

Prognosis

The prognosis for a full recovery is excellent if the underlying source of iron or blood loss is corrected and the patient receives iron supplementation.

What You DO

Treatment

Medical and nursing care is directed toward correcting the underlying source of iron or blood loss whenever possible and replenishing iron stores in the body. Ferrous sulfate is commonly given by mouth in doses of 300 mg 1 to 3 times daily until blood tests reveal normal levels of iron and hemoglobin.

Nursing Responsibilities

The nurse should do the following:
- Encourage patients to take iron preparations as instructed, and help them manage side effects, such as constipation or nausea.
- Caution patients to avoid using antacids or H2-receptor blockers with iron.
- Counsel patients to decrease their activities and conserve energy until the anemia has improved. Offer assistance with daily activities as needed, and help patients obtain assistance at home after discharge, when necessary.
- Dietary counseling is recommended. Foods high in iron include liver, fortified cereals and grains, dried apricots, raisins, meats, poultry, eggs, fish, and green leafy vegetables.

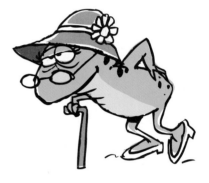

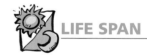
LIFE SPAN

Older patients and those with comorbid conditions should be monitored for cardiopulmonary complications. Children, pregnant women, and patients with cardiac disease are most at risk to develop serious complications from anemia.

What IS Sickle Cell Anemia?

Sickle cell disease (SCD) is a group of inherited blood disorders characterized by abnormal hemoglobin (HbS) that causes the red blood cells to become distorted and sickled when exposed to conditions of low oxygenation.

Pathogenesis

SCD is caused by an autosomal recessive mutation in the hemoglobin beta gene found on chromosome 11. In order to develop this disease, a person must inherit one copy of the gene from each parent. If a person has only one copy of the abnormal gene, he or she is said to have the sickle cell trait. In most cases, people who carry only the trait are asymptomatic.

The sickling process may be precipitated by conditions of low oxygenation or stress. Circumstances that cause oxygenation to decrease include vigorous physical exercise, flying in poorly pressurized airplanes, respiratory infections, and anesthesia. Other precipitating events include cold water, cold temperatures, and hypoxia. In many cases, no causative event can be identified.

A person with SCD has red cells that are more rigid and with irregular shapes, which causes them to become trapped in small vessels and eventually cause blockages of normal blood flow. The abnormal red cells have a shorter life span than healthy red cells and are often broken up and destroyed, which causes the patient to be anemic. Blockages of blood flow cause pain because of tissue ischemia and eventually will cause permanent organ damage. These painful episodes are called sickle cell crises.

At-Risk Populations

On a global basis, SCD is the most common form of anemia. It is most commonly found in people of African, Mediterranean, Middle Eastern, and Indian origin. The trait is thought to convey a survival advantage in areas where malaria is endemic, because red blood cells that are infected by the parasite sickle and then die. In the United States, SCD is most commonly found in people of African descent.

What You NEED TO KNOW

Clinical Manifestations

Children born with the disease usually do not have symptoms until after 6 months of age because they are protected by residual fetal hemoglobin in their circulation. Children and adolescents may have delays in growth and sexual maturity and are often underweight. Some individuals may be completely asymptomatic unless they are experiencing a vasoocclusive crisis. When symptoms occur they include pallor, fatigue, and decreased exercise tolerance. If hemolysis is present the patient may be jaundiced. Tissue hypoxia caused by vessel occlusion causes severe pain in the long bones, the chest, the back, the abdomen, and the joints.

Patients experiencing a sequestration crisis may have massively enlarged spleens. This is due to a sudden trapping of red blood cell components by the visceral organs, especially the spleen and liver. Repeated sequestration crises affecting the spleen may cause shrinking and atrophy of the spleen, with the eventual development of impaired immunity.

The sickling process is thought to cause bone marrow infarction in some patients, with subsequent release of fat emboli into the blood stream. The fat emboli cause acute chest syndrome, characterized by fever, cough, increased respiratory rate, and chest pain.

Repeated infarcts of bone tissue may cause aseptic necrosis, especially on the heads of weight-bearing bones such as the femurs, and may cause osteomyelitis and osteoporosis. Poor circulation to soft tissue predisposes patients to the development of leg and foot ulcers that are often difficult to heal. Infarctions in the eye can cause vision loss. Each sickle cell crisis causes more damage to vital organs.

Prognosis

With appropriate care, the average life expectancy is 42 to 48 years of age. Sadly, because this disease is so disabling, many people who have it are unable to attend school or maintain employment, which makes it difficult for them to obtain adequate health care.

> !
> - Acute chest syndrome is a medical emergency that requires immediate treatment in order to save the patient from acute respiratory distress and possible death.
> - The microvascular infarctions characteristic of this disease may damage every organ system. Patients have increased risk for stroke and cardiac damage including heart failure, pulmonary hypertension, and cor pulmonale.

What You DO

Treatment

Currently there is no cure for this disease, although research trials involving bone marrow transplant have shown promising results. Some patients obtain better control of their disease with the administration of hydroxyurea, an antineoplastic drug shown to decrease sickling in many individuals.

Medical therapy emphasizes control and prevention of complications associated with this disease. Acute pain crises are usually treated in the in-patient setting with intravenous opioids such as morphine sulfate and hydromorphone. Chronic persistent pain may be treated with a variety of drugs, including sustained release doses of oral morphine, nonsteroidal antiinflammatory drugs (NSAIDs), and tricyclic antidepressants. Nonpharmacologic measures used to control pain include physical therapy, transcutaneous electrical nerve stimulation (TENS), and hypnosis.

Blood transfusions may be given routinely to decrease the levels of HbS within the circulation and improve the oxygen-carrying capacity of the blood in situations such as stroke or general anesthesia. Acute chest syndrome is treated with antibiotics, analgesics, oxygen, and transfusions when indicated.

All possible measures should be taken to prevent infection in the patient with sickle cell disease. Most individuals are started on routine penicillin prophylaxis during infancy. Patients should receive the pneumonia vaccine at age 2 and have a booster at age 5. Any infection must be treated promptly with broad-spectrum antibiotics.

Nursing Responsibilities

When caring for patients with sickle cell disease, the nurse must be prepared to address the physical and psychologic effects of a chronic and painful illness. Patients and their family members should be taught how to do the following:

- Maintain adequate hydration to decrease blood viscosity and decrease sickling.
- Avoid exposure to temperature extremes, particularly cold environments. Cold environments can cause vascular constriction and increase the risk for sickling.

- Avoid strenuous activities that will increase physiologic oxygen demands.
- Abstain from tobacco. Tobacco will cause vasoconstriction and worsen sickling.
- Avoid exposure to potentially contagious illnesses, because infection may trigger a sickle cell crisis.
- Cope with mental and emotional stress.

Most patients with sickle cell disease are hospitalized repeatedly for acute pain crises. When caring for these individuals, the nurse should realize that patients who are dealing with chronic pain may not exhibit any of the behaviors that denote pain such as flinching, grimacing, or moaning. When gathering data to establish a plan of care, ask the patient to rate his or her pain using a numerical or graphical scale, and then ask what level of pain control would be satisfactory for that person. (Because many sickle cell patients have suffered organ and musculoskeletal damage, they may never be completely free of pain.) Ask patients what they have done to relieve pain crises in the past. Because these patients often have dealt with chronic pain for years, they may have developed a tolerance for opioids and require larger than normal doses in order to obtain adequate pain relief.

As a part of daily care, routinely assess the patient for evidence of complications associated with SCD. Depending upon risk factors and the level of HbS present in the circulation, neurologic exams may need to be done every 8 hours, especially if the patient has had a prior stroke.

Listen carefully to the patient's heart and lungs. Changes in breath sounds, breathlessness, and decreased exercise tolerance may be indicative of cardiac impairment. Decreased capillary oxygen levels, peripheral cyanosis, cough, and breathlessness are indicators of possible acute chest syndrome. Inspect the skin for evidence of nonhealing wounds on a routine basis. Report all abnormalities to the health care provider so that appropriate treatment may be initiated.

Because of the enormous psychologic toll of this disease, remember to address the patient's emotional concerns. Reassure the patient suffering a pain crisis that his or her pain will be addressed. Give the patient time to seek clarification regarding his or her questions and concerns. Adolescents with SCD may benefit from attending a support groups composed of their peers, especially if it offers exposure to others who are coping successfully with their illness.

Do You UNDERSTAND?

DIRECTIONS: Circle the correct answer.

1. Sickle cell disease is a form of anemia that is caused by
   a. An autosomal dominant gene.
   b. An autosomal recessive gene.
   c. An X-lined recessive gene.
   d. A Y-linked dominant gene.
2. Patients with SCD almost never have symptoms until
   a. After 6 months of age.
   b. After 2 years of age.
   c. After 5 years of age.
   d. After adulthood.
3. Patients with SCD should be encouraged to
   a. Restrict sodium.
   b. Restrict fluid intake.
   c. Maintain adequate hydration.
   d. Engage in vigorous exercise.
4. A patient with SCD complains of breathlessness, chest pain, and a cough. The nurse should first
   a. Do a thorough physical assessment.
   b. Initiate oxygen.
   c. Obtain an order for analgesics and a cough suppressant.
   d. Evaluate the patient's hydration status.

What IS a Myeloproliferative Disorder?

Myeloproliferative disorders are malignancies of the hemopoietic stem cells or immature blood cells. The hemopoietic stem cells, from which all blood cells originate, are normally found in the bone marrow. Various influences on stem cells normally cause them to differentiate or grow into RBCs, WBCs, or platelets.

Answers: **1.** b; **2.** a; **3.** c; **4.** a.

Pathogenesis

Myeloproliferative disorders result from a lack of these cells (**aplasia**), when the growth of these cells is exaggerated, or from ineffective proliferation (i.e., the cells are present in large numbers but fail to function properly). Because the most basic cell of the blood system is affected, these disorders can frequently evolve from one disorder to another, and symptoms can overlap.

The cause of myeloproliferative disease in most patients is never identified. Some association with the development of these diseases and previous exposure to radiation or chemotherapeutic treatment may be present.

At-Risk Populations

Although these diseases can occur in middle-aged individuals, older patients are most at risk for developing myeloproliferative diseases.

What You NEED TO KNOW

Clinical Manifestations

Clinical symptoms of these diseases are related to the cell line (RBC, WBC, or platelets) that is most affected. Diseases involving the RBCs will have symptoms reflective of low or high oxygen levels in the blood. These diseases frequently mimic megaloblastic anemias and occur mainly in the older population. When the WBCs are affected by disease, the symptoms reflect altered immunity, and persistent or unusual infections may occur. Platelets are involved in the clotting of blood, and a lack of platelets can result in bleeding. Excess platelets can lead to unusual and dysfunctional clotting, which will be reflected in the symptoms. An excess number of any type of cell can result in hyperviscosity or thick, sludgelike blood with associated symptoms. Although one cell line tends to be predominantly affected by a myeloproliferative disorder, the other cell lines are also affected, and a combination of symptoms will likely be present. Examples of myeloproliferative disorders include myelofibrosis and polycythemia vera.

Prognosis

Without treatment, patients with myelofibrosis will ultimately die of bone marrow failure. In some cases, the disease may transform into a type of leukemia that is often refractory to treatment. Currently, a bone marrow transplant is the only known cure for patients with this disorder, with disease-free intervals of up to 15 years having been recorded.

Patients with polycythemia vera, which is characterized by an abnormal excessive production of blood cells, may benefit from periodic therapeutic phlebotomies and the administration of myelosuppressive drugs such as hydroxyurea and busulfan.

What You DO

Treatment

Supportive care and prevention of infections is the mainstay of therapy for this population. Patients with myelofibrosis will require frequent transfusions of RBCs and platelets, and will need to be monitored closely for signs of infection.

Nursing Responsibilities

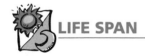
LIFE SPAN

Older patients with cardiopulmonary or renal disease will require careful evaluation during repeated transfusions for symptoms of fluid overload and other complications.

The nurse should do the following:
- Instruct patients carefully on methods of preventing infection and bleeding, as well as signs and symptoms that indicate the need for medical intervention.
- Help patients learn to manage adverse effects and complications of their disease and treatment regimen.
- Administer RBCs and platelets, when ordered.

Do You UNDERSTAND?

DIRECTIONS: **Circle all potential symptoms that may be observed in the patient with a myeloproliferative disorder.**

Bruises   Headache

Temperature elevations   Chest pain

Chills   Fatigue

Pallor   Dyspnea

References

Barker LR, Burton JR, Zieve PD: *Principles of ambulatory medicine*, ed 5, Baltimore, 1999, Williams & Wilkins.

Hillman RS, Ault KL: *Hematology in clinical practice*, New York, 1998, McGraw-Hill.

Kotter ML and Osguthorpe, SG: Alterations in oxygen transport. In Copstead, LC and Banasik, JL *Pathophysiology*, St Louis, 2005, Elsevier Saunders.

Lungstrom N, Emerson R: Alterations in hemostasis and blood coagulation. In Copstead LC and Banasik JL *Pathophysiology*, St Louis, 2005, Elsevier Saunders.

Merahn S: *PDxMD Hematology and Oncology*, Philadelphia, 2003, Elsevier Science.

Moake JL: Thrombotic thrombocytopenia purpura today, *Hosp Pract* 34(7):53, 1999.

Muszkat M et al: Ticlopidine-inducted thrombotic thrombocytopenia purpura, *Pharmacotherapy* 18(6):1352, 1998.

Petersen KL: Diagnosing polycythemia vera, *J Am Acad Nurs Pract* 11(11):485, 1999.

Tezcan H et al: Bone marrow, *Transplant* 21(1):105, 1998.

NCLEX® Review

Section A

1. ITP is more common in what population?
   1 Children
   2 Young adults
   3 Pregnant women
   4 Older adults

2. Which of the following factors may adversely affect the clotting process?
   1 Liver disease
   2 Renal failure
   3 H2-receptor blockers
   4 Antibiotic therapy

3. Which of the following drugs should patients with bleeding disorders avoid?
   1 Antibiotics
   2 Antacids
   3 Nonsteroidal antiinflammatory drugs
   4 Antifungal medications

4. Which organ system can be adversely affected by thrombotic thrombocytopenia purpura?
   1 Pulmonary
   2 Cardiac
   3 Renal
   4 Liver

Section B

5. Which of the following vitamins are required for synthesis of erythrocyte precursors?
   1 B_{12}
   2 Vitamin A
   3 Vitamin D
   4 Folic acid and vitamin C

6. Pallor in the dark-skinned individual can be detected
   1 On the palms of the hands.
   2 On the chest.
   3 In the whites of the eyes.
   4 On the lips.

7. Vitamin B_{12} deficiency usually results from a lack of
   1 Calcium.
   2 Iron.
   3 Intrinsic factor.
   4 Sunlight.

8. Folate deficiency anemia is frequently observed in what group?
   1 Older adults
   2 Alcoholics
   3 Menstruating women
   4 Infants

9. Sickle cell disease is a(n) _____ disease.
   1 autosomal dominant
   2 autosomal recessive
   3 X-linked
   4 Y-linked

10. Pain crises associated with sickle cell disease are due to
    1 Decreased coagulation.
    2 Tissue ischemia.
    3 Inadequate inflammatory response.
    4 Decreased production of cytokines.

NCLEX® Review Answers

Section A

1. **1** Idiopathic thrombocytopenia purpura is most commonly observed in children, although it may occur in any age group. In contrast, thrombotic thrombocytopenia purpura is occasionally present in pregnant women.

2. **1** Liver disease can adversely affect the clotting process, because it is ordinarily responsible for synthesis of clotting factors. Renal failure can cause anemia, but does not adversely affect platelet count or clotting components. Antibiotic therapy does not usually adversely affect clotting function.

3. **3** Nonsteroidal antiinflammatory drugs can decrease platelet aggregation; therefore they should be avoided by people with clotting disorders. Some antacids include copious amounts of aspirin, and these should be avoided as well. Normally, however, antacids, antibiotics, and antifungal medications are safe for people with clotting disorders.

4. **3** Renal failure can be present in patients with thrombotic thrombocytopenia purpura. Problems with the liver, the pulmonary system, and the cardiac system are not directly caused by thrombotic thrombocytopenia purpura.

Section B

5. **4** Folic acid and vitamin C are necessary for synthesis of erythrocyte precursors. B_{12} is needed for DNA synthesis. Vitamin A is needed for visual acuity. Vitamin D is needed for creation of strong bones and teeth.

6. **1** Pallor may be detected on the palms of the hands of dark-skinned individuals. The chest, the lips, and whites of the eyes will not show pallor in a dark-skinned person.

7. **3** B_{12} deficiency results from a lack of intrinsic factor. Osteoporosis is caused by a calcium deficiency. A lack of iron causes iron deficiency anemia. Rickets results from a lack of exposure to sunlight.

8. **2** Folate deficiency is most frequently observed with alcoholics who do not maintain an adequate diet. Older adults are at most risk for vitamin B_{12} anemia. Menstruating women most frequently have iron deficiency anemia. Infants are not at risk for anemia. Breast-fed infants absorb folate from their mothers. For infants who are bottle-fed, most formulas are fortified with folate.

9. **2** Patients with sickle cell disease must inherit one copy of the gene from each of their parents. An autosomal dominant genetic disorder requires only one copy of a gene from one parent. People who have a single copy of the gene for sickle cell disease are said to have sickle cell trait, but generally don't have symptoms of the disease. X- and Y-linked genetic disorders are inherited via the sex chromosomes, which is not the case with sickle cell disease.

10. **2** Sickle cell pain crises are the result of inadequate oxygen delivery to the tissue by defective, sickled red blood cells. This causes tissue ischemia.

Notes

Alterations in Blood Flow and Blood Pressure

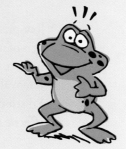

What You WILL LEARN

After reading this chapter, you will know how to do the following:

- ✔ Describe the impact of elevated serum lipid levels on the vascular system.
- ✔ Correlate atherosclerosis with the development of coronary artery and cerebrovascular disease.
- ✔ Recognize the signs and symptoms of peripheral vascular disease.
- ✔ Identify nursing interventions for a patient with vascular disease.
- ✔ Discuss the implications of hypertension on health and wellness.
- ✔ Develop a plan of care for a patient with hypertension.

This chapter provides information on the body's vascular system, including related diseases and disorders that can adversely affect the vital function of the heart and extremities. Without an effectively functioning vascular system, cardiac function can be compromised, and a potential exists for loss of limb and life. An understanding of both the normal and the abnormal hemodynamic and metabolic processes can help the nurse develop strategies for patients at risk and optimize their ability to recover from disorders affecting blood pressure and blood flow.

The vascular system is composed of three components: arterial, venous, and lymphatic conduits. Arteries carry oxygenated blood to organs under high pressure. Arterial disorders cause impaired delivery of nutrients and oxygen. Veins return unoxygenated blood to the heart within a low-pressure system, whereas lymphatic channels carry the waste products of metabolism back to the vascular system. Venous disorders adversely impact the outflow of capillary blood, return of blood to the heart, and removal of tissue waste products. Although each of these components has a distinct purpose, the normal function of other components can adversely affect each component.

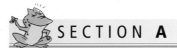

SECTION **A**

DISORDERS OF ARTERIAL CIRCULATION

Arterial disorders generally result from a mechanical obstruction or increased resistance to blood flow. Although the causes are varied, atherosclerotic occlusive disease is the most common cause of arterial obstruction. A variety of nonatherosclerotic arterial disorders exists; however, these are less common. An understanding of some of these diseases and disorders is essential for their evaluation and the care of the adult patient.

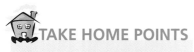

What ARE Hyperlipidemia and Hypercholesterolemia?

The terms **hyperlipidemia** and **hypercholesterolemia** refer to abnormally elevated blood levels of lipids and cholesterol.

Pathogenesis

Cholesterol is derived from two sources. The liver makes some cholesterol, and the rest is derived from eating animal products. Cholesterol and other fats cannot dissolve in the blood, thus they have to be transported by special carriers. These carriers are called lipoproteins— low-density lipoprotein cholesterol (LDL-C), or "bad" cholesterol. When deposited along the vessel walls, these fats can cause clogging. High-density lipoprotein cholesterol (HDL-C), or "good" cholesterol carries fats away from arteries. HDL-C also has antioxidant and profibrinolytic

TAKE HOME POINTS

HDL-C plays an important role in reverse–cholesterol transport, carrying LDL-C to the liver, where it is biodegraded and excreted.

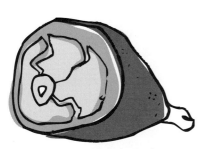

A source of cholesterol.

properties, in addition to transporting key apolipoproteins, which mediate triglyceride metabolism.

Abnormalities in lipid metabolism are manifested as a variety of clinical features. The most common clinical consequences of disorders of lipid metabolism include premature atherosclerosis, acute pancreatitis, and xanthoma formation (i.e., lipid deposits in the skin or tendons).

Causes of hyperlipidemia include both a genetic predisposition (primary hyperlipidemia) and several secondary disorders. Secondary disorders include hypothyroidism, nephrotic syndrome, obstructive liver disease, and diabetes mellitus. In addition, chronic alcohol abuse, estrogen therapy, and some other drugs can cause secondary disorders.

At-Risk Populations

Total cholesterol levels above 240 mg/dL indicate a high risk for heart attack and stroke. Additionally, an HDL-C less than 40 mg/dL or LDL-C over 100 mg/dL is associated with an increased risk of cardiovascular disease.

Because abnormal lipid metabolism tends to be hereditary, a positive family history should send up a red flag. Patients with sedentary lifestyles, obesity, and diets high in fat are also at risk.

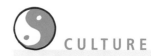

CULTURE

Abnormalities in lipid metabolism are commonly observed in industrialized societies because of the high fat content of the diet.

What You NEED TO KNOW

Clinical Manifestations

Frequently, no physical signs of hyperlipidemia are present other than abnormally elevated serum markers found in conjunction with a routine physical examination. However, signs of atherosclerosis, such as angina or intermittent claudication in middle-aged patients, can be the first warning of a problem.

Acute pancreatitis and lipid deposits in the skin or tendons (**xanthoma**) are also signs, particularly in the patient who does not follow a wellness-focused program.

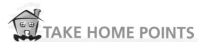

TAKE HOME POINTS

Symptoms of ischemic disease can be the first indication of hyperlipidemia.

Prognosis

Early intervention focusing on primary prevention yields the best results. In most situations, aggressive treatment is commonly associated with the lowering of cholesterol and lipids, and a slowing in the progression of atherosclerosis. However, adherence to a healthy lifestyle plays a key role.

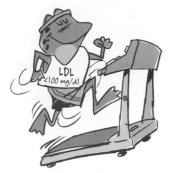

Regular exercise, with a diet low in saturated fat, can reduce cholesterol to desirable levels.

TAKE HOME POINTS

- Lowering total cholesterol levels to 160 to 199 mg/dL and LDL-C to less than 100 mg/dL is associated with a reduction in the rates of myocardial infarction and death from atherosclerosis.
- Diets low in saturated fat and cholesterol and exercise are the mainstay of primary prevention and treatment.

What You DO

Treatment

A diet low in saturated fat and cholesterol, in addition to regular exercise, is the mainstay of treatment. In patients who are overweight, reducing caloric intake to attain desired weight should also be included.

When diet and exercise fail in patients with risk factors for heart disease, more aggressive management using pharmacologic drugs is always indicated. The goal is to reach low LDL-C and high HDL-C levels. However, the desired LDL-C level depends on the risk factor profile of each patient. The general guidelines are as follows:

- An LDL-C less than 160 mg/dL in patients with one or no risk factors for primary prevention.
- An LDL-C less than 130 mg/dL in patients with two or more risk factors for primary prevention.
- An LDL-C less than 100 mg/dL in patients for secondary prevention.

The drugs of first-choice for elevated LDL-C are HMG CoA reductase inhibitors—the "statin" drugs. These drugs require medical follow-up and monitoring of liver function on a regular basis.

In recent years, patients who are not candidates for statin therapy, or those who have marginally elevated LDL-C or triglyceride levels may be prescribed fish oil capsules (i.e., omega-3 fatty acids) and red yeast rice (a drug, not a food product). Much like for the statin drugs, these over-the-counter products still require monitoring of liver function and lipid levels on a regular basis.

Nursing Responsibilities

A major focus of nursing responsibility is to promote an accurate understanding regarding the ways in which diet and exercise decrease total cholesterol and increase HDL-C. The nurse is in a strategic position to facilitate patient education and discussion regarding primary and secondary prevention of diseases associated with hypercholesterolemia. The nurse should recognize that older adult patients who are overweight may need a restrictive diet in order to maintain adequate weight and to improve overall health status.

- Counsel the patient about cardiovascular morbidity and mortality, providing information about specific problem areas, including the following:
  1. *Obesity:* Maintain ideal weight; set realistic goals, and remain active.
  2. *Smoking:* Reduce or eliminate nicotine use; participate in smoking cessation programs.
  3. *Hypertension:* Obtain regular blood pressure measurements; maintain diet, activity, and compliance with medication regimens.
  4. *Diabetes mellitus:* Monitor blood glucose regularly; maintain diet, activity, and medication regimen as prescribed.
  5. *Poor diet:* Follow reduced cholesterol and saturated-fat diet; limit caffeine and alcohol intake.
  6. *Stress:* Identify triggers for stressful situations and appropriate interventions to modify reactions.
- Explain the purpose, administration guidelines, side effects, and special instructions regarding all prescribed medications.
- Determine methods of facilitating compliance with drug therapy. Monitor for adverse effects associated with cholesterol-lowering drugs, especially decreased liver function and muscle weakness.
- Counsel the patient on the importance of regular follow-up with health care providers and monitoring of serum lipid levels and liver function.

Do You UNDERSTAND?

DIRECTIONS: **In the space provided, write the letter that corresponds to the word or phrase that completes each statement.**

_____ 1. A direct relationship exists between levels of _____ and the risk of coronary artery disease.
  a. LDL-C
  b. Triglycerides
  c. HDL-C
  d. LDL-C and total cholesterol

_____   2. _____ plays
an important role in reverse–cholesterol transport.
   a. LDL-C
   b. Apolipoproteins
   c. HDL-C
   d. Nicotinic acid

_____   3. The mainstay of treatment for hyperlipidemia is/are
_____.
   a. Statin drugs
   b. Diet
   c. Diet and exercise
   d. Dietary supplements

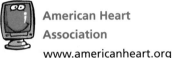

American Heart Association
www.americanheart.org
National Institute of Neurologic Diseases and Stroke
www.ninds.nih.gov
Society for Vascular Nursing
www.svnnet.org

What ARE Atherosclerosis and Arteriosclerosis?

Atherosclerosis and arteriosclerosis affect arterial blood vessels. Arteriosclerosis is a thickening and loss of vessel wall elasticity that results in luminal narrowing. Atherosclerosis is a common form of arteriosclerosis in which there is a build-up of cholesterol laden plaque.

Pathogenesis

Atherosclerosis is a complex condition that develops over a lifetime. Through a process called atherogenesis, fatty plaques (**atheromas**) are deposited on the artery walls, causing luminal narrowing (**stenosis**). When stenosis is severe and the body fails to adapt, the blood supply to tissues decreases, depriving them of oxygen. The patient will then develop symptoms resulting from ischemia. Ischemia can also result from obstruction, itself resulting from embolization of microemboli or atheromatous debris distally.

Because of damage over time, fats, cholesterol, fibrin, platelets, cellular debris, and calcium are deposited in the intimal wall of the vessels. These substances stimulate intimal cells to produce other substances that contribute to further accumulation of plaque. As the intimal wall thickens, the diameter of the artery becomes even more narrow to the extent that blood flow significantly decreases or stops.

At-Risk Populations

The incidence of atherosclerosis has been reliably predicted based on certain risk factors:

- Age: for men, 45 years or older; for women, 55 years or older or those with premature menopause without estrogen replacement therapy
- Family history of premature atherosclerotic disease (father, brother, or son with history of myocardial infarction before age 55; or mother, sister, or daughter before age 65)
- Cigarette smoking
- Blood pressure of 140/90 mm Hg or higher measured on two or more occasions
- HDL-C cholesterol less than 40 mg/dL or LDL-C cholesterol over 130 mg/dL
- Diabetes mellitus with a fasting blood sugar of 126 mg/dL or higher

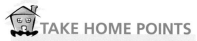

TAKE HOME POINTS

The exact cause of atherosclerosis is unknown; however, certain risk factors are thought to play an important role. These factors include
- Elevated levels of lipids in the blood.
- High blood pressure.
- Cigarette smoking.

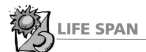

LIFE SPAN

Coronary artery disease in women and older adults may have an atypical presentation.

What You NEED TO KNOW

Clinical Manifestations

Signs and symptoms of atherosclerosis reflect tissue ischemia. Therefore, when tissue oxygen demands are not met, the following manifestations are likely to occur:

- Coronary arteries: angina, heart failure, or myocardial infarction; atypical presentations of coronary ischemia may be manifested as dyspnea, fatigue, syncope, confusion, and abdominal or back pain
- Cerebrovasculature: transient ischemic attack (TIA) or stroke
- Extremities: intermittent claudication or gangrene

Prognosis

The prognosis for patients with atherosclerosis is highly individual and depends on underlying health, number of risk factors, and the severity of disease.

Early identification of persons at risk and modification of risk factors through compliance with treatment regimens generally result in positive outcomes. However, as the severity of disease progresses and more organs become involved, the prognosis becomes grave.

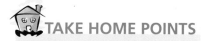

TAKE HOME POINTS

Modifying risk factors through diet, exercise, blood pressure control, and smoking cessation can improve prognosis. The prognosis for atherosclerosis is related to the severity of the disease.

What You DO

Treatment

Treatment of atherosclerosis is directed at modification of risk factors and symptom management. Drugs that inhibit platelet aggregation are frequently used to minimize thrombus formation, which frequently occurs because of plaque rupture.

Nursing Responsibilities

The nurse plays a key role in facilitating patient education focusing on primary prevention of atherosclerosis and secondary prevention of its sequelae. The nurse should do the following:

- Educate the patient about risk-factor modification and associated reduction in cardiovascular morbidity and mortality.
- Provide direction and collaborate with the patient regarding realistic dietary and exercise prescriptions.
- Provide information about smoking cessation.
- Discuss the individual patient's ischemic symptoms, focusing on contributing events and interventions that are likely to lead to an improvement.
- Define situations in which emergency assistance should be used (by calling 911).
- Educate the patient about strategies for stress management.
- Discuss methods to facilitate compliance with medication regimens such as cholesterol-lowering drugs and antihypertensives, and those that improve blood flow.
- Reinforce the importance of regular follow-up with health care providers and monitoring of appropriate laboratory tests (e.g., serum cholesterol levels, electrocardiogram data).

LIFE SPAN

Older adults who are underweight may need a less restrictive diet in order to maintain adequate weight and improve overall health status. Anxiety, frustration, depression, and fear of dying are frequently prevalent in homebound older adults.

Do You UNDERSTAND?

DIRECTIONS: **Match Column A with Column B.**

	Column A	Column B
_____	1. Treatment associated with minimizing microemboli	a. Cholesterol-lowering drugs
_____	2. Responsible for atheroma	b. Atherogenesis
_____	3. Primary prevention of atherosclerosis	c. Ischemia
_____	4. Cause of gangrene	d. Antiplatelet drugs
		e. Modification of risk factors
		f. Cholesterol

What IS Peripheral Vascular Disease?

Peripheral vascular disease (PVD) is a term commonly used to designate atherosclerotic occlusive disease involving arteries that supply the extremities.

Pathogenesis

Atherosclerosis is a complicated process that develops over a lifetime. As a result of atherosclerotic deposits in the vessels, narrowing of the arterial lumen (stenosis) occurs. Generally, signs and symptoms do not develop until an artery has narrowed by 60% or more. Although any peripheral artery can be affected, the branches of large- or medium-sized vessels of the lower extremities are most commonly involved.

Atherosclerotic occlusive disease is the primary cause of PVD. Infrequently, an inflammatory process (e.g., vasculitis) triggers the localized development of atherosclerosis.

Answers: 1. d; 2. b; 3. e; 4. c.

TAKE HOME POINTS

- The severity of PVD is a predictor of cardiovascular mortality.
- Modification of risk factors plays an essential role in the treatment of PVD. Aggressive management is generally reserved for limb-loss situations or when quality of life is greatly compromised.

At-Risk Populations

Several risk factors increase the chances of developing PVD. The risk is compounded when more than one factor is present. Risk factors include the following:

- Hyperlipidemia and hypercholesterolemia accelerate atherogenesis and increase blood viscosity, thereby increasing the risk of occlusion.
- Cigarette smoking is associated with a profound acceleration in atherosclerosis. Smoking restricts blood flow by causing vasoconstriction and promoting coagulation.
- Diabetes mellitus complicates the clinical presentation of PVD. Not only is diabetes associated with accelerated atherogenesis, but also the disease progression is atypical, with distal arteries being the first to manifest symptoms.
- Hypertension doubles the risk of symptomatic PVD.

What You NEED TO KNOW

Clinical Manifestations

TAKE HOME POINTS

- Cramping or fatigue occurs in muscles distal to the diseased segment when oxygen demands exceed supply.

Early signs of PVD can include pain, changes in appearance, or changes in sensation in the foot or leg. Pulses can be diminished, weak, or absent. Pain generally falls into two categories: intermittent claudication or limb-threatening ischemia. Other symptoms may include a cold limb with dry skin, loss of normal body hair, and ulcerations and dark discolorations that usually begins at the toes.

Intermittent claudication, the most common symptom, is characterized by muscle cramping or weakness triggered by exercise. Muscle cramping occurs distal to the obstruction, signifying insufficient blood flow to meet the demands of exercise. Increase in severity of symptoms indicates significant progression of disease. The activity that triggers intermittent claudication and the amount of rest that alleviates it are typically consistent in an individual patient.

Limb-threatening ischemia occurs when blood flow is insufficient at rest, the result of a severe arterial stenosis or complete obstruction. The patient typically develops burning pain, ulceration, or peripheral neuropathy, most commonly in the toes or the forefoot. Pain generally occurs when lying down, which can keep the patient awake at night (gravity increases blood flow to the feet when upright). This type of ischemic discomfort is called rest pain, which occurs acutely (**embolization** or **thrombosis**) or as a chronic progression of intermittent claudication.

Symptoms of PVD range from mild to severe and do not always correlate directly with the degree of stenosis. When arterial occlusion is acute, the signs and symptoms are obvious—pain, pallor, pulselessness, paresthesia, and paralysis (i.e., the "5 Ps").

Acute arterial occlusion requires emergency treatment. However, thrombosis of an arterial segment following years of progressive narrowing is usually associated with less severe symptoms because of the development of compensatory collateral pathways over time.

Chronic changes in appearance can include loss of hair over the lower legs, thickening of toenails, and muscular wasting. Changes may also occur in sensation, such as paresthesia or burning.

> The "5 Ps" signal an impending loss of limb. *Pain, pallor, pulselessness, paresthesia, and paralysis usually indicate an acute thrombosis.*

Prognosis

The prognosis for patients with PVD is highly individualized and depends on underlying health and the severity of disease. Early identification of individuals at risk and modification of risk factors through compliance with treatment regimens may slow progression of the disease.

What You DO

Treatment

Similar to other atherosclerotic diseases, treatment is aimed at palliation and secondary prevention. Structured walking programs have been found to be beneficial because they tend to increase the pain-free walking distance over time.

> The patient's blood supply is frequently sufficient to maintain tissue but not adequate for healing.

Recent advances in potent antiplatelet drugs with vasodilatory properties (**pentoxifylline** and **cilostazol**) now offer patients with intermittent claudication increased pain-free walking distances. Invasive techniques such as balloon angioplasty, stent placement, and bypass surgery are reserved for patients with symptoms that significantly affect quality of life and for patients in limb-loss situations.

Nursing Responsibilities

Primary goals in caring for the patient with PVD are directed at improving level of function and facilitating understanding of self-care measures. The nurse should do the following:

- Educate the patient regarding these practices:
    1. Modification of risk factors such as smoking cessation, weight control, control of hypertension and diabetes mellitus, and compliance with a low-fat, low-cholesterol diet
    2. Relaxation techniques, stress management, and fostering hope and spirituality
    3. Avoidance of leg crossing when sitting, prolonged sitting, and wearing of constricting garments
    4. Wearing of properly fitting footwear
    5. Daily inspection of feet and good hygiene, including the use of emollients
    6. Participation in a walking program (Exercise tolerance should be documented using specific measured distances. Walking distance should be increased in small increments with stops when pain occurs; resume after rest and pain relief. Walking should be timed [e.g., 20 to 30 minutes actual walking time] rather than using distance as a guide.)
    7. Notification of health care provider immediately when changes in color, temperature, or sensation or break in skin integrity are noticed
- Affected limbs should be kept warm, but local heat should never be applied because poorly oxygenated tissue is much more susceptible to burns and injury. Patients with limited mobility and joint flexibility may need help with foot care.
- In assessing patients, an important point to remember is that PVD is a slow process. Therefore a sudden change in symptoms, such as the 5 Ps, should alert the nurse to an emergent situation.

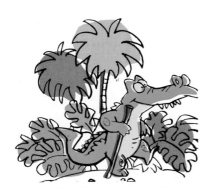

Walking for vascular health.

Do You UNDERSTAND?

DIRECTIONS: **Circle the best answer.**

_____ 1. Instructions to a patient with PVD should include which of the following?
   a. Daily inspection of skin and feet
   b. Ways to participate in a walking program
   c. Avoidance of walking when pain occurs
   d. Immediate reporting of a decrease in pain-free walking distance

_____ 2. First-line therapy for the patient with PVD includes which of the following?
   a. Balloon angioplasty, stent placement
   b. Bypass surgery
   c. Vasodilation and antiplatelet drugs

What IS Raynaud's Phenomenon?

The term *Raynaud's disease* is used to imply a benign syndrome; no demonstrable cause is present, although *Raynaud's phenomenon* is used in the presence of an underlying immunologic, pathologic source. Raynaud's phenomenon is a vasospastic disorder. Vasospasm refers to a sudden decrease in the internal diameter of a blood vessel.

Pathogenesis

Raynaud's phenomenon is characterized by episodic vasospasm of the arteries of the fingers and toes in response to exposure to cold or emotional stress. Patients may have normal vessels with an exaggerated response to stimuli. However, approximately 60% of patients have a normal vasoconstrictive response to stimuli with underlying digital artery occlusion. Of this latter group, most individuals have an immunologic or connective tissue disorder, such as systemic sclerosis.

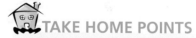

TAKE HOME POINTS

Raynaud's is frequently associated with systemic sclerosis (previously known as scleroderma). Raynaud's phenomenon occurs almost exclusively in women.

Answers: 1. a, b, d; 2. c.

The causes of Raynaud's phenomenon include the following:

- Exaggerated vasoconstrictive response to stimuli
- Underlying digital artery occlusion
- Excessive use of potent vasoconstrictive drugs (e.g., ergotamine tartrate)

At-Risk Populations

Women with the following disorders should be considered at risk:

- Peripheral arterial occlusive disease
- Connective tissue disorder, particularly systemic sclerosis
- Migraine headaches treated with ergot drugs

TAKE HOME POINTS

- Symptoms of Raynaud's phenomenon are precipitated in response to cold or emotional stress.
- Treatment of Raynaud's phenomenon is directed at symptom control (i.e., limiting symptom triggers and administering calcium channel blockers).

What You NEED TO KNOW

Clinical Manifestations

Raynaud's phenomenon is characterized by blanching of the digits and numbness with little pain. These signs and symptoms are followed by cyanosis after prolonged warming and, finally, reactive hyperemia with intense erythema and burning pain.

Prognosis

The prognosis is generally good. However, approximately 10% of patients with underlying occlusive disease eventually develop gangrene.

What You DO

Treatment

Treatment for Raynaud's phenomenon is primarily palliative, focusing on avoidance or removal of stimuli known to evoke symptoms.

Calcium channel blockers (e.g., nifedipine) can also provide benefit because of their vasodilatory effects. However, if pain and circulatory problems persist, more aggressive treatment regimens may be needed to increase regional blood flow (e.g., sympathectomy, spinal cord stimulation, acupuncture).

Nursing Responsibilities

Nursing responsibilities for the patient with Raynaud's phenomenon include the following:

- Teach patients to avoid stimuli likely to provoke vasospasm, including protecting the extremities from cold (e.g., wearing gloves, avoiding cold exposure) and reducing catecholamine release through active participation in stress-management programs.
- Encourage patients to stop smoking because of the vasoconstrictor effect of nicotine.

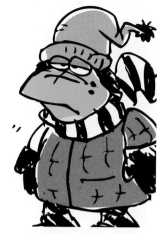

Avoid the cold.

Do You UNDERSTAND?

DIRECTIONS: Match Column A with Column B.

	Column A	Column B
_____	1. Associated with redness and burning pain	a. Raynaud's phenomenon
_____	2. Responsible for pallor and numbness	b. Raynaud's disease
_____	3. Benign vasospastic syndrome	c. Hyperemia
_____	4. Vasoconstrictive response associated with a connective tissue disease	d. Vasoconstriction
		e. Systemic sclerosis

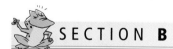 **SECTION B**

DISORDERS OF THE VENOUS CIRCULATION

The venous circulation consists of peripheral and central components. The central component includes veins from the intraabdominal and intrathoracic organs, which continuously return blood to the heart.

Answers: 1. c; 2. d; 3. b; 4. a.

The peripheral component, located primarily in extremities, contains valves that facilitate blood transport to the central venous system by modulating pressure effects under changing conditions. This section deals primarily with disorders either directly related to disease involving the peripheral venous system or related to effects of the central venous system on the extremities.

What IS Venous Stasis?

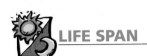

LIFE SPAN

Pregnancy frequently causes temporary venous stasis during the second and third trimesters of pregnancy. This stasis frequently manifests itself visibly as varicose veins and edema.

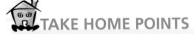

TAKE HOME POINTS

The patient confined to bed or chair is at increased risk for venous stasis.

Venous stasis includes all conditions associated with slow flow or stagnation of blood within venous circulation. These conditions include impaired mobility of extremities, heart failure, extrinsic compression of veins by masses (e.g., tumors, abscesses, lymph nodes), and decreased arterial flow (e.g., severe hypotension or hypovolemic shock).

Pathogenesis

Venous stasis occurs in response to either an overabundance or decreased removal of fluid. The following factors are common causes of venous stasis:

- Sedentary lifestyle
- Compression of blood vessels (i.e., obesity, abdominal mass)
- Heart failure
- Chronic venous disease

At-Risk Populations

Patients with heart failure or a history of venous disease, such as varicose veins or chronic venous insufficiency, and those with sedentary lifestyles are at risk for venous stasis. In addition, obesity and pelvic masses are frequently associated with venous stasis because of compression of the great veins of the abdomen.

What You NEED TO KNOW

Clinical Manifestations

Mild ankle swelling is generally the first sign of venous stasis. With progression, the patient is likely to manifest dilatation of subcutaneous veins. Patients may complain of mild discomfort, described as lower extremity heaviness or painful varicose veins.

Watch for swelling.

Prognosis

When identified early and treated effectively, the prognosis is excellent. Failure to identify the cause of venous stasis can lead to significant morbidity and mortality.

What You DO

Treatment

Treatment is directed at identifying the cause of venous stasis and management of swelling. Elevation and activity are the simplest methods to reduce extremity swelling. Pneumatic compression devices are commonly used in hospitals as primary prevention in those at risk, particularly for the surgical patient. Graduated compression stockings can also be used, particularly when the cause cannot be cured (chronic venous insufficiency).

Swollen legs can be helped by elevation higher than the patient's heart.

Nursing Responsibilities

Because venous stasis is frequently preventable, health care providers should pay particular attention to body positioning and encourage physical activity. The nurse should do the following:

- Be knowledgeable regarding the use of pneumatic compression devices and stockings.
- Teach the patient primary prevention and symptom alleviation. Education should focus on the following:
  1. Encouraging good skin care:
     - Checking skin daily for cracking or breakdown
     - Washing daily with mild soap
     - Using emollients, when necessary
     - Wearing clean stockings daily

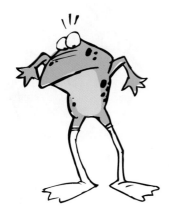

2. Staying active (e.g., walking, structured exercise program)
3. Maintaining ideal weight or weight loss
4. Avoiding leg crossing when sitting, prolonged sitting, and wearing of constricting garments
5. Preventing injury
6. Providing guidelines about what symptoms to report to health care providers

! Some brands of compression stockings contain latex, which can cause life-threatening allergic reactions in susceptible individuals.

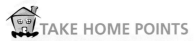

TAKE HOME POINTS

Elevation of the extremity above the level of the heart is the most effective position to decrease swelling.

! Inappropriate use of pneumatic compression devices and stockings can cause serious injury, such as obstruction of venous or arterial circulation.

Do You UNDERSTAND?

DIRECTIONS: **Indicate which statements are *true* (T) and which are *false* (F). If false, correct the statement in the margin space to make it true.**

_____ 1. Venous stasis can result from an ovarian tumor.

_____ 2. Lower extremity fatigue can be the first sign of venous stasis.

_____ 3. Walking is an effective method of preventing venous stasis.

_____ 4. Constipation can cause venous stasis.

_____ 5. Improperly fitted compression stockings can cause venous stasis.

What IS Chronic Venous Insufficiency?

Chronic venous insufficiency refers to the syndrome characterized by lower extremity edema, stasis dermatitis, and ulceration.

Pathogenesis

Chronic venous insufficiency results from persistently high pressures in deep venous circulation. The high pressures result from incompetent venous valves that are unable to facilitate normal flow from the periphery to central venous circulation. This condition leads to congestion and an alteration in the microcirculation, which causes further changes in the

Answers: 1. T; 2. F, Nocturnal swelling is generally the first sign of venous stasis; 3. T; 4. T; 5. T.

skin and subcutaneous tissues. Hemoglobin and other protein waste materials are deposited in subcutaneous tissue. These deposits subsequently result in increased pigmentation and increased oncotic pressure, which attracts additional fluid. Without treatment, obstruction of lymphatics further complicates the clinical course.

The majority of cases are related to the aftermath of deep venous thrombosis. However, other factors, such as congenital absence of or incompetent venous valves, may contribute.

At-Risk Populations

Patients with a history of deep venous thrombosis are at the greatest risk for venous insufficiency. However, individuals with varicose veins who have experienced repeated bouts of superficial thrombophlebitis should also be considered at risk.

What You NEED TO KNOW

Clinical Manifestations

Nocturnal swelling is generally the first symptom of chronic venous insufficiency, but the condition usually becomes progressive and irreversible. A brawny (i.e., reddish-brown) pigmentation (stasis dermatitis) of the lower leg can occur, along with secondary varicosities and ulceration. These ulcerations are not usually painful unless they are infected or involve deep tissues. Itching and burning sensations have been reported. Recurrent phlebitis and thrombosis are common.

Prognosis

Effective management of swelling and maintenance of skin integrity are possible when treated early. Recurrent phlebitis and thrombosis occur frequently and result in progressive deterioration. In rare cases, after many years, chronic ulceration can undergo malignant transformation. Lymphedema can be a late complication.

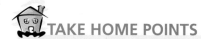

TAKE HOME POINTS

- Reddish-brown pigmentation (stasis dermatitis) of the lower leg is commonly found in patients with chronic venous insufficiency. Venous ulcers are usually not painful.
- Minor breaks in skin integrity frequently progress to ulceration.
- Compression therapy and wound care are both necessary to effectively treat venous stasis ulcerations.

What You DO

Treatment

Compression therapy, periodic elevation of the legs, and avoidance of trauma are the mainstays of management. Good skin care, including the use of emollients, is essential in preventing breaks in skin integrity. Wound care must be included when venous insufficiency is complicated by ulceration. When ulceration is present, compression therapy becomes a necessary adjunct to wound care, primarily because sustained pressures will prevent wound healing. Compression therapy may be ordered in the form of elastic bandages, graduated compression stockings, or a pneumatic compression pump.

Nursing Responsibilities

Patient education is essential in both the treatment and the prevention of complications associated with chronic venous insufficiency. The nurse should do the following:
- Be knowledgeable about the use of pneumatic compression devices and compression stockings.
- During patient encounters, document skin appearance, characteristics of ulcers (when present), the current treatment regimen, and patient compliance.
- Educate the patient to facilitate primary prevention and symptom alleviation. Education should focus on the importance of
  1. Staying active (e.g., walking, structured exercise program).
  2. Maintaining ideal weight or weight loss.
  3. Avoiding leg crossing when sitting, prolonged sitting, and wearing of constricting garments.
  4. Skin care:
     - Check skin daily for cracking or breakdown.
     - Wash daily with mild soap using lukewarm water.
     - Avoid soaking legs in bathtub.
     - Use emollients, when necessary.
  5. Injury prevention:
     - Avoid bumping and bruising legs.
     - Do not go barefoot.
     - Avoid shaving with razor or hair-remover creams.
     - Avoid excess heat or cold exposure.

6. Wound care instructions, including adverse effects.
7. Compression therapy instructions, including adverse effects.
   • Wear clean stockings daily.
   • Always wear stockings while awake.
   • Apply stockings first thing in morning.
   • Discard stocking when elastic is lost (approximately every 6 months).
   • Provide guidelines about what to report to health care providers:
8. Changes in skin (e.g., ulceration, dermatitis)
9. Changes in wound (e.g., pain, discharge, redness)

Do You UNDERSTAND?

DIRECTIONS: **Circle the best answer.**

_____   1. Compression therapy promotes healing of venous ulcers by
   a. Promoting tissue oxygenation and nutrient exchange.
   b. Protecting the area from further injury.
   c. Removing waste products.
   d. Increasing venous pressure.

_____   2. Interventions that minimize the sequelae associated with deep venous thrombosis include:
   a. Walking.
   b. Wearing compression stockings during the day.
   c. Avoiding sitting for prolonged periods.
   d. Soaking legs in a hot tub to relieve discomfort.

American Society of Hypertension
www.ash-us.org
National Heart, Lung and Blood Institute
www.nhlbi.nih.gov/index.htm

Answers: 1. a; 2, a, b, and c.

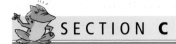

SECTION C

HYPERTENSION

Hypertension (HTN) is a disorder of blood pressure (BP) regulation. HTN refers to an abnormally elevated BP over a sustained period: above 120 mm Hg systolic or above 80 mm Hg diastolic. HTN is associated with vascular damage and increased cardiovascular morbidity and mortality.

HTN is the most commonly treated disease that involves an abnormal function of blood vessels. However, in more than 80% of cases, the exact cause is unknown. In a smaller percentage of cases, the cause are diseases of the kidney or the adrenal glands, and certain tumors.

What IS Essential HTN?

Essential, or primary HTN, refers to an abnormally elevated BP in which the exact cause cannot be defined.

Pathogenesis

HTN is a multifactorial condition in which one of the factors in the BP equation must change: peripheral resistance or cardiac output. Regulation of BP involves a complex interaction among the kidneys, the central nervous system and peripheral nervous system, and the vascular endothelium. A variety of organs, such as the adrenal and pituitary glands, also play a role. The heart responds to many of the changes mediated by these systems, secreting hormones both locally and systemically. These hormones interact with substances produced elsewhere to regulate BP levels.

Hypotheses for the cause of HTN include:

- Increased renal resorption of sodium, chloride, and water related to natriuretic hormone, which is an inherited defect in sodium transport.
- Increased activity of the renin-angiotensin-aldosterone system, resulting in extracellular fluid volume expansion and increased systemic vascular resistance.

- Increased sympathetic nervous system activity related to autonomic nervous system dysfunction.
- Decreased vasodilation of the arterioles related to vascular endothelium dysfunction.
- Insulin resistance, which can be the reason for the common association of HTN, type 2 diabetes mellitus, glucose intolerance, obesity, and hypertriglyceridemia.

Major risk factors for cardiovascular problems in the patient with HTN include tobacco abuse, hyperlipidemia, diabetes mellitus, advanced age, and a family history of premature cardiovascular disease (female relatives under age 65 and male relatives under age 55); men and post-menopausal women are at higher risk as well.

At-Risk Populations

Populations at risk for essential HTN include individuals with a positive family history, advanced age, obesity, and a sedentary lifestyle. Certain environmental factors have also been identified as contributing to the development of HTN. These factors include stress, excessive intake of sodium and alcohol, and the presence of sleep apnea.

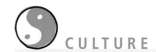

CULTURE

The increased incidence of HTN in African Americans has been attributed to an increased prevalence of salt sensitivity.

What IS Secondary HTN?

Secondary HTN is the result of an identifiable abnormality.

Pathogenesis

The pathophysiologic nature of secondary HTN varies and is dependent on the specific abnormality. Although several disorders are responsible for causing HTN, the physiologic mechanisms all lead to increased vascular resistance and can be categorized as follows:
- Increased renin secretion
- Increased aldosterone production
- Increased stimulation of angiotensin receptors
- Increased catecholamine production

Causes of secondary forms of HTN include the following:
- Renal vascular HTN: decreased renal perfusion stimulates the involved kidney to release renin

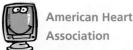

American Heart Association

www.americanheart.org

National Heart Lung and Blood Institute—Clinical Practice Guidelines

http://www.nhlbi.nih.gov/guidelines/hypertension/jncintro.htm

- Primary aldosteronism: excess aldosterone, usually a result of an adrenal tumor, causes sodium retention
- Pheochromocytoma: adrenal medulla tumor that secretes massive amounts of catecholamines
- Cushing's syndrome: excess cortisol production that increases angiotensin II and catecholamine release
- Hyperthyroidism: increased release of thyroid hormone, which stimulates catecholamine surge
- Estrogen-induced HTN: high estrogen, which causes increased generation of angiotensin II

At-Risk Populations

Certain factors increase the risk for secondary HTN, which include alcohol consumption of more than three drinks per day; history of cocaine, amphetamines, hormones, and immunosuppressive drug use; history of genitourinary or renal disease; pregnancy; presence of a neurologic disorder such as increased intracranial pressure, quadriplegia, and Guillain-Barré syndrome; and the presence of an endocrine disorder involving the adrenal, pituitary, thyroid, or parathyroid glands.

Both essential and secondary hypertensive patients are at risk for target organ damage (TOD) and cardiovascular disease (CCD). Patients in high-risk categories include those with a history of heart diseases (e.g., left ventricular hypertrophy, heart failure, angina, myocardial infarction, and prior coronary revascularization) and TIA or stroke (e.g., peripheral arterial disease, nephropathy, or retinopathy).

What You NEED TO KNOW

Essential HTN

Clinical Manifestations. HTN is generally an asymptomatic disease until a cardiovascular complication occurs. However, vague complaints, early morning occipital headache, fatigue, epistaxis, and dizziness can be early signs. Reproducible measurements of systolic BP over 140 mm Hg or diastolic over 90 mm Hg are consistent with a diagnosis of HTN. The Seventh Report of the Joint Committee on the "Detection, Evaluation, and Treatment of Hypertension" (JNC VII) summarizes the stages of HTN as shown in the following table:

Category	SBP		DBP
Normal	<120	and	<80
Pre-HTN	120-139	or	80-89
Stage 1	140-159	or	90-99
Stage 2	≥160	or	≥100

SBP, Systolic blood pressure; *DBP,* diastolic blood pressure; *HTN,* hypertension.

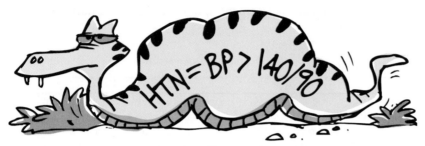

Symptom of hypertension.

Prognosis

Effective control of BP in the asymptomatic phase significantly reduces overall cardiovascular morbidity and mortality. In the United States, HTN is a leading cause of ischemic coronary and cerebrovascular disease, the second leading cause of end-stage renal disease, and the leading cause of heart failure and hemorrhagic stroke. In addition, a direct relationship exists between increasing systolic and diastolic BP levels with the incidence of coronary heart disease mortality.

Secondary HTN

Clinical Manifestations. Only 5% to 10% of patients present with a secondary cause of hypertension. However, findings that suggest secondary HTN include absence of family history and poor control on a triple-medication regimen with good compliance, or physical findings suggestive of drug abuse or neurologic, renal, or endocrine etiologic factors.

Prognosis. The prognosis is directly related to early identification of the secondary cause and effective treatment.

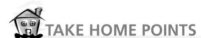
TAKE HOME POINTS

- A direct relationship exists among increasing BP and risk factors, target organ damage, and cardiovascular disease.
- A strong association exists between dietary sodium intake and BP. A stepwise approach has been adopted for pharmacologic management of HTN.

What You DO

Treatment

The goal of essential and secondary hypertensive management is to prevent death and complications by lowering and maintaining BP at 140/90 mm Hg or lower. The JNC VII has defined a BP goal of 130/85 mm Hg for patients with diabetes mellitus or with proteinuria greater than 1 gram per 24 hours. In addition, to treatment of the specific cause of secondary HTN, the same stepwise approach used to treat essential HTN is adopted. Management options for HTN are outlined in the following table.

Risk Stratification and Treatment

BP Stages	Risk Group A[1]	Risk Group B[2]	Risk Group C[3]
High-normal	Lifestyle modification	Lifestyle	Lifestyle modification
Stage 1	Lifestyle modification therapy[4] (up to 6 months)	Lifestyle	Medication modification (up to 12 months)
Stages 2 and 3	Medication therapy[4]	Medication	Medication therapy[4]

BP, Blood pressure; *CCD*, cardiovascular disease; *TOD*, target organ damage.
[1]No risk factors and no TOD or CCD.
[2]At least one risk factor, not including diabetes; no TOD or CCD.
[3]TOD or CCD and/or diabetes, with or without other risk factors.
[4]Lifestyle modification should be adjunctive therapy for all patients on medication therapy.

Lifestyle modifications associated with lowering BP include weight reduction, decreasing dietary sodium to no more than 2.4 grams of sodium or 6 grams of sodium chloride per day, increasing consumption of fruits and vegetables (to at least 4 servings per day), increasing physical activity to 30 to 45 minutes for 4 times per week, moderation of alcohol consumption, stress management, and smoking cessation.

Many antihypertensive drugs are available and may be used in combination. These include thiazide diuretics, beta blockers, calcium channel blockers, angiotensin converting enzyme (ACE) inhibitors, angiotensin II receptor blockers (ARB II), alpha-beta ganglionic blockers, alpha$_1$ blockers, and central adrenergic inhibitors.

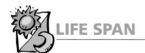

TAKE HOME POINTS

- Initial treatment of HTN targets lifestyle modification. Physical activity should begin at 10 to 15 minutes per day, 3 to 4 times per week, with gradual increase to 30 to 45 minutes, as tolerated in advanced age.

LIFE SPAN

Older adults should begin an exercise regimen under the supervision of a qualified health care provider. Exercise should be mild at first and gradually increased as the patient's tolerance improves. Underweight older adults may require a less restrictive diet to maintain weight status.

Nursing Responsibilities

Because compliance is essential to effective management, nursing responsibilities deal primarily with patient education including the following:

- Regular visits with a health care provider to monitor BP and adherence to treatment regimen are vital to good control of HTN. See the patient back according to the following schedule*:

In 1 week if patient is in stage 3
In 1 month if patient is in stage 2
In 2 months if patient is in stage 1
In 1 year if systolic BP is 130 to 139 mm Hg and diastolic BP is 85 to 89 mm Hg
In 2 years if systolic BP is less than 130 mm Hg and diastolic BP is less than 85 mm Hg

- Signs and symptoms of HTN
- Modifiable risk factors:

Smoking cessation
HTN—regular BP monitoring
Diet—low sodium, low saturated fat and cholesterol, plenty of fresh fruits and vegetables; limited alcohol
Exercise—goal of 30 to 40 minutes per day, 4 times per week
Weight loss

- Drug regimen that includes purpose, dose, adverse effects, and special considerations
- Guidelines to improve patient compliance with antihypertensive therapy include the following:
  1. Integrate medication-taking into routine activities of daily living.
  2. Anticipate side effects; adjust therapy to prevent or minimize side effects.
  3. Encourage positive attitude about achieving therapeutic goals and stress management.
  4. Consider using a nurse case management approach.

*Joint National Committee: The Seventh Report of the Joint National Committee on prevention, detection, evaluation, and treatment of high blood pressure, *U.S. Department of Health and Human Services,* NIH publication No. 03-5233.

Do You UNDERSTAND?

DIRECTIONS: **In the space provided, write the letter(s) that correspond to the word or phrase that either answers the question or completes the statement.**

_____ 1. With BP measurements repeatedly in the range of 130 to 140 mm Hg systolic and 86 to 90 mmHg diastolic, appropriate management of the patient with diabetes includes which of the following?

a. Lifestyle modification and continued monitoring of BP in 1 month

b. Lifestyle modification and antihypertensive medication

c. Risk-factor modification and continued monitoring of BP

d. Continued monitoring of BP

_____ 2. TOD as a result of HTN can be manifested as

a. Intermittent claudication.

b. An aortic aneurysm.

c. Superior vena cava syndrome.

d. Renal failure.

DIRECTIONS: **Match Column A with Column B.**

Column A

_____ 3. Increased renin secretion

_____ 4. Increased stimulation of angiotensin II

_____ 5. Primary aldosteronism

_____ 6. Massive catecholamine release

Column B

a. Pheochromocytoma

b. Adrenal tumor

c. Hyperparathyroidism

d. Estrogen therapy

e. Renal vascular HTN

What IS Accelerated HTN?

Accelerated HTN—occasionally called malignant HTN—represents an urgent situation because of the risk of progressive TOD and its implications for the cardiovascular, renal, and central nervous systems. Although no specific BP measurement is used to define accelerated HTN, it rarely occurs at levels below 160/110 mm Hg.

Pathogenesis

Accelerated HTN occurs when an acute or sustained elevation in BP causes rapid or progressive TOD, particularly in the cardiovascular, renal, and central nervous systems.

Accelerated HTN frequently indicates a secondary form of HTN, which is particularly true when BP control is difficult to achieve despite patient compliance with an adequate and appropriate triple-medication regimen. Although noncompliance with antihypertensive medication therapy or any of the secondary forms of HTN can cause accelerated HTN, renal vascular HTN is the most common etiologic factor.

Renal vascular HTN occurs in response to renal ischemia. Renal ischemia is most commonly a result of renal artery stenosis, but it may also occur because of dissection of the aorta adjacent to the kidneys. Renal vascular HTN results from increased peripheral vascular resistance induced by increased amounts of renin released from an ischemic kidney. Suppression of renin secretion in the uninvolved kidney occurs as a compensatory response, thus serum renin levels remain normal.

At-Risk Populations

Individuals who are at increased risk for accelerated HTN include young or middle-aged patients with HTN and patients who suddenly cease antihypertensive medication therapy.

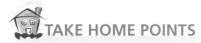
TAKE HOME POINTS

- Accelerated HTN rarely occurs below BP levels of 160/110 mm Hg.
- In accelerated HTN, BP is sufficiently elevated to cause acute vascular injury in vital organs.
- Renal vascular HTN is a common cause of accelerated HTN.

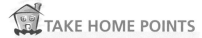
TAKE HOME POINTS

Symptoms of accelerated HTN can progress to a hypertensive crisis.

What You NEED TO KNOW

Clinical Manifestations

The clinical manifestations of accelerated HTN include the following:
- Elevated BP, typically over 160/110 mm Hg
- Heart—chest pain, dyspnea

- Central nervous system—headache, fluctuating mental status
- Retinal—retinal hemorrhage, papilledema
- Gastrointestinal—nausea, vomiting
- Renal—azotemia, oliguria, and proteinuria

Prognosis

Without treatment, most patients die from accelerated HTN within 6 months. With effective treatment, 5-year survival rates of over 70% are possible. Acute causes of death include acute renal failure, hemorrhagic strokes, and heart failure.

What You DO

Treatment

The goal of treatment is to lower the BP slowly, over a 6- to 24-hour period. Although treatment is usually initiated with an intravenous antihypertensive drug, a combination of oral and parenteral drugs is frequently used. The choice of drug is based on rapidity of action, ease in administration, and propensity for side effects. Addressing the secondary cause of HTN is equally important because antihypertensive medication therapy alone is frequently ineffective.

Nursing Responsibilities

Nursing care focuses on rapidly assessing the patient's baseline status, securing intravenous access, and facilitating admission to a critical care unit. Initial blood and urine specimens should be collected and antihypertensive medication therapy begun immediately. Abrupt falls in BP should be avoided but the goal is to lower the diastolic BP to approximately 110 mm Hg. Pressure reduction may need to be even less if signs of tissue ischemia develop (i.e., arrhythmias, chest pain, or changes in neurologic status).

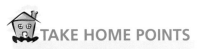

TAKE HOME POINTS

Treatment of accelerated HTN focuses on reducing BP slowly using a combination of drugs.

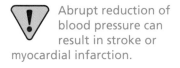

Abrupt reduction of blood pressure can result in stroke or myocardial infarction.

Do You UNDERSTAND?

DIRECTIONS: **Indicate which statements are *true* (T) and which are *false* (F). If false, correct the statement in the margin space to make it true.**

_____ 1. Diastolic BP is more important than systolic in accelerated HTN.

_____ 2. Renal artery revascularization is an important component of managing renal vascular HTN.

_____ 3. Dropping the systolic BP from 280 to 160 mm Hg in a 30-minute period in an 80-year-old patient is likely to cause a TIA or stroke.

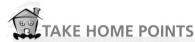

TAKE HOME POINTS

Both the elevated pressure and the rapidity in rise indicate the severity of vascular injury.

What IS a Hypertensive Crisis?

A hypertensive crisis is a situation in which a severe elevation in BP and a rapid or progressive deterioration in the function of the central nervous system, heart, kidneys, or hematologic system occur simultaneously.

Pathogenesis

In this condition, the BP is elevated to the extent that immediate vascular damage is threatened. A persistent diastolic pressure above 140 mm Hg is associated with acute vascular damage in most individuals. However, the rapidity of the rise can be a more important factor than the absolute level itself. If the pressure is not reduced rapidly, cerebral edema worsens with resultant acute herniation of the brain stem.

Causes of hypertensive crisis include hypertensive encephalopathy, increased intracranial pressure, increased systemic peripheral vascular resistance, and excessive circulating catecholamines.

At-Risk Populations

Circumstances that place patients at risk for a hypertensive crisis include the following:
- Accelerated HTN
- Intracerebral hemorrhage
- Head injury
- Ischemic stroke
- Acute aortic dissection (particularly when renal arteries are involved)
- Acute left ventricular failure
- Conditions that cause increased catecholamine circulation (e.g., pheochromocytoma, hyperthyroidism)

What You NEED TO KNOW

Clinical Manifestations

Symptoms are usually dramatic; however, some patients are relatively asymptomatic, despite markedly elevated BP levels and extensive organ damage. However, when pressures are sufficiently high to cause encephalopathy, the following clinical features are frequently present:
- *Central nervous system:* confusion, decreased level of consciousness, headache, visual disturbances, weakness, seizures, and nystagmus
- *Cardiac:* prominent apical pulse and heart failure
- *Renal:* oliguria and azotemia
- *Gastrointestinal:* nausea and vomiting
- *Hematologic:* hemolytic anemia and intravascular coagulation

Prognosis

Without immediate treatment, patients in hypertensive crisis die quickly from brain damage.

What You DO

Treatment

In a hypertensive crisis, the BP must be rapidly reduced within 1 hour. Because of the risk to life, an intravenous drug is always used. Sodium nitroprusside and nitroglycerin are two of the more commonly used drugs; however, other drugs are available.

> ⚠ Failure to lower BP may result in death. Patients who are undergoing treatment for a hypertensive crisis must be carefully monitored in an intensive care setting to decrease the risk of inadvertent hypoperfusion of vital organs.

Nursing Responsibilities

Nursing responsibility focuses on rapidly assessing the patient's baseline status, securing intravenous access, and facilitating critical-care monitoring. Initial blood and urine specimens should be collected and antihypertensive therapy begun simultaneously. Pressure reduction must be accomplished as rapidly as possible.

Do You UNDERSTAND?

DIRECTIONS: **Indicate which statements are *true* (T) and which are *false* (F). If false, correct the statement in the margin space to make it true.**

_____ 1. Dissection of the infrarenal abdominal aorta is likely to cause a hypertensive crisis.

_____ 2. Combinations of intravenous and oral drugs are used to treat hypertensive crisis.

_____ 3. Dropping the diastolic BP slowly over 3 hours from 180 to 100 mm Hg is an acceptable plan in patients with hypertensive crisis.

References

Adult Treatment Panel II: Summary of the second report of the National Cholesterol Education Program expert panel on detection, evaluation, and treatment of high blood cholesterol in adults, *JAMA* 269:3015, 1993.

American College of Physicians: Guidelines for using serum cholesterol, high-density lipoprotein cholesterol, and triglycerides as screening tests for the prevention of coronary heart disease in adults, *Ann Intern Med* 124:515, 1996.

Bisognana JD: Malignant hypertension, 2005, URL http://www.emedicine.com/MED/topic1107.htm.

Black HR, Barkris GL, Elliott WJ: Hypertension: epidemiology, pathophysiology, diagnosis, and treatment. In Fuster V, Alexander RW, O'Rourke RA, editors: *Hurst's: the heart*, ed 10, New York, 2001, McGraw-Hill.

Dormandy JA: Circulation-enhancing drugs. In Rutherford RB, editor: *Vascular surgery*, ed 5, Philadelphia, 2000, WB Saunders.

Eaton L: Cardiovascular function. In Lueckenotte AG, editor: *Gerontologic nursing*, ed 2, St Louis, 2000, Mosby.

Fahey VA, McCarthy WJ: Arterial reconstruction of the lower extremity. In Fahey VA, editor: *Vascular nursing*, ed 3, Philadelphia, 1999, WB Saunders.

Hiatt WR, Cooke JP: Atherogenesis and the medical management of atherosclerosis. In Rutherford RB, editor: *Vascular surgery*, ed 5, Philadelphia, 2000, WB Saunders.

Johnston KW: Upper extremity ischemia. In Rutherford RB, editor: *Vascular surgery*, ed 5, Philadelphia, 2000, WB Saunders.

Joint National Committee: The Seventh Report of the Joint National Committee on prevention, detection, evaluation, and treatment of high blood pressure, *U.S. Department of Health and Human Services, JAMA.* 2003;289:(doi:10.1001/jama.289.19.2560).

McCowen KC, Blackburn GL: Obesity, weight control, and cardiovascular disease. In Wong ND, Black HR, Gardin JM, editors: *Preventive cardiology*, New York, 2000, McGraw-Hill.

Monetta GL, Nehler MR, Porter JM: Pathophysiology of chronic venous insufficiency. In Rutherford RB, editor: *Vascular surgery*, ed 5, Philadelphia, 2000, WB Saunders.

Norris KC, Francis CK: African Americans. In Wong ND, Black HR, Gardin JM, editors: *Preventive cardiology*, New York, 2000, McGraw-Hill.

Ryan P: Facilitating behavior change in chronically ill persons. In Miller JF, editor: *Coping with chronic illness*, ed 3, Philadelphia, 2000, FA Davis.

Schroeder PS, Miller JF: Profiles of locus of control and coping in persons with peripheral vascular disease. In Miller JF, editor: *Coping with chronic illness*, ed 3, Philadelphia, 2000, FA Davis.

Smeltzer SC, Bare BG: Management of patients with coronary vascular disorders. In Brunner, Suddarth, editors: *Textbook of medical-surgical nursing*, ed 9, Philadelphia, 2000, Lippincott.

Sumner DS: Evaluation of acute and chronic ischemia of the upper extremity. In Rutherford RB, editor: *Vascular surgery*, ed 5, Philadelphia, 2000, WB Saunders.

Tripp TR: Laboratory and diagnostic tests. In Lueckenotte AG, editor: *Gerontologic nursing*, ed 2, St Louis, 2000, Mosby.

Walsh ME, Rice KL: Venous thrombosis and pulmonary embolism. In Fahey VA, editor: *Vascular nursing*, ed 3, Philadelphia, 1999, WB Saunders.

Wong ND, Kashyap ML: Cholesterol and lipids. In Wong ND, Black HR, Gardin JM, editors: *Preventive cardiology*, New York, 2000, McGraw-Hill.

Wright JT, Hammonds VC: Hypertension: epidemiology and contemporary management strategies. In Wong ND, Black HR, Gardin JM, editors: *Preventive cardiology*, New York, 2000, McGraw-Hill.

Zierler RE, Sumner DS: Physiologic assessment of peripheral arterial occlusive disease. In Rutherford RB, editor: *Vascular surgery*, ed 5, Philadelphia, 2000, WB Saunders.

NCLEX® Review

Section A

1. High-density lipoproteins benefit the circulation because they
   1 Increase the diameter of blood vessels.
   2 Improve elasticity of the vessels.
   3 Carry fat away from arteries.
   4 Inhibit platelet activity.

2. Which of the following diseases contribute to the development of hyperlipidemia?
   1 Hyperthyroidism
   2 Diabetes mellitus
   3 Pancreatitis
   4 Malnutrition

3. Patients who have two risk factors for cardiovascular disease but do not have actual cardiac disease should strive for an LDL-C at what level?
   1 100 mg/dL or less
   2 Less than 130 mg/dL
   3 Less than 160 mg/dL
   4 Less than 190 mg/dL

4. The patient with vascular disease should be instructed to avoid
   1 Caffeine.
   2 Excessive heat.
   3 Nonsteroidal antiinflammatory drugs (NSAIDs).
   4 Sunlight.

5. Initial signs and symptoms of Raynaud's phenomenon include
   1 Persistent erythema and swelling of the hands.
   2 Poor capillary refill in the toes.
   3 Blanching of the fingers.
   4 Pain and itching of the fingertips.

Section B

6. Venous stasis can be a consequence of all of the following *except*
   1 Heart failure.
   2 Compression of veins by masses.
   3 Increased arterial flow.
   4 Severe hypotension.

7. Pneumatic compression devices are used in hospitals to prevent
   1 Venous dilation.
   2 Venous stasis.
   3 Venous ulcers.
   4 Venous distention.

8. What lifestyle changes do *not* help minimize the effect of venous stasis?
   1 Engaging in regular structured exercise
   2 Maintaining ideal body weight
   3 Preventing injury to the lower extremities
   4 Avoiding salt in the diet

9. Why is compression therapy helpful in the treatment of venous ulcers?
   1 It protects the area from further injury.
   2 It prevents infection.
   3 It improves tissue perfusion and prevents further swelling.
   4 It dissolves blood clots.

10. Risk factors contributing to the development of venous stasis include all of the following *except*
    1 Obesity.
    2 Sedentary lifestyle.
    3 Coagulation defects.
    4 Abdominal mass.

Section C

11. Antihypertensive drugs should never be discontinued suddenly because of the risk for
    1 Renal damage.
    2 Angina.
    3 Accelerated hypertension.
    4 Severe hypotension.

12. Which of the following factors contribute to the development of hypertension?
    1 Inadequate intake of calcium
    2 Excess intake of alcohol
    3 Depression
    4 Inadequate intake of potassium

13. Poorly controlled hypertension contributes to the development of
    1 Embolic strokes.
    2 Coronary artery disease.
    3 Migraine headaches.
    4 Peripheral vascular disease.

14. Measures to reduce blood pressure to healthy levels include which of the following?
    1 Eating foods high in protein
    2 Avoiding sources of stress
    3 Minimizing tobacco use
    4 Reducing body weight

15. The best diet for a person with hypertension includes
    1 Low sodium, low potassium, and with liberal fluids.
    2 Low sodium, fresh fruits, and vegetables.
    3 Foods that are high in saturated fat and low in cholesterol.
    4 Foods that are low in fat and moderate amounts of alcohol.

NCLEX® Review Answers

Section A

1. **3** High-density lipoproteins carry fat away from arteries. High-density lipoproteins have no effect on the diameter or elasticity of blood vessels. Drugs can inhibit platelet activity, but lipoproteins do not.

2. **2** People with diabetes tend to experience problems with lipid metabolism, which can contribute to hyperlipidemia. Hypothyroidism contributes to hyperlipidemia, not hyperthyroidism. Pancreatitis can occur as an indirect consequence of hyperlipidemia but does not, in and of itself, elevate lipid levels. Patients who are malnourished tend to have low, not elevated, lipid levels.

3. **2** Patients who have risk factors should keep their LDL level at 130 mg/dL or less. Patients who have already had cardiovascular disease should strive to keep their LDL-C level at 100 mg/dL or lower. Patients with LDL-C levels over 130 mg/dL are considered to be at increased risk for cardiovascular disease.

4. **4** Heat causes vasodilation and thus it is not a contraindication. Caffeine causes vasoconstriction and thus is contraindicated for the patient with vascular disease. Sunlight does not affect vascular disease, unless excessive exposure to sunlight is involved, which causes vasodilation. NSAIDs are not contraindicated in patients with vascular disease.

5. **3** A classic symptom of Raynaud's phenomenon is bluish-white blanching of one or more fingers. Raynaud's phenomenon does not initially cause redness or swelling. Burning pain typically occurs after circulation has been restored, but the fingertips do not itch.

Section B

6. **3** Increased arterial flow does not contribute to venous stasis. Heart failure, compression of veins by masses, and severe hypotension contribute to venous stasis.

7. **2** Pneumatic compression devices are used to prevent venous pooling in the hospitalized, immobilized patient. Pneumatic compression devices do not help venous dilation, venous ulcers, or venous distention.

8. **4** Avoiding salt in daily diet does not affect venous stasis. Engaging in regular structured exercise, maintaining ideal body weight, and preventing injury to the lower extremities can decrease the effect of venous stasis and should be a part of routine patient teaching.

9. **3** Compression therapy reduces swelling and improves oxygenation of tissue, which promotes healing. Occlusive dressings are used to protect venous ulcers from further damage or infection. Compression therapy does not dissolve blood clots; medication is required.

10. **3** Coagulation defects do not contribute to the development of venous stasis. Obesity, a sedentary lifestyle, and abdominal masses contribute to venous stasis.

Section C

11. **3** Suddenly discontinuing antihypertensive drugs can result in a malignant hypertension, not hypotension. Renal damage and angina can be an indirect consequence of the malignant hypertension, but do not ensue as a result of stopping drug therapy.

12. **2** Excess consumption of alcohol in conjunction with other risk factors is most likely to cause hypertension. Electrolyte (e.g., calcium, potassium) imbalances do not generally affect blood pressure. Depression can indirectly cause a stress response, which can then elevate blood pressure.

13. **2** Poorly controlled hypertension causes damage to the vascular endothelium and increases the workload of the heart, both of which contribute to coronary artery disease.

14. **4** Weight reduction is the most efficient way to reduce blood pressure. Eating foods high in protein increases the consumption of animal fat, which is known to contribute to the development of hypertension. For most patients, stress cannot be avoided, but they can learn techniques and strategies for coping with stress. Tobacco use should be eliminated to decrease blood pressure; merely reducing consumption does not lower blood pressure.

15. **2** A diet that is low in sodium, with liberal amounts of fresh fruits and vegetables, is most desirable for the patient with hypertensive disease. Patients with hypertension may need to avoid excess fluids, particularly when they have cardiac disease in conjunction with hypertension. Diets high in saturated fat and even moderate alcohol consumption have both been shown to contribute to hypertension.

Notes

Alterations in Cardiovascular Function

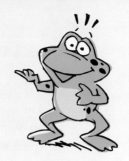

What You WILL LEARN

After reading this chapter, you will know how to do the following:

- ✔ Discuss the different causes of cardiovascular disease.
- ✔ Identify modifiable and nonmodifiable risk factors that contribute to the development of cardiovascular disease.
- ✔ List assessment findings commonly seen in patients with cardiovascular disease.
- ✔ Establish a prioritized plan of care for patients with cardiovascular disease.

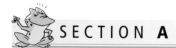

SECTION A

DISORDERS RESULTING FROM STRUCTURAL DEFECTS

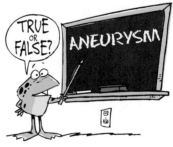

Let's learn the signs.

What IS an Aortic Aneurysm?

An aortic aneurysm is a defect causing dilation or ballooning of the aorta. Aneurysms may occur anywhere within the aorta and are classified according to their location. An aneurysm that occurs within the ascending aorta or within the aortic arch is known as a thoracic aneurysm.

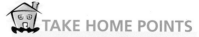

TAKE HOME POINTS

An aortic aneurysm is a defect that causes dilation or ballooning of the aorta.

205

An aneurysm that occurs within the descending aorta in the abdominal area is known as an abdominal aortic aneurysm.

Pathogenesis

The aorta is susceptible to aneurysms because the vessel is under constant pressure. A true aneurysm involves weakening of all three layers of the vessel wall. The three layers of the aorta include the innermost layer (tunica intima), the middle layer (tunica media), and the outermost layer (tunica adventitia). A false aneurysm involves weakening of one or two layers of the aortic wall. Many false aneurysms result from a tear in one or two vessel layers.

A dissecting aneurysm occurs when blood accumulates in the vessel layers. The most common cause of an aortic aneurysm is atherosclerosis. The accumulation of plaque weakens the walls of the aorta, causing them to tear and bulge, which forms an aneurysm. Hypertension is also a contributing factor because the high pressure further stresses the aorta. Other causes include syphilis and any type of infection that affects the aorta.

At-Risk Populations

There are several risk factors that contribute to aneurysms. Atherosclerosis and hypertension are the highest risk conditions associated with aortic aneurysms and are found in 50% of individuals with an aortic aneurysm. Other risk factors include Marfan's syndrome, congenital defects, and coarctation of the aorta. Marfan's syndrome is a genetic disorder characterized by a breakdown of the collagen fibers of the aorta; a fusiform aneurysm develops, which affects the thoracic ascending aorta.

> A dissecting aneurysm is a life-threatening condition. As blood accumulates within the layers, the layers separate and tear away from each other, spreading down the entire aorta.

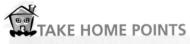

TAKE HOME POINTS

The primary causes of aneurysms include atherosclerosis and hypertension.

What You NEED TO KNOW

Clinical Manifestations

The signs and symptoms of aortic aneurysms vary, depending on the location of the defect. Most patients with an aneurysm are asymptomatic until the aneurysm begins to tear and leak. A large thoracic aneurysm can cause stridor when it presses on the trachea. An abdominal aortic aneurysm can cause a pulsating abdominal mass that can be visualized or felt.

A tear that occurs in one of the layers of the arterial wall is known as a dissection, a major complication of an aneurysm. Blood leaks in between the layers of the aneurysm and expands along an area of the aorta. The thoracic ascending area is the most common place for a dissecting aortic aneurysm, primarily because this area is under the greatest pressure from the left ventricle ejecting blood.

Clinical manifestations of a dissecting aneurysm occur suddenly, producing a sudden onset of severe chest pain that radiates to the neck and back. Initially, the blood pressure is elevated; then it will drop rapidly from the sudden loss of blood as the aorta dissects. The patient develops signs and symptoms associated with hemorrhagic shock, including tachycardia, hypotension, cold and clammy skin, decreased urine output, and weak or thready peripheral pulses. When the body experiences a decrease in the circulating volume, baroreceptors located in the carotid arteries and the aorta stimulate the sympathetic nervous system, thus producing the symptoms of hemorrhagic shock. These receptors sense the low blood pressure and stimulate the sympathetic nervous system. The stimulation causes constriction of arterioles in the body, shunting blood flow to the brain and heart. Because blood flow to the kidneys is also shunted away, the vasoconstriction produces the cool skin, weak pulse, and decreased urine output. Paralysis of the lower extremities can occur when an abdominal aortic aneurysm dissects into the area where the spinal arteries branch. A dissecting thoracic ascending aortic aneurysm near the aortic valve can tear and damage the aortic valve or cause a myocardial infarction from bleeding, sending clots through the coronary arteries. The coronary arteries originate from the base of the aorta.

> A dissecting aneurysm is an emergency situation and represents the most critical aspect of nursing care for a patient, largely because the patient looses blood quickly, resulting in immediate death. An aneurysm located in the thoracic ascending aorta or aortic arch produces the greatest signs and symptoms of hemorrhagic shock. Occasionally, the patient has symptoms that mimic an acute myocardial infarction (MI).

Prognosis

The prognosis depends on the location and size of the aneurysm. Sudden rupture of an aneurysm can be fatal, particularly when the aneurysm is large. Emergency surgery after a rupture carries a mortality rate in excess of 50%.

What You DO

Treatment

Treatment for an aneurysm is surgical repair. The aneurysm is excised and a synthetic graft sewn in its place. Surgery is usually performed when the aneurysm is greater than 5 cm; smaller aneurysms are usually not at risk for dissection or rupture. Abdominal aneurysms can also be

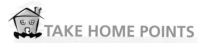
TAKE HOME POINTS

Surgical repair is necessary for aneurysms larger than 5 cm because of the risk of dissection and rupture.

repaired by a less invasive approach called endovascular repair. The procedure involves placing a graft within the aorta via the femoral artery, thus avoiding a surgical incision. Other indications for surgery include the following:

- Progressive increase in size
- Symptoms causing cerebral or coronary ischemia
- Pain
- Pericardial tamponade (i.e., blood leaking into the pericardial sac)
- Leaking, threatened, or actual rupture
- Visceral ischemia

Nursing Responsibilities

Prompt treatment and emergency surgery are required. The nurse must remain with the patient and administer intravenous fluids, such as normal saline or Ringer's lactate. Blood transfusions must be given to maintain the systolic blood pressure between 100 and 120 mm Hg or a mean arterial pressure between 60 and 80 mm Hg. A blood pressure in this range maintains adequate tissue perfusion (oxygen and nutrients supplied to the tissues) and helps prevent further dissection or rupture of the aneurysm.

A urine output of at least 30 mL per hour or 0.5 mL/kg/hr should also be maintained; if urine output falls, acute renal failure can result. In addition, the patient should not be given anything by mouth in anticipation of surgery. Several nursing interventions are required in caring for a patient with an aortic aneurysm. The nurse should do the following:

- Avoid palpating an abdominal pulsating mass to prevent rupture of the aneurysm.
- Report any signs and symptoms of dissection immediately to the health care provider, and prepare the patient for emergency surgery.
- Evaluate circulation in all extremities by assessing for color, temperature, capillary refill, and quality of pulse. A leaking thoracic aneurysm will decrease circulation to all extremities; an abdominal aneurysm will impair circulation to the lower extremities.
- Administer antihypertensive drugs if the patient with an aneurysm is hypertensive. If antihypertensive drugs taken by mouth are ineffective, intravenous formulations that dilate arteries may be given. The drugs commonly used include nitroprusside, nitroglycerin, fenoldopam, and labetalol.

Do You UNDERSTAND?

DIRECTIONS: **In the space provided, write the letter that corresponds to the phrase that answers each question.**

_____ 1. A patient who is diagnosed with a thoracic aneurysm suddenly complains of severe chest and neck pain and is anxious. What is the first nursing intervention for this patient?
   a. Administer pain drug
   b. Assess vital signs
   c. Administer intravenous fluids
   d. Call the health care provider

_____ 2. Your patient has a dissecting abdominal aneurysm. The vital signs are as follows: blood pressure, 150/70 mm Hg; pulse, 120 beats per minute (bpm); urine output, 35 mL/hr. What is the most important intervention for this patient?
   a. Administer intravenous fluids.
   b. Administer a vasoconstrictor to increase the blood pressure.
   c. Administer a vasodilator to decrease the blood pressure.
   d. Place the patient supine.

_____ 3. Maintaining a urine output more than 30 mL/hr for a patient with a dissecting aneurysm is important for what reason?
   a. To prevent acute renal failure
   b. To prevent renal hemorrhage
   c. To reduce pressure on the aneurysm
   d. To prevent further bleeding from the aneurysm

_____ 4. What type of aneurysm will produce profound shock?
   a. Descending aortic aneurysm
   b. Abdominal aortic aneurysm
   c. Abdominal saccular aneurysm
   d. Ascending aortic aneurysm

Answers: 1. b; 2. c; 3. a; 4. d.

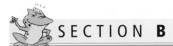

SECTION B

ENDOCARDIAL AND VALVULAR HEART DISEASE

What IS Valvular Heart Disease?

Valvular heart disease is damage to the structure of one or more of the heart valves resulting from a variety of diseases and conditions. Valvular heart disease usually affects the mitral or aortic valve. Valvular heart disease can affect the tricuspid and pulmonic valve, but such damage is rare and is usually congenital when it occurs. A variety of congenital or acquired conditions can cause valvular heart disease including the following:

- Ischemia (MI)
- Infection (endocarditis)
- Inflammation (rheumatic fever)
- Calcification
- Trauma

Because rheumatic fever frequently causes valvular heart disease, further discussion is warranted. Rheumatic fever is an abnormal immune or inflammatory response to group A beta-hemolytic streptococcus. Rheumatic fever has a 3% chance of developing as a result of a streptococcal infection. Typically, this type of streptococcal infection occurs in either the skin or the throat ("strep throat"). Toxins that are produced from streptococcus stimulate the immune system. The antibodies produced by the immune system to attack the bacteria also attack the connective tissues of the heart. All layers of the heart can be affected, resulting in inflammation of the endocardium (endocarditis), the myocardium (myocarditis), or the pericardium (pericarditis). The valves are affected when endocarditis occurs because of the inflammation of the innermost layer of the heart where the heart valves are located. One or more of the valves become inflamed, and vegetative lesions develop on the valve leaflets. Eventually, as the inflammatory response resolves, the affected valve or valves develop scar tissue, which alters the shape of the valve. When the valve leaflets become rigid and deformed, the condition is then referred to as rheumatic heart disease. This condition develops

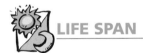

LIFE SPAN

In children, rheumatic fever can affect the heart, the joints, the skin, and the central nervous system. During the acute stages, the patient may have inflammation of the valves, the myocardium, and the pericardium, as well as cardiac enlargement **(cardiomegaly)** and heart failure. Narrowing of the valves **(stenosis)** may eventually require surgical intervention.

after acute or repeated episodes of rheumatic fever. Recurrent episodes of rheumatic fever typically occur within 5 years of the initial episode.

Pathogenesis

Two types of general structural damage can occur in valvular heart disease: stenosis and incompetence. When a valve is stenotic, narrowing within the orifice occurs when the valve opens. Narrowing presents a problem because flow of blood from behind the valve is restricted through the valve. As a result, excess blood remains in the chamber behind the valve. Narrowing also creates resistance against which the heart chamber must pump. The chamber pumping through the stenosed valve must work harder than normal to push blood through the narrow opening. Eventually the walls of the chamber behind the stenosed valve become thickened and enlarged (hypertrophy) as a result of the excess blood remaining in the chamber and because of having to pump with an increased force.

An incompetent valve is one in which the leaflets "flap back" and cause the valve to partially open when it should be closed. Such a valve allows blood from the chamber in front of the valve to leak back into the chamber behind the valve. Insufficiency and regurgitation are the terms used to describe the back flow of blood from the incitement valve. Excess blood builds up in the chamber behind the valve and the chamber eventually thickens (hypertrophies).

All types of valvular heart disease will eventually lead to heart failure and pulmonary congestion as the conditions worsen. The most common types of valvular heart disease are summarized in the following text.

The murmur associated with valvular heart disease is heard because of the turbulent blood flow that occurs when it is passing through a stenosed valve or is regurgitating through an incompetent valve. The sound is usually a swishing or blowing sound.

A murmur can be heard either during the first heart sound (systole) or during the second heart sound (diastole). A murmur heard during systole is referred to as a systolic murmur, and a murmur heard during diastole is referred to as a diastolic murmur. A systolic murmur may represent either aortic stenosis or mitral insufficiency. The murmur can be aortic stenosis because, during systole, the left ventricle is ejecting blood through the aortic valve. A systolic murmur can be a result of mitral insufficiency because, during systole, the mitral valve should be closed. However, when the valve is incompetent, blood from the left ventricle regurgitates through the mitral valve during systole.

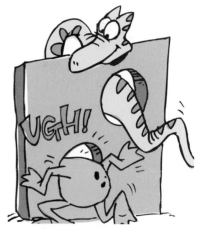

Narrowed valves can block the flow of blood.

A diastolic murmur indicates either mitral stenosis or aortic regurgitation. The murmur may indicate mitral stenosis because, during diastole, blood is leaving the left atrium and passing into the left ventricle. A diastolic murmur can also be a result of aortic insufficiency because, during diastole, the aortic valve should be closed. However, when the valve is incompetent, the blood regurgitates from the aorta back into the left ventricle.

Mitral Stenosis. During diastole, blood flow from the left atrium to the left ventricle decreases. This causes a decrease in cardiac output, because the left ventricle ejects less blood to the body than is normal. Blood backs up from the left atrium to the pulmonary system and can cause pulmonary edema or pulmonary hypertension as a result of the increased pressure in the pulmonary system. Because of the high pressure in the pulmonary system, the left atrium eventually enlarges, and right ventricular failure results.

Mitral Insufficiency or Regurgitation. During systole, some of the blood from the left ventricle regurgitates into the left atrium. This results in a decrease in cardiac output, because the left ventricle ejects less blood than is normal. Because blood backs up from the left atrium to the pulmonary system, pulmonary congestion and right ventricular failure can result. Eventually, left ventricular hypertrophy and left atrial enlargement occur.

A prolapsed mitral valve is a type of mitral insufficiency and occurs when one or both of the valve cusps flap into the left atrium during systole.

> ⚠ All four of the valve disorders ultimately lead to heart failure without treatment or when the condition worsens.

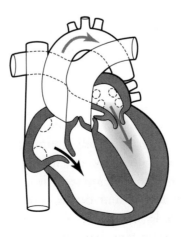

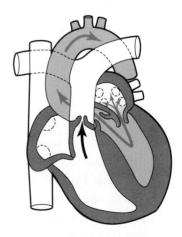

MITRAL STENOSIS   MITRAL INSUFFICIENCY

Aortic Stenosis. During systole, the left ventricle is unable to eject all of the blood through the narrow opening of the aortic valve, causing a decrease in blood flow to the systemic circulation. Because not all of the blood is able to pass through the narrowed aortic valve, cardiac output decreases. Left ventricular hypertrophy results because of the excess blood remaining in the ventricle and because the left ventricle has to pump harder to get blood through the narrow opening in the aortic valve. Blood eventually backs up into the left atrium and then into the pulmonary system, and right ventricular failure can result because of the increased pressure within the pulmonary system.

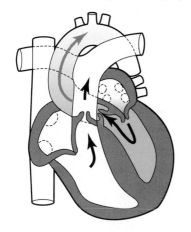 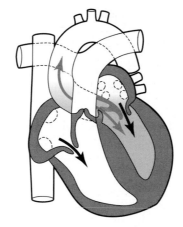

AORTIC STENOSIS   AORTIC INSUFFICIENCY

Aortic Insufficiency or Regurgitation. During diastole blood regurgitates back from the aorta into the left ventricle. This results in a decrease in cardiac output, because not all of the blood passes through the aorta into the systemic circulation. Left ventricular hypertrophy, increased pulmonary congestion, and right ventricular failure can result.

At-Risk Populations

Any individual with a valvular defect is at risk for cardiac complications. Patients with minor structural defects may be asymptomatic until they develop a coexisting illness or stressor that adversely affects cardiac function. Risks for valvular heart disease include atherosclerosis, myocardial infarction, endocarditis, rheumatic fever, hypertension, and pulmonary disease causing pulmonary hypertension (high pressure within the pulmonary arteries).

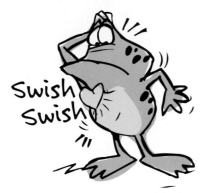

Cardiac murmurs can cause a blowing or swishing sound.

What You NEED TO KNOW

Clinical Manifestations

Clinical manifestations of valvular heart disease depend on the nature and severity of the particular valve disorder. Patients can be asymptomatic with only mild stenosis or insufficiency of the valve. Primary symptoms of left ventricular failure include dyspnea on exertion, crackles in the lungs, a nonproductive cough, weakness, and fatigue. As the condition worsens, pulmonary edema can develop. Eventually, if right ventricular failure results, then symptoms such as jugular vein distention, hepatomegaly, and peripheral edema will occur. Patients with mitral stenosis can develop atrial arrhythmias (i.e., abnormal cardiac rhythms originating from the atria) because of the enlarged left atrium. A patient with detectable valvular heart disease usually has a murmur that can be auscultated. The murmur results because of turbulent blood flow either through a stenosed valve or regurgitating back from an incompetent valve.

Prognosis

The prognosis for recovery from valvular heart disease depends on the severity of the defect, the presence of coexisting diseases that can adversely affect cardiac function, and the patient's access to prompt and appropriate medical care.

What You DO

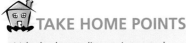

TAKE HOME POINTS

Valvular heart disease is treated with drugs. Surgery to repair or replace the valve is indicated for patients experiencing symptoms of heart failure.

Treatment

Several drugs are used to treat valvular heart disease. Treatment includes primarily the management of heart failure. Digoxin is given to increase myocardial contractility and slow the heart rate. Diuretics are used to reduce excess fluid, thus the weakened ventricles will have less blood to pump. An angiotensin converting enzyme (ACE) inhibitor is also used because it dilates systemic arterioles, which decreases the pressure within the vessels, and relieves symptoms of heart failure. This reduction in pressure decreases the resistance against which the weakened left ventricle has to pump during systole.

Valve surgery is the treatment of choice for patients experiencing symptoms of heart failure or when the left ventricle is at risk for failure. Valves can be either replaced or repaired. Three types of reconstructive surgery can be performed. Open commissurotomy is typically performed for mitral stenosis, which involves incising fused leaflets and removing calcium deposits on the valve. An annuloplasty is typically performed for mitral insufficiency, which involves the insertion of a ring to reduce the size of a dilated mitral valve. A valvuloplasty involves a variety of techniques used to repair valves, such as patching damaged portions of a valve or removing excess tissue or calcium deposits on a valve. Valve replacement surgery is performed for a severely damaged valve that cannot be repaired. The valve is removed and replaced with either a tissue or prosthetic valve.

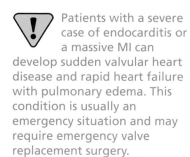

Patients with a severe case of endocarditis or a massive MI can develop sudden valvular heart disease and rapid heart failure with pulmonary edema. This condition is usually an emergency situation and may require emergency valve replacement surgery.

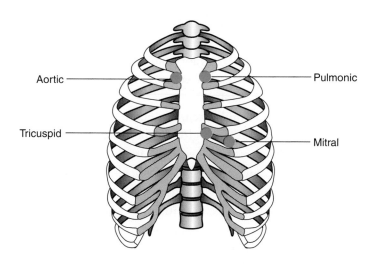

Aortic

Pulmonic

Tricuspid

Mitral

TAKE HOME POINTS

Murmurs are best heard over the following areas:

Type of murmur	Location to auscultate
Aortic	2nd intercostal space, right sternal border
Pulmonic	2nd intercostal space, left sternal border
Tricuspid	5th intercostal space, left sternal border
Mitral	5th intercostal space, midclavicular line

Nursing Responsibilities

The nurse caring for a patient with valvular heart disease should be able to recognize the basic heart murmurs associated with the specific disorder. Auscultating for murmurs is a difficult skill and must be practiced. The best way to become familiar with murmurs is to always auscultate heart sounds on patients with known valvular heart disease. For example, if you read in the history and physical examination that the patient has aortic stenosis, auscultate the heart sounds and listen for the murmur. Become familiar with the circulation of blood through the heart, and know which valves should be opened and closed during systole and diastole.

The following list highlights simple steps in auscultating for murmurs:

- Listen for the first or systolic heart sound (S_1) and then for the second or diastolic heart sound (S_2).
- Determine whether the murmur occurs during the first or second heart sound and whether it is a systolic or diastolic murmur.
- Listen over the four points on the precordium where each valve is best heard. If you hear the murmur louder in the area over a specific valve, that valve is likely to be damaged.
- Determine whether the valve has stenosis or insufficiency by assessing whether the murmur is systolic or diastolic.
  1. Auscultate both heart sounds.
  2. Listen for a murmur during the first heart sound to know that the murmur is systolic.
  3. Listen over the four areas of heart sounds, and determine if the murmur is loudest over the aortic area.
  4. If so, the patient likely has aortic stenosis because (a) the murmur is systolic, and (b) the left ventricle is pumping blood through the aorta during systole.
- Teach patients and family members about early treatment of skin and throat infections. When group A beta-hemolytic streptococcus infection is left untreated, rheumatic fever may result. Antibiotic therapy is a mainstay of treatment. Penicillin is the drug of choice although erythromycin or clindamycin can be used if the patient is allergic to penicillin. Teaching must include the importance of completing antibiotic therapy as prescribed.
- Assess for signs and symptoms of heart failure and report these immediately to the health care provider; symptoms can indicate worsening of the valve dysfunction. Signs and symptoms of heart failure include shortness of breath, crackles, dyspnea on exertion, jugular vein distention, peripheral edema, and weight gain.
- Notify the health care provider if the patient becomes hypotensive and the skin becomes cool and clammy. These symptoms indicate that the left ventricle is failing significantly and insufficient blood is being pumped to the body.
- Report signs and symptoms of pulmonary edema. It is an emergency situation that can lead to respiratory failure. Signs and

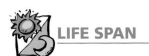

LIFE SPAN

Appropriate antibiotic therapy is particularly important for children to decrease the risk of cardiac complications in adulthood.

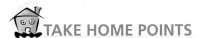

TAKE HOME POINTS

Patients with valvular heart disease should receive prophylactic antibiotics before any invasive procedure, including dental work, to prevent endocarditis.

symptoms of pulmonary edema include severe labored breathing, tachycardia, crackles in all lung fields, and pink, frothy sputum.

• Report any fever to the health care provider immediately; endocarditis may be the cause of the fever. Turbulent blood flow through damaged valves increases the risk for patients to develop endocarditis.

Do You UNDERSTAND?

DIRECTIONS: **In the space provided, write the letter that corresponds to the phrase that answers each question.**

_____ 1. Which statement by a patient with rheumatic fever indicates that further teaching is required?

a. "I will need to take antibiotics for 10 days and for 5 years after my diagnosis."

b. "I only need to take antibiotics for 10 days."

c. "I will need to take a dose of an antibiotic for 5 years to prevent the infection from returning."

d. "I should not miss any doses of the antibiotics."

_____ 2. Which one of the following statements defines an incompetent valve?

a. It has a narrow opening

b. The valve leaflets are fused and unable to open

c. The leaflets flap backward when the valve should be closed

d. The leaflets flap inward when the valve should be open

Answers: 1. b; 2. c.

Monitor preload and afterload.

TAKE HOME POINTS

Heart failure is the most common cause of mortality in cardiac disease and is responsible for one third of deaths as a complication of MI.

What IS Heart Failure?

To understand heart failure, the nurse must first understand the cardiac cycle, including the concepts of preload and afterload.

The cardiac cycle is made up of two phases: diastole and systole. During diastole the ventricles fill with blood from the atria. **Preload** refers to the amount of stretching imposed on the myocardial fibers by blood coming into the heart at the end of diastole. The amount of blood the left ventricle ejects into the circulation is known as **cardiac output.** Specifically, cardiac output is the amount of blood that is ejected expressed in liters per minute. Normal cardiac output in the adult is 4 to 8 liters per minute. Preload is important because it affects cardiac output.

During the second phase of the cardiac cycle (systole), the ventricles eject blood. The left ventricle ejects blood through the aorta to systemic arteries; the right ventricle ejects blood through the pulmonary artery into the lungs. These arteries create resistance that the ventricles must overcome **(Afterload).** The resistance depends on the diameter of the vessels. If the vessels are dilated, pressure and resistance decreases. If the vessels are constricted (narrowed), pressure and resistance increases. Left ventricular afterload is important because it directly affects the cardiac output.

Heart failure occurs when the heart muscle fails to pump a sufficient amount of blood to meet the complex metabolic demands of the body. A complex clinical syndrome develops that is characterized by dyspnea and fatigue secondary to structural and functional changes in the heart which occurs in the milieu of neurohormonal activation and cytokine release.

Heart failure can be either an acute or a chronic condition. Acute heart failure occurs suddenly. Persons with chronic heart failure can develop episodes of acute heart failure when treatment is ineffective or when a sudden illness develops. Chronic heart failure develops slowly and progressively with retention of sodium and water. Several conditions can result in heart failure: atherosclerosis, hypertension, MI, valvular heart disease, cardiomyopathy, arrhythmias, and circulatory overload.

Pathogenesis

Two basic types of heart failure have been identified: left ventricular failure and right ventricular failure. The most common type is left ventricular failure. In most cases, primary left ventricular failure will lead to secondary right ventricular failure. These patients are said to have biventricular failure because both ventricles fail.

With left ventricular failure, the left ventricle is weak and unable to pump all of its blood into systemic circulation. A reduction in cardiac output results because of the decreased amounts of blood ejected by the left ventricle. The weak left ventricle is unable to empty all of its blood from the chamber, thus an increase in left ventricular preload is present. The residual volume of blood makes emptying all of the left atrium's blood into the left ventricle during diastole difficult. The left atrium now overfills, and the pulmonary veins are unable to return all of the blood from the pulmonary arteries into the left atrium. The buildup of blood in the pulmonary arteries causes congestion and increases pressure within the vessels. The high pressure eventually forces fluid from the pulmonary arteries into the alveoli, and fluid enters the lungs. At this point, the patient develops pulmonary symptoms such as crackles, dyspnea, and an increase in respiratory rate.

Right ventricular failure follows left ventricular failure. The right ventricle becomes involved because the high pressure and congestion within the pulmonary system prevents the right ventricle from emptying all of its blood through the pulmonary artery. The right ventricle overfills with blood, and now the right atrium is unable to empty all of its blood into the right ventricle. The veins throughout the body that return blood to the heart via the superior and inferior vena cava into the right atrium are unable to return all of the blood, and venous congestion results. The patient now develops systemic symptoms, such as jugular vein distention and peripheral edema. High pressure and excess fluid in the veins causes edema because high pressure forces fluid into the space between the vascular space and tissues **(interstitial space).**

When heart failure occurs, various neurohormonal mechanisms respond to the low cardiac output. These compensatory attempts actually worsen heart failure. Low cardiac output stimulates the sympathetic nervous system, resulting in tachycardia and vasoconstriction of the systemic arteries. The increase in heart rate increases myocardial oxygen demand and shortens diastole. Decreasing the time for the ventricles

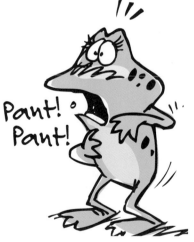

Loss of breath.

to fill with blood during diastole further decreases cardiac output. Vasoconstriction of the systemic arteries occurs in order to shunt blood flow to the brain and the heart. This compensatory mechanism increases the systemic vascular resistance (afterload) the weak left ventricle has to pump against. Indications of peripheral vasoconstriction include weak, intermittent (thready) or nonpalpable peripheral pulses, cool skin, diaphoresis, and decreased or absent urine output. The neurotransmitters released cause more vasoconstriction; these include vasopressin from the pituitary gland and endothelin from the endothelial cells lining the blood vessels.

A decrease in blood flow to the kidneys stimulates the renin-angiotensin-aldosterone system (RAAS), which causes additional systemic vasoconstriction and causes the kidneys to retain sodium and water. The decreased blood flow to the kidneys triggers the kidneys to release an enzyme, renin. Once renin is released, it stimulates the formation of angiotensin converting enzyme (ACE), which converts angiotensin I to angiotensin II. Angiotensin II produces several detrimental effects in the presence of heart failure. Angiotensin II is a very potent vasoconstrictor, so it increases left ventricular afterload. It also stimulates thirst, making a person in acute decompensated heart failure drink despite the fluid over-load. Angiotensin II stimulates release of aldosterone from the adrenal gland. Aldosterone causes the kidneys to retain fluid and sodium which results in a decreased urine output.

In acute decompensated heart failure there is increase in volume and pressures within the ventricles and the atria. The increase in volume and pressure activates a counterregulatory mechanism that attempts to counteract the RAAS. The increase in volume and pressure stimulates the release of natriuretic polypeptides into the circulation. A-type natriuretic polypeptide is released from the atria; B-type natriuretic polypeptide is released from the ventricles; and C-type from the endothelial cells within blood vessels. Natriuretic polypeptides cause systemic vasodilation and increases urine output, which are opposite effects from that of the RAAS. Unfortunately, during acute decompensated heart failure, the RAAS is more powerful than natriuretic polypeptides and overrides those counterregulatory mechanisms.

Over time, heart failure will result in left ventricular hypertrophy (enlarged left ventricle) from the ventricle pumping against continuous high pressure within the systemic circulation. The myocytes eventually become enlarged developing an abnormal shape and restricting effective contraction of the myocardium. The change in shape of the myocytes is known as remodeling.

Heart failure is classified several ways. It can be classified as acute or chronic, with acute occurring when acute symptoms are present and chronic where there are slow progressive symptoms, but the heart failure is compensated. Heart failure can be classified as systolic or diastolic failure. The majority of heart failure is systolic failure, where the left ventricle is unable to eject sufficient blood during systole. Diastolic failure is less common and involves a stiff or rigid left ventricle, which decreases the left ventricle's capability to stretch back during diastole and fill with sufficient blood. A common classification system used to classify heart failure comes from the New York Heart Association and is based on patient symptoms.

Class I—no signs of failure

Class II—symptoms with exertion

Class III—dyspnea with less than ordinary level of activities

Class IV—symptoms when at rest, severe limitations on activities

At-Risk Populations

A variety of diseases and conditions place people at risk for heart failure. These conditions include MI, arrhythmias, cardiomyopathy, and valvular heart defects. Other conditions adversely affecting the pumping action of the heart include systemic hypertension, chronic obstructive pulmonary disease, and thyrotoxicosis.

What You NEED TO KNOW

Clinical Manifestations

Clinical manifestations of heart failure are related to low cardiac output and the presence of left or right ventricular failure. The lower the cardiac output, the stronger the sympathetic response. Signs and symptoms include tachycardia, decreased urine output, dark amber urine, weak pulses, and cool skin. As mentioned, pulmonary symptoms reflect left ventricular failure, and systemic symptoms indicate right ventricular failure. If both pulmonary and systemic symptoms are present, the person is in biventricular failure.

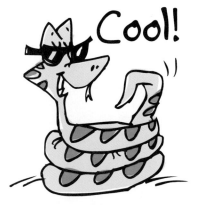

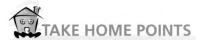
TAKE HOME POINTS

Signs and symptoms of heart failure include tachycardia, decreased urine output, dark amber urine, weak pulse, and cool skin.

The two most dangerous complications of heart failure are pulmonary edema and cardiogenic shock. If treatment is not implemented immediately, respiratory arrest will follow.

Heart Failure

Pulmonary Symptoms Associated with Left-Sided Heart Failure	Systemic Symptoms Associated with Right-Sided Heart Failure
• Tachypnea, dyspnea	• Jugular vein distention
• Pulmonary crackles	• Peripheral edema
• Restlessness (from hypoxemia)	• Hepatomegaly

Pulmonary edema occurs as the result of acute left ventricular failure. Fluid builds up in the pulmonary vessels to the extent that the fluid forces its way from the capillary bed into the alveoli. The fluid literally "drowns" the patient. Clinical manifestations of pulmonary edema include extreme dyspnea and tachypnea, tachycardia, restlessness or agitation, sense of impending doom and panic, severe crackles in all lung fields, and pink, frothy sputum. The sputum is pink because some blood enters the alveoli from the capillary vessels. Pulmonary edema can be reversed when appropriate treatment is initiated in a timely manner. An immediate intravenous dose of a loop diuretic such as furosemide, bumetanide, or torsemide will reverse pulmonary edema if administered in a timely fashion.

Cardiogenic shock is a complication of heart failure, with a 75% to 95% mortality rate. This emergency situation occurs at either the end stage of chronic heart failure or suddenly after a massive MI. In cardiogenic shock, less than 20% of the myocardium is contracting normally. The left ventricle is unable to eject sufficient blood to deliver oxygen to the body (low tissue perfusion). This condition is a state of shock because shock, by definition, is a decrease in circulating volume insufficient to provide oxygen and nutrients to the tissues. Clinical manifestations of cardiogenic shock include hypotension (systolic blood pressure less than 90 mm Hg) and sympathetic symptoms such as tachycardia, cold and diaphoretic skin, weak, thready pulse, and little or no urine output.

Prognosis

Despite recent treatment advances, patients with heart failure have poor survival rates. Of those who survive the first acute episode of failure, 50% die within 5 years. Mortality rates are increased in men, older adults, and those with underlying heart disease.

What You DO

Treatment

A variety of drugs are used to treat heart failure; each aimed at reducing preload and afterload and increasing contractility. ACE inhibitors are a mainstay of treatment and are used to counteract the RAAS by inhibiting ACE thus preventing the conversion of angiotensin II. By blocking the formation of angiotensin II, systemic vasodilation results thus reducing afterload. If a person is unable to take an ACE inhibitor, an angiotensin II receptor blocker may be given. These drugs block the effect of angiotensin II through inhibition at the receptor site.

Loop diuretics are used to pull fluid from the alveoli and reduce the circulating volume, thereby reducing preload. Nitroglycerin is also used to reduce preload because it primarily dilates veins. When veins are dilated, less blood returns to the heart, and thus the ventricles fill with less blood. When dilation occurs, the pressure decreases within systemic arteries, resulting in a decrease in resistance or left ventricular afterload. Nesiritide, a recombinant form of B-type natriuretic peptide, is an intravenous drug used to treat acute decompensated heart failure. The drug overpowers the RAAS by causing systemic vasodilation and increases urine output. Beta-adrenergic blockers, such as metoprolol, may also be used to prevent tachycardia and prevent remodeling. For acute decompensated heart failure, where there is low perfusion (decreased urine output, decreased blood pressure, etc), inotropic drugs such as dobutamine and milrinone may be used. These drugs increase the force of contraction of the myocardium.

TAKE HOME POINTS

Treatment of heart failure includes drugs such as diuretics, ACE inhibitors, inotropic drugs, and beta-adrenergic blockers.

Nursing Responsibilities

The nurse should be aware that all patients with chronic heart failure have the potential to develop acute heart failure. The nurse must be alert to early signs and symptoms of an acute episode, which include worsening of symptoms (e.g., increasing dyspnea), increasing heart rate, and development or worsening of crackles. These crackles are best auscultated in the posterior bases of the lungs because fluid gravitates to the lowest areas of the lungs.

Urine output is the best and most sensitive indicator of cardiac output. Urine output declines before changes in blood pressure or pulse are

When the crackles are auscultated higher than the posterior bases of the lungs, an acute episode of heart failure is occurring and a diuretic is needed immediately to prevent pulmonary edema.

observed. When blood flow to the kidneys is sufficient, tissue perfusion is also sufficient, thus urine output is maintained. The nurse must also immediately report when the patient's urine output averages less than 30 mL/hour or 0.5 mL/kg/hr, an indication that cardiac output is decreased to the point of diminishing organ perfusion. When cardiac output drops, blood flow to the kidneys is immediately shunted away.

Nursing care centers on preventing acute episodes and preventing complications and therefore the nurse should do the following:

- Maintain the patient in a semi-Fowler's to a high-Fowler's position to reduce preload. Venous return is reduced with the head in an upright position.
- Give drugs as ordered, and do not omit doses. Drugs such as nitroglycerin, ACE inhibitors, and diuretics decrease the systolic blood pressure and can cause hypotension. These drugs should be withheld only when the systolic pressure is less than the parameter ordered by the health care provider, such as 100 or 110 mm Hg. If a patient is on nothing by mouth status (NPO) in anticipation of surgery or a procedure, the nurse should check with the health care provider about administering drugs with small sips of water. The patient may develop acute heart failure or pulmonary edema in surgery or during a procedure if the drugs are not administered.
- Check the potassium level before administering a loop diuretic, which increases the excretion of potassium. Hypokalemia can be dangerous because it causes abnormal ventricular rhythms (ventricular arrhythmias).
- Limit fluid intake by mouth and minimize intravenous fluids used for drugs that reduce preload.
- Maintain strict intake and output measurements. The intake should balance the output, or the output should exceed the input if the patient has acute heart failure.
- Daily weights are necessary to assess whether the patient is retaining fluid. A weight gain of more than 2.5 pounds in 1 day indicates fluid retention. A low-sodium diet should also be maintained to help prevent fluid retention.

Do You UNDERSTAND?

DIRECTIONS: **Fill in the blanks to complete the following statements.**

1. Heart failure occurs when the _____
   _____ fails to pump sufficient blood to meet the needs of the
   body.

2. A weak left ventricle will result in an increase in left ventricular
   _____.

3. A congested left ventricle will eventually causes the person to
   experience _____ because of congestion within
   the pulmonary vessels.

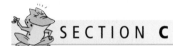

SECTION C

MYOCARDIAL DISORDERS

What IS Cardiomyopathy?

Cardiomyopathy is a group of disorders affecting the heart muscle
(**myocardium**). Cardiomyopathy impairs the heart's ability to fill and
eject blood efficiently. The myocardium should normally be able to
stretch and fill with enough blood, and then contract strongly enough
to eject blood out of the chambers. The three basic types of these
disorders are dilated, hypertrophic, and restrictive cardiomyopathy. The
types of cardiomyopathy can be further grouped as either primary or
secondary.

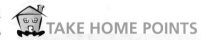

TAKE HOME POINTS

The term cardiomyopathy refers
to a group of disorders that affect
the myocardium, resulting in
decreased ability of the heart to fill
and eject blood efficiently.

Answers: **1. myocardium (or heart muscle); 2. preload; 3. breathlessness.**

Pathogenesis

The cause of primary cardiomyopathy is unknown (idiopathic). Secondary types are a result of other cardiac or noncardiac causes. These are causes of secondary cardiomyopathy:

- Ischemic (coronary artery disease)
- Valvular heart disease
- Severe hypertension
- Alcohol abuse
- Autoimmune disease
- Drugs (some antineoplastic drugs)

The two most common types of secondary cardiomyopathy result from ischemia and hypertension. Ischemic cardiomyopathy occurs from either a massive MI or from multiple MIs. Ischemia from an infarction causes necrosis of the myocardium. When a significant amount of the myocardium is affected, the muscle is unable to fill and contract as efficiently as it should. Chronic severe hypertension causes cardiomyopathy because of the high pressure within the arterioles. Without treatment, the left ventricle has to pump against the high vascular pressure for years. Eventually, the left ventricle enlarges and weakens from being overworked, and the myocardium fails.

Dilated cardiomyopathy consists of severe dilation, which reduces ventricular contractility. The reduction in contraction by the ventricles, particularly the left ventricle, decreases cardiac output and causes heart failure. Most cases of dilated cardiomyopathy are idiopathic, with the other cases resulting from ischemia, cardiotoxic drugs, alcohol, and postpartum conditions. When present, and for reasons unknown, dilated cardiomyopathy in the postpartum patient usually develops 3 to 4 months after delivery.

Hypertrophic cardiomyopathy involves an abnormal thickening of the interventricular septum. The septum becomes greatly thickened to the extent that the left ventricle chamber size is significantly decreased. Occasionally, the septum enlarges asymmetrically within the left ventricle and blocks the outflow of blood from the left ventricle into the systemic circulation **(idiopathic hypertrophic subaortic stenosis [IHSS])**. Usually, survival for hypertrophic cardiomyopathy is long-term.

Restrictive cardiomyopathy occurs when the myocardium becomes rigid and loses compliance, which presents a problem during diastole, primarily because the ventricles are unable to stretch adequately while filling with blood. As a result, the left ventricle fills with a reduced amount

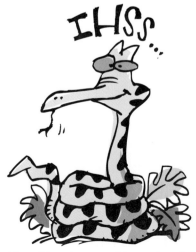

Idiopathic hypertrophic subaortic stenosis.

of blood, thus decreasing cardiac output. Typically, infiltrative diseases of the myocardium, such as amyloidosis, hemochromatosis, and glycogen storage disease, cause restrictive cardiomyopathy. Prognosis is poor, and death usually results from either arrhythmias or heart failure.

At-Risk Populations

Cardiomyopathy can develop in anyone with cardiovascular disease or certain immune-mediated disorders such as rheumatic fever. Risk factors for cardiovascular disease include smoking, obesity, dyslipidemia, and hypertension.

What You NEED TO KNOW

Clinical Manifestations

Clinical manifestations of all types of cardiomyopathy are those associated with heart failure, including shortness of breath **(dyspnea),** fatigue, dyspnea on exertion, crackles, and peripheral edema. Abnormal heart rhythms **(arrhythmias)** are common in all types of cardiomyopathy.

Prognosis

The prognosis for dilated cardiomyopathy depends on the degree of left ventricular function, because left ventricular failure is the primary cause of death. Most deaths occur within 5 years after diagnosis.

What You DO

Treatment

Treatment varies with each type of cardiomyopathy but is aimed at optimizing cardiac output (i.e., the amount of blood the left ventricle pumps to the systemic circulation). For dilated cardiomyopathy, digoxin, dobutamine, and amrinone are used to increase the myocardial contractility, and diuretics are used to reduce excess fluid. ACE inhibitors are used to relieve symptoms of heart failure and dilate the systemic arteries, resulting in decreased pressure within the arteries.

The reduced pressure decreases the workload of the left ventricle because the left ventricle now has less pressure against which to pump during systole. Nitroglycerin is used because it dilates both arteries and veins. Veins return blood from the body to the heart. When veins are dilated, blood pools in the peripheral veins, which decreases the amount of blood returning to the heart. The workload of the myocardium is reduced because the heart now has less blood to pump than is normal.

Treatment for hypertrophic cardiomyopathy includes the use of beta-adrenergic blockers. These drugs inhibit the beta-receptors of the heart to decrease the heart rate. The decreased rate gives more time for the ventricles to fill, which ultimately increases cardiac output.

No definite treatment for restrictive cardiomyopathy exists, other than treating symptoms of heart failure. Beta-adrenergic blockers are occasionally used to increase ventricular filling time, as is the case with hypertrophic cardiomyopathy.

Nursing Responsibilities

Knowing which type of cardiomyopathy the patient has is important because treatment will vary. The most important aspects of nursing care required for a patient with any type of cardiomyopathy are monitoring and treating heart failure.

- Place the patient in a semi-Fowler's to a high-Fowler's position. When the head of the bed is up, venous return to the heart is decreased, thus reducing the workload of the heart.
- Report any episodes of acute heart failure, such as worsening of dyspnea, crackles, increased heart rate, and jugular vein distention. Pulmonary edema, which is an emergency situation requiring prompt treatment, should be reported immediately.

Special considerations for patients with IHSS are needed. Vasodilating drugs and inotropic drugs (drugs that increase contractility)—treatments of choice for most cardiomyopathies—can be dangerous for patients with IHSS. Drugs that reduce venous return to the heart (e.g., nitroglycerin) and drugs that increase contractility (e.g., digoxin, dobutamine, amrinone) should be avoided because these drugs cause an obstruction of the outflow tract (i.e., area from the left ventricle through the aorta), and blood from the left ventricle is blocked and restricted from leaving the left ventricle.

Negative inotropic drugs (i.e., drugs that decrease contractility) can be used to prevent obstruction of blood from the left ventricle through the

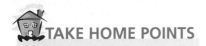

TAKE HOME POINTS

Treatment of cardiomyopathy is aimed at maximizing and supporting cardiac output and preventing acute episodes of heart failure.

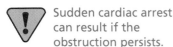

Sudden cardiac arrest can result if the obstruction persists.

aorta. Commonly used drugs include beta-adrenergic blockers and disopyramide.

Intravenous inotropic drugs are used during acute decompensated heart failure for most types of cardiomyopathies except IHSS. The nurse must be familiar with preparation, safe dose ranges, action, and precautions for the drugs. The most common intravenous inotropic drugs used are dobutamine and milrinone.

TAKE HOME POINTS

Dobutamine
- Action: Stimulates B_1 receptors
- Precautions: Increases workload of myocardium; worsens myocardial ischemia

Milrinone (Primocor)
- Action: Positive inotrope; relaxes vascular smooth muscle
- Precautions: Arrhythmias, angina, thrombocytopenia

Do You UNDERSTAND?

DIRECTIONS: **Fill in the blanks by unscrambling the letters. (Not all the words may be used.)**

1. Dobutamine should be used with caution because it can worsen myocardial _____.
2. Drugs that increase _____ should be avoided in patients with IHSS.
3. Vasodilating drugs are helpful in the treatment of cardiomyopathy because they decrease _____.

   misheca   *clicartitnoty*
   prouefis   *reacadc kradolow*

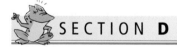

SECTION D

PERICARDIAL DISORDERS

What IS Pericarditis?

Pericarditis is inflammation that occurs within the pericardium. The pericardium is a double-walled membranous sac surrounding the heart. The area between the outer layer (**parietal pericardium**) and the inner layer (**visceral pericardium**) is the pericardial cavity or sac. This cavity

Answers: 1. ischemia; 2. contractility; 3. cardiac workload.

contains approximately 10 to 30 mL of fluid (**pericardial fluid**) which creates a smooth and frictionless atmosphere for the pumping heart.

Pathogenesis

The inflammatory response in pericarditis causes fibrin to be deposited in the pericardium, with the subsequent development of edema and thickening of the pericardial membrane. Pericarditis can be an acute or chronic condition. Acute pericarditis is a condition that suddenly occurs, usually secondary to an infection, a MI, or trauma. Acute pericarditis usually responds to treatment and is resolved without problems. However, some patients can develop recurrent episodes of acute pericarditis. Chronic pericarditis is a slow and progressive process during which the pericardium transforms into scar tissue. The pericardium becomes extremely thick, up to 10 times the normal thickness. The scar tissue of the pericardium limits or constricts the movement of the pericardium; thus chronic pericarditis is frequently referred to as constrictive pericarditis.

Pericardial disease is usually secondary to another disorder. The two most common pericardial disorders are pericarditis and pericardial effusion. A pericardial effusion is a condition in which fluid, exudate, or blood accumulates within the pericardial sac. A pericardial effusion can occur from any of the conditions that cause pericardial disease and can be associated with either acute or chronic pericarditis. A pericardial effusion can develop suddenly, or slowly, as with chronic pericarditis. Pericardial effusion associated with trauma involves blood leaking into the pericardial sac and usually occurs with chest trauma caused by the steering wheel in a motor vehicle accident or after any type of cardiac surgery. Pericardial effusions associated with pericarditis involve the accumulation of fluid in the pericardial sac. Small pericardial effusions usually do not present a problem.

A large pericardial effusion is a problem if the pericardial sac fills with too much fluid or blood. The heart's movement is restricted, and vessels unable to fill and contract, which results in the ejection of less blood than is normal. When the amount of fluid or blood severely impairs the heart's movement, the condition is referred to as a **cardiac tamponade.** This condition is an emergency situation because cardiac output is severely diminished, and cardiogenic shock results because the left ventricle is unable to eject sufficient blood to supply oxygen to the tissues.

At-Risk Populations

Pericarditis is not limited to an age group or population and may occur at any time as a consequence of other conditions and disease processes.

Conditions that place a patient at risk for pericarditis include connective tissue disorders, cancer, infections (particularly of the heart and lungs), trauma, amyloidosis, drugs, acute MI, and end-stage renal failure. Common causes of chronic pericarditis include tuberculosis, cancer, and amyloidosis.

What You NEED TO KNOW

Clinical Manifestations

Chest pain is the main clinical manifestation of acute pericarditis. The patient is typically uncomfortable and restless. Differentiating pericardial chest pain from ischemic chest pain is important. Chest pain associated with pericarditis is usually persistent and unrelieved by nitroglycerin or opioids. The pain is relieved only by an antiinflammatory drug, such as a nonsteroidal antiinflammatory drug (NSAID). Inspiration or cough frequently aggravates the chest pain and can be relieved after the patient sits up. Most patients will also have fever. Patients who have had an MI can develop pericarditis, usually within 24 to 48 hours after the infarction **(Dressler's syndrome).** These patients complain of persistent chest pain, and nitroglycerin is ineffective. An electrocardiogram (ECG) may show ST segment elevation on all or most leads. This widespread ST elevation represents inflammation of the pericardium.

A pericardial friction rub may be auscultated when assessing heart sounds in a patient with acute pericarditis. A "creaky" or "leathery" sound is usually heard with each heartbeat. A pericardial friction rub should not be confused with a pleural friction rub, which indicates inflammation of the pleura. When auscultating heart sounds, feel the patient's pulse at the same time; when the rub is heard with the pulse, the sound is a pericardial friction rub. Another way to differentiate a pericardial friction rub from a pleural friction rub is to have the patient stop breathing for a few seconds; if you still hear the rub, then the sound is a pericardial friction rub.

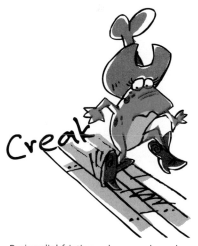

Pericardial friction rubs sound creaky.

Clinical manifestations of chronic pericarditis are those associated with diastolic heart failure such as peripheral edema, crackles, fatigue, and shortness of breath. Jugular vein distention, dyspnea on exertion, generalized edema, and hepatomegaly are frequently observed in the presence of chronic pericarditis.

Clinical manifestations of a pericardial effusion depend on the amount of fluid or blood in the pericardial sac. Typically, the patient is asymptomatic until the fluid impairs cardiac output. When the cardiac output is impaired, the patient will have signs and symptoms associated with heart failure. In severe cases, when cardiac tamponade develops, signs and symptoms are distinct. Severe jugular vein distention is present with a cardiac tamponade. Heart sounds are muffled and frequently cannot be auscultated. Pulsus paradoxus is also a classic sign of cardiac tamponade. Pulsus paradoxus is a condition in which the cardiac output and blood pressure are decreased more during inspiration than they are during expiration. This condition occurs because venous return to the right ventricle is increased during inspiration. This increase in volume adds further pressure to the left ventricle, along with the pericardial fluid.

When clinical manifestations of cardiogenic shock are present symptoms such as hypotension, tachycardia (usually 120 or greater), weak and thready peripheral pulses, cool and clammy skin, and diminished or absent urine output are noted.

Prognosis

Any form of pericarditis can result in a pericardial effusion. Eventually, if it is not recognized and treated appropriately the accumulation of fluid will restrict the heart's ability to fill with blood.

What You DO

Treatment

Treatment of acute pericarditis is aimed at reducing the inflammation. NSAIDs are the drugs of choice, and improvement is usually rapid. If no response to NSAIDs is forthcoming, and no infection is present, steroids are used. When bacterial pericarditis is suspected, intravenous antibiotics are administered.

Treatment for chronic pericarditis involves surgery. The surgical procedure is a pericardectomy, which involves excision of the pericardium to allow movement of the pericardium. Some centers perform laser pericardectomy, during which laser slits are made in the pericardium.

Treatment of a pericardial effusion involves removal of the fluid or blood when the fluid produces symptoms. A pericardiocentesis is a nonsurgical procedure that is performed to evacuate the pericardial fluid.

When cardiac tamponade occurs with pericardial effusion, removal of the fluid must be performed immediately, or the condition will be fatal.

The procedure involves inserting a needle into the pericardial sac. The heart may be visualized with the use of either an echocardiogram or a cardiac catheterization to facilitate correct placement of the needle. Surgical drainage is typically performed on patients with trauma or a tumor because the surgery allows for repair of any damage from trauma, and a biopsy can be obtained from tumors.

Nursing Responsibilities

The nurse must know several important aspects of the care of patients with pericardial disease. The nurse should do the following:

- Recognize signs and symptoms of increasing pericardial effusion and cardiac tamponade. These signs and symptoms must be reported to the health care provider immediately. If treatment is not implemented promptly, the condition can be fatal.
- Be alert for signs and symptoms of cardiogenic shock, jugular vein distention, and pulsus paradoxus. Assess for pulsus paradoxus by taking the patient's blood pressure during inspiration and again during expiration. Pulsus paradoxus is present when the systolic blood pressure during inspiration is 10 mmHg or lower than during expiration.
- Monitor for the occurrence of acute pericarditis following an acute MI and following cardiac surgery. These patients usually complain of continuous chest pain 24 to 48 hours after the infarct or surgery and are extremely uncomfortable. The pain is unrelieved by nitroglycerin and opioids. Measures to help alleviate pain include administering NSAIDs as ordered (with food to prevent gastrointestinal ulcers), and keeping the patient in an upright position.

Pulmonary complications, such as atelectasis and pneumonia, can result because the intensified pain with inspiration prevents the patient from taking deep breaths. To optimize breathing, do the following:

- Assist the patient with the use of an incentive spirometer and with deep-breathing exercises.
- Maintain the patient in a high-Fowler's position to promote lung expansion, and administer pain drugs as ordered.

To prevent cardiac complications, watch for clinical manifestations of increasing pericardial effusion or a cardiac tamponade.

Signs and symptoms of cardiac tamponade include faint muffled heart sounds, distention of the jugular veins, and pulsus paradoxus. These symptoms must be reported to the health care provider immediately. Other signs and symptoms include a pericardial friction rub and heart failure.

Do You UNDERSTAND?

DIRECTIONS: **Fill in the blanks to complete the following statements.**

1. The condition that causes the formation of scar tissue within the pericardium is known as _____ pericarditis.

2. Chest pain associated with acute pericarditis can be differentiated from pain associated with myocardial ischemia in that it is not relieved by _____.

3. A patient after cardiac surgery develops hypotension, jugular vein distention, tachycardia, cold and clammy skin, and muffled heart sounds. The patient most likely has developed cardiac _____.

4. Chronic pericarditis diminishes cardiac output because it causes _____.

5. A pericardial friction rub can be auscultated when a patient is _____.

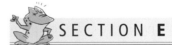

SECTION E

ISCHEMIC HEART DISEASE

Journals of the American Heart Association
http://www.ahajournals.org/

American Heart Association
http://www.americanheart.org/

What IS Coronary Artery Disease?

Coronary artery disease (CAD) is the leading cause of death from heart disease. CAD affects the coronary arteries by causing narrowing within the lumen of the artery.

Pathogenesis

CAD is a progressive condition in which fat and fibrin are deposited along arterial walls. These deposits of fat and fibrin are known as plaque. Vessels eventually become thickened and hardened. The lumen of the vessels becomes narrow and blood flow through the lumen restricted. As a result, the tissue distal to the narrowing becomes ischemic. CAD causes two ischemic heart conditions: angina and myocardial infarction. All arteries can be affected, in addition to the coronary arteries, such as the cerebral, carotid, renal, and peripheral arteries. Significant occlusions within cerebral or carotid arteries place the person at risk for a stroke.

Three stages have been theorized in the development of plaque in atherosclerosis. The first stage is the fatty streak stage, during which streaks of fat form on the vessel walls. The second stage is the fibrous plaque stage, during which plaque is formed and lipids are accumulated. The third stage is the advanced stage, during which the plaque becomes hardened or calcified.

Angina is a symptom of CAD that occurs when a coronary artery becomes temporarily occluded. Blood flow is blocked to the area of the myocardium (heart muscle) distal to the location in which the coronary artery is supplying blood. The occlusion associated with angina causes the myocardium to become ischemic but does not cause necrosis.

MI occurs when a coronary artery becomes completely blocked (occluded). Inflammation and stress on the coronary arteries causes plaque to rupture. When plaque ruptures, platelets become activated and adhere to the ruptured site to stop the bleeding. Platelets help to form a clot, and it is this clot that results in total occlusion of the coronary artery. The complete occlusion blocks blood flow to more distal areas of the myocardium (heart muscle), which eventually results in necrosis of the myocardium. Less common causes of an MI include spasms of the artery, aortic aneurysm, and dissection, which occurs when the arterial wall is torn from a cardiac catheterization procedure and the torn piece blocks the coronary artery.

Three stages, frequently referred to as zones, of myocardial damage take place during an MI. A zone of ischemia occurs when the myocardium becomes ischemic and injured cells are viable. The zone of injury occurs when cells have a significant reduction in blood flow in a myocardial region. The zone of infarction is characterized by cellular death and muscle necrosis. Damage in the zone of infarction is irreversible.

Irreversible myocardial damage occurs 6 hours after the onset of the infarction or occlusion. The myocardium becomes distended, pale, and cyanotic after an infarction. The infarcted area of the myocardium forms into scar tissue over 3 to 4 weeks; the healing process of the myocardium is complete after 6 weeks.

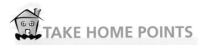

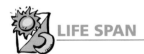

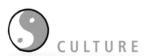

Two basic types of MIs have been identified: transmural and subendocardial. A transmural infarction causes necrosis of all three layers of the heart; the endocardium, myocardium, and epicardium. A subendocardial infarction involves only the endocardium. MIs can also be classified as either a Q wave or a non–Q wave infarct as identified on an ECG. A Q wave infarct occurs when the ECG shows ST segment elevation during the infarct, and then deep Q waves appear after the infarct. A non–Q wave infarct occurs when the ECG shows ST segment depression, and Q waves do not appear after the infarct.

An MI can affect any surface area of the myocardium, depending on which coronary artery is occluded. The areas of the myocardium that can be affected include the front of the heart (anterior wall), the side of the heart (lateral wall), the undersurface of the heart (inferior wall), and the back of the heart (posterior wall). The coronary arteries and the areas of the heart where an infarct would occur when the vessel becomes blocked are listed below in the Prognosis section.

At-Risk Populations

A variety of risk factors are associated with CAD. Nonmodifiable risk factors include age, gender, family history, and race. Modifiable risk factors include elevated serum lipids, hypertension, smoking, impaired glucose tolerance, diets high in saturated fat, cholesterol, calories, sedentary lifestyle, obesity, oral contraceptive use, psychologic stress, personality type, and coping skills.

Cholesterol levels have a significant correlation with CAD. Persons with levels greater than 270 mg/dL have 4 times the risk of developing CAD than those with lower levels. Elevated triglycerides also contribute to CAD. Substances known as lipoproteins transport cholesterol and triglycerides in the body. Very low–density lipoproteins (VLDL) carry triglycerides to the vessels where they accumulate. Low-density lipoproteins (LDL), the "bad" lipoproteins, carry cholesterol to vessels, and the cholesterol accumulates within the arterial walls. High-density lipoproteins (HDL), conversely, are "good" lipoproteins because they carry cholesterol away from tissues to the liver where it is metabolized. This process prevents cholesterol from building up within the arteries. Elevated HDL levels are associated with a lower risk of developing CAD.

What You NEED TO KNOW

Clinical Manifestations

Clinical manifestations of angina include pain in the chest, neck, arms, jaw, or back. The pain results from the ischemia and typically lasts from 30 seconds to 30 minutes. Women tend to have more atypical pain and stomach (**epigastric**) pain than men. Factors that can precipitate angina include exercise, exertion during cold weather, emotional upset, and sexual activity.

Stable angina begins gradually, reaches maximal intensity in minutes, and then dissipates. Stable angina can be precipitated by activity or hypertension. Unstable angina is more intense than stable angina and is described as pain rather than discomfort. Usually, treatment requires more than nitroglycerin alone. Unstable angina can remain in a stable pattern or result in a new onset of severe angina. Unstable angina can also be precipitated by activity or hypertension.

Variant, or Prinzmetal's angina, is a result of coronary vasospasm, a spasm that occurs within the coronary artery, temporarily closing off the artery. This type of angina may or may not have an atherosclerotic lesion. Variant angina frequently occurs at rest. Smoking, alcohol, sudden temperature change, and cocaine use can precipitate a variant angina attack.

Silent ischemia is myocardial ischemia without the patient experiencing symptoms of angina and may be associated with less severe ischemia. Persons who may experience silent ischemia include women, persons with diabetes, and those experiencing high stress. Persons with diabetes may have silent ischemia because of the presence of neuropathy and be unable to feel the pain.

> **!** Silent ischemia is associated with an increased risk of MI and sudden cardiac death.

The main clinical manifestation of MI is pain in the chest, arms, neck, jaw, or epigastric area. The pain is different from angina in that it is not temporary and it is not relieved by nitroglycerin. Profuse sweating (**diaphoresis**) is present in almost all MI cases. Nausea is frequently present, and vomiting indicates a severe infarction because blood is being shunted from the gastrointestinal tract as a result of a significant decrease in cardiac output. A sudden onset of heart failure or pulmonary edema may indicate a moderate to severe MI.

Several complications can occur from an MI. Arrhythmias occur in 95% of all MIs. Inflammation of the pericardium (**pericarditis**) can

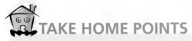

occur 24 to 48 hours after the infarct. Rupture of the ventricular septum and papillary muscle rupture can occur and will cause death in most cases.

Prognosis

The prognosis for angina is positive if the patient is willing to modify behaviors, thus decreasing the chance of further angina attacks. Severe angina attacks may be relieved with nitroglycerin.

The prognosis for recovery from an MI depends on the area and extent of damage to the myocardium, the presence of preexisting organ disease, and access to prompt medical care. Anterior wall infarcts have occlusion of the left anterior descending artery and are associated with twice the mortality of inferior wall infarcts. Anterolateral wall infarcts have occlusion of the circumflex branch. Inferior wall infarcts have occlusion of the right coronary artery. Posterior wall infarcts have occlusion of the circumflex branch.

What You DO

Treatment

Treatment of angina and an MI is aimed at increasing coronary perfusion (coronary blood flow and oxygen) and decreasing the myocardial workload. The myocardial workload (**myocardial oxygen demand**) is a general term used to describe the extent to which the myocardium must work to pump blood. The harder the myocardium has to pump, the more oxygen it requires. When angina occurs, the myocardial oxygen demand is reduced because oxygen to the myocardium is already compromised.

Nitroglycerin is the drug of choice in treating angina because it increases coronary perfusion and reduces the myocardial oxygen demand. Nitroglycerin increases coronary perfusion because it dilates the large coronary arteries. In addition, nitroglycerin reduces the myocardial oxygen demand because it dilates systemic veins and arteries. By dilating the veins, preload is reduced; by dilating the arteries, afterload is also reduced. A reduction in preload decreases the myocardial oxygen demand because the ventricles do not have to eject as forcefully as when they are filled with less blood. A reduction in afterload decreases the myocardial oxygen demand because a reduction in arterial pressure reduces the resistance against which the left ventricle must pump.

Other drugs used to reduce the myocardial oxygen demand are beta-adrenergic blockers, calcium channel blockers, and ACE inhibitors. Beta-adrenergic blockers decrease the heart rate and force of contraction, thereby reducing the myocardial oxygen demand. As the heart rate increases, the myocardial oxygen demand also increases. Beta-adrenergic blockers also reduce stress within the coronary arteries and reduce blood pressure by causing dilation of the arteries, thus decreasing the chance for plaque rupture and MI. These drugs have become the mainstay for treatment in patients with CAD and angina. If beta-adrenergic blockers are contraindicated for patients, calcium channel blockers may be used. Calcium channel blockers block the flow of calcium into the myocardium, thus myocardial contractility is reduced. Calcium channel blockers also dilate arteries and reduce pressure within the arteries. ACE inhibitors are used for patients who develop heart failure.

Other drugs are used to prevent clot formation in the area of the coronary artery that has plaque. Because most of the clot is made up of platelets, antiplatelet aggregation drugs are used. Antiplatelet drugs inhibit platelets from agglutinating or "clumping" together. Antiplatelet drugs include aspirin and clopidogrel. Heparin or low–molecular weight heparin may be used to help prevent clot formation. Low–molecular weight heparin is used in patients with unstable angina or non–Q wave MI.

Treatment of an acute myocardial infarction (AMI) involves reestablishing blood flow to the myocardium, particularly during the "6-hour window," but preferably within 2 hours. Some of the damage to the myocardium can be reversed if blood flow is returned within 6 hours after the onset of symptoms. One way to establish blood flow is to dissolve the clot within the coronary artery that is producing the complete occlusion. Administering a thrombolytic drug accomplishes this task. Thrombolytics dissolve clots throughout the body, including the clot causing the MI. Common drugs used are tissue plasminogen activators (tPa). An emergency percutaneous transluminal coronary angioplasty (PTCA) with stent placement can also be performed if personnel and equipment are available within 90 minutes after the cardiac event. This procedure involves taking the patient to the cardiac catheterization laboratory. The cardiologist places a catheter into the coronary artery and inflates a balloon on the end of the catheter until the coronary artery is open. If the patient with an MI has multiple vessel disease, an emergency coronary artery bypass graft (CABG) surgery may be performed. The surgery should take place within the 6-hour window because complications of a CABG surgery significantly increase after that time.

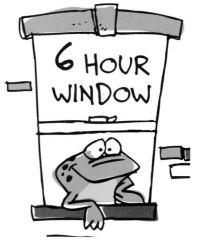

Window of opportunity.

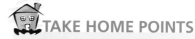

Treatment of angina and MI is aimed at increasing coronary perfusion and decreasing the cardiac workload. The nurse should report hypotension immediately, and drug dosages may be adjusted. Additionally, watch for bradycardia with use of beta-adrenergic and calcium channel blockers. A heart rate less than 60 beats per minute should be reported to the health care provider.

Nursing Responsibilities

Nurses must be aware of several important points when caring for a patient with angina or an MI. The nurse should begin immediate treatment and monitoring measures, including the following:

- Administration of oxygen, low-dose aspirin, nitroglycerin, and morphine, and placement on a cardiac monitor. An ECG should be obtained and evaluated and base line laboratory studies done.
- Maintain the systolic blood pressure less than 135 mm Hg to decrease the afterload, which, in turn, decreases myocardial oxygen demand. Many of the drugs used for ischemic heart disease—such as nitroglycerin, beta-adrenergic blockers, calcium channel blockers, and ACE inhibitors—decrease blood pressure.
- Watch for signs and symptoms of heart failure in more extensive MIs. Signs and symptoms include dyspnea, pulmonary crackles, jugular vein distention, and tachycardia.
- Monitor for cardiogenic shock that can occur with a massive infarct. Signs and symptoms of cardiogenic shock include hypotension, tachycardia, cool and clammy skin, weak peripheral pulses, and decreased urine output.
- Give drugs as ordered, and be certain that doses are not omitted. Drugs such as nitroglycerin, ACE inhibitors, and beta-adrenergic blockers can decrease the systolic blood pressure and can cause hypotension. Administer morphine sulfate for relief of ischemic pain that is not relieved by nitroglycerin. The drugs should be held only when the systolic pressure is less than the parameter ordered by the health care provider, such as 100 or 110 mm Hg. When a patient is NPO in anticipation of surgery or a procedure, check with the health care provider about administering the drugs with small sips of water. The patient may develop acute angina or infarction in surgery or during a procedure if the drugs are not given.
- Obtain a 12-lead ECG when a patient with ischemic pain does not obtain relief with nitroglycerin. The 12-lead ECG should be examined for ST segment elevations, which indicates an AMI. A 12-lead ECG is needed because it records conduction throughout the heart 12 different ways, each representing a different surface area of the heart. A single-lead cardiac monitor, frequently used in telemetry units or in the cardiac care units, records conduction traveling only one way in the heart, thus only one surface area of the heart is reflected. If an infarction occurs in another area, one not represented by the lead, no changes will be observed.

- Maintain bed rest with bedside commode privileges; using a commode results in less straining compared with a bedpan.
- Maintain semi-Fowler's position to decrease preload.
- Provide a clear liquid diet during acute anginal attacks and for the first 24 hours after AMI. Food increases the gastrointestinal tract's demand for oxygen. A weakened myocardium has to pump harder to get blood flow to the gastrointestinal tract.
- Maintain a quiet environment and administer antianxiety drugs as ordered when the patient is anxious. Anxiousness and an increase in heart rate increase the myocardial oxygen demand.
- Patient education is directed toward maintaining optimal cardiovascular health after discharge, including activity restrictions, dietary modifications, and the need for continuing health care and evaluation.

Do You UNDERSTAND?

DIRECTIONS: Fill in the blanks by unscrambling the letters.

1. High levels of _____ reduces the occurrence of coronary artery disease. *(DHL)*

2. The type of angina that frequently occurs at rest and usually results from coronary vasospasms is known as _____ _____ angina. *(travian)*

3. _____ can result when the contractility of the myocardium is significantly diminished after an MI. *(iodraccenig cohsk)*

4. A patient with unstable angina complains of chest pain to the nurse. After administering nitroglycerin, the patient does not obtain relief. The most important intervention is for the nurse to _____ _____. *(binato na gec)*

Answers: 1. HDL; 2. variant; 3. cardiogenic shock; 4. obtain an ECG.

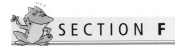

SECTION F

ARRHYTHMIAS

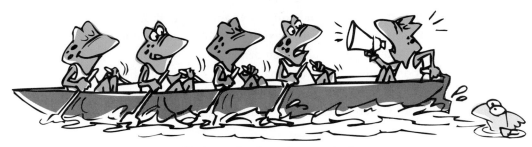

Work together for optimum output.

To understand arrhythmias, the way in which a normal rhythm of the heart is produced must be examined. For the atria and ventricles to fill and contract, proper timing and synchronization must exist between the atria and the ventricles. The conduction system of the heart is responsible for facilitating proper timing and synchronization. The conduction system is made up of specialized cells that produce electrical impulses throughout the atria and the ventricles. These electrical impulses produce perfect timing of contractions between the atria and ventricles.

Specialized cells that make up the conduction system are present throughout the heart. Pacemaker cells initiate electrical impulses. The sinoatrial (SA) node of the right atrium is the normal pacemaker of the heart, and produces a rate of 60 to 100 beats per minute. Conducting cells carry the electrical impulses from the SA node to the left atrium and through the ventricles. The conduction cells then stimulate the muscle cells, and these cells cause contraction of the myocardium. The normal pathway of the conduction system is illustrated on page 243.

Conduction of the electrical impulses through the heart produces a normal sinus rhythm (NSR), as well as normal heart rate and stroke volume. The heart rate is the number of times the heart contracts per minute; the stroke volume is the amount of blood the left ventricle ejects with each contraction. When the heart rate is too slow, the left ventricle will not pump as much blood as is needed by the body. The formula for cardiac output is:

$$\text{heart rate (HR)} \times \text{stroke volume (SV)} = \text{cardiac output}$$

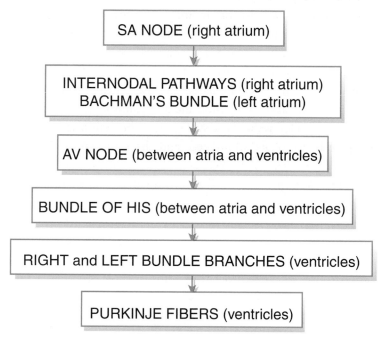

Pathway of the conduction system.

What IS an Arrhythmia?

Arrhythmias are any rhythm that is not an NSR. Some arrhythmias can be faster or slower compared with the NSR. Other arrhythmias are abnormal rhythms produced by conducting cells that produce electrical impulses outside of the normal conduction system. These abnormal conducting beats are referred to as ectopic beats.

A variety of arrhythmias exist. Four common types of arrhythmias are sinus tachycardia, sinus bradycardia, atrial fibrillation, and premature ventricular contraction.

Pathogenesis

Sinus Tachycardia. Sinus tachycardia is a normal rhythm; however, the rate is greater than 100 beats per minute but usually less than

150 beats per minute. The cause of sinus tachycardia is not a conduction problem with the heart, but rather, various problems outside of the conduction system. Any condition that increases the pulse rate will cause sinus tachycardia.

Sinus Bradycardia. Sinus bradycardia is a normal rhythm; however, the rate is less than 60 beats per minute. Causes of sinus bradycardia include drugs, severe hypoxemia, and acute MI. Stimulation of the vagus nerve can also cause sinus bradycardia. The vagus nerve is a parasympathetic nerve, thus when it is stimulated, the heart rate decreases. Common factors that cause vagal stimulation include vomiting, retching, bearing down, and bowel movements. Usually, after the action is stopped, the vagus nerve is no longer stimulated, and the heart rate increases to a normal rate.

Atrial Fibrillation. Atrial fibrillation is an abnormal rhythm originating from an ectopic beat in the atria. The atrial ectopic site becomes the primary pacemaker of the heart and conducts at an extremely fast rate, making the atria quiver rather than contract. The rhythm of atrial fibrillation is regularly irregular; an irregular pulse can be palpated. Common causes of acute atrial fibrillation include stimulants such as coffee and tobacco, myocardial ischemia, acute heart failure, cardiomyopathy, chronic obstructive pulmonary disease, drugs (e.g., theophylline, isoproterenol), and cardiac surgery.

Premature Ventricular Contractions. Premature ventricular contractions (PVCs) originate from an ectopic focus in the ventricles. Common causes of PVCs include an acute MI or ischemia, hypoxemia, and drugs that irritate the heart.

At-Risk Populations

Sinus Tachycardia. Many conditions stimulate the sympathetic nervous system, which results in sinus tachycardia. Common conditions include heart failure, hypoxemia, fever, pain, shock, hemorrhage, hypovolemia, and anxiety. Drugs can cause sinus tachycardia also, including theophylline and any drug that stimulates the sympathetic nervous system, such as alpha- and beta-adrenergic drugs. Adrenergic drugs include epinephrine, norepinephrine, dopamine, dobutamine, and over-the-counter decongestants and phenylephrine. Atropine can also cause sinus tachycardia.

Sinus Bradycardia. Patients at the highest risk for sinus bradycardia include those who have had an acute MI, particularly an inferior wall infarct, and those taking various cardiac drugs. Commonly used cardiac

---

⚠ Sinus bradycardia can be a dangerous rhythm if the heart rate is insufficient to provide adequate cardiac output.

🏠 TAKE HOME POINTS

- Always assess for an underlying cause of sinus tachycardia such as fever, hypotension, pain, drugs, and so on.
- Watch patients with angina or MI who develop sinus tachycardia because the increased heart rate increases myocardial oxygen demand, which in turn can cause chest pain.

drugs associated with sinus bradycardia include digoxin, beta-adrenergic blockers, calcium channel blockers, and any antiarrhythmic drug. Severe hypoxemia can cause a sudden bradycardia, which usually leads to cardiopulmonary arrest. Immediate action is therefore required to resolve the hypoxemia.

Sinus bradycardia can be a normal condition for athletes or persons who exercise regularly. A person who exercises regularly increases venous return to the heart. Eventually, this increase in venous return causes the left ventricle to strengthen and enlarge. The increase in size allows the left ventricle to hold more blood, thus increasing the stroke volume. Because the stroke volume is increased, a normal heart rate is unnecessary to have an adequate cardiac output, thus the heart rate slows.

Atrial Fibrillation. The most common causes of atrial fibrillation are ischemic heart disease, rheumatic fever, and hyperthyroidism. In atrial fibrillation, the atrium does not contract normally during diastole. As a result, the atrium is unable to empty all of its blood into the ventricles. This pooling of blood in the atria forms clots. These clots can eventually break loose and cause a pulmonary embolus, a stroke, or a bowel infarct. Atrial fibrillation can be an acute problem or a chronic rhythm and is the most common type of chronic arrhythmia.

Premature Ventricular Contractions. The causes of PVCs are numerous. Any form of heart disease can cause PVCs, such as ischemic heart disease or cardiomyopathy. The most common metabolic causes include hypoxemia, hypokalemia, acidosis, and a low magnesium level. Drugs that can cause PVCs include digoxin, theophylline, adrenergic drugs, and certain antiarrhythmic drugs.

What You NEED TO KNOW

Clinical Manifestations

Sinus Tachycardia. The clinical manifestations of sinus tachycardia are palpitations and a rapid pulse rate.

Sinus Bradycardia. A patient with sinus bradycardia may not have any symptoms if cardiac output is sufficient. Patients with reduced cardiac output frequently experience weakness, dizziness, fainting, chest pain, hypotension, diaphoresis, cool and clammy skin, and decreased level of consciousness.

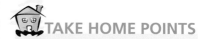

TAKE HOME POINTS

- Sinus bradycardia is an emergency situation if the patient is symptomatic. Atropine or a transcutaneous pacemaker should be available.
- When severe hypoxemia causes bradycardia, cardiopulmonary arrest will usually follow unless the hypoxemia is corrected. High-risk patients include those with a tracheostomy and those with any type of respiratory disorder.
- Because the heart rate of a patient with atrial fibrillation is regularly irregular, the nurse must take the pulse for one full minute to get an accurate pulse rate.
- Be alert for stroke, pulmonary embolus, and bowel infarction in patients with atrial fibrillation. Clinical manifestations of stroke include weakness or paralysis of any of the extremities, slurred speech, sudden unconsciousness, and facial or eyelid droop. Clinical manifestations of a pulmonary embolus include sudden chest pain, difficulty breathing, tachycardia, diaphoresis, and hypoxemia. Clinical manifestations of a bowel infarct include abdominal pain, abdominal distention, and hypoactive or absent bowel sounds, and vomiting.

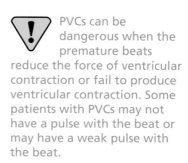

PVCs can be dangerous when the premature beats reduce the force of ventricular contraction or fail to produce ventricular contraction. Some patients with PVCs may not have a pulse with the beat or may have a weak pulse with the beat.

Atrial Fibrillation. Most patients with atrial fibrillation are asymptomatic. A regularly irregular pulse may be palpated or heard on auscultation of the apical pulse.

Premature Ventricular Contractions. Most patients with PVCs have no symptoms. Some may complain of feeling a "skipped beat." When a patient is having frequent PVCs, an irregular pulse can be palpated.

Prognosis

Sinus Tachycardia. The prognosis for sinus tachycardia is usually good, because after the underlying problem is corrected, the sinus tachycardia is resolved.

Sinus Bradycardia. The prognosis for sinus bradycardia can be poor when the heart rate is insufficient to produce an adequate cardiac output. Tissues will not receive sufficient oxygen if the heart is not pumping at the required rate.

Atrial Fibrillation. The prognosis for atrial fibrillation is fair to poor because of the risk for clot formation. These patients are at risk for stroke, pulmonary embolus, and ischemic bowel disease.

Premature Ventricular Contractions. The prognosis for patients with PVCs is usually good, provided the PVCs do not progress to more lethal ventricular arrhythmias. Ordinarily, when metabolic conditions are corrected or irritating drugs are discontinued, the PVCs will stop.

What You DO

Treatment

Sinus Tachycardia. The treatment for sinus tachycardia includes determining and treating the underlying cause. For example, if the patient has hypoxemia, oxygen should be given to the patient. Sinus tachycardia usually does not, in and of itself, present a problem unless the patient has ischemic heart disease. An increase in heart rate increases the myocardial oxygen demand, and the ischemic myocardium can become overworked. These patients will develop chest pain or acute heart failure with sinus tachycardia.

Sinus Bradycardia. Treatment of sinus bradycardia is needed only when the person is symptomatic or fails to tolerate the slow rate. Signs and symptoms of a person who is not tolerating sinus bradycardia include hypotension, chest pain, cool and clammy skin, dizziness, fainting, or confusion. Treatment for sinus bradycardia includes administration of intravenous atropine or insertion of a pacemaker. Atropine inhibits the parasympathetic response, thus the heart rate increases. A pacemaker is an electronic device used to artificially stimulate conduction within the heart. Pacemakers can be temporary or permanent.

Atrial Fibrillation. Treatment for atrial fibrillation includes the use of antiarrhythmics and synchronized cardioversion. Common antiarrhythmic drugs include diltiazem, digoxin, amiodarone, and adenosine. Synchronized cardioversion is used when the heart rate is greater then 120 beats per minute and antiarrhythmic drugs have been ineffective. Synchronized cardioversion is a procedure in which an electrical voltage is sent through the heart that is synchronized with ventricular contraction. The voltage is sent from electrical paddles placed on the chest.

Premature Ventricular Contractions. PVCs are treated only when the patient is symptomatic, such as in the presence of hypotension, chest pain, cool and clammy skin, dizziness, fainting, or confusion. Treatment includes use of antiarrhythmics such as amiodarone and lidocaine.

Nursing Responsibilities

The nurse should have some familiarity with interpreting basic arrhythmias on an ECG. The ECG device measures electrical currents of the heart. Electrical impulses are picked up by electrodes placed on the skin and are recorded on graph paper. Be aware that an ECG is a diagnostic test that measures only electrical conduction. The nurse must also be aware that a wide range of normal ECG patterns exists. In other words, a normal sinus rhythm can appear slightly different in each patient; however, when a patient develops any of the signs and symptoms of an arrhythmia, the nurse should do the following:

- Evaluate the patient's tolerance of the abnormal rhythm.
- Assess for signs of decreased tissue blood flow (perfusion), such as cool and clammy skin, weak or thready pulses, decrease in urine output, and capillary refill greater than 3 seconds.
- Report any signs of intolerance to the health care provider immediately.

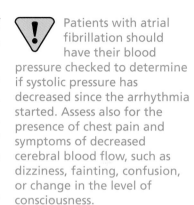

Patients with atrial fibrillation should have their blood pressure checked to determine if systolic pressure has decreased since the arrhythmia started. Assess also for the presence of chest pain and symptoms of decreased cerebral blood flow, such as dizziness, fainting, confusion, or change in the level of consciousness.

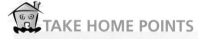

TAKE HOME POINTS

Steps for assessing a patient who develops any of the four arrhythmias:
- Check vital signs—pulse and blood pressure
- Assess for chest or cardiac ischemic pain
- Assess for decrease in cerebral perfusion
- Assess for decrease in tissue perfusion

SINUS TACHYCARDIA

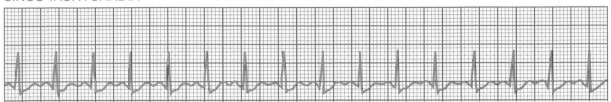

(Redrawn from Cohn EG, Gilroy-Doohan M: Flip and see ECG, Philadelphia, 1996, WB Saunders.)

Sinus Tachycardia

- Determine the underlying cause, such as drugs, fever, anxiety, or acute heart failure.
- Carefully monitor patients with ischemic heart disease because the increase in heart rate can cause chest pain or precipitate an MI.

SINUS BRADYCARDIA

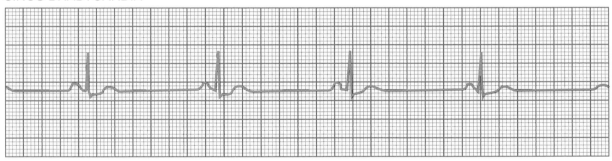

(Redrawn from Cohn EG, Gilroy-Doohan M: Flip and see ECG, Philadelphia, 1996, WB Saunders.)

Sinus Bradycardia. The nurse must be aware that sinus bradycardia should be treated only when the person is symptomatic, especially when the person has any type of ischemic heart disease. If atropine is given to a patient with ischemic heart disease who is not symptomatic, the increase in heart rate can increase the myocardial oxygen demand too much and ischemia can result. An important point to remember is that the faster the heart rate is, the more oxygen the heart will require. A person with ischemic heart disease may be unable to supply the additional oxygen needed; therefore the nurse should do the following:

- Immediately assess the patient's tolerance of the slow rate, and prepare for emergency treatment, because sinus bradycardia can progress to a cardiac arrest.
- Keep atropine at the bedside, even when the patient is asymptomatic, in case the patient suddenly becomes symptomatic.
- Always check the apical pulse rate before giving cardiac drugs that commonly cause bradycardia, such as beta-blockers, calcium channel blockers, and digoxin.
- The clinical manifestations of ischemic heart disease include a sudden onset of chest pain, dyspnea, tachycardia, and hypoxemia. A pulmonary embolus can occur when a clot from the atria breaks loose and lodges in a branch of the pulmonary artery.

ATRIAL FIBRILLATION

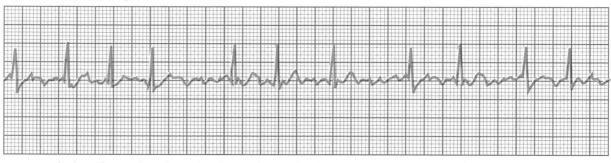

(Redrawn from Paul S, Debra J: The nurse's guide to cardiac rhythm interpretation, Philadelphia, 1996, WB Saunders.)

Atrial Fibrillation. Be alert for thrombotic episodes ("throwing clots") in patients with atrial fibrillation. The person may also develop a cerebral vascular stroke or "brain attack" if a clot enters the cerebral arteries. Clinical manifestations include weakness or paralysis of extremities on one side of the body, slurred speech, facial droop, aphasia, or unresponsiveness in severe strokes. The patient may also develop an ischemic bowel from a clot entering the mesentery. Clinical manifestations include abdominal distention, abdominal pain, hypoactive or absent bowel sounds, and shock. The nurse should do the following:

- Suspect atrial fibrillation when a patient has a regularly irregular pulse.

- Immediately report when a patient with atrial fibrillation also has tachycardia (pulse greater than 100 beats per minute). The fast heart rate along with the atrial fibrillation increases the risk for clot formation and decreases cardiac output.
- Administer anticoagulants as ordered to prevent clot formation. The most common drug used is warfarin. Report any signs of bleeding.
- Watch patients after cardiac surgery for sudden development of atrial fibrillation. The pulse rate is usually fast in these patients (150 to 200 beats per minute).

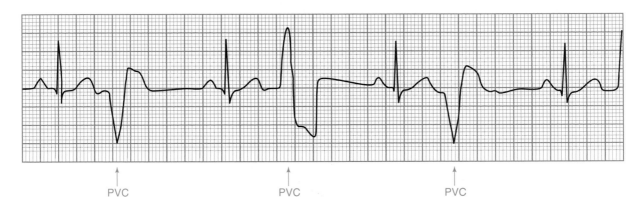

(Redrawn from Chernecky C et al: Real-world nursing survival guide: ECGs and the heart, Philadelphia, 2002, WB Saunders.)

Premature Ventricular Contractions

- Report frequent occurrences of PVCs, such as more than 5 episodes per minute, particularly in the patient with an acute myocardial infarction. The PVCs can cause a lethal rhythm called ventricular fibrillation in which the ventricles quiver and the patient has no pulse.
- When a patient suddenly develops PVCs, determine possible causes such as hypoxemia, drugs, or acute myocardial ischemia.

Do You UNDERSTAND?

DIRECTIONS: **Fill in the blanks to complete the sentences using the words listed below. Words are only used once, and not all words are used.**

1. The _____ is the pacemaker of the heart.
2. The _____ are responsible for contraction of the ventricles.
3. Sinus tachycardia can be hazardous when the patient has _____ _____ disease.
4. Sinus bradycardia can be normal for _____.

ischemic heart	atrioventricular node
Purkinje fibers	sinoatrial node
athletes	

References

Lewis SM, Heitkemper MM, Dirksen SR: *Medical-surgical nursing: assessment and management of clinical problems*, ed 5, St Louis, 2000, Mosby.

Manning WJ: Pericardial disease. In Goldman L, Bennett JC, editors: *Textbook of medicine*, ed 21, Philadelphia, 2000, WB Saunders.

NCLEX® Review

Section A

1. Which of the following conditions carries no increased risk for aneurysms?
   1 Viral pneumonia
   2 Marfan's syndrome
   3 Atherosclerosis
   4 Hypertension

2. Which symptom suggests a thoracic aneurysm?
   1 Hoarseness
   2 Substernal pain
   3 Pulsating abdominal mass
   4 Epigastric pain

3. Signs and symptoms of a dissecting aneurysm include all of the following *except:*
   1 Pallor
   2 Falling blood pressure
   3 Rapid, bounding pulse
   4 Decreased capillary refill

4. Causes of secondary cardiomyopathy include which of the following?
   1 Alcohol
   2 Hypotension
   3 Renal failure
   4 Pericardial effusion

5. The type of cardiomyopathy that involves abnormal thickening of the interventricular septum is _____ cardiomyopathy.
   1 Dilated
   2 Hypertrophic
   3 Restrictive
   4 Ischemic

6. Which medications should be avoided in patients with IHSS?
   1 Beta-adrenergic blockers
   2 Atropine
   3 Nitroglycerin
   4 Epinephrine

Section B

7. Which infectious organism contributes to the development of valvular heart disease?
   1 *Staphylococcus aureus*
   2 Group A beta-hemolytic streptococci
   3 *Pneumocystis carinii*
   4 *Pseudomonas aureus*

8. Which of the following describes an incompetent valve?
   1 Fails to open appropriately during the cardiac cycle
   2 Fails to close appropriately during the cardiac cycle
   3 Leaves too little blood in the chamber behind the valve
   4 Causes increased cardiac output

9. Stenosis of the mitral valve may result in
   1 Decreased cardiac output and atrophy of the left atrium.
   2 Pulmonary hypertension only.
   3 Atrophy of the left atrium only.
   4 Decreased cardiac output and pulmonary hypertension.

Section C

10. Chronic pericarditis is the result of repeated inflammation that
    1 Damages the myocardium
    2 Causes stenosis of the valves
    3 Causes scar tissue in the pericardium
    4 Leads to thinning of the pericardial sac

11. Which complication may be observed first as a consequence of pericarditis?
    1 Ventricular bradycardia
    2 Decreased cardiac output
    3 Hypertension
    4 Bounding peripheral pulses

12. Pulsus paradoxus associated with pericardial effusion occurs as a result of
    1 Increased filling of the ventricles.
    2 An irregular heart beat.
    3 Decreased filling of the ventricles.
    4 Stenosis of the coronary vessels.

Section D

13. Nitroglycerin is used for ischemic heart disease because it
    1 Increases afterload and decreases preload.
    2 Decreases afterload and increases preload.
    3 Dilates coronary arteries and decreases preload and afterload.
    4 Dilates coronary arteries and increases preload and afterload.

14. A patient with a myocardial infarction 2 days ago is NPO in anticipation of a coronary angiogram. The patient is scheduled to receive nitroglycerin and a beta-adrenergic agent. Which of the following should the nurse do?
    1 Hold the drugs until the patient returns from the procedure.
    2 Call the health care provider to determine whether the medications can be given with sips of water.
    3 Maintain the patient NPO.
    4 Administer one half of the medications.

15. Which symptom would suggest that a patient is experiencing angina rather than a myocardial infarction?
    1 Pain in the chest that does not respond to nitroglycerin
    2 Diaphoresis
    3 Abnormal cardiac rhythms
    4 Pain in the chest that is relieved by nitroglycerin

16. What diet should be provided for a patient who is experiencing an acute myocardial infarction?
    1 Clear liquid
    2 Low sodium
    3 Bland
    4 Regular

Section E

17. Medications that primarily dilate veins will decrease
    1 Preload.
    2 Tissue oxygenation.
    3 Contractility.
    4 Afterload and contractility.

18. With heart failure, left ventricular preload is
    1 Decreased.
    2 Increased.
    3 Unchanged.
    4 Decreased, then increased.

19. Signs and symptoms of compensation for acute heart failure include a(n):
    1 Decrease in pulse rate.
    2 Strong and bounding pulse.
    3 Increase in urine output.
    4 Increase in pulse rate.

20. The nurse is caring for a patient diagnosed with heart failure. During the initial assessment, the nurse auscultated crackles in the bases of the lungs. Three hours later, the nurse auscultates crackles in the apices and bases of the lungs. The nurse knows that the change in assessment indicates
    1 Improvement in left ventricular failure.
    2 Worsening of left ventricular failure.
    3 No change in left ventricular failure.
    4 A need for fluids.

Section F

21. A patient is vomiting and suddenly develops sinus bradycardia with a heart rate of 40 beats per minute. The cause of the bradycardia is most likely related to
    1 Hypoxemia.
    2 Vagal stimulation.
    3 Myocardial ischemia.
    4 Dehydration.

22. A patient with atrial fibrillation complains of abdominal pain, and the abdomen is distended and firm. The nurse suspects
    1 Congestive heart failure.
    2 Appendicitis.
    3 A bowel infarct.
    4 Pulmonary embolus.

23. A patient develops sinus bradycardia with a heart rate of 45 beats per minute. The nurse should first perform which of the following?
    1 Administer atropine
    2 Notify the health care provider
    3 Prepare for a pacemaker
    4 Assess blood pressure

24. Which statement regarding premature ventricular contractions (PVCs) is *true*?
    1 PVCs may or may not produce a pulse.
    2 PVCs always produce a pulse.
    3 PVCs never produce a pulse.
    4 PVCs are always treated.

25. Anticoagulants are frequently administered for patients with
    1 Sinus bradycardia.
    2 Sinus tachycardia.
    3 Atrial fibrillation.
    4 Premature ventricular contractions (PVCs).

NCLEX® Review Answers

Section A

1. **1** Viral pneumonia does not affect the integrity of the vessel wall, thus the risk of aneurysm is not increased. Marfan's syndrome, hypertension, and atherosclerosis affect the integrity of the vessel walls and cause decreased elasticity, tearing, and eventual rupture in some cases.

2. **1** Hoarseness can occur when a large thoracic aneurysm presses on the trachea. Substernal pain is associated more frequently with angina or esophagitis. An abdominal aortic aneurysm can cause a pulsating mass that can be seen or felt. Epigastric pain may be a result of angina, gastric ulcers, or gastroesophageal reflux disease.

3. **3** A dissecting aneurysm will cause loss of intravascular volume, which would cause a weak, thready pulse or loss of palpable peripheral pulses. Pallor, falling blood pressure, and decreased capillary refill are reflective of loss of perfusion as a result of declining intravascular volume.

4. **1** Chronic alcohol abuse causes damage to the myocardial fibers. Hypotension has no direct adverse affect on the heart. Renal failure can cause arrhythmias but does not damage the myocardium. Pericardial effusion interferes with the pumping action of the heart.

5. **2** Hypertrophic cardiomyopathy involves abnormal thickening of the interventricular septum. The septum is large to the extent that the size of the left ventricle is significantly decreased. Dilated cardiomyopathy causes the ventricle to enlarge to the extent that the ventricle is unable to contract effectively. In restrictive cardiomyopathy, the myocardium becomes rigid and loses its elasticity. Ischemic cardiomyopathy is caused by necrosis of the myocardium.

6. **3** Vasodilating agents such as nitroglycerin should not be used because they cause an obstruction of the outflow tract, blocking the ejection of blood from the left ventricle. Beta-adrenergic blockers can be helpful in the treatment of restrictive cardiomyopathy. Epinephrine causes vasoconstriction and raises blood pressure, which would increase the cardiac workload. Atropine stimulates heart rate, increasing cardiac workload.

Section D

7. **2** Group A beta-hemolytic streptococci have been shown to trigger an inappropriate inflammatory response that can cause damage to the heart, skin, joints, and kidneys. This phenomenon has not been documented with other infectious organisms, such as *S. aureus, Pneumocystis carinii,* or *Pseudomonas aureus.*

8. **2** An incompetent valve is one that fails to close completely during the cardiac cycle, which allows blood to leak backwards into the heart and causes a build up of blood in the chamber behind the valve. A valve that fails to open appropriately is described as stenotic. Inadequate blood flow within the heart leads to decreased, not increased, cardiac output.

9. **4** Blood flow from left atrium to left ventricle decreases, ultimately providing the left ventricle with less blood to eject. Blood backs up from the left atrium into the pulmonary system, causing pulmonary hypertension because of increased pressure. Blood backing into the left atrium causes hypertrophy, not atrophy.

Section C

10. **3** Chronic pericarditis is the result of repeated inflammation that causes scar tissue in the pericardium. Chronic pericarditis does not damage the myocardium or cause valve stenosis, because pericardial disease involves only the pericardial tissue. Chronic pericarditis does not lead to thinning of the pericardial tissue; recurrent episodes of inflammation lead to thickening and stiffening of the pericardial tissue.

11. **2** Scar tissue of the pericardium inhibits ventricles' ability to stretch and fill with blood, thus lowering cardiac output. Decreased cardiac output leads to hypotension, not hypertension. Bounding peripheral pulses are not observed with decreased cardiac output. The heart initially beats more rapidly, not more slowly (as in ventricular tachycardia or ventricular bradycardia) in an attempt to compensate for poor cardiac output.

12. **3** Pulsus paradoxus associated with pericardial effusion occurs as a result of decreased filling of the ventricles. Fluid in the pericardial sac interferes with the filling of the ventricles—decreasing, not increasing, filling. An irregular heart rate does not cause changes in blood pressure during inspiration and expiration, nor does stenosis of the coronary vessels.

Section D

13. **3** Nitroglycerin is used for ischemic heart disease because it dilates coronary arteries, which decreases preload and afterload. Dilating the coronary arteries and veins decreases the myocardial oxygen demand. Increasing afterload or preload places more stress on the myocardium.

14. **2** The patient, NPO in anticipation of an angiogram, may need to receive medications. The nurse should call the health care provider to determine whether the medications can be given with sips of water. Failure to give cardiac medications can cause acute angina or infarction to develop during a procedure.

15. **4** Cardiac pain resulting from an infarction is not relieved by nitroglycerin. Angina does not cause diaphoresis or arrhythmias. Nitroglycerin relieves cardiac pain resulting from angina.

16. **1** Clear liquid diet should be given during acute anginal attacks and for the first 24 hours after an acute MI to decrease the gastrointestinal tract's demand for oxygen. A low sodium, bland, or regular diet would increase the gastrointestinal tract's demand for oxygen and is contraindicated.

Section E

17. **1** Medications that dilate veins decrease preload. Dilated vessels improve perfusion and oxygenation. Decreasing contractility causes heart failure to worsen.

18. **2** Because of the inadequate pumping action of the heart, the weakened ventricle is unable to completely empty the chamber, leading to an increase in left ventricular preload in heart failure.

19. **4** During early stages, the heart is able to compensate by increasing the number of contractions (pulse rate). Eventually, the pumping ability of the myocardium declines, resulting in heart failure. With decreased cardiac output, blood flow is shunted away from the kidneys, resulting in decreasing urine output.

20. **2** The change in location of the crackles indicates worsening left ventricular failure. Increasing crackles are a reflection of left ventricular failure that is causing congestion of the pulmonary vessels, forcing fluid into the alveoli. Fluids should be restricted in heart failure.

Section F

21. **2** Vomiting is a common stimulant of the vagus nerve. Vagus nerve stimulation can lead to sinus bradycardia. No indication that the patient has hypoxemia or myocardial ischemia is present; thus, in this case, these symptoms would not be from sinus bradycardia. Dehydration causes sinus tachycardia.

22. **3** Abdominal pain and distention are signs and symptoms of a bowel infarct. Tachycardia, decreased urine output, dark amber urine, weak pulses, and cool skin are characteristics of heart failure. Lower right quadrant abdominal pain and fever are characteristics of appendicitis. Sudden chest pain, difficulty breathing, tachycardia, diaphoresis, and hypoxemia are characteristics of pulmonary embolus.

23. **4** In a patient with sinus bradycardia, assessment to determine whether he or she is symptomatic is imperative. No treatment is necessary if the patient is asymptomatic including absence of hypotension. Atropine is administered only when the patient is hypotensive or symptomatic. Notifying the health care provider and preparing the patient for a pacemaker is premature. Assessment is needed before intervention.

24. **1** PVCs may or may not produce a pulse. PVCs are usually not treated if the patient is experiencing no symptoms.

25. **3** Patients with atrial fibrillation are at high risk for stroke, bowel infarct, and pulmonary embolus because of thrombus formation. Therefore anticoagulants are the treatment of choice. Sinus bradycardia, sinus tachycardia, and PVCs do not cause clot formation and thus do not necessitate anticoagulant therapy.

Notes

Alterations in Respiratory Function

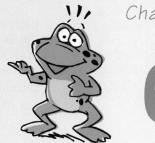

What You WILL LEARN

After reading this chapter, you will be know how to do the following:

- ✔ Differentiate between restrictive, obstructive, and infectious lung diseases.
- ✔ Describe the physical manifestations most commonly associated with restrictive and obstructive lung diseases.
- ✔ Identify predisposing factors for lung disease.
- ✔ Identify complications of restrictive, obstructive, and infectious lung diseases.
- ✔ Discuss priority nursing interventions for the patient with lung disease.

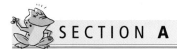

SECTION A

RESTRICTIVE LUNG DISEASES

Respiratory disorders can adversely affect quality of life and impair people's ability to care for themselves, work, and socialize with others. Restrictive lung diseases are a consequence of inflammatory conditions that affect lung tissues, causing the tissues to stiffen and become noncompliant. This chapter provides an overview of the various diseases and disorders that commonly affect the lungs and respiratory system.

What IS Sarcoidosis?

Sarcoidosis is a disorder that currently has no known cause. This disease can affect every part of the body, but the most commonly affected areas include the lungs, the skin, the eyes, the lymph nodes, and the liver. It is characterized by inflammation of the tissue in affected organs. The inflammatory process produces small lumps or granulomas in the affected areas. A granuloma is an accumulation of inflamed cells. In many cases the disease is self-limiting and subsides spontaneously without treatment. The disease is thought to be the result of an increased cellular immune response to a persistent antigen that the body is unable to destroy. This illness is characterized by the accumulation of T lymphocytes (a specialized type of white cell that is active in the immune response), mononuclear phagocytes, granulomas in epithelial tissues, and changes in the structure of affected organs. Depending on the degree of involvement, these accumulations of abnormal cells (lesions) ultimately interfere with normal organ function, particularly the lungs.

Research indicates that the disease likely has both immunologic and genetic components. In approximately 15% of patients, the disease appears to be genetic. Causative agents can be infectious or noninfectious. Various infectious organisms are considered as contributing factors, including mycobacteria, fungi, and spirochetes. Environmental compounds that may contribute to the disease include beryllium, organic dusts (e.g., peanut or wheat dusts), and inorganic compounds (e.g., clay).

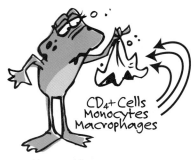

CD4+ Cells
Monocytes
Macrophages

Abnormal immune response.

Pathogenesis

Sarcoidosis begins with an accumulation of CD4+ cells, monocytes, and macrophages within the targeted tissue. These cells secrete cytokines that maintain and promote the inappropriate inflammatory process. Monocytes and macrophages begin to differentiate and form a ring around the inflamed areas, eventually evolving into granulomas. If the inflammatory process persists, the affected tissue will eventually become scarred and fibrotic.

At-Risk Populations

Sarcoidosis has been found in both genders and nearly all ages and races throughout the world. Cases of sarcoidosis have been seen within families, which is suggestive of environmental and genetic factors. In the

United States, African Americans are more frequently and severely affected with sarcoidosis than Caucasians, and these individuals tend to be younger than Caucasians with the disease. In Europe, the disease is most common among people in Sweden and among Irish women. On a worldwide basis, nearly 80% of patients with the disease are Caucasian. In children, the disease is usually self-limiting and can resolve within 2 to 3 years.

What You NEED TO KNOW

Clinical Manifestations

Sarcoidosis can be acute, subacute, or chronic in nature. Patients with sarcoidosis tend to have depressed cell-mediated immunity with a decreased number of circulating T lymphocytes. Many patients are asymptomatic and are diagnosed incidentally with a chest x-ray film.

When symptoms occur, they tend to be related to the organ system involved. Wheezing, breathlessness, cough, and chest pain are commonly observed when lungs are involved. Nodules, papules, and plaques are frequently present with skin involvement. When the disease affects the eyes, patients experience a sensitivity to light, excessive tearing, and visual changes. Involvement of the peripheral lymph nodes is common, particularly in the cervical, axillary, epitrochlear, and inguinal areas. These nodes tend to be mobile, with a firm, rubbery texture when palpated.

Constitutional symptoms include fever, fatigue, anorexia, chills, and night sweats. The disease tends to be unpredictable and can either follow a chronically progressive course, or have periods of exacerbation interspersed with periods of remission. Other symptoms include weight loss; skin rashes with local pain; burning, itching eyes; chest pain; cough; and an irregular heart beat. Complications associated with sarcoidosis include diabetes insipidus, hypercalcemia and hypercalciuria (which may cause kidney stones), and hydronephrosis and subsequent renal failure.

Prognosis

Even individuals with subacute or fluctuating forms of sarcoidosis generally experience some residual organ dysfunction. The prognosis for the disease depends largely on the clinical manifestations and behavior of the disease. Acute pulmonary sarcoidosis can present with or without symptoms of pulmonary dysfunction or demonstrable abnormalities on radiologic examination. Sarcoidosis may subside without treatment, or it may respond well to a comparatively brief course of steroids. Disease that persists for 2 years or longer is considered chronic.

Patients with the chronic form frequently experience progressive pulmonary dysfunction. The prognosis of pulmonary sarcoidosis appears to be correlated with the presence or absence of other symptoms. Patients who have erythema nodosum, arthritis, and fever at the time of diagnosis tend to have a better prognosis than persons who have skin lesions, splenomegaly, or bone involvement. Patients who are severely affected may experience progressive dyspnea with the eventual development of cor pulmonale and death.

Sarcoidosis appears to have a poorer prognosis for African American patients and for those who are diagnosed after the age of 40. In the United States, 10% of patients with sarcoidosis will die of the disease.

What You DO

Treatment

Goals of therapy are directed toward decreasing inflammation that impairs organ function, preventing pulmonary damage, and decreasing distressing symptoms. When patients are first seen with mild symptoms and normal pulmonary function tests, they are typically placed under ongoing medical observation to monitor for disease progression.

When patients have organ involvement, particularly of the eyes, the skin, the heart, the lungs, and the central nervous system, treatment is indicated. To preserve organ function, corticosteroids are administered to suppress the acute inflammation. Patients may need a low dose of prednisone for up to 1 year to prevent a recurrence of symptoms.

Patients who fail to respond to corticosteroids or who cannot tolerate the adverse effects of these drugs may require alternate therapy with immunosuppressive agents. Some of the drugs proven useful in the treatment of sarcoidosis include methotrexate, azathioprine, and pentoxifylline, although these drugs also have significant adverse effects and require close monitoring by a health care provider.

Nursing Responsibilities

In the acute-care setting, nurses must be prepared to monitor and evaluate for evidence of progressive disease. The nurse should do the following:

- Establish a baseline physical assessment and then monitor for changes in status, particularly of the respiratory, cardiac, and neurologic systems. Careful physical assessment is particularly important when the patient is undergoing a steroid taper.

- Design a plan of care to alleviate distressing symptoms. Patients who have severe dyspnea and hypoxia may require oxygen and aggressive respiratory therapy with aerosolized bronchodilators. Plan patient-care activities to minimize oxygen demands, and help the patient conserve energy as much as possible.

- Administer prescribed steroids accurately and on time. Minimize toxicities and adverse effects associated with steroid therapy as much as possible. Inspect the patient's mouth daily for evidence of oral candidiasis, particularly when therapy is being given with nebulized corticosteroids. Give steroids with meals to decrease gastric irritation. Seek an order for an antiulcer drug.

- Monitor lab results routinely for possible hyperglycemia, particularly when a family history of diabetes and hypercalcemia is present.

- Inform the patient about the desired therapeutic effects and potential adverse effects and toxicities associated with treatment.

- Help the patient learn to manage adverse effects of drug therapy competently before discharge.

- Explain and be certain that the patient understands that even when the disease appears to be in remission, a potential for recurrence is always present.

- Alert the patient about possible signs and symptoms of recurrence that require medical evaluation and follow-up. All patients with sarcoidosis should be evaluated by an ophthalmologist every 6 months because of the possibility of eye involvement, which may lead to blindness if untreated.

National Heart Lung and Blood Institute
Facts about Sarcoidosis
http://www.nhlbi.nih.gov/health/public/lung/other/sarcoidosis/

Do You UNDERSTAND?

DIRECTIONS: **Choose the correct answer to each of the following questions and write the corresponding letter in the space provided.**

_____ 1. Sarcoidosis is thought to be a result of which of the following?
   a. Decreased immune response
   b. Defective genes
   c. Infectious organisms
   d. An overactive immune response

_____ 2. In the United States, sarcoidosis has the highest incidence in which population?
   a. Native Americans
   b. Asians
   c. African Americans
   d. Caucasians

_____ 3. A symptom typically associated with skin involvement in sarcoidosis is which of the following?
   a. Vesicles
   b. Plaques
   c. Local pain
   d. Pruritus

_____ 4. Drugs used in the treatment of sarcoidosis include which of the following?
   a. Antineoplastics
   b. Corticosteroids
   c. Cytotoxic drugs
   d. Interferon

What IS Pulmonary Fibrosis?

The term *pulmonary fibrosis* is used to describe a group of lung diseases characterized by thickening and scarring of interstitial tissue in the lungs. The interstitium is the wall between the alveoli of the lungs. Damage to

Answers: 1. d; 2. c; 3. b; 4. b.

this tissue decreases the ability of oxygen to travel from the alveoli across the damaged membrane into the bloodstream. Other terms used to describe this process include *interstitial lung disease*, idiopathic pulmonary fibrosis, usual interstitial pneumonia, acute interstitial pneumonia, and cryptogenic fibrosing alveolitis. Pulmonary fibrosis is associated with many different diseases and conditions; however, it can also arise without any apparent cause or explanation.

Pathogenesis

Pulmonary fibrosis is the result of an exaggerated inflammatory response in lung tissue. As the inflammatory response progresses, pulmonary tissue is infiltrated by lymphocytes and plasma cells. Mononuclear cells begin to accumulate in the alveoli. The alveolar sacs become thickened, scarred, and are eventually destroyed, leading to the formation of large cysts within the lungs and enlarged bronchioles.

Pulmonary fibrosis can result from many different causes and conditions and is frequently observed with connective tissue disorders such as scleroderma, rheumatoid arthritis, and systemic lupus erythematosus. Drugs and certain medical therapies can also cause this condition, as will exposure to certain organic and inorganic agents in the environment. Dilantin, amiodarone, and some antineoplastic drugs can cause pulmonary damage. In some cases, the cause of pulmonary fibrosis is unknown. This group of disorders can also have a genetic component.

At-Risk Populations

This disorder is thought to occur in approximately 5 per 100,000 people in the United States. Individuals with connective tissue diseases and autoimmune disorders have an increased risk for pulmonary fibrosis. In addition, anyone who experiences long-term exposure to inhaled air-borne agents (e.g., coal dust, glass particles, asbestos, and wheat chaff) is at high risk for lung disease.

Many occupations are known to carry an increased risk of lung disease, including coal mining, farming, and those involving steel and heavy metal industries. Individuals in high-risk occupations who are exposed to air pollution have a high cumulative risk for developing pulmonary disease.

People who work in occupations known to have respiratory hazards must be provided with the appropriate protective devices to safeguard their health. Examples of these protective measures include special air-filtering systems and particulate respirator masks. Workers in hazardous

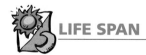

TAKE HOME POINTS

Pulmonary fibrosis causes permanent damage to lung tissue and ultimately results in respiratory failure.

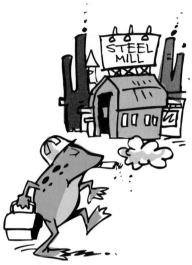

Increasing the risk for lung disease.

LIFE SPAN

Idiopathic pulmonary fibrosis (pulmonary fibrosis of an unknown cause) is diagnosed most frequently in patients 40 to 60 years of age.

environments may also need to have their work schedule modified to reduce the duration of their exposure and will benefit from training in safety measures to decrease their risk of exposure. Anyone exposed to occupational hazards will require vigilant screening by a qualified health care provider to detect early signs and symptoms of pulmonary changes when the disease is most likely to respond to treatment.

What You NEED TO KNOW

Clinical Manifestations

Gradually increasing breathlessness is the most common presenting complaint of pulmonary fibrosis. Some patients also complain of fever, fatigue, weight loss, and diffuse muscle and joint pain. Other symptoms include a dry, nonproductive cough; rapid, shallow breathing (**tachypnea**); clubbed finger tips; inspiratory crackles; and dyspnea on exertion.

In early stages of pulmonary fibrosis, chest x-rays show a characteristic "ground glass" appearance, which is frequently described as *diffuse interstitial infiltrates*. As the disease progresses, cysts form within lung tissue and cause a honeycombed appearance on x-rays, which typically indicates a poor prognosis.

Prognosis

The prognosis varies to some extent, depending on the probable cause of the disorder and the amount of lung damage sustained. When the initial inflammatory response that damaged the lungs can be halted or controlled, some patients experience a stabilization of their disease but will require life-long treatment.

Patients who have interstitial lung disease associated with other diseases such as lupus may respond favorably to steroids. After scarring of pulmonary tissue has occurred, the process is irreversible. The prognosis for patients with idiopathic pulmonary fibrosis is poor, with a mean survival of 5 to 7 years after diagnosis.

What You DO

Treatment

Corticosteroids are the primary treatment available for pulmonary fibrosis, but they appear to help only 10% to 20% of patients and, in some cases, may even be harmful. These drugs are given in an attempt to suppress the inflammatory process and prevent further lung damage. Patients most likely to respond to this therapy include those with limited lung damage or those who have coexisting diseases, such as lupus or mixed connective tissue disorders. Other pharmacologic measures that appear to benefit some patients include immunosuppressant drugs such as cyclophosphamide and azathioprine. In cases in which the causative agent can be identified, the patient must be removed from that environment immediately to decrease the risk for further lung damage.

Generally, supportive measures such as supplemental oxygen and respiratory therapy will be required to help maintain respiratory function. For patients who fail to respond to conventional therapy and show progressive disease, lung transplant may be a lifesaving alternative.

Nursing Responsibilities

For the patient with pulmonary fibrosis the nurse should do the following:

- Help the patient learn ways to cope with progressive respiratory disease and to maintain optimal respiratory function. The patient must be protected from factors such as infection that can further compromise respiratory function.
- Advise the patient with pulmonary disease that influenza and pneumococcal vaccinations are desirable to reduce the risk of a respiratory infection.
- Teach patients who are receiving medical therapy for their respiratory disease the proper way to self-administer medications and to manage potential adverse effects of corticosteroid therapy.
- Teach patients how to use hand-held metered dose inhalers and nebulizer machines when necessary.
- Carefully assess respiratory function on a routine basis.
- Document and report evidence of declining respiratory status, including abnormal (**adventitious**) breath sounds, increased respiratory rate, cyanosis, complaints of increased breathlessness, and decreased oxygen

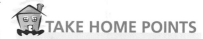

TAKE HOME POINTS

Medical management of this disease is directed toward preventing further inflammation and scarring of lung tissue with corticosteroids and immunosuppressive agents. Nursing management is directed toward maintaining optimal respiratory function and oxygenation, as well as preventing complications.

saturation levels. Patients with severe respiratory involvement must also be evaluated for evidence of cardiac compromise, including gallops (an abnormal heart rhythm) and peripheral edema.

- Organize activities and nursing care to minimize the patient's oxygen demands.
- Offer assistance with personal care as necessary.
- Promote relaxation, rest, and comfort, because stressors such as anxiety and pain increase the patient's oxygen requirements.
- Position the patient to promote maximal lung expansion, and remove noxious agents from the environment that may cause further respiratory compromise.
- Prohibit visitors from smoking in the patient's environment. Instruct family and caregivers that highly aromatic aerosolized compounds such as cleaning solutions and perfumes can exacerbate respiratory distress.

Some patients benefit from carefully supervised exercise training, which will decrease dyspnea upon exertion and improve exercise tolerance. Patients experiencing severe respiratory distress may require frequent respiratory treatments and high doses of oxygen. Continuous positive airway pressure machines (CPAP) may provide an alternative to endotracheal intubation and ventilatory support, and may also help improve the patient's exercise tolerance. Some breathless patients obtain partial relief from a fan blowing across their face. Improvement of nutritional status by means of intravenous hyperalimentation may also help improve function of the respiratory muscles, even when done on a short-term basis. Low doses of parenteral morphine can help relieve the sensation of air hunger that many patients with end-stage disease experience. Nebulized morphine may help diminish feelings of severe dyspnea and suffocation, particularly for patients in the terminal phases of respiratory disease.

Do You UNDERSTAND?

DIRECTIONS: **Fill in the blanks to complete the following statements.**

1. _____ is an early symptom of pulmonary fibrosis.

2. Patients with pulmonary disease should be immunized with _____ and _____ vaccines.

3. List three measures that can be used to help a patient who is experiencing respiratory distress.

   _____

   _____

   _____

What IS a Pleural Effusion?

The pleural space contains 5 to 10 mL of serous fluid, which serves as a lubricant between the visceral and parietal pleura. This lubrication allows the layers of the pleura to slide smoothly across one another, facilitating expansion of the lungs with respiration. Ordinarily, this fluid enters the pleural space from the capillaries that line the parietal pleura. The fluid is then resorbed by the capillaries in the visceral pleura and is also taken up into the lymphatic system. The term *pleural effusion* refers to an excess accumulation of fluid within the pleural space, which can ultimately restrict the movement of the lungs within the chest cavity.

Patients who have experienced chest trauma or undergone lung surgery may develop an accumulation of blood within the pleural cavity (hemothorax). A severe infection is evidenced by purulent pleural fluid (empyema) and a high white blood cell count, thus the fluid must be drained and the condition treated. In cases of obstruction or trauma to the thoracic duct, pleural fluid can be thick and white. This leakage of lymph (chyle) from the thoracic duct is called a *chylothorax*.

Pathogenesis

Four possible mechanisms behind pleural effusions have been identified:
- Increased hydrostatic pressure
- Reduced capillary pressure
- Increased capillary permeability, resulting from infection or trauma
- Impaired lymphatic function and drainage, usually from obstruction by tumor

Pleural effusion occurs as a consequence of a variety of diseases and disorders. Transudative effusions are frequently observed in conjunction with heart failure (HF), cirrhosis of the liver, and nephritic syndrome. All of these diseases tend to cause increased venous and hydrostatic pressure. The hypoalbuminemia associated with hepatic and renal disease can also cause decreased oncotic pressure.

Exudative effusions occur as a result of a change in permeability of the pleural capillary membranes. These effusions tend to occur in conjunction with infectious and inflammatory processes such as pneumonia and tuberculosis. Other causes include lung abscesses subsequent to surgery, pancreatitis, esophageal rupture, rheumatologic diseases, and malignancies.

At-Risk Populations

Any individual with the diseases and disorders previously listed is at risk for a pleural effusion. In cases of malignancy, patients with certain types of tumors, especially of the lungs, the breast, and lymphatic tissue, appear to have an increased risk for developing malignant pleural effusions.

What You NEED TO KNOW

Clinical Manifestations

Small effusions can be asymptomatic. Early symptoms of effusion include decreased strong vocal vibrations (tactile fremitus) and dull or flat percussion notes heard when examining the chest. Patients may also complain of chest pain with deep inspiration. Large effusions tend to restrict chest expansion, causing complaints of dyspnea during exertion and a nonproductive cough. Uneven chest expansion may be noted and breath sounds are usually decreased.

Prognosis

Recovery from a pleural effusion depends on the nature of the event that caused the effusion and the overall status of the patient. When the underlying disease process that caused the effusion can be reversed or cured, many patients recover. Without treatment, pleural effusions can lead to fibrosis and scarring, with subsequent respiratory compromise.

Effusion resulting from rupture of the esophagus can be serious because of the tendency of organisms from the gastrointestinal tract and mouth to colonize in the lung and set up local inflammation and infection. Prompt treatment with surgical closure of the esophageal defect is required.

For patients with a primary diagnosis of cancer, pleural effusions are usually a result of advancing disease. Malignant effusions frequently recur and may require repeated drainage and treatment to maintain respiratory function.

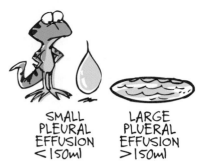

SMALL PLEURAL EFFUSION <150ml   LARGE PLUERAL EFFUSION >150ml

Larger effusions require treatment.

What You DO

Treatment

Small pleural effusions (150 mL of fluid or less) may resolve without treatment. Larger effusions are likely to cause respiratory distress and require prompt treatment. Large effusions must be drained to improve the patient's respiratory status. Microscopic examination of the pleural fluid also provides valuable information about the cause of the effusion and is helpful in establishing a diagnosis.

To provide immediate relief, the health care provider may perform a thoracentesis and remove up to 1500 mL of pleural fluid. This procedure involves inserting a long, thin catheter into the pleural cavity and draining the accumulated fluid. For larger or recurrent effusions, a chest tube may be inserted and connected to gentle suction to drain the fluid and promote reexpansion of the lung. In the acute-care setting, both procedures are done at the patient's bedside.

Depending on the cause of the effusion, concurrent management and treatment of underlying disease processes must also take place. For example, the patient with cardiac disease may require oxygen, diuretic therapy, and vasoactive drugs to improve and stabilize cardiac function.

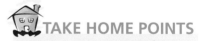 **TAKE HOME POINTS**

Medical treatment is directed toward resolving the underlying cause or causes of the effusion. Measures to provide symptom relief include thoracentesis, insertion of chest tubes, and, occasionally, pleurodesis. Nursing care emphasizes maintaining optimal respiratory function for the patient, assessing for changes in respiratory function, and assisting with therapeutic procedures.

In patients with underlying malignancies, effusions tend to recur, unless the pleural space is obliterated. This treatment is called pleurodesis and is performed by instilling an irritating agent into the pleural cavity. Various agents have been used, including nitrogen mustard, sterile talc, bleomycin sulfate, and doxycycline. These drugs are usually instilled through a large-bore chest tube and allowed to remain in place for 2 to 4 hours, depending on the preference of the health care provider. During this time, the patient must be helped to turn from side to side and positioned in Trendelenburg and reverse Trendelenburg position, thus helping the drug to coat all the pleural surfaces. When possible, the patient's cancer must also be adequately treated.

Nursing Responsibilities

For the patient with a pleural effusion the nurse should do the following:

- Frequently assess and evaluate the patient's lungs:
  1. Listen carefully for decreased breath sounds or a pleural rub.
  2. Percuss the lungs and assess for decreases in tactile fremitus, which can indicate an expanding pleural effusion.
  3. Use a pulse oximeter to obtain capillary oxygen levels, and notify the health care provider of declining trends in readings.
- Plan activities and nursing care to minimize oxygen demands.
- Provide supplemental oxygen, when indicated.
- Place frequently used objects within convenient reach of the patient, and offer assistance with personal care, such as hygiene and toileting.
- When the patient requires drainage of the effusion, explain the procedure to the patient and gather the appropriate equipment. Be sure that a procedural consent is obtained from the patient.
- For a thoracentesis, the patient may be positioned either leaning over a tray table or in a side-lying position, depending on the status of the patient, the location of the effusion, and the health care provider's preference.
- When a chest tube insertion is performed, place the patient in either a supine or a side-lying position, and administer analgesics for the procedure as ordered. Be prepared to help maintain sterile technique for the procedure and receive specimen tubes as fluid is removed.
- The chest tube must be secured with a heavy occlusive bandage to prevent air from entering the chest cavity and should be securely taped to prevent the tube from becoming accidentally dislodged.

Document the amount and characteristics of the drainage from the chest tube on the patient's intake and output records.

- Perform regular assessments of the patient's respiratory status. Assess the integrity of the chest tube and suction at least every 2 hours and with each patient contact. Remember to assess the patient's level of comfort routinely after the chest tube is inserted. Patients with poor pain control after chest tube placement tend to have inadequate lung expansion and are consequently at risk for further respiratory complications.

- For patients requiring pleurodesis, assist with the procedure and rotate the patient according to the directions of the health care provider. Because the procedure involves instillation of an irritating substance, the patient should be medicated with the appropriate analgesic before the procedure and assessed for adequate pain control on an ongoing basis. Some agents used for pleurodesis may also cause low-grade fevers, which can be readily treated with acetaminophen. As mentioned previously, maintaining adequate pain control is imperative to help the patient regain optimal respiratory function.

Do You UNDERSTAND?

DIRECTIONS: **Indicate which statements are *true* (T) and which are *false* (F). If false, correct the statement in the margin space to make it true.**

1. _____ The pleural space normally contains 5 to 10 mL of pleural fluid.

2. _____ Blood within the chest cavity is called an empyema.

3. _____ Chest tubes must be secured with a heavy bandage to prevent accidental dislodging of the chest tube and air from entering the chest cavity.

What IS Acute Respiratory Distress Syndrome?

Acute respiratory distress syndrome (ARDS) is a consequence of injury to lung tissue that damages the alveolar-capillary membrane. Various clinical conditions are associated with the development of ARDS including severe traumatic injury, direct contusions to the lungs, head injury, sepsis, near drownings, aspiration of gastric contents, smoke inhalation, and narcotic overdoses. Usually this syndrome develops quickly, often within a few hours after the triggering event.

Pathogenesis

Injury to the epithelial cells within the lungs causes increased permeability of the capillary-alveolar membranes, with consequent movement of blood cells, serum, and plasma proteins into the alveoli and interstitial spaces. Damage to cells of the alveoli causes the accumulation of fluid, decreases surfactant activity, and leads to hyaline membrane formation. Gas exchange is impaired, the lungs lose their resilience and elasticity, and profound hypoxia results. Even in patients who recover from this syndrome, there is often residual pulmonary fibrosis, with subsequent life-long pulmonary insufficiency.

At-Risk Populations

ARDS is always a consequence of secondary lung injury and can occur in adults and children. Conditions that predispose a patient to this syndrome include aspiration, exposure to drugs and toxins, systemic infections, trauma, shock, and severe hypovolemia. The common factors shared by all of these precipitating events are hypoperfusion and/or hypoxia of lung tissue.

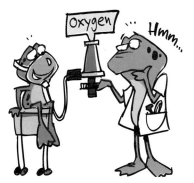

Hint: It could be ARDS.

What You NEED TO KNOW

Clinical Manifestations

In otherwise healthy individuals, the onset of ARDS is usually rapid and characterized by rapidly increasing severe respiratory distress. Because the lungs are stiffening and losing compliance, the individual will become tachypneic in order to compensate. The tachypnea will lead to acute respiratory alkalosis. Initially, chest x-rays will appear normal, but as the syndrome progresses they will show bilateral consolidation of lung tissue because the alveoli are filling up with fluid. Further symptoms include cyanosis, a productive cough, and increased use of accessory muscles. Hypoxemia will become refractory and severe as alveoli lose function and collapse.

Prognosis

Chances for recovery from this syndrome depend upon the patient's overall status, including the presence or absence of underlying health conditions and the factors that caused the initial lung injury. Estimates of mortality associated with this condition range from 50% to 85%. The highest mortality rates are seen with sepsis. Of patients who recover from this syndrome, 50% will have permanent lung damage. The remaining survivors may take up to a year to recover normal lung function.

What You DO

Treatment

ARDS is a life-threatening condition and necessitates prompt recognition and treatment if the patient is to survive. Goals of therapy are to maintain oxygenation and to support the function of vital organs until the precipitating event has been resolved and the lungs have had a chance to heal. In the acute stages, patients usually require respiratory support with endotracheal intubation and a ventilator. In order to maximize their chances for survival, patients with ARDS should be cared for in an intensive care unit.

Nursing Responsibilities

Carefully assess and monitor all patients with respiratory failure who are in a high-risk category for the development of ARDS. Symptoms of ARDS may be less dramatic in patients who have underlying comorbid conditions or diseases such as asthma, chronic obstructive pulmonary disease, or diabetes. Detection of this syndrome in the early stages may protect a patient from subsequent, more severe lung injury associated with worsening hypoxia.

In an emergency setting, act quickly to stabilize the patient. Anticipate the need for the following:

- Cardiac monitoring
- Pulse oximetry to measure capillary oxygen levels
- An intravenous (IV) site to give fluids to patients who are hypovolemic or hypotensive
- Oxygen therapy to keep oxygen saturation levels at or above 90%

After the patient is admitted, the nurse should do the following:

- Carefully monitor intake and output, because fluid overload may worsen ARDS.
- Prepare for endotracheal intubation and ventilator support if the patient shows evidence of respiratory fatigue or acidosis.
- Monitor ventilator settings when applicable to decrease the risk of barotraumas (damage to the lungs caused by high-pressure ventilation).
- Place the patient in a prone position if hypoxemia is refractory to other measures.
- Provide emotional support to patients, their family, and significant others because fear and anxiety may exacerbate feelings of respiratory distress.

Do You UNDERSTAND?

DIRECTIONS: **Fill in the blanks or circle the appropriate answer.**

1. In the space provided, identify at least 3 potential causes of ARDS.
   _____, _____, and
   _____

2. Your patient suffered a fracture to his femur and several broken ribs in a motor vehicle accident several hours ago. When performing a physical assessment, you note that his respiratory rate has increased to 26 per minute, and his pulse is elevated. The nurse should first
   a. Notify the physician of the change in the patient's status.
   b. Obtain a pulse oximetry reading.
   c. Inspect the patient's nail beds for cyanosis.
   d. Place the patient on oxygen by nasal cannula.

3. Increased levels of airway pressure for a patient who is on a ventilator may result in
   a. Hypoxia.
   b. Barotrauma.
   c. Collapse of alveoli.
   d. All of the above.

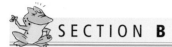

SECTION **B**

INFECTIOUS LUNG DISEASES

The respiratory tract is one of the most frequent sites for infection because every breath taken exposes an individual to potential pathogens. The pathogens may be carried on dust, smoke, or droplets from other individuals with infectious illnesses. This section discusses some of the most common infections of the upper and the lower respiratory tract.

What IS an Upper Respiratory Tract Infection?

Upper respiratory tract infections (URI), frequently referred to as common colds, are the most common type of infections that affect humans. The infection can attack any part or the entire upper respiratory tract, including the nose, sinuses, throat, larynx, and trachea.

Pathogenesis

In most cases, a virus causes the common cold. Viral infections can be spread through the air or contracted by a person's touching contaminated surfaces. Because of the many different viral strains, developing complete immunity to viral infections is nearly impossible. Occasionally, bacterial organisms can also cause URIs but are much less common as causative agents. URIs usually occur more frequently in the fall and winter, primarily because this is the time during which people congregate indoors.

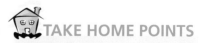
TAKE HOME POINTS

Viruses cause most URIs and do not respond to antibiotics.

Answers: 1. sepsis, trauma, shock, aspiration, or ingestion of drugs or toxic agents; 2. b; 3. b.

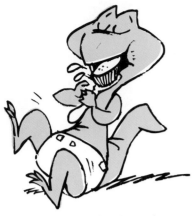

Make sure those hands are clean!

At-Risk Populations

Anyone can contract a URI, although some individuals are more susceptible than others. Individuals who smoke, have a previous history of lung disease or hematolymphatic disorders, or who are undergoing immunosuppressive therapy are all highly susceptible to respiratory infections. Because of their decreased immune status, the very young and the very old have an increased risk for respiratory infections. Young children are likely to "catch" a cold because of their poor hand-washing habits and their tendency to put things in their mouth.

What You NEED TO KNOW

Clinical Manifestations

The pathogen triggers an inflammatory response with subsequent swelling of the mucous membranes. These membranes secrete a serous or mucopurulent exudate. Purulent discharge in the nose, the mouth, or the throat is suggestive of a bacterial rather than a viral infection. Other symptoms of a URI include sneezing, nasal stuffiness, a sore and irritated throat, fatigue and malaise, and a low-grade fever.

Prognosis

Debilitated or susceptible individuals may experience longer periods of infection, or they may have secondary complications, including bronchitis, sinusitis, and pneumonia.

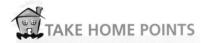

TAKE HOME POINTS

In most cases, a viral respiratory infection is self-limiting and subsides within a week.

What You DO

Treatment

No cure for the common cold is available. The risk of contracting a viral infection can be decreased through good hand-washing practices. Because the disease is self-limiting, most health care providers recommend rest, a sensible diet, and maintaining adequate hydration. A variety of over-the-counter and prescription drugs including decongestants, antihistamines, and anticholinergic preparations may be used to make the cold sufferer more comfortable. Some research indicates that zinc lozenges can shorten the duration of a viral infection. Antibiotics are inappropriate for colds unless the patient has a secondary bacterial infection, in addition to the cold virus. Rest has been shown to significantly shorten the duration of a cold.

Nursing Responsibilities

Most colds can be managed at home. However, the nurse should do the following:

- Encourage the patient with a cold to rest, keep warm, and drink plenty of liquids.
- Remind the patient to practice meticulous hand washing, to cover the nose and mouth when coughing or sneezing, and to use disposable tissues rather than a handkerchief.
- Advise patients who have a history of hypertension, thyroid disorders, or cardiovascular disease to consult with their health care provider or pharmacist before using over-the-counter cold remedies.

Do You UNDERSTAND?

DIRECTIONS: **Indicate which statements are *true* (T) and which are *false* (F). If false, correct the statement in the margin space to make it true.**

1. _____ Most viral infections of the respiratory tract cause purulent nasal discharge.
2. _____ The very young and very old are at increased risk for viral respiratory infections.

What IS Sinusitis?

Sinusitis is a bacterial infection of the sinuses and the paranasal sinuses that typically occurs after viral rhinitis. Acute sinusitis lasts 3 weeks or less. Subacute sinusitis lasts 3 weeks to 3 months, and chronic sinusitis persists for 3 or more months. Fungal infections of the sinuses may occur in patients who are immunocompromised.

Answers: 1. F. Nasal discharge may be discolored in both viral and bacterial infections, however, bacterial infections may cause purulent nasal discharge; 2. T.

Pathogenesis

Viral rhinitis leaves the sinus mucosa inflamed and edematous, which impairs and obstructs the normal drainage of the sinus cavities, which then forms an ideal location for proliferation of pathogens.

At-Risk Populations

Individuals who have frequent upper respiratory infections are more likely to have sinusitis. This disorder is rarely seen in children less than 1 year of age. Patients at risk for fungal sinusitis include those with diabetes, cancer, liver disease, and renal failure, and those undergoing chronic immunosuppressive therapy such as organ transplant patients.

What You NEED TO KNOW

Clinical Manifestations

Symptoms associated with sinusitis include purulent nasal discharge, facial tenderness when palpated, headache (particularly when leaning forward), cough, and sore throat.

Prognosis

With appropriate treatment, most patients recover completely.

What You DO

Treatment

Treatment of sinusitis is directed toward the restoration of normal sinus drainage. Increasing fluids and using humidity at bedtime will help to keep the sinus passages moist. Additionally, patients with acute or chronic sinusitis should irrigate their sinuses 2 to 4 times daily using an isotonic solution of saline. Any prescribed nasal steroids should be used following one of the irrigations. For the patient who suffers from allergies that contribute to sinusitis, leukotriene inhibitors (e.g., montelukast) and steroid nasal sprays may be used. Various drugs such as antihistamines and decongestants, may be used. In the presence of infection, prompt treatment with antibiotics and antifungals are necessary. Patients with chronic severe sinusitis that does not respond to saline nasal irrigations or pharmacologic measures may require sinus surgery to restore normal drainage of the sinus cavities.

Nursing Responsibilities

Patient education is one of the most important aspects of nursing care for the individual with sinusitis. The nurse should do the following:

- Teach the patient the proper technique for nasal irrigations and for use of nasal steroid sprays.
- Explain the importance of taking antibiotics as prescribed and over-the-counter medications appropriately.
- Instruct patients to drink lots of fluids and to use a humidifier or vaporizer in their home to keep secretions thin and watery to improve sinus drainage.
- Warm, moist compresses to the sinuses will help to relieve pain.
- Have patients seek immediate medical help if they develop high fever, or changes in vision or mental status, as these may be indications that the infection has spread beyond the sinus cavities.

Do You UNDERSTAND?

DIRECTIONS: **Fill in the blanks to complete the following statements.**

1. Acute sinusitis is most often treated with: (1) _____;
   (2) _____; (3) _____;
   (4) _____; and _____, if indicated.

2. Patients with chronic, recurrent sinusitis may need _____ _____ to facilitate sinus drainage and to clear our infection.

3. Hydration and humidity are important for the patient with sinusitis so as to: _____ _____.

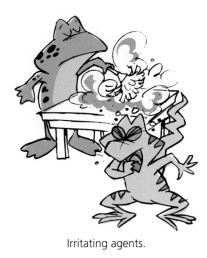

Irritating agents.

What IS Bronchitis?

Pathogenesis

Acute bronchitis is an inflammation of the bronchial tree caused by an infectious organism or irritating agents such as smoke, dust, pollen, or chemical irritants. Chronic bronchitis is characterized by repeated attacks of acute bronchitis, lasting for at least 3 months, over a 2-year period. Both types of bronchitis are the result of an inflammatory process. An inflammatory response in the bronchial tubes leads to swelling and mucus production. Excess accumulations of mucus within the airways provide a favorable environment for bacterial growth.

At-Risk Populations

Patients who have had a recent URI, influenza, or other infectious diseases can develop bronchitis. Smokers, individuals who are exposed to respiratory irritants, or those who are debilitated, malnourished, or with a compromised immune system are also at risk for this disorder.

What You NEED TO KNOW

Clinical Manifestations

Signs and symptoms of bronchitis include fever, painful persistent cough that may or may not be productive, chest tightness, a runny nose, sore throat, muscle aches, chest pain, and general malaise. Symptoms can be present for up to 10 days, but the cough can persist for several weeks.

Prognosis

With appropriate care, persons without other underlying diseases will recover fully without residual lung damage. In weakened or debilitated individuals, bronchitis can evolve into pneumonia. Chronic bronchitis tends to have more serious long-term consequences and can cause chronic obstructive pulmonary disease (see Section C in this chapter).

What You DO

Treatment

Acute viral bronchitis is treated with rest and palliative measures. Patients may benefit from inhaling moist air and increased intake of liquids to help dilute thick, sticky (viscous) respiratory secretions. Prescription or over-the-counter expectorants or antitussive drugs can also be helpful, depending on the patient's condition. Patients with documented bacterial infections or those who are extremely debilitated may require antibiotic and respiratory therapy. Antibiotic therapy does not improve the outcome or shorten the duration of the illness in people who are otherwise healthy. No cure for chronic bronchitis is available. Patients with this disorder will require supportive care and must be instructed to avoid contagious respiratory illnesses and environmental irritants that may exacerbate their condition.

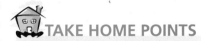

TAKE HOME POINTS

Unlike most URIs, bronchitis may require treatment with antibiotics in some patients.

Nursing Responsibilities

Nursing measures for the patient with bronchitis are directed toward relieving symptoms, improving comfort, and decreasing the risk for future recurrences. The nurse should do the following:

- Encourage the patient to maintain adequate hydration to dilute respiratory secretions.
- Administer expectorants and mucolytic drugs as ordered to promote mobilization of secretions.
- Position the patient to promote effective coughing, and monitor the color and character of pulmonary secretions. Inhalation of warm or cold steam can help loosen secretions.
- Administer antibiotics on time.
- Ensure that the patient understands the importance of taking antibiotics for the prescribed length of time.
- Teach patients to avoid exposure to environmental irritants and contagious persons with colds or influenza. The patient who smokes should be urged to stop and referred to a smoking cessation program for further assistance.

Do You UNDERSTAND?

DIRECTIONS: **Fill in the blanks to complete the following statements.**

1. Bronchitis can occur after a(n) _____ respiratory tract infection.

2. Chronic bronchitis can lead to _____ _____.

3. Hydration is important for the patient with bronchitis to _____ _____ respiratory secretions.

What IS Pneumonia?

Pathogenesis

Pneumonia is an inflammatory process that can involve all or part of the lungs and is a consequence of infection within the respiratory tract. Many different pathogens, including bacteria and viral and fungal organisms, can cause pneumonia. In most cases, pathogenic organisms are inhaled into the upper airway and spread to the parenchyma of the lungs. Pneumonia may also result as a consequence of aspiration of irritating substances, such as food or gastric contents. Affected tissues become edematous, altering the ability of the lungs to maintain oxygenation.

Typically, pneumonia is categorized according to the causative event or pathogen. Most pneumonias are classified as either a community-acquired pneumonia (CAP) or a hospital-acquired pneumonia (HAP). CAP is defined as an infection that became symptomatic before the patient was hospitalized or within 2 days after hospitalization. HAP occurs 2 or more days after admission to the hospital setting.

At-Risk Populations

Pneumonia is more likely to cause complications in people with underlying chronic diseases. People with compromised immune systems, such as patients undergoing transplant or antineoplastic therapy, are at risk.

Answers: 1. upper; 2. chronic obstructive pulmonary disease; 3. dilute.

Other risk factors include cystic fibrosis, diabetes mellitus, bronchial obstruction, and altered levels of consciousness. Because the placement of an enteral feeding tube increases the risk of aspiration of gastric contents, patients with these devices are at increased risk for aspiration pneumonia. Pneumonia can also as the result of a blood-borne infection from an infected site elsewhere in the body **(hematogenous spread).**

What You NEED TO KNOW

Clinical Manifestations

The signs and symptoms vary, depending on the individual, the severity of the infection, and the causative organism. Common complaints include high fever of abrupt onset, cough, malaise, and breathlessness. Patients may also complain of chills, sweats, pleuritic chest pain, and purulent, blood tinged, or rust-colored sputum. A physical examination may reveal wheezes, crackles or rhonchi, dullness on chest percussion, egophony, a pleural friction rub, tachypnea, and changes in levels of consciousness. Bacterial pneumonias tend to be characterized by a rapid, sudden onset of symptoms.

Prognosis

The prognosis of pneumonia is highly variable and depends on the immune status, age, and underlying health of the patient, as well as the timeliness and availability of appropriate treatment. Frail, immunocompromised, or debilitated individuals are most likely to succumb to this infection. Without antibiotic therapy, 30% of patients will succumb to their illness. Before the advent of antibiotics, pneumonia was one of the leading causes of death in the United States.

What You DO

Treatment

Antimicrobials are the mainstay of therapy for pneumonia. Individuals who are otherwise in good health and under 60 years of age can be successfully treated on an outpatient basis with macrolide antibiotics,

 People who have had a stroke or seizure, received general anesthesia, or who use alcohol to excess lack the normal cough or gag reflexes that serve to protect the airway and, consequently, have an increased risk for aspiration and bronchial obstruction. Pneumonia is now the sixth leading cause of death in the United States.

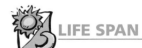 **LIFE SPAN**

Older individuals may show few of the symptoms commonly associated with pneumonia but may have changes in behavior and mental status.

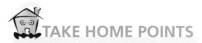 **TAKE HOME POINTS**

Pneumonia must be treated promptly with the appropriate therapy to decrease the risk of dying from this illness.

such as erythromycin or azithromycin. People with comorbid illnesses, such as cardiovascular disease, may require hospitalization and treatment with intravenous antibiotics. Patients with viral or fungal pneumonias will require treatment with the appropriate therapy, particularly if they are immunocompromised. Supportive measures to improve oxygenation include nebulized respiratory therapy, chest physiotherapy, and supplemental oxygen. Acutely ill patients may require respiratory support with a mechanical ventilator.

Nursing Responsibilities

Nursing care for the patient with pneumonia places priority on maintaining oxygenation and treating the underlying cause of the infection. The nurse should do the following:

- Assess the patient carefully for evidence of respiratory distress, and report abnormal respirations and oxygen saturation levels promptly to the health care provider.
- Position the patient to optimize lung expansion, and encourage the patient to turn, cough, and deep breathe frequently.
- Administer antibiotics as scheduled, and monitor for therapeutic response to treatment.
- Collaborate with respiratory therapists to help the patient obtain maximal benefit from treatments.
- Schedule activities requiring exertion after treatments.
- Mobilize the patient as much as possible to avoid further respiratory complications associated with inactivity.
- Teach the patient the proper way to correctly self-administer medications and about the symptoms that indicate the need for medical intervention.
- Assess the patient for risk factors, such as a smoking history or occupational exposure to respiratory irritants, that may have to be modified or eliminated.

Do You UNDERSTAND?

DIRECTIONS: **Indicate which statements are *true* (T) and which are *false* (F). If false, correct the statement in the margin space to make it true.**

1. _____ Patients with decreased levels of consciousness are not at risk for pneumonia.
2. _____ Pneumonia can be lethal, particularly when the individual is frail or debilitated.
3. _____ Patients with pneumonia should always be kept on strict bed rest to decrease oxygen demands.

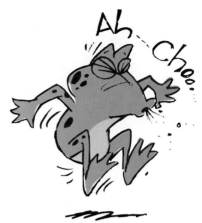

Sneezing can spread tuberculosis.

What IS Tuberculosis?

Tuberculosis (TB) is an infectious disease caused by the organism *Mycobacterium tuberculosis*. This organism can affect any area of the body but usually invades the lungs. TB is spread via aerosolized droplets from a person with the infection. The droplets are spread by activities such as laughing, coughing, and sneezing. TB is spread neither by hand-to-hand contact nor by contact with infected items in the environment.

Pathogenesis

After the droplets are inhaled, they are picked up by macrophages in the lungs and moved to hilar lymph nodes. Macrophages can engulf and contain the organism and may interact with T lymphocytes to form granulomas. The residual effect of the initial infection is a healed, hardened lesion called a Ghon complex. These patients will have a positive TB skin test. As these lesions heal, the infection may either progress or become dormant. Bone and joints may be involved, as well as the kidneys and adrenal glands. Reactivation of TB can occur years later if the patient has decreased immune function.

Answers: 1. T; 2. T; 3. F. Keeping a patient on bedrest contributes to atelectasis and worsening pneumonia and increases oxygen demands. The priority is on maintaining oxygenation.

At-Risk Populations

TB is prevalent in Native American, Hispanic, and Asian populations. Patients with human immunodeficiency virus (HIV) are highly vulnerable to tuberculosis. Other risk factors include homelessness, living in crowded conditions (e.g., prisons, mental hospitals), or living in countries with poor housing and sanitation. A large portion of TB cases diagnosed in the United States are among immigrants from Asian and Latin American countries.

What You NEED TO KNOW

Clinical Manifestations

Most patients are asymptomatic during the early stages. As the disease progresses, patients experience weight loss, night sweats, fever, cough, chest pain, and bloody sputum (hemoptysis).

Prognosis

Most patients recover fully from the disease when they receive adequate treatment, particularly during the early stages of the disease. In patients with HIV, tuberculosis tends to progress rapidly if left untreated.

What You DO

Treatment

Medical management of TB involves the use of drug therapy. Because a growing worry over drug-resistant TB exists, a combination of four drugs is usually required to treat the disease. First-line drugs used in the treatment of TB include isoniazid, rifampin, pyrazinamide, and ethambutol. To cure the disease, therapy must be continued consistently for at least 6 to 9 months. Patients with known exposure to TB may undergo preventive therapy (chemoprophylaxis) to keep them from developing the disease. In most cases, this therapy may be accomplished with daily doses of isoniazid. Usually, TB therapy can be successfully accomplished on an outpatient basis.

⚠ Patients who take their drugs inconsistently or skip doses are at risk for developing a drug-resistant strain of the disease. Multi–drug resistant strains of TB have been transmitted to health care workers as well as other patients. Personnel caring for the patient with active TB must wear an individually fitted, disposable particulate dust-mist respirator mask.

Nursing Responsibilities

The nurse should treat all patients who fall in a high-risk category and have symptoms of possible TB as potentially contagious, and take the appropriate protective measures. Any patient suspected of having TB should be placed on isolation precautions immediately. Other interventions include the following:

- Impress on all patients the importance of taking anti-TB therapy on time and for the duration ordered. Patient noncompliance with therapy is thought to be a major factor in developing drug-resistant tuberculosis. Directly observed therapy (DOT) may be necessary for patients at risk for noncompliance, which means that the patient must take their medication in the presence of a qualified health care provider.

- Help the patient identify measures to cope with the therapy and minimize adverse effects. Many antitubercular drugs have adverse effects and are poorly tolerated.

- Place the hospitalized patient in respiratory isolation for at least 2 weeks after the start of therapy. Untreated patients with active disease who are coughing require placement in a negative pressure room that filters and exchanges the air with outside air. Isolation should be maintained until the patient demonstrates clinical improvement and has had three negative sputum cultures on 3 different days. Personnel caring for patients with active TB must use special respirator face masks that offer protection from contaminated respiratory droplets. Conventional face masks are not adequate protection when caring for the patient with active disease.

Do You UNDERSTAND?

DIRECTIONS: Complete the following activities.

1. Identify the two major differences between pneumonia and tuberculosis. _____

_____

2. Summarize safety measures that should be used when caring for a TB patient with active disease. _____

_____

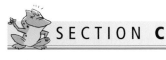

SECTION C

OBSTRUCTIVE LUNG DISEASES

Chronic obstructive pulmonary disease (COPD) is a respiratory disorder characterized by gradual reduction in the ability to exhale air. COPD is frequently used as an umbrella term to refer to a variety of respiratory diseases that cause obstruction of the airways. Other terms that may be used to refer to this disorder include chronic obstructive airway disease (COAD) and chronic obstructive lung disease (COLD). A variety of diseases can lead to this condition, including chronic bronchitis, asthma, and emphysema. This section will provide an overview of these diseases.

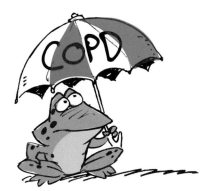

The wide umbrella of COPD.

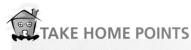

TAKE HOME POINTS

Chronic bronchitis is a result of exposure to respiratory irritants such as tobacco smoke or a respiratory infection, such as a virus.

What IS Chronic Bronchitis?

Pathogenesis

Chronic bronchitis is characterized by excessive production of mucus with a chronic cough that lasts 3 months of the year for 2 or more consecutive years. Chronic bronchitis is usually a result of prolonged exposure to respiratory irritants, particularly tobacco smoke, air pollution, toxic

Answers: **1.** Tuberculosis can affect other tissues and organs in the body, as well as the lungs. Tuberculosis requires significantly longer treatment than does pneumonia; **2.** Use negative-pressure isolation rooms with air-filtration system. All personnel in direct contact with the infected patient should wear a particulate respirator mask.

fumes, and dust. The irritating agents produce a chronic inflammation that causes swelling and thickening of the lining of the bronchioles, along with enlargement of the mucus-producing glands. Repeated or prolonged inflammation eventually results in scarring and damage to the mucociliary lining of the respiratory tract. The small airways become distorted and begin to close prematurely when the patient exhales, causing air to be trapped within the lungs. Eventually the small airways are destroyed.

At-Risk Populations

Smoking and exposure to second-hand smoke are the two major causes of chronic bronchitis. COPD and associated respiratory disorders tend to run in some families, suggesting a genetic component in the development of this disorder.

Respiratory infections may be fatal for patients with severe COPD.

What You NEED TO KNOW

Clinical Manifestations

Patients with chronic bronchitis have a persistent, productive cough, particularly after a night's sleep. Frequently, the mucus is purulent because of a superimposed respiratory infection. The thick, sticky mucus associated with this disorder is a favorable breeding ground for pathogens. Recurrent infections cause further damage and scarring of the lungs. As the disease progresses, patients experience increased severe coughing, chest congestion, and shortness of breath. Patients with advanced disease can experience right-sided heart failure and chronic severe hypoxia. With progressive disease, patients will develop a barrel-shaped chest and clubbed fingertips.

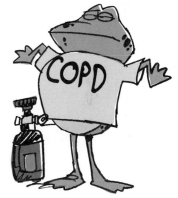

Progressive COPD can lead to a "barrel chest".

Prognosis

The outcome of chronic bronchitis depends on the presence of other, concurrent health problems, such as heart disease, and the patient's access to and ability to comply with medical therapy. Few patients develop serious airway obstruction, but they may be disabled to the extent that they are unable to hold a job and have poor quality of life. In most cases, patients die from complications of this disease rather than the disease itself, particularly heart failure and respiratory infection.

What You DO

Treatment

Medical therapy is directed toward slowing the progression of the disease and maintaining respiratory function. The single most important and effective intervention for chronic bronchitis is to convince the patient who is still smoking to stop.

Inhaled bronchodilators are useful for patients with chronic bronchitis. Systemic and inhaled glucocorticoids are frequently used to reduce the inflammatory response. Glucocorticosteroids are discussed later in this section.

Continuous oxygen has also been shown to prolong life in patients with low arterial oxygen levels because it decreases the risk for development of pulmonary hypertension and right-sided heart failure. In some cases, noninvasive positive pressure ventilation is helpful for individuals with poor oxygenation. Patients with respiratory compromise also benefit from pulmonary rehabilitation, which will improve their level of fitness and exercise tolerance. Lung-reduction surgery has been shown to improve respiratory function in some patients and is the subject of ongoing research.

Nursing Responsibilities

For the patient with chronic bronchitis, the nurse should do the following:

- Help the patient cope with this disease with extensive education and support. Provide the patient with comprehensive written and verbal information about medications, as well as the signs and symptoms of infection that require medical intervention.
- Instruct the patient in the proper use of metered dose inhalers (MDIs). Older or debilitated patients can have difficulty using an inhaler correctly and may require a spacer—a device that attaches to the inhaler that helps dispense the nebulized medicine.
- Teach patients the importance of avoiding potential sources of respiratory infection.
- Encourage patients to receive influenza shots annually, as well as vaccinations for pneumonia.

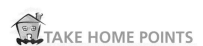

TAKE HOME POINTS

Care for most patients with chronic bronchitis successfully takes place in the outpatient setting, although many patients undergo frequent hospitalization for treatment of distressing symptoms and respiratory infections.

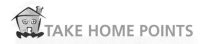

TAKE HOME POINTS

Cessation of smoking and avoidance of second-hand smoke is a vital part of the treatment of bronchitis.

Do You UNDERSTAND?

DIRECTIONS: **Indicate which statements are** *true* **(T) and which are** *false* **(F). If false, correct the statement in the margin space to make it true.**

1. _____ Chronic bronchitis is characterized by thick, bloody sputum.
2. _____ Chronic bronchitis is primarily a disease of smokers.
3. _____ Patients with chronic bronchitis usually have a nonproductive cough.

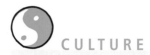

CULTURE

People with an alpha$_1$-antitrypsin deficiency usually develop severe emphysema in their 30s and 40s, particularly when they smoke.

What IS Emphysema?

Pathogenesis

Emphysema is a chronic, progressive lung disease characterized by enlargement of distal air spaces in the lungs and destruction of the alveoli. Two types of emphysema have been identified. Centrilobular emphysema is strongly correlated with cigarette smoking. Panlobular emphysema tends to run in families.

Emphysema is a disease primarily of smokers. Irritating substances in cigarette smoke damage the epithelial lining of the alveoli, which causes a release of inflammatory mediators. Those who smoke have increased numbers of neutrophils and macrophages in their lungs. Smoking increases the availability and activity of elastase, an enzyme that is capable of digesting lung tissue. Smoking releases free radicals that inhibit the activity of protective agents in the lungs, contributing to further lung damage. Because of a genetic deficiency, some persons are unable to secrete a protein called alpha$_1$-antitrypsin, which minimizes the damage caused by elastase.

At-Risk Populations

People who began smoking at an early age or those who have a deficiency of alpha$_1$-antitrypsin are at the greatest risk for emphysema.

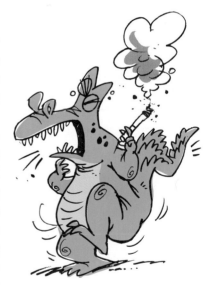

TAKE HOME POINTS

Emphysema is a chronic, progressive pulmonary disease that is caused by smoking.

Answers: 1. F. Chronic bronchitis is characterized by the production of excessive, thick mucus; 2. T; 3. F. Patients with chronic bronchitis usually have a persistent, productive cough, particularly after a night's sleep.

What You NEED TO KNOW

Clinical Manifestations

Gradually increasing breathlessness, particularly with exertion, is the hallmark of emphysema. Ultimately, the patient will be breathless at rest, with a prolonged expiratory phase of the respiratory cycle. Patients with emphysema tend to be chronically malnourished because eating increases their oxygen demands. Malnutrition causes loss of muscle mass, including the respiratory muscles, which leads to further decline in respiratory function. Patients are typically barrel-chested and breathe through pursed lips to open distal airways.

Prognosis

Emphysema is a progressive, incurable disease. Most patients die of respiratory acidosis and coma, heart failure, or massive pneumothorax.

TAKE HOME POINTS

Emphysema is characterized by gradually increasing breathlessness with obstruction and reduction of exhaled air. Most emphysema patients eventually become oxygen-dependent and require treatment with bronchodilators and steroids.

What You DO

Treatment

Treatment for emphysema focuses on maintaining respiratory function and preventing complications of the disease. Bronchodilators and glucocorticosteroids are the mainstay of treatment. Patients with emphysema benefit significantly from respiratory therapy treatments. Most individuals will require supplemental low-flow oxygen at some point in their illness.

Nursing Responsibilities

For the patient with emphysema, the nurse should do the following:
- Help the breathless patient minimize oxygen demands by spacing out care and activities requiring exertion to provide adequate rest periods, and placing frequently used items within convenient reach.
- Help the patient explore and develop strategies to maintain self-care ability, particularly after discharge from the hospital setting.
- Make sure the patient or the caregiver understand how to use hand-held MDIs or nebulizer machines when appropriate.

- Provide five to six nutrient-dense, high-calorie meals each day to help maintain nutritional status.
- Assist patients who are severely disabled and who require assistance with activities of daily living at home to find home care assistance. Placement in an extended-care facility may be necessary when no other source of assistance is available.
- For additional nursing care measures, see the sections on asthma and bronchitis in this chapter.

Do You UNDERSTAND?

DIRECTIONS: **Provide answers to the following statements.**

1. Summarize the difference between chronic bronchitis and emphysema. _____

_____

2. List useful education topics for the patient with COPD.

_____

_____

What IS Asthma?

Pathogenesis

Asthma is a respiratory disorder that has three main characteristics: recurring episodes of airway obstruction, hypersensitive ("twitchy") airways that narrow in response to certain stimuli, and inflammation of the airways. This hyperresponsiveness often occurs after exposure to agents that would not bother a person without asthma. Inflammation of the bronchioles causes further hyperresponsiveness to other stimuli, ultimately resulting in episodes of airflow obstruction. Most people with asthma experience greater obstruction of airflow during the expiratory phase of breathing. Asthma attacks can range in severity from mild

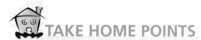

TAKE HOME POINTS

Asthma is frequently associated with allergies but may be of unknown origins.

Answers: **1.** Chronic bronchitis is characterized by chronic inflammation that causes swelling and thickening of the lining of the bronchioles, along with enlargement of the mucus-producing glands. Emphysema is characterized by destruction of the alveoli. **2.** smoking cessation, avoidance of respiratory infection, signs and symptoms of respiratory infection.

Certain drugs can cause asthmalike responses in susceptible individuals. These drugs include aspirin, nonsteroidal antiinflammatory drugs, and propranolol. Repeated asthma attacks can cause permanent changes in the pulmonary structure, with subsequent respiratory compromise and impairment.

shortness of breath to respiratory failure and death. Various agents can trigger the inflammatory response associated with asthma, including dust, animal dander, pollen, and perfume.

Research indicates that respiratory viruses, gastroesophageal reflux disease, and chronic sinusitis also trigger the inflammatory response. Other causes include extreme physical or emotional stress, cold or dry air, air pollutants (e.g., cigarette smoke, automobile emissions), and some foods (e.g., eggs, fermented alcohol). Forty percent of asthma is triggered by exercise.

Inflammation causes the production of cytokines within the lining of the bronchial tree. These substances prolong and amplify the inflammatory process within the airways. As a consequence of inflammation, collagen is deposited below the basement membrane of the bronchial lining, which causes thickening of the airway walls. In poorly controlled chronic asthma, overgrowth of glands and secretory cells that line the bronchial tree results, which causes further thickening of the airway walls and excess secretion of mucus. Some patients may have chronic asthma, with varying ranges of symptoms and respiratory compromise. With disease progression, the epithelial lining of the airways is lost, causing increased airflow resistance and further hyperresponsiveness to stimuli. Hypersecretion of mucus and hyperresponsive airways cause blocked areas in the lungs with subsequent hypoxia and inadequate gas exchange.

Asthma attacks typically have two separate phases. The early phase occurs in reaction to the presence of a precipitating event or irritant. Mast cells in the bronchial lining release histamine, leading to contraction of the smooth muscles within the respiratory tree, swelling of the lining, and secretion of mucus. This phase tends to last approximately 2 hours. Without treatment, the inflammatory response will continue, which stimulates the release of other cytokines that support and prolong the inflammatory reaction. The late phase of asthma typically begins several hours after the triggering event and can evolve into severe respiratory compromise, unless the appropriate treatment is initiated. Asthma may lead to permanent damage to the airways, particularly if inadequately treated.

At-Risk Populations

The prevalence of asthma on a worldwide basis has increased by 30% in the last 20 years. The reason for this increase is unknown. Asthma that occurs in children is usually a result of allergies. In adults, the cause of asthma is frequently unknown.

LIFE SPAN

Asthma can occur at any time in life, although it is generally more common under the age of 25. Many people with childhood asthma outgrow the condition as they reach adulthood. The condition may return later in adulthood, typically in late middle age or later.

Asthma is more common in African Americans than in Caucasians. Asthma appears to be most common in industrialized countries and appears to occur most frequently in socially and economically disadvantaged groups.

What You NEED TO KNOW

Clinical Manifestations

Breathlessness, severe cough, wheezing, and chest tightness are the hallmarks of asthma. Many patients also have thick, tenacious mucus that is difficult to clear from airways. A patient with mild asthma may be asymptomatic between attacks. Many people with more severe disease live in a chronic asthmatic state with varying degrees of respiratory compromise.

Prognosis

With appropriate treatment, most people with asthma live a normal life span. African Americans are 3 times more likely to die from asthma than Caucasians.

 Status asthmaticus—a severe form of asthma that does not respond to normal treatment—is characterized by severe bronchospasm, mucous plugs, and increased airway resistance. Status asthmaticus is life-threatening and requires immediate medical care.

What You DO

Treatment

The goals of asthma management are to eliminate or control symptoms, maintain normal respiratory function, and minimize adverse effects and complications associated with both the disease and its therapy. Treatment is directed toward decreasing the inflammation and bronchospasm associated with this disease. Patients who work in farming, animal husbandry, mining, and steel production may need to seek other employment that minimizes their exposure to respiratory irritants. Patients with asthma should also be examined and treated for sinusitis and gastroesophageal reflux disease, both of which contribute to the development of asthma.

Pharmacologic measures include oral and inhaled bronchodilators and antiinflammatory drugs. Short- and long-acting $beta_2$ adrenergic agonists are useful in treating symptoms and have a rapid effect, particularly when given by inhaler. Long-acting $beta_2$ adrenergic agonists such as salmeterol are given on a routine, twice-a-day schedule to prevent symptoms

⚠ Patients who have no breath sounds, those using accessory muscles to breathe, and those who have tachypnea and tachycardia are in danger of respiratory arrest and require immediate emergency medical intervention.

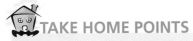

TAKE HOME POINTS

People with asthma may need to modify their home environment, lifestyle, and work setting to control their disease.

from occurring. The bronchodilating drug theophylline—a methylxanthine derivative—is also useful for some people with asthma, although it has a narrow therapeutic margin and may be poorly tolerated. Leukotriene antagonists help to interrupt the inflammatory response that leads to changes in the airways.

Glucocorticoids such as prednisone are highly effective in controlling inflammation. Eliminating or minimizing the chronic inflammation associated with severe asthma is important to prevent permanent structural damage to the lungs. Patients must be instructed that up to one year of steroid therapy may be required before an improvement in symptoms and pulmonary function is observed. For chronic use, these drugs have serious systemic effects that must be carefully considered when designing a plan of care. For some patients, adverse effects can be minimized and symptoms can be adequately controlled with the use of inhaled steroids.

Many patients with asthma, particularly older adults, have a decreased perception of breathlessness and may not seek medical help until they become desperately ill.

Parents of young children who are highly allergic (atopic), may need to modify the home environment.

Nursing Responsibilities

For the patient with asthma, the nurse should do the following:
- Maintain and support adequate respiratory function. Carefully evaluate the patient's respiratory status, and promptly report adverse changes to the patient's health care provider.
- Provide the patient with detailed information about asthma drugs and signs and symptoms that require medical intervention.
- Teach drug-dependent patients to keep an extra supply of their asthma drugs available at all times and not to allow their prescriptions to run out.
- Instruct the patient with exercise-induced asthma to use their bronchodilation drug before anticipated exertion to improve exercise tolerance and minimize breathlessness.
- Evaluate the home and work environment for possible asthma triggers, and help the patient develop strategies to eliminate them.
- Advise patients who smoke to stop immediately. Provide assistance in the form of counseling, behavior modification, and referral to a smoking cessation support group. Patients should encourage friends and family not to smoke around them or in their home, because second-hand smoke frequently triggers an asthma attack.

Several strategies are available that can help the asthmatic patient in modifying the home environment. Carpets, curtains, and upholstered furniture frequently retain dust and residue from dust mites and insects. Whenever possible, carpets should be removed and replaced with rugs that can be easily laundered. Drapes should be replaced with blinds or shades. Down pillows should be replaced with hypoallergenic fiber pillows, and pillows and mattresses must be covered with impermeable, hypoallergenic material. All bedding, including blankets, must be laundered frequently in hot water. Ideally, a new home should be found for all pets, because animal dander and excrement can also be a source of allergy. When the patient is unwilling to comply with this restriction, all pets must be kept out of the patient's bedroom, and someone else in the household should assume responsibility for grooming the pet and cleaning up after it.

Do You UNDERSTAND?

DIRECTIONS: **In the space provided, write the letter(s) that correspond(s) to the word or phrase that answers each question. More than one answer may be chosen.**

_____ 1. Asthma can be caused by which of the following?
    a. Air pollution
    b. Food
    c. Warm, moist air
    d. Animal dander

_____ 2. In what population does asthma typically occur?
    a. Under the age of 25
    b. Over the age of 50
    c. Of all ages

_____ 3. Drugs that are useful in the treatment of asthma include which of the following?
    a. Bronchodilators
    b. Diuretics
    c. Steroids

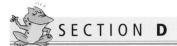

SECTION **D**

PULMONARY MALIGNANCIES

Cancer can affect nearly any tissue in the body. Cancer is classified and described according to the location in which it first appears (the primary site), the type of cell involved, the size of the tumor, whether the tumor has spread to other parts of the body (metastasized), and the way cells appear under the microscope. This section will discuss lung cancer, the second most common type of cancer.

Lung cancer is the most commonly occurring fatal cancer in the United States and is now the leading cause of cancer deaths in both men and women. Over 90% of tumors arising in the lungs are malignant. The rising incidence of lung cancer over the last 70 years is directly linked to increased rates of tobacco use and air pollution.

What IS Lung Cancer?

A direct correlation with tobacco exposure is seen in 85% to 90% of all lung cancers. Prolonged exposure to respiratory irritants causes changes in the mucociliary lining of the lungs. Lung cancer is thought to be the result of repeated exposure to irritating substances in the environment, leading to inflammatory changes that eventually undergo malignant transformation. These substances are inhaled as part of the air. Most lung cancers originate in the epithelial lining of the lungs and bronchioles—the parts of the lungs that are exposed to ambient air and inhaled agents. Environmental carcinogens that contribute to the development of lung cancer include asbestos and radon. Up to 15% of lung cancer cases are thought to be the result of occupational exposure to carcinogens. Genetic changes also contribute to the development of lung cancer.

After cessation of smoking, 15 years may be required for lung tissue to return to normal. Research indicates that for women who smoke, a longer time may be required for their lungs to return to presmoking status.

Pathogenesis

Two main types of lung cancer have been identified: small cell lung cancer (SCLC) and non–small cell lung cancer (NSCLC). The various types of lung cancer have different patterns of growth and respond differently to treatment.

SCLC grows rapidly and has, in many cases, already spread to other areas of the body by the time of diagnosis. SCLC usually responds well to antineoplastic therapy or radiation, but the response is short-lived. SCLC has the poorest survival rates of all lung cancers.

NSCLC comprises 80% of lung cancers. The subcategories of NSCLC include squamous cell carcinoma, adenocarcinoma, and large cell carcinoma. Squamous cell cancers tend to originate in the central part of the chest and grow rapidly, but they are less likely to spread to other areas of the body. For this reason, squamous cell tumors have the greatest potential for cure of all the lung tumors, although overall survival rates remain poor. Adenocarcinomas tend to arise in the peripheral regions of the lungs, a location in which they frequently invade the lymphatics and then spread to other areas of the body, particularly the brain, bone, and the liver (metastasize). Large cell tumors tend to behave in a manner similar to that of adenocarcinomas.

At-Risk Populations

In most cases, carcinogenic agents in the tobacco combustion stream cause lung cancer. Smokers who use filtered, low-nicotine, low-tar cigarettes tend to inhale more deeply and, consequently, they have more tumors originating in the periphery of the lungs. People who smoke and who are exposed to other carcinogens, such as asbestos (found in old building insulation) and radon, have an incrementally higher risk of contracting the disease.

Environmental agents contributing to the development of lung cancer include silica, cadmium, chromium, and coal dust. Occupations that entail exposure to respiratory irritants also convey an increased risk for lung cancer. These high-risk jobs include mining, some aspects of farming, and work in refineries and steel mills. The presence of multiple risk factors increases the overall risk for developing lung cancer. For example, miners who smoke have 20 times the risk of developing lung cancer when compared with a similar group of nonsmokers.

Women who smoke are more likely to develop lung cancer than men who smoke an equal amount. People who begin smoking at a younger

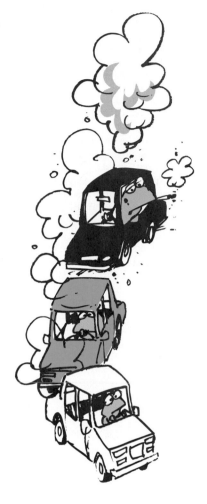

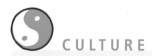

CULTURE

Lung cancer is the most commonly occurring fatal cancer in the United States and is now the leading cause of cancer deaths in both men and women. Over 90% of tumors arising in the lungs are malignant. The rising incidence of lung cancer over the last 70 years is directly linked to increased rates of tobacco use and air pollution.

TAKE HOME POINTS

- Lung cancer is caused by prolonged exposure to respiratory irritants. Tobacco is responsible for 85% of all lung cancers.
- The risk for lung cancer increases with the amount and duration of the individual's smoking history. People who begin smoking before the age of 15 have a greater risk of developing lung cancer compared with those who begin after the age of 25. People with the highest incidence of lung cancer began smoking before the age of 17, inhale deeply, and smoke half a pack or more cigarettes per day. Lung cancer among nonsmokers can be attributed, at least in part, to exposure to cigarette smoke during childhood and adolescence. At least 3000 nonsmokers per year die from lung cancer that developed as a consequence of exposure to second-hand smoke.

age are more likely to develop lung cancer than those who acquire the habit later in life. Patients who have received alkylating drugs and/or radiation therapy to the lungs for treatment of other malignant diseases are at increased risk for the development of lung cancer.

A small percentage of the population is genetically predisposed to the development of lung cancer. People who live in heavily industrialized areas with high levels of air pollution are also at risk for the disease.

What You NEED TO KNOW

Clinical Manifestations

Most lung cancers have **metastasized** by the time the disease is diagnosed. The signs and symptoms of the disease vary according to the size of the lung tumor, its location, and the number of other organs that are affected.

Patients with tumors in the central portion of the chest tend to present with coughing, shortness of breath, and persistent respiratory infections. Because many patients have a history of chronic lung disease, they may disregard the symptoms and fail to seek medical help. Breathlessness (dyspnea) may also be due to obstruction of an airway by tumor, or from accumulations of fluid in the pleural space or pericardial sac (pleural or pericardial effusions). As the tumor progresses, the presenting symptoms become increasingly severe, and the patient may cough up blood (**hemoptysis**) and experience stridor and wheezing.

When the tumor is sufficiently large to compress the superior vena cava, the patient may have swelling of the face, neck, torso, arms, and hands (**superior vena cava syndrome**). Tumors that involve the thoracic nerves can cause pain in the shoulder that radiates down the arm. Patients who are hoarse and have trouble speaking or swallowing may have tumor involvement of the laryngeal nerve or compression of the esophagus. Tumors located in the peripheral area of the lungs may invade the pleura and chest wall, causing severe pain and difficulty breathing. Lung tumors can also invade and destroy bony tissue, causing pathologic fractures and subsequent pain.

Some tumors also have the ability to secrete substances that disrupt the electrolyte and metabolic balance of the body. Of patients with SCLC, 11% will develop syndrome of inappropriate antidiuretic hormone (SIADH). Tumor cells create vasopressin, resulting in sodium loss and water retention. These patients experience decreased reflexes, confusion, lethargy, nausea, and vomiting, or they may be asymptomatic. Secretion of a substance that mimics the action of the parathyroid hormone, known as parathormone-related protein, can cause hypercalcemia and subsequent loss of appetite, as well as increased nausea, vomiting, constipation, and mental confusion.

Prognosis

The prognosis for lung cancer is poor for a variety of reasons. In most cases, the tumor is diagnosed when the disease has already spread to other parts of the body, substantially decreasing the likelihood of cure. Because most patients with this disease have a history of smoking, they tend to have other smoking-related problems, such as cardiovascular disease or respiratory compromise, which can disqualify them from aggressive but potentially curative therapies. Of those diagnosed with lung cancer, 13% of men and 17% of women survive 5 years after their diagnosis.

For patients with NSCLC, surgical excision of the tumor can be curative for some patients. The 5-year survival rate for patients with lung cancer that is diagnosed early is approximately 80%; however, most patients with lung cancer have metastatic disease at the time of diagnosis. For every eight patients diagnosed with lung cancer, only one will survive 5 years.

What You DO

Treatment

Currently, the three major therapies available for lung cancer are surgery, radiation therapy, and antineoplastic therapy. The overall status of the patient must be evaluated carefully before the start of treatment. Excision of the lung mass can offer prolonged survival and even a cure when the patient has a single lesion. Radiation therapy may be given in conjunction with surgery or antineoplastic therapy to control local disease. When tumor is obstructing airways or eroding mucosa, radiation therapy helps relieve breathlessness or hemoptysis. Radiation is also helpful in treating metastatic disease, particularly in bone or brain tissue.

Antineoplastic drugs are given to treat metastatic lung tumors that are too advanced to be treatable with surgery or radiation therapy. Drugs that are commonly used to treat lung cancer include cisplatin,

TAKE HOME POINTS

Nonsmoking wives of smokers have 3 times the risk of developing lung cancer than women who live with nonsmokers.

carboplatin, ifosfamide, paclitaxel, gemcitabine, topotecan, and navelbine. Antineoplastic therapy offers limited benefit to most lung cancer patients, in many cases extending life expectancy only a few additional months.

Nursing Responsibilities

Care of the patient with lung cancer is directed toward helping the patient withstand the rigors of treatment and providing supportive and palliative care when active treatment is no longer an option. All patients and health care providers must understand the effects of disease and treatment and be familiar with strategies to manage treatment and disease-related complications. The nurse should do the following:

- Extensively monitor patients who are recovering from lung surgery to decrease the risk of further respiratory compromise. These individuals will often have chest tube drainage, incisions and severe pain, all of which must be addressed in order to maintain adequate oxygenation and gas exchange.
- Take proactive measures such as the use of incentive spirometers, respiratory therapy treatments, thoracentesis, oxygen therapy, diuretics, and steroids, when required.
- Remove respiratory irritants from the environment.
- Encourage diaphragmatic breathing.
- Keep a bedside fan blowing across the patient's face.
- Keep the ambient air cool and moist.
- Plan care around the patient's radiation and antineoplastic therapy treatments to allow for rest periods. Both treatment modalities can cause extreme fatigue, loss of appetite, difficulty eating and swallowing, changes in gastrointestinal tract function, with damage to skin and normal tissues within the radiation field.
- Position the patient upright to help relieve dyspnea.
- Monitor the patient who is receiving antineoplastic therapy for evidence of immunosuppression related to the effects of drugs on hematopoietic cells. Anemia, neutropenia, and thrombocytopenia are likely to occur, particularly if the patient is also receiving radiation therapy.
- Protect the patient who is undergoing antineoplastic therapy from infection.
- Encourage the patient to report his or her pain. Collaborate with other health care providers to establish a plan of care that manages, rather than treats, pain and other distressing symptoms.

Plate 1

Aspects of the Disease Process (Etiology, Pathogenesis, Clinical Manifestations)

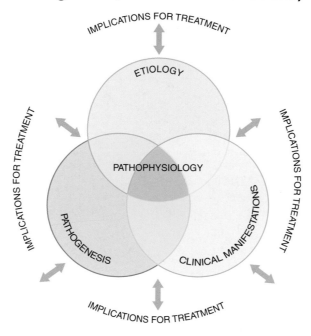

Plate 2

Alarm Reaction Responses from Increased Sympathetic Activity

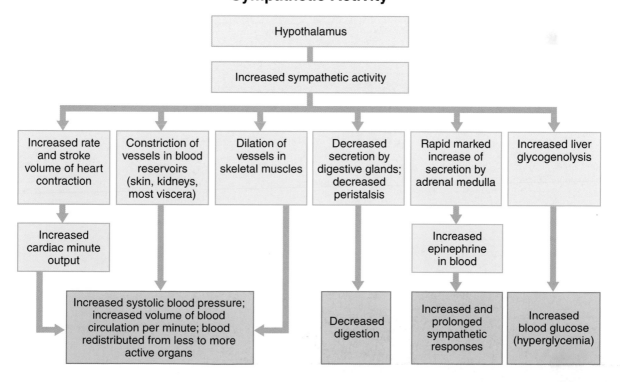

Plate 3

Effects of Excessive Stress on Target Organs and Organ Systems

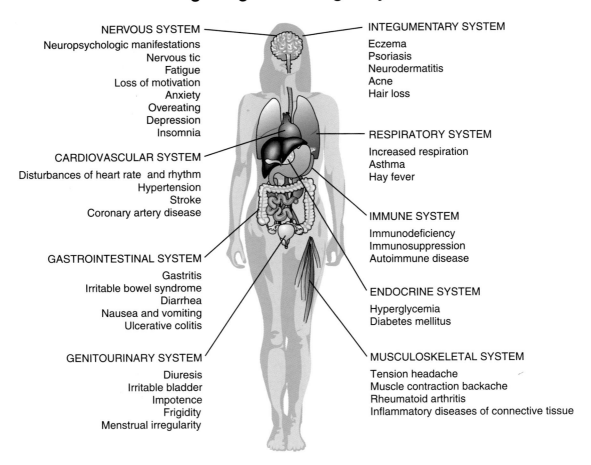

NERVOUS SYSTEM
Neuropsychologic manifestations
Nervous tic
Fatigue
Loss of motivation
Anxiety
Overeating
Depression
Insomnia

CARDIOVASCULAR SYSTEM
Disturbances of heart rate and rhythm
Hypertension
Stroke
Coronary artery disease

GASTROINTESTINAL SYSTEM
Gastritis
Irritable bowel syndrome
Diarrhea
Nausea and vomiting
Ulcerative colitis

GENITOURINARY SYSTEM
Diuresis
Irritable bladder
Impotence
Frigidity
Menstrual irregularity

INTEGUMENTARY SYSTEM
Eczema
Psoriasis
Neurodermatitis
Acne
Hair loss

RESPIRATORY SYSTEM
Increased respiration
Asthma
Hay fever

IMMUNE SYSTEM
Immunodeficiency
Immunosuppression
Autoimmune disease

ENDOCRINE SYSTEM
Hyperglycemia
Diabetes mellitus

MUSCULOSKELETAL SYSTEM
Tension headache
Muscle contraction backache
Rheumatoid arthritis
Inflammatory diseases of connective tissue

Plate 4

Theoretical Steps in the Development of Cancer

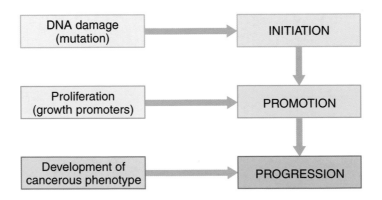

DNA damage (mutation)	→	INITIATION
Proliferation (growth promoters)	→	PROMOTION
Development of cancerous phenotype	→	PROGRESSION

Plate 5

Integrated Function of Immune Components

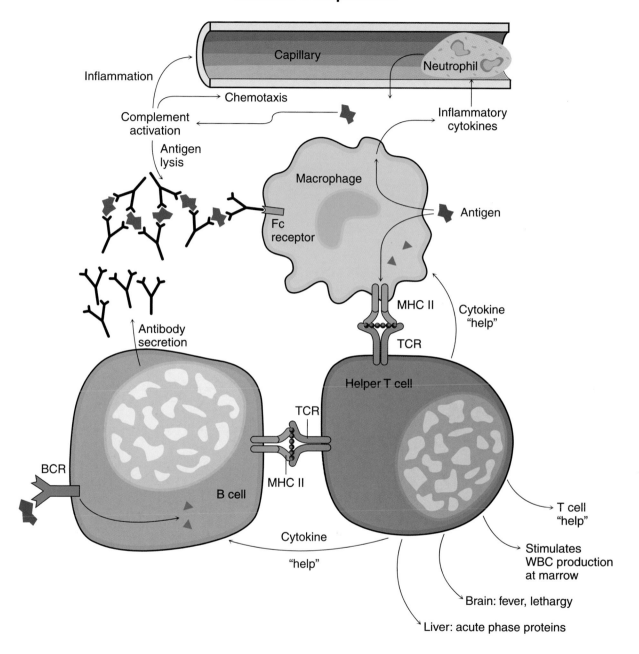

Plate 6

Renin-Angiotensin-Aldosterone System

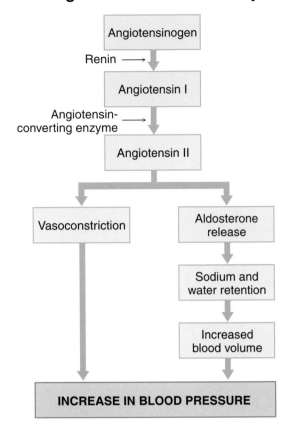

Plate 7

Conduction System of the Heart

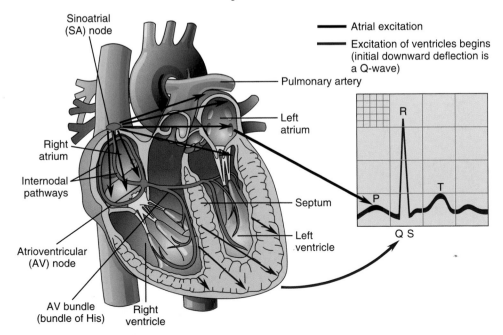

Plate 8

Summary of Events After Myocardial Infarction

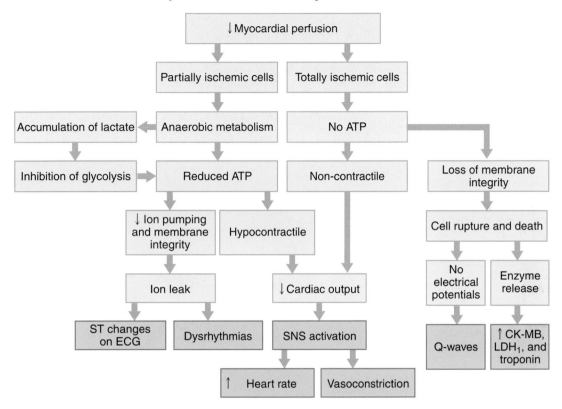

Plate 9

Pathophysiology of Nephrotic Syndrome

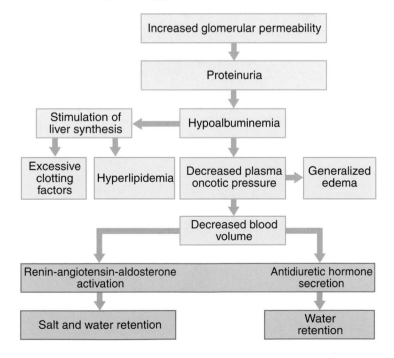

Plate 10

Pathogenesis of Acute Pancreatitis

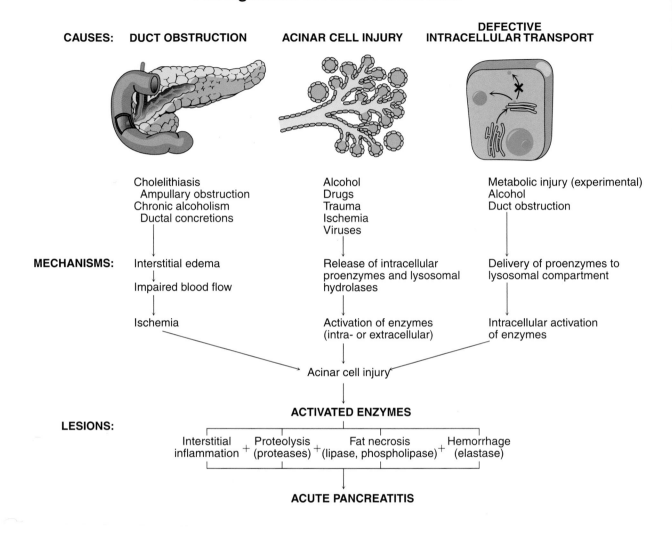

CAUSES: **DUCT OBSTRUCTION**   **ACINAR CELL INJURY**   **DEFECTIVE
INTRACELLULAR TRANSPORT**

Cholelithiasis
  Ampullary obstruction
Chronic alcoholism
  Ductal concretions

Alcohol
Drugs
Trauma
Ischemia
Viruses

Metabolic injury (experimental)
Alcohol
Duct obstruction

MECHANISMS:

Interstitial edema

Impaired blood flow

Ischemia

Release of intracellular
proenzymes and lysosomal
hydrolases

Activation of enzymes
(intra- or extracellular)

Delivery of proenzymes to
lysosomal compartment

Intracellular activation
of enzymes

Acinar cell injury

ACTIVATED ENZYMES

LESIONS:

Interstitial
inflammation + Proteolysis
(proteases) + Fat necrosis
(lipase, phospholipase) + Hemorrhage
(elastase)

ACUTE PANCREATITIS

Plate 11

Negative-Feedback Loop

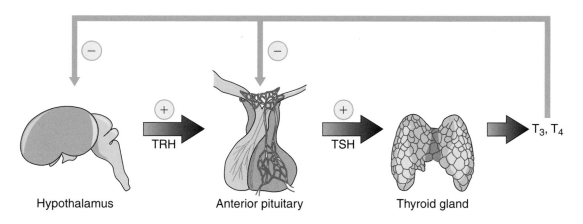

Hypothalamus   Anterior pituitary   Thyroid gland

TRH   TSH T_3, T_4

Plate 12

Syndrome of Inappropriate Antidiuretic Hormone (SIADH)

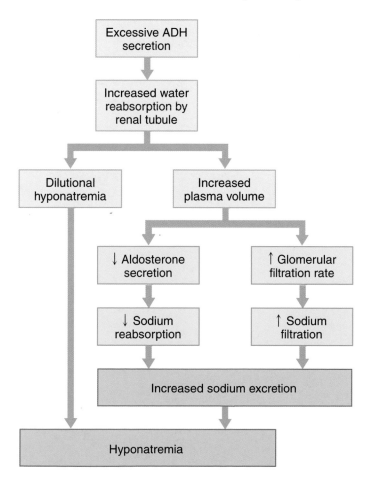

Excessive ADH secretion

Increased water reabsorption by renal tubule

Dilutional hyponatremia

Increased plasma volume

↓ Aldosterone secretion

↑ Glomerular filtration rate

↓ Sodium reabsorption

↑ Sodium filtration

Increased sodium excretion

Hyponatremia

Plate 13

Glaucoma

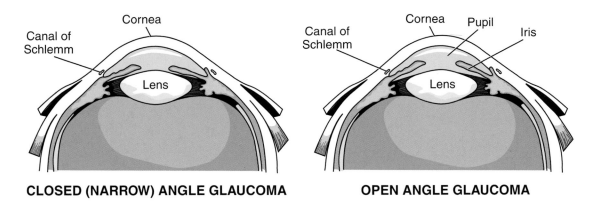

CLOSED (NARROW) ANGLE GLAUCOMA   **OPEN ANGLE GLAUCOMA**

Plate 14

Pathogenesis of Osteoarthritis

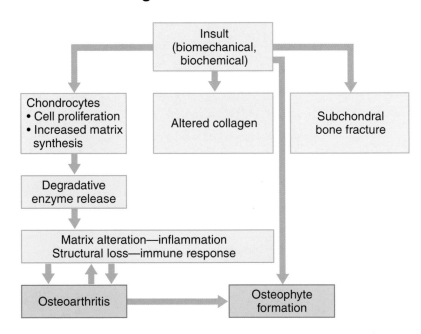

- Monitor patients for evidence of disabling depression or hopelessness, and prepare to intervene on their behalf. Patients and their caregivers frequently require intense emotional support. Some individuals benefit from counseling with a social worker, chaplain, or psychiatrist. Further benefit can also be obtained by the judicious use of antidepressant drugs.
- Educate the public regarding the dangers of smoking, and motivate people who smoke to stop. Young people and nonsmokers must be targeted for educational programs before they actually start to smoke. Nurses can also be politically active and support public legislation that limits the sale and use of tobacco products.

Do You UNDERSTAND?

DIRECTIONS: **Provide answers to the following questions.**

1. What type of lung cancer has the greatest potential for cure?
   _____

2. What are three environmental agents that contribute to the development of lung cancer? _____
   _____

3. What are two side effects associated with radiation therapy?
   _____

References

Celli BR: Diseases of the diaphragm, chest wall, pleura, and mediastinum. In Goldman L, Bennett JC, editors: *Cecil textbook of medicine*, ed 21, Philadelphia, 2000, WB Saunders.

Colice GL, Rubins JB: Practical management of pleural effusions: when and how should fluid accumulations be drained? *Postgrad Med* 105(7):67, 1999, URL http://www.postgradmed.com/issues/1999/ 06_99/colice.htm.

Day MW: Caring for patients with pleural effusions, *Nursing* 28(10):56, 1998, URL http://www.findarticles.com/cf_0/m3231/n10_v28/ 21224629/print.jhtml.

Egan JJ: New treatments for pulmonary fibrosis? *Lancet* 354:1839, 1999, URL http://www.findarticles.com/cf_0/m0833/9193_354/58061352/print.jhtml.

Answers: 1. squamous cell carcinoma; 2. radon, asbestos, chromium; 3. fatigue, skin damage.

Flannery M: Nursing care of the client with lung cancer. In Itano JK, Taoka KN, editors: *Core curriculum for oncology nursing*, ed 4, St Louis, 2005, Elsevier Saunders.

Jenkins TW: Sarcoidosis. In Buttaro TM et al, editors: *Primary care: a collaborative approach*, St Louis, 1999, Mosby.

Kelly K: Lung cancer. In Wood ME and Philips GK, editors: *Hematology/oncology secrets*, ed 3, Philadelphia, 2003, Hanley & Belfus.

Knop CS: Lung cancer. In Yarbro CH, Frogge MH, Goodman M, editors: *Cancer nursing: principles and practice,* ed 6, Sudbury, 2005, Jones and Bartlett.

Lewis SM: Nursing management of lower respiratory disorders. In Lewis SM, Heitkemper MM, Dirksen SR, editors: *Medical-surgical nursing: assessment of clinical problems*, St Louis, 2000, Mosby.

Lindsey LP, Thielvodt D: Non-small cell lung cancer. In Miaskowski C, Buchsel P, editors: *Oncology nursing: assessment and clinical care*, St Louis, 1999, Mosby.

Macklin LA, Bullock BL: Altered pulmonary function. In Bullock BA, Henze RL, editors: *Focus on pathophysiology*, Philadelphia, 1999, Lippincott–Williams and Wilkins.

Magaldi MC: Nursing care of patients with lower respiratory disorders. In Monahan FD, Neighbors M, editors: *Medical-surgical nursing: foundations for clinical practice*, Philadelphia, 1998, Lippincott.

Michaelson JE: Idiopathic pulmonary fibrosis, *Chest*, 2000, URL http://www.findarticles.com/cf_0/m0984/3_118/66188599/print.jhtml.

Toews GB: Interstitial lung disease. In Buttaro TM et al, editors: *Primary care: a collaborative approach*, St Louis, 1999, Mosby.

Turino GM: Respiratory diseases. In Goldman L, Bennett JC, editors: *Cecil textbook of medicine*, Philadelphia, 2000, WB Saunders.

NCLEX® Review

Section A

1. The interstitium is the
   1 Lining of the thoracic cavity.
   2 Outermost covering of the lungs.
   3 Wall between the alveoli.
   4 Outer membrane of the heart.

2. Signs and symptoms of pulmonary fibrosis include which of the following findings?
   1 Productive cough
   2 Slow, labored respirations
   3 Tachypnea
   4 Pallor

3. Corticosteroids are given to treat lung disease in an attempt to:
   1 Support the immune response.
   2 Decrease scarring of lung tissue.
   3 Increase the inflammatory response.
   4 Increase scarring of lung tissue.

4. Which individual has the highest risk for pulmonary disease?
   1 Nonsmoker who works on a farm
   2 Nonsmoking housewife
   3 Smoker who works in a boutique
   4 Smoker who works in a steel mill

Section B

5. Identify the statement that is *not* true.
   1 Bronchitis is always a result of an infectious organism.
   2 Chronic bronchitis can lead to the development of COPD.
   3 Bronchitis usually subsides in 10 days.
   4 Patients with bronchitis can benefit from inhaling warm, moist air.

6. Which drug should *not* be given to treat a common cold?
   1 Antitussives
   2 Antihistamines
   3 Antibiotics
   4 Expectorants

7. Which topic would *not* be appropriate to teach the patient with chronic bronchitis?
   1 Avoidance of people with upper respiratory infections
   2 Avoidance of smoke and respiratory irritants
   3 Signs and symptoms of respiratory infection
   4 Decreasing fluid intake

8. Which of the following conditions is a risk factor for infectious respiratory disease?
   1 Obesity
   2 Dermatitis
   3 Immunocompromise
   4 Allergies

9. Which of the following is *not* a risk factor for pneumonia?
   1 Impaired level of consciousness
   2 Sedentary lifestyle
   3 Diabetes mellitus
   4 Cystic fibrosis

Section C

10. Which symptom is typically observed with chronic bronchitis?
    1 Severe, prolonged, nonproductive cough lasting 3 months or more
    2 Prolonged, productive cough lasting 3 months or more for 2 consecutive years
    3 Chest pain
    4 Weight gain

11. In children, asthma is usually a result of which of the following?
    1 Exposure to temperature extremes
    2 Blockages in distal airways
    3 Allergies
    4 Dilation of distal airways

12. Chronic bronchitis is *not* a result of
    1 Stress
    2 Exposure to a respiratory irritant
    3 Smoking
    4 Virus

13. Which dose of oxygen would be safest for a patient with emphysema?
    1 35% by face mask
    2 2 L per minute by nasal cannula
    3 100% by nonrebreather face mask
    4 10 L per minute by nasal cannula

Section D

14. The most curative treatment for single lesion lung cancer is which of the following?
    1 Radiation therapy
    2 Surgery
    3 Chemotherapy
    4 Antineoplastics

15. Which individual has the greatest risk for developing lung cancer?
    1 Nonsmoking spouse of a smoker
    2 65-year-old person who has smoked for 50 years
    3 Nonsmoker with a family history of lung cancer
    4 65-year-old person who has smoked for 20 years

16. Which symptom is *not* suggestive of lung cancer?
    1 Thick, tenacious yellow sputum
    2 Bloody sputum
    3 Localized chest pain
    4 Persistent cough

17. A patient with lung cancer presents with swelling of the face, arms, and hands. This is probably a result of which of the following?
    1 Fluid retention
    2 Vascular damage
    3 Compression of the superior vena cava
    4 Compression of the inferior vena cava

NCLEX® Review Answers

Section A

1. **3** The term *inter* means between and refers here to the membrane or wall between the alveoli. The membranes that cover the lungs and the thoracic cavity are called the visceral and parietal pleura. The pericardium is the outer membrane of the heart.

2. **3** Tachypnea is a common sign of pulmonary fibrosis. A productive cough is observed in the presence of an underlying infection. Slow, shallow respirations are more likely to be observed in diabetic coma, neurologic damage, and drug-induced respiratory depression. Pallor is a reflection of inadequate perfusion or anemia.

3. **2** Corticosteroids suppress the inflammatory response, thereby decreasing scarring and fibrosis of lung tissue. Supporting the immune response, in this case, causes more scarring and inflammation of lung tissue.

4. **4** Any smoker is at increased risk for cardiovascular and pulmonary disease. The risk increases exponentially when the smoker is also exposed to other substances that are harmful to lung tissue, such as air pollution or heavy metals. Therefore a smoker who also works in a steel mill is at a higher risk for developing pulmonary disease compared with a smoker who works in a boutique.

Section B

5. **1** Bronchitis is caused not only by an infectious organism, but also by a chronic irritation from environmental agents such as dust or smoke. Chronic bronchitis can lead to the development of COPD. Bronchitis usually subsides in 10 days. Bronchitis patients can benefit from inhaling warm, moist air.

6. **3** Antibiotics are ineffective against viral organisms, such as the common cold. Antitussives, antihistamines, and expectorants help alleviate the discomfort that the patient with the common cold experiences.

7. **4** Fluid intake should be increased in patients with chronic bronchitis. The patient with chronic bronchitis should be counseled to avoid contact with people who have URIs, to avoid smoke and respiratory irritants, and to recognize the signs and symptoms of respiratory infection.

8. **3** Immunocompromise decreases the individual's ability to fight off URIs. Obesity, dermatitis, and allergies are not risk factors for developing URIs.

9. **2** A sedentary lifestyle, in and of itself, is not a risk factor for pneumonia. An impaired level of consciousness, diabetes mellitus, and cystic fibrosis are all risk factors for pneumonia.

Section C

10. **2** Prolonged productive cough lasting 3 months or more for 2 consecutive years is typically observed in the chronic bronchitis patient. A nonproductive cough is highly unusual for a true bronchitis patient. Patients with bronchitis may experience chest pain but only because of repeated prolonged coughing spasms. Most patients with obstructive lung disease lose weight because increased oxygen demands make eating difficult.

11. **3** Allergies frequently cause asthma in children. Exposure to temperature extremes can cause an asthma attack but does not cause asthma. Airways are blocked as a consequence of asthma. Distal airways are enlarged when patients have emphysema, not asthma.

12. **1** Stress has not been directly correlated with the development of bronchitis, although it can precipitate asthma in some individuals. Exposure to respiratory irritants, smoking, and respiratory viruses can cause bronchitis.

13. **2** The best oxygen treatment for emphysema patients would be 2 liters per minute by nasal cannula. Oxygen 35% by face mask, 100% by nonrebreather face mask, and 10 liters per minute by nasal cannula decreases the respiratory drive.

Section D

14. **2** Surgery is the most effective cancer treatment only when a single lesion is present. Radiation is used in conjunction with surgery or antineoplastic therapy to attempt a cure or to prolong life. Radiation is especially helpful with metastatic cancers in the bones or the brain. Chemotherapy or antineoplastic treatment usually prolongs life only a short time and does not offer opportunity for a cancer cure.

15. **2** A 65-year-old smoker who has smoked for 50 years began smoking before the age of 15 and is most likely to contract lung cancer. People who begin smoking before the age of 15 have a greater risk of developing lung cancer than do those who begin after the age of 25. Therefore the 65-year-old person who has been smoking 20 years began smoking well after his teenage years and has less of a chance of contracting lung cancer than does his 65-year-old counterpart who started smoking at age 15. Nonsmoking spouses of smokers have 3 times the risk of developing lung cancer compared with spouses who live with nonsmokers. Only a small percentage of the population may be genetically predisposed to the development of lung cancer.

16. **4** A persistent cough is not necessarily an indicator of lung cancer. Cough can indicate other respiratory diseases, such as bronchitis and asthma. Thick, tenacious, yellow sputum, bloody sputum, and localized chest pain all point to lung cancer.

17. **3** A lung cancer tumor large enough to compress the superior vena cava causes the patient's face, arms, and hands to swell. Fluid retention can cause any area of the patient's body to appear swollen. Vascular damage causes swelling only of the face, arms, and hands if the damage is localized to these areas and is not related to lung cancer.

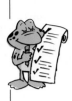

Notes

Alterations in Endocrine Function

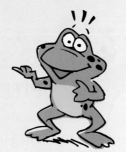

What You WILL LEARN

After reading this chapter, you will know how to do the following:

- ✔ Compare and contrast the causes and effects of hypopituitarism and hyperpituitarism.
- ✔ Discuss the pathogenesis of syndrome of inappropriate antidiuretic hormone (SIADH).
- ✔ Explain how SIADH and diabetes insipidus are alike and how they are different.
- ✔ Explain the differences in signs and symptoms of hypothyroidism and hyperthyroidism.
- ✔ Discuss the effects of hyposecretion and hypersecretion of the adrenal medulla and adrenal cortex.
- ✔ Differentiate the signs and symptoms of hypoglycemia from hyperglycemia.
- ✔ Explain the mechanisms responsible for Kussmaul respirations in the patient with diabetes.
- ✔ Discuss the mechanisms associated with gestational diabetes.
- ✔ Discuss the difference between type 1 and type 2 diabetes.
- ✔ Identify populations that are most likely to develop diabetes.
- ✔ Describe nursing interventions for patients with diabetes.

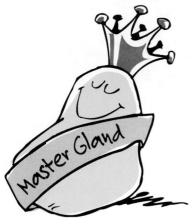

Introducing the master pituitary gland.

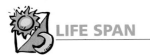

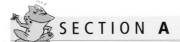

SECTION **A**

PITUITARY DISORDERS

The pituitary gland and hypothalamus, as parts of the central nervous system, are responsible for many endocrine functions. The pituitary gland, known as the master gland of the endocrine system, is located at the base of the brain and is attached to the hypothalamus. The pituitary gland is divided into the anterior and posterior lobes.

The anterior lobe of the pituitary gland secretes six important hormones: human growth hormone (HGH), thyroid-stimulating hormone (TSH), adrenocorticotropic hormone (ACTH), prolactin, follicle-stimulating hormone (FSH), and luteinizing hormone (LH). These hormones are responsible for regulation of growth, development, and proper functioning of other endocrine glands. In addition, these hormones are vital for the growth, maturation, and reproduction of the individual.

The posterior lobe stores and secretes two hormones: oxytocin and antidiuretic hormone (vasopressin). Antidiuretic hormone is responsible for reducing urine formation. Oxytocin acts as a powerful stimulant to the uterus, particularly toward the end of pregnancy.

Hormones are chemical messengers that are transported in body fluids. A single hormone can exert a variety of effects in different tissues, or several hormones can regulate a single body function. Water-soluble hormones combine with receptors on the surface of the cell membrane to exert their effects. Fat-soluble hormones permeate the cell membrane to combine with receptors found in the nucleus of the cell. Every cell contains approximately 2000 to 100,000 hormone receptor sites.

Anterior Pituitary Disorders

What IS Hypopituitarism?

Pathogenesis

Hypopituitarism is a generalized condition of the anterior lobe of the pituitary gland that is caused by partial or total failure of the pituitary gland's vital hormones—ACTH, TSH, LH, FSH, HGH, and prolactin.

At-Risk Populations

Any disorder that leads to obstruction or constriction (vasospasm) of the artery supplying blood to the pituitary gland leads to tissue death (necrosis) and loss of pituitary hormones. After tissue death, the pituitary gland swells, which further interrupts the blood supply. Causes of the reduction in blood supply fall into nine categories, known as the "nine I's" of hypopituitarism:

1. **I**nvasive (most common)—pituitary tumors, central nervous system tumors, carotid aneurysm
2. **I**nfarction—postpartum necrosis, pituitary stroke, malformation of pituitary blood vessels
3. **I**nfiltrative—sarcoidosis, hemochromatosis
4. **I**njury—head trauma, child abuse
5. **I**mmunologic—white blood cell invasion of pituitary gland, sickle cell disease, diabetes mellitus
6. **I**atrogenic—surgery, radiation therapy
7. **I**nfectious—fungal infections, tuberculosis, syphilis
8. **I**diopathic—familial
9. **I**solated—deficiency of anterior pituitary

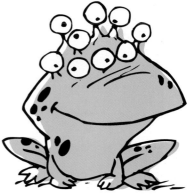

The "nine I's" (eyes) of hypopituitarism.

What You NEED TO KNOW

Clinical Manifestations

The signs and symptoms of hypopituitarism vary depending on the hormones affected. Hypopituitarism usually starts with hypogonadism or gonadotropin failure (decreased FSH and LH). There will be signs of hypofunction of target glands. For example, when all of the hormones are absent, the patient experiences retarded growth from lack of HGH, cortisol deficiency from the lack of ACTH, thyroid hormone deficiency from the lack of TSH (hypothyroidism), diabetes insipidus (although rare) from the lack of ADH, and gonadal failure (hypogonadism), and loss of secondary sex characteristics from the absence of FSH and LH (secondary amenorrhea, impotence, infertility, decreased libido, lactation failure, failure of secondary sexual characteristics to develop). Laboratory testing will confirm hormonal deficiencies. Radioimmunoassay of pituitary and target gland hormones is often done. A computerized tomography (CT) scan or magnetic resonance image (MRI) of the head may help

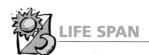

LIFE SPAN

The risk of hypopituitarism is increased during pregnancy because of the pituitary gland's increased size and large blood supply. Hypopituitarism in postpartum women results in loss of breast milk because of the absence of prolactin.

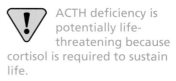

ACTH deficiency is potentially life-threatening because cortisol is required to sustain life.

to identify the cause of the deficiency. Radiographs of the chest, the skull, the hands, and the wrists may be done to determine bone age. Pathologic findings include destruction of the anterior pituitary and atrophy of the adrenal cortex, the thyroid, and the gonads.

Prognosis

Hypopituitarism can be acute or chronic with a variable, but guardedly favorable, course with hormone replacement therapy. Patients with post-partum hypopituitarism may have complete or partial recovery. Patients with ACTH deficiency must be on drug therapy for life to compensate for the lack of cortisol. Blindness and adrenal crisis are possible complications of hypopituitarism, and life-long drug therapy may be necessary.

What You DO

Treatment

The treatment of hypopituitarism involves removal of the cause and replacement of hormones. Surgical removal of the pituitary (hypophysectomy) may be needed when the disorder is due to a pituitary tumor. Drugs are used to replace the missing hormones and include growth hormone to treat HGH deficiency, glucocorticosteroids for correcting ACTH deficiency, thyroid hormones to treat thyroid hormone deficiency, and sex hormones to correct the decreased functional activity of the gonads.

Nursing Responsibilities

The nursing responsibilities for the patient with hypopituitarism are directed toward the problems that result from deficiency at the target organ (e.g., thyroid, adrenal glands, and gonads). The nurse should do the following:

- Encourage the patient to verbalize concerns about body image and self-concept.
- Administer hormonal replacement drugs as prescribed, which may include hydrocortisone, levothyroxine, androgens or cyclic estrogens, or HGH (for treating dwarfism and in selected adult patients).
- Teach the patient and family about the prescribed drug therapy and the importance of continued follow-up and adherence to therapy.

- Encourage patients to wear medical identification that states they have hypopituitarism and will require hormonal replacement therapies during stressful events.
- If hospitalized, stress the importance of additional cortisone at times of any major physical stress (e.g., fever above 101° F, acute illness, surgery).
- Encourage an active physical exercise program.
- A diet high in calories and protein should be consumed.
- Monitor laboratory test results at 3- and 12-month intervals to ensure drug therapy is at a safe level.

Do You UNDERSTAND?

DIRECTIONS: **Indicate in the space provided whether the site of secretion for each hormone is the anterior pituitary (A) or the posterior pituitary (P).**

_____ 1. Growth hormone
_____ 2. Prolactin
_____ 3. Antidiuretic hormone
_____ 4. Thyroid-stimulating hormone
_____ 5. Follicle-stimulating hormone
_____ 6. Adrenocorticotropic hormone
_____ 7. Oxytocin
_____ 8. Luteinizing hormone

What IS Hyperpituitarism?

Pathogenesis

Increased activity of the pituitary gland, particularly secretion of HGH and prolactin, causes hyperpituitarism. The disorders that result from the increased secretion of HGH include acromegaly and gigantism, as well as abnormal milk secretion **(galactorrhea).**

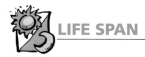
LIFE SPAN

Acromegaly, an uncommon disorder, appears more frequently in women than it does in men and is diagnosed most frequently between ages 40 and 60.

Answers: 1. A; 2. A; 3. P; 4. A; 5. A; 6. A; 7. P; 8. A.

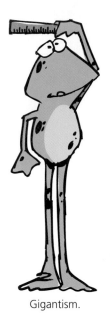

Gigantism.

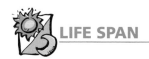

LIFE SPAN

In children, overproduction of HGH stimulates growth of long bones and results in an unusually tall individual. **Gigantism** is due to excessive pituitary secretion occurring before puberty and before the epiphyses of long bones close. When the abnormality is extreme, the individual can reach a height of 8 feet or more, although the body proportions are usually normal.

Acromegaly is due to excessive secretion of human growth hormone and is characterized by progressive enlargement of the head and face, the hands and feet, and the thorax. The most common cause of acromegaly is continuous hormonal secretion from a primary HGH-secreting pituitary tumor (**adenoma**). An unpredictable pattern develops with the excess secretion levels, which stimulates growth. In the adult, connective tissue and the bony matrix multiplies, which results in the enlargement of facial features and long bones. Secretion of HGH is also increased during exercise, hypoglycemia, stress, and nervous-system stimulation.

The metabolic effects of HGH on the renal tubules contribute to high levels of phosphates in the blood. Carbohydrate intolerance and an increased metabolic rate are present. Blood glucose levels elevate, followed by insulin resistance. Diabetes mellitus develops when the pancreas cannot secrete sufficient insulin to offset the effects of HGH.

At-Risk Populations

Patients who are most at risk for hyperpituitarism are those who have a pituitary adenoma. Approximately one third of patients with HGH abnormalities have glucose intolerance, and one half of these patients develop diabetes mellitus. Of all pituitary adenomas, 30% secrete sufficient prolactin to cause galactorrhea, and approximately 25% of those secrete excesses of both HGH and prolactin.

What You NEED TO KNOW

Clinical Manifestations

In adults whose bone growth has stopped, a gradual enlargement and coarsening of facial features, hands, and feet is observed. Early signs include increased metabolism and strength and excessive sweating. The patient experiences joint pain, weakness, visual disturbances, and signs and symptoms of diabetes mellitus.

Female patients with excessive prolactin levels develop abnormal milk secretion in the nonlactating breast, cessation of menses (**amenorrhea**), and vaginal dryness. Male patients with excessive prolactin levels experience a loss of interest in sex and an inability to obtain and sustain an erection. Depression, anxiety, headaches, and vision loss occur in both genders.

Prognosis

Without treatment, hyperpituitarism—specifically acromegaly—is a slow, progressive disease associated with decreased life expectancy.

What You DO

Treatment

Treatment of patients with acromegaly or excessive prolactin secretion consists of radiation or surgical removal of the pituitary gland (**hypophysectomy**). Adjunctive drug therapy with a dopamine receptor agonist (e.g., bromocriptine) can be used for patients with excessive prolactin. The use of bromocriptine can reduce prolactin levels in 90% of patients. Octreotide, a growth hormone analog, is effective in reducing HGH levels in 60% to 80% of patients.

Gigantism can be corrected only through early diagnosis in childhood and surgical removal of a portion of the pituitary gland or through radiation therapy.

Nursing Responsibilities

Nursing care of the patient with hyperpituitarism is most frequently related to perioperative care. The nurse should do the following:

- Assess the patient's expectations involving the surgery, educational needs related to diagnosis and treatment regimen, and the available support system.
- Obtain baseline vital signs.
- Perform perioperative neurologic assessments that include pupil equality and reactivity to light; handgrip; level of consciousness; orientation to time, place, and situation; appropriate response to stimuli; and visual acuity and visual fields.
- Teach the patient and family about the diagnosis, the surgical intervention, and the drug therapy that are required after surgery.
- Instruct the patient to avoid sneezing, coughing, and bending over from the waist to avoid disrupting the surgical site. Instruct the patient how to change the nasal drip pad used postoperatively to collect nasal discharge.
- Support changes in patient's self-image and self-concept.

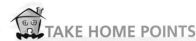

TAKE HOME POINTS

Patients who have had their pituitary gland completely removed or destroyed with radiation therapy must take hormone replacements, particularly cortisone, for the remainder of their lives.

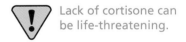

Lack of cortisone can be life-threatening.

- Administer glucocorticoids as ordered during the perioperative period to help the patient tolerate the stress of surgery and the absence of cortisol.

Do You UNDERSTAND?

DIRECTIONS: **Match Column A with Column B.**

Column A	Column B
_____ 1. Hyperpituitarism	a. A benign tumor in which the cells form a recognizable glandular structure or in which the cells are derived from glandular epithelium
_____ 2. Adenoma	b. Surgical removal of a portion or all of the pituitary gland; indicated when there is a tumor of the gland
_____ 3. Prolactin	c. An anterior pituitary hormone that controls general growth of the skeleton and influences metabolism
_____ 4. Growth hormone	d. An anterior pituitary hormone that promotes the growth of breast tissue and stimulates and sustains milk production during the postpartum period
_____ 5. Hypophysectomy	e. A condition from pathologically increased activity of the pituitary gland, especially growth hormone or prolactin

Answers: 1. e, 2. a, 3. d, 4. c, 5. b.

Posterior Pituitary Disorders

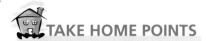

What IS Syndrome of Inappropriate Antidiuretic Hormone?

Pathogenesis

Syndrome of inappropriate antidiuretic hormone (SIADH) involves low serum sodium levels (hyponatremia) with inappropriately elevated urine osmolality. In SIADH there is a secretion of excessive amounts of antidiuretic hormone (ADH) from the posterior pituitary gland and other areas outside the pituitary gland. The resulting abnormal sodium excretion leads to dilutional hyponatremia. Total body sodium levels may be normal or near normal. Total body water is usually increased.

The most common cause of excessive production of ADH is carcinoma; the carcinoma produces additional ADH. Tumors associated with SIADH include carcinoma of the tongue, the lung, the duodenum, the pancreas, and the connective tissues, as well as leukemia, lymphoma, and Hodgkin's diseases. A transient SIADH can follow pituitary surgery or the use of certain drugs (e.g., barbiturates, general anesthetics, vincristine, nicotine, morphine, diuretics, and synthetic hormones). These drugs serve either to simulate ADH release or to enhance the physiologic effects of ADH.

ADH is normally released in response to elevated serum concentrations and a decrease in extracellular fluid volume. ADH increases the kidney's permeability to water, thus promoting resorption and a decrease in urine output. In SIADH, ADH is not inhibited by the low concentration of solutes in the extracellular fluid.

Continual release of ADH causes water retention from renal tubules and collecting ducts. Extracellular fluid volume increases with a dilution of serum sodium. Hyponatremia suppresses renin and aldosterone secretions. The result of hyponatremia is a suppression of renin and aldosterone, causing a decrease in the resorption of sodium by the renal tubules.

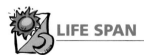

At-Risk Populations

Patients with SIADH are usually found in the hospital setting, where the incidence can be as high as 35%. Patients who are at risk for SIADH include those with a history of carcinoma of lung, duodenum, brain, bladder, pancreas, or prostate. Patients with an infection of the brain, brain trauma, or infectious processes of the lungs are also at risk. Patients who are taking certain drugs (e.g., morphine, diuretics, barbiturates, nicotine) that serve either to stimulate ADH release or to enhance its effects can also be predisposed to SIADH.

What You NEED TO KNOW

Clinical Manifestations

The signs and symptoms of SIADH are related to the onset and severity of low serum sodium levels. Some patients may be totally asymptomatic, but those who have a rapid decrease in serum sodium level from 140 to 130 mEq/L complain of thirst, impaired taste, anorexia, dyspnea on exertion, fatigue, and dulled mentation. Severe gastrointestinal symptoms such as nausea and vomiting appear with a drop in serum sodium from 130 to 120 mEq/L. Other manifestations include headache, irritability, lethargy, restlessness, confusion, edema (rare), decreased deep tendon reflexes, seizure, and coma.

A serum sodium level below 115 mEq/L produces confusion, lethargy, muscle twitching, seizures, coma, and, occasionally, irreversible neurologic damage.

Laboratory testing shows a normal or low blood urea nitrogen (BUN) and creatinine. Urine osmolality is over 200 mOsm/kg, and urinary sodium concentration exceeds 20 mEq/L. There will be an elevated serum concentration of ADH and a low uric acid level. Imaging is not usually required for diagnosis.

Prognosis

The prognosis of SIADH depends on the cause and the sodium level. Resolution of SIADH usually occurs within 3 days. The prognosis is poor for patients who have carcinoma of the lung. Seizures and coma can contribute to chronic brain dysfunction.

What You DO

Treatment

Treatment for SIADH includes identifying and treating the underlying cause. SIADH ordinarily resolves with the correction of hyponatremia. No drug is available that suppresses sources of ADH coming from outside the posterior pituitary gland. Although the mechanism is unknown, demeclocycline inhibits the action of pituitary-secreted ADH at the renal tubules, thus producing a nephrogenic diabetes insipidus. The drug takes 1 week to start working; therefore it is not used for acute patient management. Lithium has been used to treat SIADH because it, too, blocks ADH at the renal tubules. The disadvantage of this drug is the risk of lithium toxicity, and it has antianabolic effects, which is of particular concern in patients with cirrhosis and congestive heart failure.

In mildly symptomatic patients (serum sodium over 125 mEq/L) a fluid restriction of 800 to 1000 mL/day may be all that is needed. For patients with acute SIADH of less than 48 hours' duration, a hypertonic saline solution may be administered along with a loop diuretic such as furosemide.

In symptomatic patients (i.e., those with seizures and coma) the very low serum sodium (less than 120 mEq/L) is treated by restricting free water to two thirds of maintenance levels (i.e., 600 to 800 mL/day), increasing oral salt intake, and correcting the serum sodium deficit with hypertonic intravenous fluids.

Nursing Responsibilities

The nurse should identify patients who are at risk for SIADH. For the patient with SIADH, the nurse should do the following:

- If the disorder will be long-term, encourage patients to wear medical identification that states they have SIADH to reduce the risk of inappropriate treatment in the case of an acute event.
- Monitor electrolytes in postoperative patients to determine if fluid intake needs restriction.
- Assess for signs and symptoms of hyponatremia through evaluation of neurologic status.
- Monitor fluid restriction to avoid exceeding daily fluid-restriction requirements.
- Obtain weight readings at the same time daily, on the same scale, and in the same type of clothing; accurately record intake and output.
- Administer drug therapy as ordered.
- Use appropriate strategies to reduce the patient's risk of injury secondary to altered neurologic status.
- Provide age-appropriate and culturally appropriate patient and family information regarding the disorder. A life-long fluid restriction may be needed.

Do You UNDERSTAND?

DIRECTIONS: Unscramble the italicized letters to form terms associated with SIADH.

1. _____
   (noedhraiydt)

2. _____
   (dutecnaiirti)

3. _____
   (mecllyoecenidc)

What IS Diabetes Insipidus?

Pathogenesis

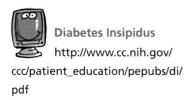

Diabetes Insipidus
http://www.cc.nih.gov/
ccc/patient_education/pepubs/di/
pdf

The hypothalamus normally produces ADH, which is stored in the posterior pituitary gland. ADH, sometimes called vasopressin, is released into the bloodstream when needed to cause the kidney tubules to resorb water. Water that cannot be resorbed is passed out of the body in the form of urine. Diabetes insipidus is caused by a defective regulation of water balance secondary to decreased secretion of, or failure of response to, vasopressin. Two types of this disorder have been classified.

In neurogenic diabetes insipidus, ADH is either missing or present at a low level. ADH synthesis or release is improperly affected by a malfunction of the posterior pituitary gland. Injury to the brain, tumors, neurosurgical operations, infections, or bleeding can affect the brain's ability to release ADH.

In nephrogenic diabetes insipidus, ADH is produced normally, but the distal tubules and collecting ducts cannot respond to the hormone's signal to resorb water. This form of the disorder can be acquired or inherited by male children.

At-Risk Populations

Patients who are at risk for diabetes insipidus include those with head injuries, patients who have had neurosurgery or pituitary tumors, or those who have had inflammation or infection of brain tissue. There have been autosomal dominant cases of diabetes insipidus, although they are usually isolated cases. Nephrogenic diabetes insipidus is usually inherited (sex-linked recessive) and is expressed primarily in males. It is rare in females. Administration of drugs that inhibit ADH release (e.g., ethanol, glucocorticosteroids, adrenergics, phenytoin, opioid antagonists, lithium) can also increase a person's risk of developing diabetes insipidus.

What You NEED TO KNOW

Clinical Manifestations

Although the two forms of diabetes insipidus are different in cause, the signs and symptoms are similar. Changes in mentation, insomnia, excessive continued thirst **(polydipsia),** weight loss, urinary frequency with a urinary output of 4 to 18 liters per day, and nighttime voiding **(nocturia)** are common. The skin and mucus membranes are cool.

Prognosis

Diabetes insipidus is usually a permanent condition, although an occasional case following trauma or tumor goes into permanent remission. The prognosis overall is excellent, depending on the underlying disorder, and as long as drug therapy is taken as prescribed. Without treatment, dehydration can lead to confusion, stupor, and coma. Dilatation of the urinary tract is probably secondary to the large volume of urine. In some patients with nephrogenic diabetes insipidus, there is an associated retardation of mental development. A subnormal growth rate may be seen.

What You DO

Treatment

Treatment of the patient with either type of diabetes insipidus includes identifying and treating the underlying cause of the disorder. Fluid intake is balanced with urinary output. ADH is replaced using intravenous, subcutaneous, or intranasal desmopressin (DDAVP) or intramuscular vasopressin. Surgical removal of the posterior pituitary gland may be required in some patients.

Nursing Responsibilities

For patients with either type of diabetes insipidus, the nurse should do the following:

- Know which patients are at risk for the disorder.
- Encourage a normal diet with free access to fluids. Infants with nephrogenic diabetes insipidus may benefit from a low-solute formula.
- Monitor for excessive urination or thirst and provide good skin and mouth care on a regular basis.
- Obtain weights at the same time daily, on the same scale, and in the same type of clothing; accurately record intake and output.
- Monitor urine-specific gravity and osmolality. Therapy is adjusted based on the urine and electrolyte concentrations and the patient's symptoms.
- Administer desmopressin intranasally twice daily in doses necessary to control polyuria or polydipsia, or parenterally in 2 divided doses. Administer any other drugs as prescribed.
- Provide age-appropriate and culturally-appropriate patient and family information regarding the disorder and the importance of adherence to drug therapy. Patient monitoring requires regular follow-up at intervals of 2 to 3 weeks initially and every 3 to 4 months later on.
- Teach the patient to avoid situations incurring a marked increased in water loss and to take fluids as dictated by thirst with no water restriction.

Do You UNDERSTAND?

DIRECTIONS: Indicate which statements are *true* (T) and which are *false* (F). If false, correct the statement in the margin space to make it true.

_____ 1. Excessive urination is known as polydipsia.

_____ 2. Patients who have diabetes insipidus are seldom thirsty.

_____ 3. Patients should be taught to call the health care provider when they are unable to balance their fluid intake with fluid output.

_____ 4. Patients need not call their health care provider when they cannot balance their fluid intake and output.

_____ 5. The lack or deficiency of ADH causes diabetes insipidus.

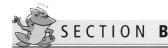

SECTION B

THYROID AND PARATHYROID DISORDERS

There are three basic types of thyroid abnormalities: enlargement of the thyroid, known as a goiter; hypofunction, known as hypothyroidism; and hyperfunction, known as hyperthyroidism. Hypothyroidism and hyperthyroidism represent disorders of thyroid hormone secretion.

Thyroid Diseases from Medline Plus
http://www.nlm.nih.gov/medlineplus/ency/article/001159.htm

What IS Hypothyroidism?

Hypothyroidism is a clinical state resulting from decreased circulating levels of free thyroid hormone or from resistance to thyroid hormone action. The term myxedema connotes severe hypothyroidism.

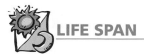

LIFE SPAN

Severe hypothyroidism in children is known as cretinism.

Answers: 1. F—excessive urination is known as polyuria; 2. F—patients are usually very thirsty; the medical term for this thirst is polydipsia; 3. T; 4. F—patients should call their health care provider to avoid dehydration; 5. T.

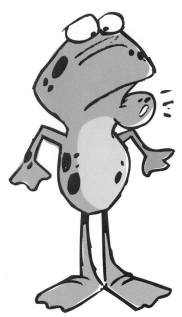

Goiters are enlarged thyroid glands.

Pathogenesis

In hypothyroidism, the production of thyroid hormones is inadequate, which results in a decrease in the basal metabolic rate. The thyroid gland may enlarge in an attempt to compensate for the inadequacy, and a goiter is formed.

Congenital defects of thyroid function, defective hormone synthesis, iodine deficiency, antithyroid drugs, or chronic autoimmune Hashimoto's disease can cause primary hypothyroidism. Surgery or radiation therapy for hyperthyroidism can also contribute to a hypothyroidism state.

Secondary hypothyroidism occurs when TSH levels are increased as a result of insufficient stimulation of a normal thyroid gland. Peripheral resistance to thyroid hormones can also cause secondary hypothyroidism.

Tertiary hypothyroidism develops when the hypothalamus fails to produce thyroid-releasing hormone (TRH) and thus no stimulation of the pituitary to secrete TSH is present. This form of hypothyroidism can be a result of a tumor or another destructive lesion in the hypothalamus.

A goiter is an enlargement of the thyroid gland. A deficiency of iodine that develops most frequently in the autumn and winter is a primary cause of endemic goiter. Sporadic goiter is related to genetic defects that result in faulty iodine metabolism, to the ingestion of large amounts of nutritional goitrogens, and to the ingestion of medical goitrogens.

Endemic goiter most frequently affects adolescents who have decreased thyroid hormones during periods of growth spurts, pregnant women, and nursing mothers who are living in iodine-deficient regions.

At-Risk Populations

Hypothyroidism affects more women than men, by a ratio of 4:1; the highest rate occurs in women between 30 and 65 years of age, with a predominant age of 40. Women over the age of 65 make up 6% to 10% of patients with hypothyroidism. Those living in the Midwest, Northwest, and Great Lakes regions, in which the soil and water are deficient in iodine, are at greater risk for developing goiter.

The ingestion of large amounts of foods that inhibit thyroxine production (**goitrogens**) such as rutabagas, cabbage, soybeans, peanuts, peaches, peas, strawberries, spinach, and radishes contributes to goiter formation. Patients who take drugs such as lithium, cobalt, aminosalicylic acid, phenylbutazone, tolbutamide, and iodine in large doses are also at risk.

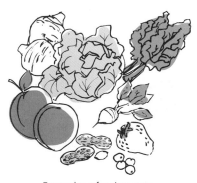

Examples of goitrogens.

What You NEED TO KNOW

Hypothyroidism

SIGNS AND SYMPTOMS	ASSOCIATED PATHOPHYSIOLOGY
Respiratory distress and dysphagia	Goiter formation
Hypoxia and mental status changes, forgetfulness, depression	Decreased cerebral blood flow
Reduced stroke volume and heart rate	Reduced cardiac output
Increased systolic blood pressure	Increased peripheral vascular resistance
Reduced urinary output, increase in total body water, low serum sodium levels	Reduced renal blood flow
Anemia	Reduced production of erythropoietin and red blood cells
Decreased appetite, weight gain, constipation; increased cholesterol and triglyceride levels with subsequent development of atherosclerosis and heart disease; decreased absorption of glucose	General slowing of gastrointestinal function; abnormalities in lipid metabolism; increased sensitivity to exogenous insulin
Sensitivity to cold; reduced inability to sweat; dry, flaky skin; brittle head and body hair; nails are slow-growing	Decreased metabolic rate and basal body temperature; reduced secretions from sweat and sebaceous glands
Delayed skeletal and soft tissue growth; delayed wound healing	Decreased protein metabolism

Clinical Manifestations

Hypothyroidism in its severe form (myxedema) is characterized by physical and mental sluggishness, obesity, hair loss, enlargement of the tongue, and thickening of the skin. Myxedematous changes in respiratory muscles lead to hypoventilation and carbon dioxide retention. Pleural effusions associated with dyspnea are possible, although patients can be asymptomatic. Complicating factors to myxedema coma include hyponatremia, hypercalcemia, secondary adrenal insufficiency, hypoglycemia, and water intoxication. Myxedema can also be brought on by the stress of surgery, infection, or noncompliance with thyroid replacement hormone therapy.

Hypothyroidism is diagnosed based not only on signs and symptoms, but also on thyroid function tests. The serum TSH becomes elevated in an attempt to compensate for low levels of thyroid hormones (A TSH greater than 0.02 international units per liter is diagnostic of primary thyroid failure). Total serum thyroxine (T_4), free thyroxine concentration (fT_4), the metabolically active form of T4, and triiodothyronine (T_3) levels are low. The radioactive iodide uptake is decreased, and TRH levels are elevated in patients with severe hypothyroidism. Anemia and elevated cholesterol, creatinine phosphokinase (CPK), lactate dehydrogenase (LDH),

> ⚠ Unrecognized and undiagnosed hypothyroidism can progress to myxedema coma, which has a mortality rate approaching 100%.

and aspartate transaminase (AST) levels may appear, and the serum sodium level may be low.

Prognosis

Most patients with hypothyroidism have a good prognosis with treatment.

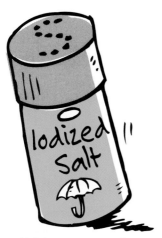

Helping prevent a goiter.

What You DO

Treatment

The primary treatment for hypothyroidism is life-long hormonal replacement therapy. The patient is encouraged to use iodized salt to ensure sufficient iodine intake. Levothyroxine sodium is the primary drug used. After therapy is started, patients will notice an improvement in their signs and symptoms within 2 to 3 weeks. Levothyroxine sodium and corticosteroids are administered intravenously to patients with myxedema coma.

Thyroid hormone replacement therapy may need adjustment should the patient become pregnant. TSH levels should be monitored monthly during the first trimester and again 6 weeks post partum. A painless, subacute inflammation of the thyroid gland may occur in the postpartum period leading to a transient hypothyroidism lasting about 3 months. Treatment with replacement therapy may be warranted. Up to 30% of patients with postpartum hypothyroidism develop permanent hypothyroidism.

The elderly and patients with cardiac disease must be started on low doses of thyroid hormone to reduce the risk of heart failure or myocardial infarction. These complications of therapy develop as a result of increasing metabolism, myocardial oxygen requirements, and, consequently, the workload on the heart.

Nursing Responsibilities

For the patient with hypothyroidism, the nurse should do the following:
- Assess the patient for manifestations of hypothyroidism and response to therapy (e.g., mental status, quality of skin and hair, subnormal temperature, bradycardia, respiratory rate, blood pressure, worsening heart failure, weight gain or loss).
- Provide instructions for a low-calorie diet until the patient's weight stabilizes within an ideal range. Weight gain develops when the

patient's appetite improves with the start of therapy, but energy levels have not yet improved. Reassure the patient that energy levels will return to normal after hormone therapy is begun.

- Encourage activity as tolerated to reduce constipation.
- Advise the patient to drink six to eight glasses of water daily and to eat high-fiber foods. A stool softener may be needed if diet and exercise are ineffective.
- Teach the patient and family the importance of life-long drug therapy, about the disease and the importance of monitoring thyroid hormone levels, the benefits and adverse effects of hormone replacement therapy, and when to contact the health care provider for assistance.
- Maintain a patent airway, administering oxygen, and intravenous fluids for the patient with myxedema coma.
- Monitor and record intake, output, and daily weights.
- Provide the patient with a comfortable, warm environment. Supply extra clothing and warm blankets when necessary.
- Administer no more than one half to one third of the usual dose when the patient requires a sedative or opioid analgesic. Reassess the patient for signs of respiratory depression or a decreased level of consciousness after drug administration.
- Monitor the sacrum, the coccyx, the elbows, the scapula, and other pressure points for evidence of redness or tissue breakdown. The edematous tissues are prone to decubitus ulcer formation.
- Turn the patient on a regular schedule. Use a pressure-reduction mattress.
- Advise the patient to take the drug at the same time every day to maintain blood levels. Taking the drug in the morning on an empty stomach will facilitate drug absorption as well as helping to prevent insomnia.

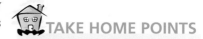

TAKE HOME POINTS

Do not administer thyroid hormone replacement drugs if the patient has had a heart attack, thyrotoxicosis, or untreated adrenal insufficiency without first contacting the health care provider.

Use the drugs cautiously in patients who have angina pectoris and other cardiovascular disorders, renal insufficiency or failure, or poor circulation.

Do You UNDERSTAND?

DIRECTIONS: Fill in the blanks to complete the following statements.

1. The primary food source of iodine is _____.
2. List five foods that can precipitate development of goiter:

   _____

   _____

   _____

   _____

   _____

What IS Hyperthyroidism?

Pathogenesis

Excessive thyroid hormone secretion **(hyperthyroidism)** can cause various thyroid disorders. Graves' disease, the most common hypersecretion condition, is an autoimmune disorder mediated by the immunoglobulin G (IgG) antibody. Thyroid-stimulating immunoglobulins (TSIs) of the IgG class are produced and bind to TSH receptors on the thyroid gland. The TSIs mimic the action of TSH and cause excess secretion of T_4 and T_3. Excessive stimulation of the sympathetic nervous system can also cause hyperthyroidism. In either case, a loss of the normal regulatory controls of thyroid hormone secretion is present. Because the action of thyroid hormones on the body is stimulation, hypermetabolism results, with increased sympathetic nervous system activity.

Overtreatment of hypothyroidism in its clinical state **(thyrotoxicosis)** with thyroid hormones can result in hyperthyroidism. Hyperthyroidism can also result from single or multiple functioning thyroid cancer **(thyroid adenoma)**.

At-Risk Populations

Hyperthyroidism is predominantly a disorder of women, affecting 1 out of every 1000 women with the peak during the third and fourth decades of life. Graves' disease tends to occur in twins. Patients who are at risk also include those who have been overtreated for hypothyroidism. Patients

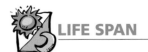
LIFE SPAN

Hyperthyroidism affects women 4 times as frequently as it does men, particularly young women aged 20 to 40 years.

Answers: 1. iodized salt; 2. rutabagas, cabbage, soybeans, peanuts, peaches, peas, strawberries, spinach, and radishes.

also at risk for hyperthyroidism include those who have a history of posterior pituitary disease, hypothalamic disease, or those who use amiodarone to treat atrial fibrillation.

When hyperthyroidism alters hypothalamic, pituitary, and gonadal metabolism before puberty, sexual development is delayed. After puberty, hyperthyroidism results in decreased libido in both men and women. Women note menstrual irregularities and decreased fertility.

What You NEED TO KNOW

Clinical Manifestations

The signs and symptoms of hyperthyroidism vary from mild to severe. Excessive amounts of thyroid hormones stimulate the cardiovascular system and increase the number of beta-adrenergic receptors. This increase leads to tachycardia and increased cardiac output, stroke volume, peripheral blood flow, and adrenergic responsiveness. Dyspnea is common in three quarters of patients with the disorder.

The metabolic rate increases significantly, leading to a negative nitrogen balance, lipid depletion, and nutritional deficiency. Weight loss occurs in about half of the patients despite a ravenous appetite. The patient will also experience loose bowel movements, heat intolerance, profuse sweating, tachycardia, and a lack of coordination. The skin becomes warm, smooth, and moist. The hair appears thin and soft.

The patient's emotions are volatile because of the turbulent activity within the body. Moods can be cyclic, ranging from mild euphoria to extreme hyperactivity, delirium, fatigue, and depression. As a consequence of the chaotic emotional state, interpersonal relationships can deteriorate. The patient may appear extremely nervous, agitated, and irritable, and have a resting tremor of the hand.

The patient with Graves' disease also exhibits an enlarged thyroid and abnormal protrusion of the eyes (**exophthalmia**). Exophthalmos appears to be an autoimmune problem of the tissues behind the eye. The patient has protruding eyes and a fixed stare resulting from the accumulation of fluids in the fat pads and muscles that lie behind the eyes. Because the eyes are surrounded by bone, edema forces the eyes forward out of their sockets, producing the typical appearance of hyperthyroidism. In children there is an acceleration of linear growth, and ophthalmic abnormalities are more common.

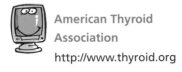

A thyroid crisis **(thyroid storm)** is an acute exacerbation of hyperthyroidism. A thyroid storm is a medical emergency that leads to life-threatening cardiac, hepatic, or renal failure.

Hyperthyroidism alters the metabolism of hypothalamic, pituitary, and gonadal hormones. It is diagnosed based on thyroid function tests. The serum TSH is decreased or undetectable in primary hyperthyroidism and elevated when excessive TSH secretion is the cause of the disorder. T_4 and T_3 levels are elevated, as is fT_4. The radioactive iodide uptake is increased. TRH levels are decreased.

Prognosis

With treatment, the prognosis for hyperthyroidism is good. Inadequate treatment of hyperthyroidism, stressors (e.g., stroke, surgery, infection, pulmonary embolism, myocardial infarction, diabetic ketoacidosis), and preeclampsia can precipitate a thyroid storm. The patient may have marked tachycardia, vomiting, and stupor. Other findings include a combination of irritability and restlessness, double vision **(diplopia)**, tremor and weakness, cough with shortness of breath, angina, and extremity edema. A high fever can develop insidiously, rising rapidly to a lethal level. Without treatment, the patient will experience vascular collapse, hypotension, coma, and death.

What You DO

Treatment

The treatment for hyperthyroidism includes antithyroid drugs, radioactive iodine therapy, iodine therapy, dietary therapy, and surgery.

Propylthiouracil (PTU) is the most commonly used antithyroid drug. Methimazole is used for children, young adults, pregnant women, and patients who are not candidates for radioactive iodine therapy or surgery.

Radioactive iodine therapy (^{131}I) is used primarily for middle-aged and older patients. The rationale for this therapy is simple: the thyroid gland is unable to distinguish between regular iodine atoms and radioiodine atoms, thus the thyroid gland picks up the radioiodine and concentrates it precisely as it would regular iodine. As a result, the cells that concentrate ^{131}I to make T_4 are destroyed by the irradiation, and thyroid hormone secretion diminishes. In most patients, hypermetabolic symptoms diminish within 6 to 12 weeks. A few patients may require a second dose. Because of the delay in drug activity, concurrent treatment with beta-adrenergic blockers may be desirable. The beta-adrenergic blockers used most frequently are propranolol and reserpine.

Iodine therapy reduces the vascularity of the thyroid gland before surgery and is prescribed to treat a thyroid storm. Iodine preparations such as potassium iodide act temporarily to prevent the release of thyroid hormones into the circulation by increasing the amount of hormone stored within the gland. When surgery is warranted, a partial thyroidectomy is most frequently used thus decreasing its size and capacity for hormone production.

> Inadvertent removal of the parathyroid glands during surgical removal of the thyroid gland can cause postoperative hypoparathyroidism manifesting as hypocalcemia.

Nursing Responsibilities

For the patient with hyperthyroidism, the nurse should:

- Provide education regarding the signs and symptoms of hyperthyroidism for persons at risk.
- Instruct the patient about the importance of a well-balanced, high-calorie diet, and discourage intake of foods that increase peristalsis and thus result in diarrhea (i.e., highly seasoned, bulky, or fibrous foods).
- Advise the patient to notify the health care provider when a weight loss of more than 2 kg (4.4 lb) occurs.
- Assign a hospitalized patient with hyperthyroidism, restlessness, and hyperactivity to a private room to promote rest and prevent being disturbed by others. Assess for signs of a thyroid storm (e.g., elevated temperature, extreme restlessness, agitation, and tachycardia). Report temperature elevations over 100° F (37.7° C).
- Direct the patient with exophthalmos to use artificial tears and eye patches as needed to prevent irritation.
- Teach the patient to stay in a cool environment, primarily because heat intolerance is common. Use lightweight linens and encourage the wearing of light, loose clothing.
- Monitor the patient who has had a thyroidectomy for weakness and hoarseness of the voice as a result of trauma or damage to the laryngeal nerve, hypocalcemia, and tetany; respiratory obstruction as a result of edema of the glottis; laryngeal nerve damage; or tracheal compression from hemorrhage.
- Maintain intake and output record for 2 to 3 days while watching for difficulty swallowing.
- Teach the patient to support the head and neck when sitting up in bed to prevent stress on the suture line. Be certain to check the patient's neck for bleeding at the front, sides, and back of the neck because blood tends to drain posteriorly.
- Emphasize the importance of routine follow-up laboratory testing.

Do You UNDERSTAND?

DIRECTIONS: Fill in the blanks to complete the following statements.

1. The best room location for a patient with hyperthyroidism who is awaiting surgery is: _____.
2. The most commonly used antithyroid drug used in the treatment of hyperthyroidism is _____.
3. In most patients, hypermetabolic symptoms diminish within _____ weeks.

What IS Hypoparathyroidism?

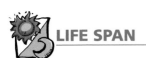

LIFE SPAN

Hypocalcemia is fairly common in the older adult and can be a result of multiple abnormalities, not hypoparathyroidism alone.

Pathogenesis

Hypoparathyroidism is the result of inadequate circulating parathyroid hormone (PTH). PTH helps regulate calcium and phosphate levels by stimulating bone resorption, the renal tubular resorption of calcium, and the activation of vitamin D. Hypoparathyroidism is characterized by hypocalcemia, resulting from a lack of PTH to maintain serum calcium levels. PTH resistance at the cellular level can also occur. This resistance is the result of a genetic defect from hypocalcemia, despite normal or high PTH levels, and is frequently associated with hypothyroidism and hypogonadism. The most common cause of hypoparathyroidism is iatrogenic; that is, accidental removal of the parathyroid glands or damage to the vascular supply of the glands during neck surgery.

At-Risk Populations

All forms of hypoparathyroidism are rare, but the disorder affects persons of all ages with those of both genders equally at risk. Hypomagnesemia, as observed in alcoholism or malabsorption, impairs PTH secretion and its action on bone and kidneys, thus increasing the risk of hypocalcemia. Other risk factors include neck trauma or surgery and carcinoma of the head and neck.

Most patients with congenital hypoparathyroidism have no family history of the disease. The pattern of inheritance is as varied as are the

Answers: 1. in a quiet room away from the nurses' station; 2. propylthiouracil; 3. 6 to 12 weeks.

kinds of genetic abnormalities that cause the disease. Children in some families are at a 50% risk for contracting the disease (dominant gene defect); others are at a risk of 25% or less (recessive gene defect).

What You NEED TO KNOW

Clinical Manifestations

The signs and symptoms of hypoparathyroidism are those of hypocalcemia. Sudden decreases in calcium concentration result in neuromuscular irritability (tetany). Tetany is characterized by tingling of the lips, the fingertips, and occasionally the feet, and by increased muscle tension, leading to paresthesias and stiffness. Patients are usually anxious and apprehensive. Painful tonic spasms of smooth and skeletal muscles of the extremities and face, as well as dysphagia (a constricted feeling in the throat), laryngospasms, and hyperactive deep tendon reflexes are also present. Accessory muscle spasm and laryngeal spasm–induced airway obstruction can compromise respiratory function. Other signs include irritability of the facial nerve when tapped (Chvostek's sign) and carpopedal spasm within 2 minutes of inflating a blood pressure cuff over systolic pressure (Trousseau's sign). The total and ionized serum calcium level is decreased (less than 8.5 mg/dL), and the serum phosphorous level is increased (greater than 5.4 mg/dL). Chronic hypoparathyroidism and thus hypocalcemia may be asymptomatic.

Prognosis

Death can result from respiratory obstruction secondary to tetany and laryngospasm if treatment is not begun rapidly. Patients with chronic hypoparathyroidism will develop calcifications of the eye and basal ganglia if treatment is delayed.

What You DO

Treatment

Vitamin D and calcium supplements are the primary treatments for hypoparathyroidism, regardless of the cause. The only exception is when inactivity of PTH is a result of hypomagnesemia, which is readily treated

⚠ An acute attack of hypoparathyroidism is life-threatening and necessitates immediate attention to airway maintenance and slow intravenous administration of calcium gluconate until tetany ceases. When the patient is awake, breathing into a paper bag can help raise serum ionized calcium levels.

with magnesium supplementation. Currently, a replacement form of PTH is unavailable. Oral vitamin D (ergocalciferol [vitamin D_2], calcitriol, 1, 25-dihydroxycholecalciferol, dihydrotachysterol) increases intestinal absorption of calcium from the diet. Along with calcium supplements (e.g., calcium carbonate, calcium lactate, calcium gluconate), vitamin D helps maintain normal blood calcium levels. Transient forms of hypoparathyroidism may not require treatment.

Life-long treatment may be required for patients with a chronic form of the disease. For some patients, a thiazide diuretic can be used to increase phosphate excretion and decrease calcium excretion.

Nursing Responsibilities

The primary objectives of treatment are to treat tetany when present and prevent long-term complications by maintaining normal serum calcium levels. As such, for the patient with hypoparathyroidism, the nurse should do the following:

- Identify patients at risk for hypoparathyroidism and periodically assess for presence of Chvostek's and Trousseau's signs.
- Maintain a patent airway, and administer intravenous calcium as needed for tetany. Monitor the electrocardiogram while administering calcium.
- Use seizure precautions because of the risk of tetany.
- Provide careful and detailed teaching about life-long maintenance therapy with oral calcium preparations, and the signs and symptoms of over-treatment (**hypercalcemia**) as well as undertreatment (**hypocalcemia**).
- Teach the patient about the importance of a high-calcium, low-phosphate diet and of avoiding foods containing oxalic acid (e.g., spinach, rhubarb), phytic acid (e.g., bran, whole grains), and phosphorus (dairy products, diet sodas). These food substances reduce calcium absorption. Green leafy vegetables and calcium supplements may be needed to normalize serum calcium levels if daily products must be avoided.
- Encourage the patient to keep follow-up appointments and to have periodic laboratory testing of serum calcium and phosphorous levels (3 to 4 times per year and as needed).
- Encourage the use of skin softeners for scaly skin.
- Use stool softeners, adequate fluids, and fresh fruits to prevent constipation associated with calcium supplements.
- Teach the patient how to distinguish between overtreatment and undertreatment.

Do You UNDERSTAND?

DIRECTIONS: Fill in the blanks by unscrambling the letters.

1. Inadvertent removal of the parathyroid glands can cause postoperative hypoparathyroidism and _____.
2. Irritability of the facial nerve when tapped is referred to as the _____ sign.
3. Carpal-pedal spasms noted when the blood pressure is taken is known _____ sign.
4. _____ must be balanced with calcium to prevent tetany.
5. _____ is caused by a sudden decrease in serum calcium levels.

    ssthvckoe   aeouustsr   aimeclacopyh   hphpssooour *muiccla*

What IS Hyperparathyroidism?

Pathogenesis

The primary disease of parathyroid glands is overactivity (**hyperparathyroidism**). There is a loss of control of the body's normal regulatory feedback mechanism on the parathyroid glands, and their ability to maintain a normal serum calcium level is disrupted, thus they make excess PTH regardless of the level of calcium.

Primary hyperparathyroidism is a result of either glandular hyperplasia of all four glands or adenoma of only one gland. The result is an unregulated increase of PTH production and release, and a subsequent rise in serum calcium levels. Secondary hyperparathyroidism occurs when the glands are hyperplastic from malfunction of another organ system. This condition is usually found in patients with chronic renal failure but can also occur with vitamin D deficiency, osteogenesis imperfecta, Paget's disease, multiple myeloma, and carcinoma with bone metastasis.

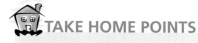

TAKE HOME POINTS

Hyperparathyroidism was first described in 1925, and the symptoms have become known as "painful bones, renal stones, abdominal groans, and psychic moans."

At-Risk Populations

Hyperparathyroidism is rare in children. Male and female adults over age 50 are most at risk, with women more frequently affected than men. Hyperparathyroidism is not related to age in patients with renal failure. The disorder occurs more frequently in temperate climates and in persons exposed to therapeutic low levels of radiation. Hyperparathyroidism is associated with drugs that include thiazide diuretics, furosemide, excessive amounts of vitamins A and D, and exogenous calcium intake. Long periods of immobilization predispose a patient to hypercalcemia.

What You NEED TO KNOW

Clinical Manifestations

⚠️ In extreme cases, the entire kidney can become calcified, taking on the characteristics of bone because of deposition of excess calcium within the tissues. Not only is this condition painful because of the presence of kidney stones; in severe cases, it can also cause kidney failure.

Some patients with hyperparathyroidism can be entirely asymptomatic. In patients with the severe form, bones can give up calcium to the extent that they become brittle and break (osteoporosis and osteopenia). This problem is even more of a concern in older patients. Bones can also have small hemorrhages within their center, which will cause bone pain.

Because the major function of the kidney is to filter and clean the blood, constant exposure of the kidney to high levels of calcium causes a collection of calcium within the renal tubules, which leads to kidney stones.

High levels of calcium in the blood can be dangerous to a number of cells, including the lining of the stomach and the pancreas. The cells of both of these organs become inflamed and painful (ulcers and acute pancreatitis).

Mental fatigue, somnolence, apathy, anxiety, depression, and psychosis are possible. Changes in the mental status observed in the older adult can be misinterpreted as senile dementia.

Diagnosis of hyperparathyroidism is made when the serum calcium level is greater than 10.2 mg/dL on three successive measurements. Elevated PTH levels and low serum phosphate levels (less than 2.5 mg/dL) are also noted.

Prognosis

The prognosis of the patient with hyperparathyroidism depends primarily on the duration and severity of the disease. The cure rate for primary hyperparathyroidism after surgical removal of the glands is greater than 95%. Secondary hyperparathyroidism carries a poor prognosis because of the primary disease state of chronic renal failure.

What You DO

Treatment

Surgical removal of the parathyroid glands is the only proven curative therapy for hyperparathyroidism. Antihypercalcemic drugs such as plicamycin and gallium nitrate lower serum calcium levels within 48 hours; their use is limited to patients with hyperparathyroidism caused by parathyroid carcinoma. Biphosphonates such as etidronate, pamidronate, and calcitonin inhibit osteoclastic bone resorption and helps normalize serum calcium levels. Estrogen or progestin therapy can reduce serum and urinary calcium levels in postmenopausal women and may retard demineralization of the skeleton. Oral phosphates can be used in patients who have normal kidney function and low serum phosphate levels to inhibit the calcium-absorbing effects of vitamin D in the intestine. Glucocorticoids can be used to reduce hypercalcemia by decreasing the gastrointestinal absorption of calcium. Diuretics can be given to increase the urinary elimination of calcium. Administration of furosemide (**Lasix**) can be helpful in well-hydrated patients to promote sodium loss and decrease renal tubular resorption of calcium.

Nursing Responsibilities

The treatment of hyperparathyroidism is directed at lowering severely elevated serum calcium levels, increasing calcium excretion, and increasing the bone resorption of calcium. Thus for the patient with hyperparathyroidism, the nurse should do the following:

- Ensure that serum calcium levels are lowered by hydration (a minimum of 3000 mL per day), and that the calcium in the urine is eliminated through the administration of furosemide.
- Administer antiresorption drugs as prescribed, and monitor for adverse effects.
- Teach the patient about the importance of adherence to drug therapy and the importance of periodic laboratory testing to be certain that the hyperparathyroid state does not redevelop.
- Instruct the patient about the importance of a diet low in calcium and vitamin D. Cranberry and prune juice make urine more acidic, thus helping to prevent renal stones. Calcium is more soluble in acid urine.
- Instruct the patient to use stool softeners, drink adequate fluids, and eat fresh fruits to prevent constipation associated with hypercalcemia.
- Strain the urine for the patient who has developed kidney stones.
- Teach about safety measures and monitor the patient's environment.
- Postoperatively monitor for signs and symptoms of transient tetany, laryngeal nerve damage, bleeding, and infection.
- Encourage ambulation as soon as possible after surgery because weight-bearing speeds the recalcification process.

Do You UNDERSTAND?

DIRECTIONS: **Fill in the blanks in the crossword puzzle below with the 4 primary complaints of patients with of hyperparathyroidism.**

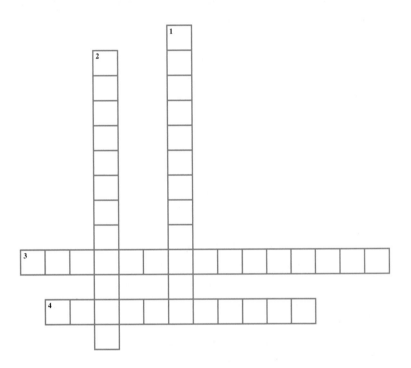

Across

3. Related to gastrointestinal distress of HPT
4. Related to hypercalciuria

Down

1. Related to low BMD
2. Related to overall symptoms of HPT

SECTION C

ADRENAL DISORDERS

The adrenal glands are small, triangular endocrine glands; one located on the top of each kidney, and are composed of two parts: the center of the gland (**medulla**) and the outer portion of the gland (**cortex**). The adrenal cortex secretes more than 30 different steroids. These steroids are divided into three major groups: the glucocorticoids, the mineralocorticoids, and the androgens. The glucocorticoids received their name because they raise blood glucose levels *(gluco)*, are produced by the adrenal cortex *(corti)*, and are made from cholesterol, which is a steroid *(oid)*. The mineralocorticoids, as their name implies, involve the concentration of minerals (**electrolytes**) in the fluid between the cells. Androgens are any steroid hormones that promote male characteristics, such as beard growth and the deepening of the voice at puberty. Many androgens are converted to estrogens elsewhere in the body.

The primary glucocorticoid is cortisol (**hydrocortisone**), which is responsible for more than 95% of all glucocorticoid activity. The most important job of cortisol is to help the body respond to stress. In addition, cortisol helps maintain blood pressure and cardiovascular function, helps slow the immune system's inflammatory response, balances the effects of insulin in breaking down sugar for energy, and regulates the metabolism of carbohydrates, proteins, and fats.

Disorders of the adrenal gland are organized into two groups: those affecting the medulla and those affecting the cortex. The disorders can be further divided into two additional groups: those that are caused by too much activity (**hyperfunction**) and those that are caused by too little activity (**hypofunction**).

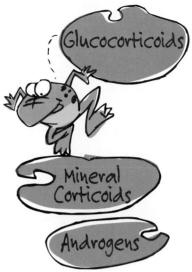

The three major groups of steroids.

National Institute of Diabetes and Diseases of the Kidney: Addison's Disease

http://www.niddk.nih.gov/health/endo/pubs/addison/addison.htm

What IS Primary Adrenal Insufficiency?

Pathogenesis

Primary adrenal insufficiency is a chronic autoimmune disorder (**Addison's disease**) that can occur as either a primary or a secondary deficit in the production of glucocorticoids and mineralocorticoids.

Primary adrenal insufficiency is a result of an autoimmune inflammation of the adrenal gland that occurs as a consequence of tuberculosis, fungal infections, or nonsecreting tumors of the adrenal cortex. The autoimmune process accounts for 75% of primary adrenal insufficiency. Basically, some factor causes the adrenal glands to produce insufficient cortisol and, occasionally, the hormone aldosterone. Infiltration of the adrenal cortex by a type of white blood cell (**lymphocyte**) is the characteristic feature. Gradual, continued destruction of the adrenal gland leads to inadequate amounts of mineralocorticoids, as well as glucocorticoids and androgens.

A lack of ACTH from the anterior pituitary gland causes secondary adrenal insufficiency. Hypofunction of the pituitary gland, surgical removal, and certain tumors of the gland eventually result in a decrease or total absence of ACTH, the hormone that triggers the release of other hormones from the adrenal cortex.

At-Risk Populations

This potentially life-threatening autoimmune disorder affects persons of all ages and occurs equally in both genders and all races. About 40% of patients with autoimmune adrenal insufficiency have a first- or second-degree relative with one of the related disorders. Individuals who are at risk for primary adrenal insufficiency include those with a history of other endocrine disorders. Persons taking glucocorticoids for more than 3 weeks who suddenly stop therapy, and those taking glucocorticoids more frequently than once every other day, are at risk. Surgical removal of the adrenal glands also increases the risk. Tuberculosis is the cause in approximately 20% of cases worldwide. Other causes include metastatic carcinomas of the lung, the breast, or the gastrointestinal tract.

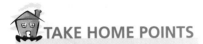
TAKE HOME POINTS

Acquired immunodeficiency syndrome (AIDS) is becoming a more common cause of adrenal insufficiency than are autoimmune processes and tuberculosis.

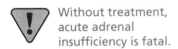
Without treatment, acute adrenal insufficiency is fatal.

What You NEED TO KNOW

Clinical Manifestations

Symptoms of adrenal insufficiency are slow and progressive, and as such they are frequently unnoticed until a stressor appears, such as illness or accident. The development of signs and symptoms appears with the loss of over 90% of both adrenal cortices. A profound drop in blood sugar occurs (**hypoglycemia**), in addition to orthostatic hypotension, cardiac irregularities (**arrhythmias**), sodium loss with potassium retention, and, when acute, volume depletion. Mental confusion, mood swings, loss of consciousness, and shock, also occurs when the condition is acute. Muscle pain and weakness, fatigue, and sudden penetrating pain in the back, the abdomen, or the legs are also present when an acute deficiency exists. An unusual darkening (bronzing) of skin folds, pressure areas, the areolae, the fingers and toes, and sun-exposed body parts also appears.

Prognosis

The patient with primary adrenal insufficiency can lead a fairly normal life with hormonal replacement therapy. Hormonal replacement therapy usually brings about a rapid recovery.

What You DO

Treatment

The treatment of primary adrenal insufficiency focuses on replacing hormones and using exogenous glucocorticoids (hydrocortisone) and mineralocorticoids (fludrocortisone). Intravenous feedings of glucose are used to prevent a severe drop in blood glucose levels when fasting is required for diagnostic studies or surgery.

The treatment goal for acute adrenal insufficiency is to prevent the morbidity and mortality associated with the crisis. After the cause of the crisis has been determined, the low blood pressure and electrolyte imbalance are quickly corrected. An isotonic intravenous solution will usually correct the volume depletion, salt depletion, and hypotension. Low blood sugar is corrected with glucose. The patient also receives oxygen, drugs to raise blood pressure (**vasopressors**) or volume expanders, and hydrocortisone.

Symptoms of acute adrenal insufficiency **(Addisonian crisis)** can occur when the patient has been under stress without appropriate hormonal replacement. Stressors include pregnancy, surgery, infection, dehydration, anorexia, fever, and emotional upheaval.

Nursing Responsibilities

For the patient with adrenal insufficiency, the nurse should do the following:

- Monitor vital signs, including orthostatic blood pressure readings and electrocardiogram tracings, when indicated.
- Provide for adequate rest periods.
- Monitor for signs and symptoms of hypoglycemia and infection.
- Obtain daily weights at the same time, on the same scale, and in the same type of clothing; accurately record intake and output.

- Implement safety measures to prevent falls and injury.
- Administer hydrocortisone and other hormone replacement therapy as ordered.
- Provide age-appropriate and culturally appropriate patient and family teaching regarding the disorder and stress-reduction strategies.

Do You UNDERSTAND?

Ms. McMahon has Addison's disease. She is worried about going home from the hospital because she is too tired to clean her house. Most of the time, she is too tired to cook dinner.

DIRECTIONS: **Place a check next to the priority nursing intervention for Ms. McMahon.**

_____ 1. Encourage Ms. McMahon to consume a diet that is high in sodium, potassium, and fats.

_____ 2. Help her divide her house cleaning and dinner preparation into small, manageable tasks that can be separated by rest periods.

_____ 3. Teach stress-reduction strategies to Ms. McMahon.

_____ 4. Arrange for a housekeeper to help Ms. McMahon.

What IS Cushing's Syndrome?

Excessive cortisol secretion leads to Cushing's disease.

Pathogenesis

Cushing's syndrome is essentially the opposite of Addison's disease. Cushing's syndrome is made up of a group of symptoms resulting from prolonged exposure of the body's tissues to high levels of the glucocorticoid hormone cortisol for long periods (hypercortisolism). Approximately 85% of patients with Cushing's syndrome have a tumor of the pituitary gland that causes excessive secretion of ACTH. Many people experience iatrogenic Cushing's because they take high-dose, long-term glucocorticoid hormones such as prednisone for asthma, rheumatoid arthritis, lupus, or other inflammatory diseases.

The signs and symptoms of Cushing's syndrome are the result of the action of cortisol. Normally, the production of cortisol follows a precise chain of events. First, the hypothalamus sends corticotropin-releasing hormone (CRH) to the pituitary gland. CRH causes the pituitary gland to secrete ACTH, a hormone that stimulates the adrenal glands. When the adrenal glands receive the ACTH, they respond by releasing cortisol into the bloodstream.

When the amount of cortisol in the blood is adequate, less CRH and ACTH is released. This mechanism ensures that the amount of cortisol released is precisely balanced to meet the body's daily needs. However, when "something goes wrong" with the adrenal glands or their regulating switches in the pituitary gland or the hypothalamus, cortisol production can go awry.

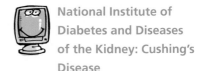

National Institute of Diabetes and Diseases of the Kidney: Cushing's Disease
http://www.niddk.nih.gov/health/endo/pubs/cushings/cushings.htm

At-Risk Populations

Cushing's syndrome affects mostly adults ages 20 to 50 years. Patients at risk for Cushing's syndrome include those with a history of a cortisol-secreting adrenal tumor, adrenal hyperplasia, or those who are receiving glucocorticoid drugs (steroids).

What You NEED TO KNOW

Clinical Manifestations

The signs and symptoms of Cushing's syndrome vary, but most people have hypertension, arrhythmias, low serum potassium levels, sodium and fluid retention, and elevated blood glucose levels (hyperglycemia). The upper body becomes obese with a rounded face and increased fat around the neck. The arms and legs are thin because of loss of muscle mass. Generalized weakness and osteoporosis are present. Men become impotent, with decreased fertility and loss of sex drive. Women develop excessive hair growth on the face, the neck, the chest, the abdomen, and the thighs. Menstrual periods can become irregular or stop. The skin is thin with bruising from even minor injuries. Purplish-pink stretch marks (atrophic striae) appear on the abdomen, the thighs, the buttocks, the arms, and the breasts.

Prognosis

Cushing's syndrome causes many other serious health problems. Without treatment, approximately 50% of patients who have Cushing's die within 5 years of the onset of the disease. The major causes of death include overwhelming infection, suicide, complications from generalized hardening of the arteries (**arteriosclerosis**), and hypertension.

What You DO

Treatment

Treatment of Cushing's syndrome is complex and depends on the specific reason for cortisol excess. Therefore differentiation among pituitary, adrenal, and ectopic causes of the excess cortisol secretion is essential for effective treatment. Generally, treatment includes removal of the adrenal gland or the causative tumor, radiation therapy, and antineoplastic therapy.

Cortisol-inhibiting drugs such as aminoglutethimide and mitotane inhibit glucocorticoid synthesis without destroying the adrenal cortex. ACTH-reducing drugs such as somatostatin may be used when the cause of the disorder is a pituitary tumor. When the cause of excess cortisol is long-term use of glucocorticoid hormones to treat another disorder, the dosage is reduced to the lowest dose that controls that disorder. After control is established, the daily dose of glucocorticoid may be doubled and given on alternate days to reduce the side effects.

Nursing Responsibilities

For the patient with Cushing's syndrome, the nurse should do the following:

- Support the patient and family during diagnostic phase of the disease.
- Take measures to prevent injury and infection.
- Keep the bed in lowest position, raising the side rails for protection.
- Assist the patient to ambulate to reduce risk of falls.
- Promote periods of mental and physical rest.
- Provide good skin care to reduce the likelihood of skin breakdown.
- Assess the patient closely for manifestations of severe hypertension (e.g., elevated blood pressure, headache, failing vision, irritability, and dyspnea).

⚠️ For patients who have had their adrenal glands removed **(adrenalectomy),** teach that life-long glucocorticoid replacement is essential to life.

- Obtain daily weights at the same time, on the same scale, and in the same type of clothing; monitor vital signs at frequent intervals.
- Obtain daily blood sugar readings via fingerstick to monitor for hyperglycemia.
- Assist in the collection of 24-hour urine specimen for free cortisol.
- Encourage a diet low in calories, carbohydrates, and sodium but with ample protein and potassium.
- Help the patient and family acquire effective coping mechanisms.
- Anticipate mood swings, and provide reassurance that physical appearance and moods will most likely return to normal after the disorder is treated.
- Administer drugs as prescribed and monitor for adverse effects.
- Provide age-appropriate and culturally-appropriate patient and family teaching regarding the disorder.

Do You UNDERSTAND?

Mr. Rodriquez is a 26-year-old elementary school teacher who is seeking the advice of his health care provider because of changes in his appearance over the last year. Mr. Rodriquez comes to the office today complaining of weight gain, particularly through his midsection, easy bruising, and edema of his feet, lower legs, and hands; he has been having increasing problems sleeping (**insomnia**). Blood pressure is 150/110; he has 2+ edema of lower extremities, striae on the abdomen, birdlike extremities with thin, friable skin, and severe acne on the face and neck.

DIRECTIONS: **Place a check next to four of the seven treatments listed below that are most appropriate for Mr. Rodriquez.**

_____ 1. Use of cortisol-inhibiting drugs

_____ 2. Removal of the causative tumor

_____ 3. Radiation therapy

_____ 4. Intravenous fluids low in sodium and potassium and high in glucose

_____ 5. Antineoplastic therapy

_____ 6. Brushing teeth twice daily

_____ 7. Driving only during daylight hours

Answers: 1, 2, 3, and 6.

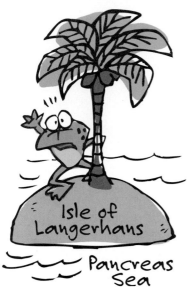

Isle of
Langerhans

Pancreas
Sea

Insulin production.

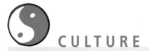

CULTURE

Type I diabetes is more prevalent in Caucasians than it is in other ethnic groups.

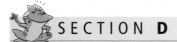

SECTION D

DIABETES

What IS Type 1 Diabetes Mellitus?

Pathogenesis

Diabetes is a metabolic disorder that causes hyperglycemia. It is classified according to the pathologic process that causes the disease to occur. Type 1 diabetes mellitus is a disorder resulting from absolute insulin deficiency and is characterized by chronic hyperglycemia and the presence of disturbances in the metabolism of carbohydrates, fats, and proteins. In the past, type 1 diabetes was known by several names, such as insulin-dependent diabetes mellitus (IDDM), juvenile-onset diabetes, brittle diabetes, or ketosis-prone diabetes. Individuals with this type of diabetes are prone to ketosis, as well as numerous other complications.

Type 1 diabetes results from the destruction of the pancreatic beta cells of the islet of Langerhans. Beta cells are responsible for the secretion of insulin. The damage results from a cell-mediated autoimmune mechanism, genetic susceptibility, or environmental factors. Environmental factors include viruses or exposure to a toxic agent. In 85% to 90% of cases, autoantibodies to the islet cells are present, which damage the pancreas. The autoantibodies can be present for years before insulin secretion is affected and symptoms appear.

Viruses such as those that cause mumps, the Coxsackie virus, and the cytomegalovirus are associated with the development of type 1 diabetes. Drugs and chemicals such as alloxan, streptozocin, pentamidine, and Vacor (a rat poison) are environmental influences.

The lack of insulin production affects the metabolism of carbohydrates, fats, and proteins. Without insulin, glucose cannot enter adipose and muscle tissues, leading to elevated blood glucose levels (**hyperglycemia**). High blood glucose levels cause osmotic fluid loss from the cells, resulting in intracellular dehydration. The dehydration stimulates the hypothalamus and consequently causes thirst (**polydipsia**). When the amount of glucose filtered by the glomeruli and resorbed by the renal tubules is exceeded, glucose spills into the urine (**glycosuria**), resulting in large amounts of osmotic fluid loss. In the absence of insulin, glucose cannot be transported into cells; thus the cells are depleted of carbohydrates, fats, and protein stores, resulting in cellular starvation and an increase in hunger **(polyphagia).** Because fats and proteins are used for energy, body tissue is lost. Osmotic diuresis **(polyuria)** causes fluid to be lost, resulting in weight loss. Fatigue is a result of the metabolic changes.

Hyperglycemia, along with the presence of the autoantibodies, indicates that the islet cells of the pancreas have been damaged to the extent that the secretion of insulin by these cells is severely inadequate or nonexistent. Destruction of 80% to 90% of the beta cells occurs before hyperglycemia is observed. Beta cell destruction causes an imbalance of the hormones produced by the islets of Langerhans. When beta cells cannot produce insulin and blood glucose levels are elevated, the alpha cells overproduce glucagon.

Glucagon is a hormone that opposes the action of insulin. When intake of food is inadequate, glucagon is released. Glucagon also stimulates the body to use alternate energy sources such as fat and protein. When no insulin is present to oppose the production of glucose, the overproduction of glucagon stimulates the new production of glucose from glycogen **(glycogenolysis)** and the production of glucose from amino acids and glycerol in the liver **(gluconeogenesis).**

In the presence of inadequate insulin, the body is unable to use carbohydrates as an energy source, and must use proteins and fats instead. This causes unintended weight loss, which is often one of the presenting complaints of patients who are newly diagnosed with diabetes. Ketones, an end-product of fat metabolism, tend to accumulate as fat is broken down by the body. Eventually acidosis will occur as a consequence of this abnormal accumulation.

At-Risk Populations

Of all cases of diabetes, 5% to 10% are type 1. Genetic predisposition increases the risk of developing type 1 diabetes. Approximately 10% of diagnosed individuals have a parent or sibling with type 1 diabetes. Type 1 diabetes occurs in 40% of individuals who had congenital rubella.

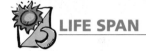

LIFE SPAN

Type 1 diabetes is one of the most common childhood diseases. Peak onset of the disorder occurs at approximately 12 years of age. Type 1 diabetes is rarely present in children younger than 1 year or adults older than 30 years.

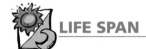

LIFE SPAN

An increased risk of developing diabetes exists after the age of 40.

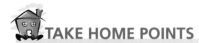

TAKE HOME POINTS

Kussmaul respirations and "fruity" **(acetone odor)** breath are the first presenting symptoms of ketoacidosis.

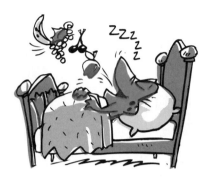

The leading cause of diabetes-related deaths is heart disease.

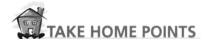

TAKE HOME POINTS

Daily insulin injections for the patient with type 1 diabetes mellitus are required for the remainder of the patient's life. Many of the complications of diabetes can be avoided if the patient maintains strict control of glucose levels with medication, diet, and exercise.

What You NEED TO KNOW

Clinical Manifestations

Classic symptoms of diabetes mellitus are polydipsia, polyphagia, and polyuria. As glucose accumulates in the blood, fluids are drawn out of the tissues into the bloodstream, causing an osmotic diuresis which results in excessive loss of electrolytes and fluids via the urine. Other clinical manifestations are fluctuations in blood glucose levels, weight loss, nausea, vomiting, abdominal pain, and fatigue. Individuals with type 1 diabetes are also prone to ketoacidosis.

The increased metabolism of fat and protein results in the increase of circulating ketones. Excess ketones decrease blood pH, causing a decrease in the bicarbonate concentration, which results in metabolic ketoacidosis. To compensate for metabolic acidosis, the lungs blow off acetone through Kussmaul respirations, giving the breath a sweet, "fruity" odor. Hypokalemia occurs in response to the metabolic acidosis. Hypovolemia can result in decreased, normal, or elevated sodium, magnesium, and phosphorus levels, depending on the extent of fluid loss. The hematocrit, hemoglobin, white blood count, serum creatinine, BUN, and serum osmolality are increased during ketoacidosis because of hypovolemia.

Prognosis

Acute or chronic complications of diabetes result in morbidity and mortality. Over 15% of patients with type 1 diabetes die by the age of 40. Most complications are the result of chronic hyperglycemia and metabolic alterations. Microvascular, macrovascular, and neuropathic insults are responsible for many of the serious complications. Periodontal disease occurs in 30% of persons with diabetes who are 19 years or older. Diabetes is the leading cause of new blindness in patients between the ages of 20 and 74 and is also the leading cause of end-stage renal failure. Other complications of uncontrolled diabetes include the following:

- Damage to the blood vessels of the retina (diabetic retinopathy) which results in blindness
- Loss of sensation, particularly in the extremities (peripheral neuropathy)
- Vascular disease, particularly coronary artery disease, peripheral vascular disease, and hypertension

- Gastrointestinal problems including diabetic gastroparesis, constipation, and diarrhea
- Impaired wound healing, chronic skin infections, foot ulcers
- Gangrene and amputation of extremities
- Impaired renal function, up to and including renal failure
- Sexual dysfunction

What You DO

Treatment

The treatment goal is to maintain near-normal blood glucose levels (**euglycemia**), avoid hypoglycemia (blood glucose of 45 to 60 mg/dL) or hyperglycemia (fasting blood glucose over 126 mg/dL), and to avoid complications. The treatment plan is individualized and specific, considering the patient's lifestyle, age, and activity level. Treatment includes strict dietary adherence, planned exercise, and daily monitoring of blood glucose levels.

Periodic measurement of glycosylated hemoglobin (A_{1c}) should be monitored to evaluate the effectiveness of the treatment plan and, if any adjustments are required, to maintain normal blood glucose levels. The A_{1c} is a reflection of blood glucose control over the previous 3 months.

Nursing Responsibilities

For the patient with type 1 diabetes, the nursing responsibilities are primarily supportive. The nurse should do the following:

- Provide information to the newly diagnosed patient and the family about the disorder and prevention, as well as the ways to reduce the risk of complications.
- Stress the importance of adherence to the treatment plan, including the technique for insulin administration, blood glucose monitoring, dietary and exercise regimes, proper foot care, and ways to recognize signs and symptoms of hypoglycemia and hyperglycemia.
- Provide instruction regarding management of diabetes during illness and any needed adjustments to dosage or diet.
- Assess the patient's psychosocial resources and provide information on support groups and community resources that are available for patients with diabetes, such as the American Diabetes Association.

The National Center for Biotechnology Information
The Genetic Landscape of Diabetes (on-line book)
http://www.ncbi.nlm.nih.gov/books/bv.fcgi?rid=diabetes.chapter.3
American Diabetes Association Home Page
http://www.diabetes.org/home.jsp
National Institute of Diabetes & Digestive & Kidney Diseases
http://www.niddk.nih.gov/

Severe hypoglycemia or hyperglycemia may be lethal! When possible, instruct other family members as well as the patient on management of the disease.

- Instruct the patient to wear MedicAlert identification.
- Encourage the patient to have annual eye and foot examinations during each visit.
- Assess A_{1c} levels quarterly to evaluate the effectiveness of the treatment plans

Do You UNDERSTAND?

DIRECTIONS: Fill in the blanks to complete the following statements.

1. Type 1 diabetes results from a (n) _____ _____ insulin deficiency.
2. The peak onset of type 1 diabetes occurs at approximately _____ years of age.
3. A metabolic complication of hyperglycemia that those with type 1 diabetes are prone to is _____.

DIRECTIONS: Fill in the letter of the best choice.

4. _____ is a common presenting symptom of Type 1 diabetes.
   a. Fluid retention
   b. Weight loss
   c. Decreased appetite
   d. Polyuria

What IS Type 2 Diabetes Mellitus?

Pathogenesis

Type 2 diabetes is characterized by a relative insulin deficit, the development of insulin resistance in peripheral tissues, and excessive glucose production by the liver. The result is similar to type 1 diabetes. In the past, type 2 diabetes was called other names, such as non–insulin-dependent diabetes mellitus (NIDDM), adult-onset diabetes, maturity-onset diabetes, or ketosis-resistant diabetes. Because symptoms tend to develop slowly, only about 50% of all cases of type 2 diabetes have actually been diagnosed. Approximately 90% to 95% of all diagnosed cases of diabetes mellitus in the United States are type 2.

Insulin resistance is associated with decreased number of insulin receptors, decreased action of glucose transporters, and increased production of glucagon. Obesity and inactivity increase insulin resistance. The insulin resistance is initially compensated for by increased insulin production. However, because the beta cells are unable to produce sufficient insulin, decreased numbers and abnormal function of beta cells result. The increased insulin resistance, decreased production of insulin, and increased production of glucagon result in hyperglycemia.

At-Risk Populations

Major risk factors for type 2 diabetes include a family history of diabetes, age 40 or above, hypertension, and a history of gestational diabetes. Approximately 85% of patients with type 2 diabetes are obese. The risk of developing type 2 diabetes is higher in the older adult and non-Caucasian populations. Type 2 diabetes is more common in the African American, Hispanic American, and Native American populations, and is more prevalent in women than it is in men.

> ⚠ The life-threatening complication common in type 2 diabetes is hyperglycemic hyperosmolar nonketotic (HHNK) coma. HHNK is characterized by severe dehydration and hyperglycemia with little or no ketosis. The production of ketone bodies, which results from lipolysis, is suppressed by the presence of endogenous insulin; thus no ketosis is present, as it is in type 1 diabetes.

What You NEED TO KNOW

Clinical Manifestations

Type 2 diabetes is an insidious disease. Initially, the patient usually has no symptoms. The patient frequently reports nonspecific symptoms, such as itching (pruritus), recurrent infections, visual changes, fatigue, and burning or prickling sensation (paresthesias). The classic symptoms of polydipsia, polyuria, and polyphagia may be present, as well as fluctuations in blood glucose levels.

Prognosis

The mortality of patients with type 2 diabetes is twice that of persons without diabetes. Life expectancy is reduced by 5% to 10% among middle-aged populations. Early detection and treatment reduces the microvascular, macrovascular, and neuropathic changes that are responsible for the retinopathy, renal, cardiovascular, and peripheral vascular complications of diabetes mellitus.

What You DO

Treatment

Like type 1 diabetes, the treatment goals for type 2 diabetes are to maintain euglycemia, correct related metabolic disorders, and avoid complications.

Drug therapy for type 2 diabetes includes the use of antidiabetic drugs such as a sulfonylurea, biguanide, alpha glucosidase inhibitor, meglitinide, and/or a thiazolidinedione. Treatment includes using a single antidiabetic drug **(monotherapy),** combination therapy using two drugs, or insulin therapy. Insulin therapy is used when oral drugs fail to maintain a near-normal blood glucose level.

Nursing Responsibilities

Patient education is important for this population because much of the treatment takes place in an outpatient setting. The nursing responsibilities for patients diagnosed with type 2 diabetes are similar to those for type 1 and primarily include being supportive and educating the patient and family in medical and nutritional therapy, using oral antidiabetic drugs or insulin when necessary, and preventing complications. Patients often need help and reinforcement when learning to modify lifestyles, including diet modification and how to monitor for complications of the disease.

TAKE HOME POINTS

- Oral antidiabetic drugs, exercise, and diet therapy are basic treatments for type 2 diabetes.
- Physiologic stressors such as infection may cause type 2 diabetics to require insulin to regain normal glucose levels.
- Obese patients with type 2 diabetes may decrease their need for drug therapy with weight loss and regular exercise.

Do You UNDERSTAND?

DIRECTIONS: Fill in the blanks to complete the following statements.

1. Type 2 diabetes accounts for _____ to _____ of all diagnosed cases of diabetes in the United States.
2. The three basic pathologic changes causing type 2 diabetes are ____
   _____,
   _____,
   and _____.
3. Type 2 diabetes is most prevalent in the ethnic or cultural groups of
   _____,
   _____,
   and _____ populations.

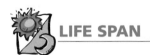

Gestational diabetes affects a small percentage of pregnancies.

What IS Gestational Diabetes Mellitus?

Pathogenesis

The onset or first recognition of gestational diabetes (GDM) occurs during pregnancy. The cause of GDM is similar to that of type 2 diabetes: tissue resistance to insulin and deficiency in insulin production.

During normal pregnancy, tissue resistance to insulin is present. Weight gain and the presence of placental hormones contribute to insulin resistance. Pregnant women require 2 to 3 times more insulin than women who are not pregnant. The deficiency in insulin production and increased tissue resistance causes glucose intolerance.

At-Risk Populations

Women at the highest risk for GDM are those who are obese, have a first-degree relative with diabetes, have a previous history of GDM, or have had infants whose birth weight exceeded 9 pounds.

LIFE SPAN

GDM affects approximately 4% of all pregnancies. Women who have had GDM are more likely to become diabetic later in life. A risk assessment for GDM should be completed at the first prenatal visit.

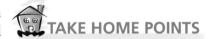

TAKE HOME POINTS

Women over 40 years of age are at risk for GDM. During pregnancy, a deterioration of glucose tolerance is present, particularly during the third trimester during which insulin needs increase significantly.

Answers: **1. 90%, 95%; 2. insulin resistance, insulin production deficiency, excessive glucose production by the liver; 3. African American, Hispanic American, Native American.**

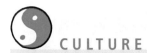

CULTURE

Women of Hispanic American, Native American, Asian American, African American, and Pacific Islander ethnic or racial groups are at greater risk for the development of GDM.

⚠️ When GDM is not treated during pregnancy, metabolic abnormalities and stillbirth of the infant can occur. An increased rate of cesarean delivery and chronic hypertension, as well as the development of diabetes later in life, are maternal complications related to GDM.

What You NEED TO KNOW

Clinical Manifestations

The signs and symptoms of GDM are similar to those of type 2 diabetes. The classic symptoms of polydipsia, polyuria, and polyphagia may be present, as well as fluctuations in blood glucose levels and fatigue. Complications of GDM are infants of high birth weight (over 4000 grams) and neonatal hypoglycemia.

Prognosis

The woman should be reassessed approximately 6 weeks after delivery and classified, according to the American Diabetes Association's diagnostic criteria, as (1) having diabetes, (2) with impaired fasting glucose, (3) with impaired glucose tolerance, or (4) as normoglycemic. GDM will reoccur in future pregnancies in as many as 90% of women.

What You DO

Treatment

All pregnant women with a family history of diabetes should be screened for gestational diabetes. Similar to type 1 and type 2 diabetes, the goal is to maintain blood sugar levels in the normal range and to prevent hypoglycemia, hyperglycemia, and complications. Treatment of GDM includes blood glucose and urine ketone monitoring, exercise, and dietary counseling. The safe use of oral hypoglycemic agents has not been determined; therefore if hyperglycemia continues, insulin therapy should be used.

Nursing Responsibilities

The nursing responsibilities for patients diagnosed with GDM are similar to those for patients with type 1 diabetes and primarily include being supportive and educating the patient and family involving medical and diet therapy, in the use of insulin when necessary, and in the prevention of complications. Women with high-risk characteristics should have their glucose tested initially and, when negative for GDM, they should be retested again at 24 to 28 weeks' gestation. Women with an average risk should be glucose-tested between 24 and 28 weeks' gestation.

Do You UNDERSTAND?

DIRECTIONS: Provide answers for the following questions.

1. How does GDM differ from type 1 diabetes? _____

    _____

2. Do all women who have GDM develop type 2 diabetes? Why or why not? _____

    _____

References

Asp AA, Kirkhorn MJ: Endocrine function, metabolism and nutrition. In Copstead LC and Banasik JL editors: *Pathophyiology*, ed 3, St. Louis, 2005 Elsevier Saunders.

American Diabetes Association: Report of the expert committee on the diagnosis and classification of diabetes mellitus, *Clinical Practice Recommendations 2000* 23(Suppl 1), 2000, [On-Line], URL http://journal.diabetes.org/FullText/Supplements/DiabetesCare/Supplement100/.

Copstead L, Banasik J: *Pathophysiology: biological and behavioral perspectives*, ed 2, Philadelphia, 2000, WB Saunders.

Fain JA: Management of clients with diabetes mellitus. In Black JM and Hawks JH: *Medical-surgical nursing: clinical management for positive outcomes*. ed 7, St Louis, Elsevier Saunders

Huether S, McCance, K: *Understanding pathophysiology*, ed 3, St Louis, 2005, Mosby.

Lewis S, Heitkemper, M, Dirksen S: *Medical-surgical nursing: assessment and management of clinical problems*, ed 5, St Louis, 2004, Mosby.

McCance K, Huether S: Pathophysiology: *The biologic basis for disease in adults and children*, St Louis, 2002, Mosby.

National Institute of Diabetes and Diseases of the Kidney: *Addison's disease*, 2004, URL http://www.niddk.nih.gov/health/endo/puds/ addison/addison.htm.

National Institute of Diabetes and Diseases of the Kidney: *Cushing's disease*, 2002, URL http://www.niddk.nih.gov/health/endo/pubs/cushings/cushings.htm.

National Institutes of Health: *Diabetes insipidus*, 1998, URL http://www.cc.nih.gov/ccc/patient_education/pepubs/di.pdf.

National Institutes of Health: *Secretion of inappropriate antidiuretic hormone*, 2003, http://www.nlm.nih.gov/medlineplus/print/ency/article/000394.htm.

Thyroid Diseases from Medline Plus: URL http://www.nlm.nih.gov/medlineplus/ency/article/001159.htm.

Answers: **1.** type 1 diabetes results from an absolute insulin deficiency, whereas GDM and type 2 diabetes both result from insulin resistance and a deficiency in insulin production; **2.** no, but they are at a higher risk for type 2 diabetes than women who have not had GDM.

NCLEX® Review

Section A

1. Which of the following is the most common cause of pituitary dysfunction?
   1 Congenital defects
   2 Drug overdose
   3 Head injury
   4 Tumor

2. The nurse is explaining diabetes insipidus to a patient with the disorder. The nurse should explain that the signs and symptoms are related to a deficiency in which hormone?
   1 ADH
   2 FSH
   3 HGH
   4 Oxytocin

3. Which laboratory values would be expected in a patient with SIADH?
   1 Serum sodium of 150 mEq/L and dilute urine
   2 Serum potassium of 5 mEq/L and dilute urine
   3 Serum sodium of 120 mEq/L and dilute urine
   4 Serum potassium of 3 mEq/L and concentrated urine

4. The nurse is caring for a 25-year-old woman admitted for diagnostic workup for acromegaly. Physical assessment would identify which of the following signs?
   1 Alopecia
   2 Growth spurt of inches in the last year
   3 Increased forehead and jaw size
   4 Orthostatic hypotension

Section B

5. Which of the following can prevent endemic goiters?
   1 Avoiding the use of harsh mouthwashes
   2 Encouraging the intake of calcium supplements with vitamin D
   3 Encouraging the use of iodized salt
   4 Restricting the intake of caffeine

6. The clinical manifestations of primary hypothyroidism are all a result of which of the following?
   1 Absence of thyroid hormones
   2 Congenital absence of the thyroid
   3 Excessive intake of iodine
   4 Thyroid enlargement

7. A patient with primary hypothyroidism asks the nurse how long the levothyroxine drug should be taken. Which of the following is the nurse's best response?
   1 For approximately 2 to 3 years
   2 For the remainder of your life
   3 Until all symptoms are under control
   4 Until the health care provider decides that the drug is no longer required

8. Hypoparathyroidism is most frequently treated with
   1 Biphosphates.
   2 Antihypercalcemic drugs.
   3 Calcium preparations and vitamin D.
   4 Normal saline administered intravenously.

9. Hyperparathyroidism is most frequently treated with:
   1 Formulations of vitamin D.
   2 Calcium preparations.
   3 Biphosphates.
   4 Thiazide diuretics.

Section C

10. Mr. Wong has been diagnosed with adrenal insufficiency and is taking a daily dose of glucocorticosteroids. You have told him to contact his health care provider if a minor illness develops. "That's silly!" he snorts. "Why should I call the doctor when I get a cough and runny nose? I can handle that myself!" What does Mr. Wong need to know?

    1 A minor illness increases the body's need for glucocorticoids. He should consult the health care provider about a temporary increase in drug dosage.

    2 A minor illness increases the body's need for mineralocorticoids. He should consult the local pharmacist for recommendations of an over-the-counter product.

    3 A minor illness decreases the body's need for mineralocorticoids. He should consult the health care provider about a temporary decrease in drug dosage.

    4 A minor illness decreases the body's need for glucocorticoids. He should consult the local pharmacist for instructions on the ways to reduce the drug dosage.

11. Patients at risk for Cushing's syndrome include those who have which of the following?

    1 Increased secretion of mineralocorticoids

    2 A history of receiving glucocorticoids

    3 Bilateral adrenal atrophy

    4 A reduced quantity of cortisol in the hypothalamus

Section D

12. What percentage of Americans are affected by type 2 diabetes?

    1 10%

    2 50%

    3 70%

    4 90%

13. Which of the following characterizes type 1 diabetes?

    1 Inadequate insulin production

    2 Insulin resistance

    3 Lack of any insulin production

    4 Obesity

14. Women who are at high risk for developing GDM include all of the following *except* those who have which of the following?

    1 First-degree relative with diabetes

    2 History of GDM

    3 Given birth to an infant whose birth weight was 6 pounds

    4 Native American heritage

NCLEX® Review Answers

Section A

1. **4** A tumor is the most common cause of pituitary dysfunction. Congenital defects can cause many types of conditions affecting all body systems. A drug overdose most likely causes neurologic, respiratory, renal, and cardiovascular problems. Head injuries can cause neurologic problems.

2. **1** Signs and symptoms of diabetes insipidus are related to deficiency of ADH. FSH deficiency reduces growth of ova and sperm. Growth hormone deficiency leads to short stature. Oxytocin deficiency results in lack of uterine contraction and lactation.

3. **3** Serum sodium levels less than 120 mEq/L produce signs and symptoms of SIADH. Potassium levels are not directly related to SIADH. A serum sodium level of 150 mEq/L indicates hypernatremia.

4. **3** High levels of growth hormone after closure of epiphyses results in increased forehead and jaw size. Alopecia is related to hereditary influences; postpartum hormonal changes; drugs; physical or psychologic stress; nutritional deficiencies; and a number of other diseases and disorders. Growth spurts are found in children and adolescents. Orthostatic hypotension is related to fluid volume deficit.

Section B

5. **3** Ingesting iodized salt will help prevent goiter, which is the result of a deficiency of iodine in the body. No relationship between goiter and the use of mouthwash exists. The use of calcium supplements with vitamin D promotes healthy bones and teeth. Restricting caffeine intake reduces the risk of gastric distress, elevated blood pressure, and faulty absorption of calcium.

6. **1** Primary hypothyroidism manifests in the absence of thyroid hormones. Congenital absence of the thyroid gland is not a primary cause of hypothyroidism. Excessive iodine intake is not considered to be a significant public health problem in the United States and Canada. Thyroid enlargement is the result of an attempt by the thyroid to increase thyroid hormone secretion.

7. **2** The patient with primary hypothyroidism lacks thyroid hormones, thus necessitating hormonal replacement for life. The other options (all instructing the patient that treatment time is finite) are not feasible if hypothyroidism is to be adequately treated and adverse effects of the disorder prevented.

8. **3** Patients with hypoparathyroidism lack calcium, thus calcium supplements are required. Biphosphates inhibit osteoclastic bone resorption and help normalize serum calcium levels. Antihypercalcemic drugs reduce calcium utilization. Intravenous normal saline further reduces serum calcium levels, contributing to adverse effects.

9. **3** Biphosphates inhibit osteoclastic bone resorption and help normalize serum calcium levels, thus normalizing circulating PTH levels and resolving hypoparathyroidism. Vitamin D, calcium, and thiazide diuretics increase serum calcium levels.

Section C

10. **1** Glucocorticoids reduce the inflammatory response. Thus the patient may be more ill than is otherwise apparent and in need of evaluation. A minor illness does not increase or decrease the need for mineralocorticoids or glucocorticoids. Lack of glucocorticoids is a life-threatening problem.

11. **2** Persons with a recent history of receiving glucocorticoids are at risk for developing Cushing's syndrome. Increased secretion of mineralocorticoids offsets glucocorticoid levels rather than increasing them. Adrenal atrophy reduces the level of glucocorticoids. Cortisol is not found in the hypothalamus.

Section D

12. **4** Type 2 diabetes occurs in 90% of Americans; 10% of Americans have type 1 diabetes; 50% and 70% are statistically incorrect options.

13. **3** Type 1 diabetes is the result of a total lack of insulin production. Insufficient insulin and insulin resistance are associated with type 2 diabetes, as is obesity.

14. **3** Birth of a 6-pound infant reduces the risk of GDM. A mother with a first-degree relative with diabetes, of Native American heritage, or with a previous history of GDM is at high risk for developing GDM. In addition, mothers who have given birth to babies with a birth weight of 9 pounds or more are at risk for GDM in future pregnancies.

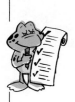

Notes

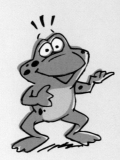

Alterations in Gastrointestinal Function

What You WILL LEARN

After reading this chapter, you will know how to do the following:

- ✔ Discuss the mechanisms that cause nausea and vomiting.
- ✔ Compare and contrast constipation with diarrhea and fecal incontinence in terms of cause and treatment.
- ✔ Discuss the relationship between gastroesophageal reflux disorder (GERD) and hiatal hernia and how symptoms of GERD can be confused with those of esophageal and gastric cancers.
- ✔ Relate the pathogenesis of peptic ulcer disease to its treatment with antibiotics and proton pump inhibitors.
- ✔ Explain the clinical manifestations of pancreatitis to its pathogenesis.
- ✔ Compare and contrast Crohn's disease and ulcerative colitis in terms of clinical manifestations and prognosis.
- ✔ List the patients who are at risk for diverticular disease and their prognosis
- ✔ Identify the treatment for gluten-sensitive enteropathy (celiac sprue).
- ✔ Compare and contrast the various types of hepatitis in terms of incubation periods and transmission routes.
- ✔ Relate the pathogenesis of cirrhosis to its clinical manifestations.
- ✔ Identify the population most at risk for cholecystitis
- ✔ Discuss how a patient who is obese can be malnourished.
- ✔ List the risk factors for colon cancer.

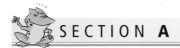

SECTION **A**

MANIFESTATIONS OF GASTROINTESTINAL DYSFUNCTION

What ARE Nausea and Vomiting?

Pathogenesis

Nausea is a subjective experience associated with many different conditions, some minor and some more serious. It is an unpleasant sensation vaguely referred to the epigastrium and abdomen, with a tendency to vomit. Retching begins with a deep breath. The glottis closes, and pressure within the chest falls, and the esophagus becomes distended. At the same time, abdominal muscles contract, creating a rise in pressure into the thorax. The lower esophageal sphincter (LES) and body of the stomach relax, but the duodenum and antrum of the stomach go into spasm. The reverse peristalsis and the pressure force chyme from the stomach and duodenum into the esophagus. Because the upper esophageal sphincter is closed, chyme does not enter the mouth. As abdominal muscles relax, the contents of the esophagus fall into the stomach. This process may be repeated a number of times before vomiting occurs.

Vomiting usually follows retching. When the stomach becomes full of gastric contents, the diaphragm is forced upward into the thoracic cavity by contractions of abdominal muscles. The high pressure within the chest forces the upper esophageal sphincter to open, and chyme is expelled from the mouth. The LES then closes. The cycle is repeated if there is a volume of chyme remaining in the stomach. Projectile vomiting is vomiting not preceded by nausea or retching. It is caused by direct stimulation of the vomiting center by lesions in the brain stem.

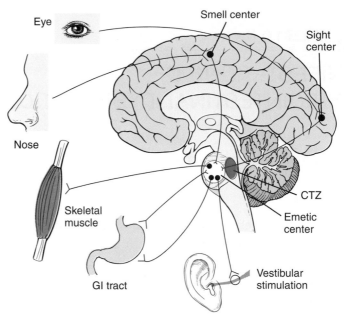

CTZ and other sites that activate the emetic center. *(From McKenry LM, Salerno E: Mosby's guide to pharmacology in nursing, ed 22, St. Louis, 2006, Mosby.)*

At-Risk Populations

Nausea and vomiting are found in a wide variety of gastrointestinal (GI) disorders, as well as conditions unrelated to GI disease such as pregnancy, infectious diseases, central nervous system (CNS) disorders, and vestibular disorders; in cardiovascular disorders such as myocardial infarction (MI) or heart failure; in metabolic derangements such as uremia and motion sickness; and with psychologic factors such as stress or fear. Although nausea and vomiting may occur with any drug, it is often associated with alcohol, aspirin, opioids, antibiotics, cardiac glycosides, antineoplastic therapy, and theophylline drugs.

The threat of pulmonary aspiration is a concern when vomiting occurs in a patient who is unconscious or who has a condition that impairs the gag reflex. Older patients and young children are at particular risk.

What You NEED TO KNOW

Clinical Manifestations

A lack of appetite (anorexia) usually accompanies nausea and is brought on by objectionable stimulation involving any of the five senses. Parasympathetic stimulation causes relaxation of the LES, an increase in gastric motility, and a pronounced increase in salivation followed by an emesis. Sympathetic activation produces tachycardia, tachypnea, and diaphoresis.

Prognosis

Nausea and vomiting are usually self-limiting events. However, when nausea and vomiting are prolonged, dehydration rapidly occurs. In addition to water, essential electrolytes (e.g., potassium, sodium, chloride, hydrogen) are also lost. As vomiting persists, there may be severe electrolyte disturbances, loss of extracellular fluid volume, decreased plasma volume, and eventually circulatory failure. Metabolic alkalosis and acidosis are possible.

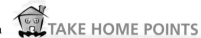

TAKE HOME POINTS

Sporadic episodes of nausea and vomiting are fairly common, but epidemic occurrences suggest environmental exposure to viral or bacterial infections or food poisoning.

What You DO

Treatment

The overall goal in treating the patient is to relieve the nausea and vomiting, maintain fluid and electrolyte balance, and return the patient to a normal fluid balance and nutrient intake.

Nursing Responsibilities

For the patient with nausea and vomiting, the nurse should do the following:

- Assess duration, frequency, and nature of nausea and vomiting; check for aggravating and alleviating factors and for signs of dehydration (e.g., lethargy, sunken eyeballs, dry mucus membranes, poor skin turgor, decreased urinary output, urine concentration) and electrolyte imbalance (e.g., hypokalemia).
- Remove visual stimuli and source of odors to avoid precipitating triggers.

- Maintain a quiet environment by restricting visitors and unnecessary activity or procedures.
- Administer antiemetic as ordered.
- Accurately record intake and output, and monitor vital signs.
- Keep the patient on nothing-by-mouth (NPO) status and give intravenous (IV) fluids, as appropriate, until nausea and vomiting have subsided. A nasogastric (NG) tube may be needed for some patients (keeping the stomach empty reduces the stimulus to vomit).
- Place the patient who cannot adequately manage self-care in a semi-Fowler's or side-lying position to prevent aspiration.
- Assist with mouth care as needed after vomiting episodes.
- Educate the patient and family as to appropriate food and fluid items to consume. Gatorade, tea or broth, dry crackers or toast, plain gelatin, and bland foods such as pasta, rice, and cooked chicken are generally well tolerated in small amounts.

Do You UNDERSTAND?

DIRECTIONS: Unscramble the italicized letters to form terms associated with nausea and vomiting.

_____ *(apesdihosi)*
_____ *(aycdiatrach)*
_____ *(patheayn)*
_____ *(aixerona)*

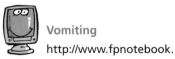

Vomiting
http://www.fpnotebook.com/GI259.htm

Constipation
http://www.fpnotebook.com/GI13.htm

Diarrhea
http://www.fpnotebook.com/GI16.htm

What ARE Constipation and Diarrhea?

Pathogenesis

Constipation is defined as infrequent defecation, a hardening or reduced caliber of stool, a sensation of incomplete evacuation, and the need to strain with bowel movements. The fundamental mechanism involves the increased length of time the stool is in the colon along with increased resorption of fluid. Regardless of the cause of constipation, prolonged

Answers: 1. diaphoresis; 2. tachycardia; 3. tachypnea; 4. anorexia

retention of stool in the rectum results in drying because of the resorption of water. The harder and drier the stool, the more difficulty it is to expel.

Diarrhea is defined as the rapid movement of fecal matter through the intestines, resulting in poor absorption of water, nutritive elements, and electrolytes, and producing abnormally frequent evacuation of watery stools. In essence, diarrhea is caused by any factor that decreases fluid resorption in the small or large intestine, increases fluid secretion (e.g., deranged electrolyte transport), alters bowel motility, or is associated with mucosal injury. Acute diarrhea is usually bacterial or viral in origin, and although it is problematic, it is not usually voluminous in nature.

At-Risk Populations

Constipation affects up to 14% of the population. Immobility, a sedentary life style and lack of regular exercise place persons at risk for constipation. Lack of access to bathroom facilities and constantly suppressing the urge to empty the bowel are other risk factors. Drugs, particularly those with anticholinergic effects, contribute to constipation.

Although avoiding laxatives in the presence of diarrhea seems all too obvious, concealed abuse of stimulant laxatives is a surprisingly frequent cause of chronic diarrhea of unknown origin. Patients at risk for chronic diarrhea are those with malabsorption syndromes, irritable bowel disease, and surgical procedures that shorten the intestinal tract or that cause rapid emptying of the stomach. The very young and older adults are most at risk.

What You NEED TO KNOW

Clinical Manifestations

Normal bowel movement patterns range from 2 to 3 evacuations per day to one per week.

The clinical manifestations of constipation involve changes in this pattern including less frequent defecations, smaller stool volumes, difficulty moving stool through the rectum, or a feeling of rectal fullness and discomfort. Hard dry stools can irritate hemorrhoids and may cause rectal bleeding. Because definitions of constipation differ greatly among patients, the disorder must be individually defined.

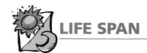

LIFE SPAN

Women with a tendency toward constipation may find the condition more troublesome during the third trimester and require dietary adjustment and supplements.

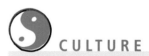

CULTURE

Diarrhea is the leading cause of death in developing countries, where daily over 10,000 children younger than 5 years of age are affected. In the United States, diarrhea accounts for 250,000 hospitalizations per year and 7.9 million office visits.

Diarrhea is accompanied by frequent and liquid bowel movements, abdominal cramps, and general weakness. The stools often contain mucus and may be blood streaked. Systemic manifestations of acute diarrhea include fever, nausea, vomiting, and malaise. Leukocytes, blood and mucus may be present in the stool depending on the cause of the diarrhea. Tenesmus, a spasmodic contraction of the anal sphincter with pain and a persistent desire to defecate and cramping abdominal pain are often present. Frequent, liquid stools can cause irritation of the skin around the anus.

Diarrhea is considered chronic if it persists for at least 2 weeks, produces over 300 grams of stool daily, or when it subsides and returns more than 2 to 4 weeks after the initial episode. In chronic diarrhea the patient is likely to be anemic and suffering from malnutrition.

Prognosis

Constipation or diarrhea that is occasional, brief, and responsive to simple measures is harmless. That which is habitual can be a life-long nuisance.

What You DO

Treatment

The goal of treatment for the patient with constipation is to return bowel activity to a pattern normal for the patient and developing an awareness of the need to establish a regular routine of elimination. Lab testing is only necessary when other disorders are being considered as the cause of constipation (e.g., a CBC to detect anemia that may indicate colorectal neoplasm; a TSH to check for hyperthyroidism).

The goal of treatment for the patient with diarrhea is to identify the underlying cause, correct dehydration, disturbances in acid-base balance, and nutritional deficiencies while maintaining fluid and electrolyte balance. Because diarrhea is a symptom rather than a disease, lab testing or diagnostic procedures may be necessary to determine the cause. Treatment is symptomatic.

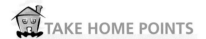

TAKE HOME POINTS

Unless there is a demonstrable organic disorder causing constipation, regular bowel elimination is largely a matter of habit. Patients with life-long tendency toward constipation often encounter increasing difficulty with advancing age. There is an increased incidence of colorectal neoplasms with age that may be associated with constipation.

Excessive concern over constipation and frequent use of laxatives can be as harmful as deliberately ignoring the need for regular elimination.

Nursing Responsibilities

For the patient with constipation, the nurse should do the following:

- Encourage regular bowel function by adhering to healthful habits of diet and exercise
- Increase dietary fiber to 15 grams/day (e.g., bran, fruit, green vegetables, and whole grain cereals and breads) and liberal fluid intake
- Help the patient develop an awareness of the need to establish a regular routine for elimination. (adequate time for evacuation in a quiet, unhurried environment, thighs flexed toward abdomen)
- Develop a bowel training program as appropriate
- Permit the patient to voice concerns of altered self-concept, anxiety, anger, and a lack of understanding about the cause and prognosis of the condition.
- Discourage routine use of laxatives and other bowel stimulants while eliminating the use of drugs that cause or worsen constipation
- Reinforce the use of bulk-forming laxatives (e.g., psyllium, methylcellulose)

For the patient with diarrhea, the nurse should do the following:

- Provide the patient with an atmosphere conducive to rest and relaxation.
- Permit the patient to voice concerns of altered self-concept, anxiety, anger, and a lack of understanding about the cause and prognosis of the condition.
- Assess duration, frequency, and nature of nausea and vomiting; aggravating and alleviating factors and for signs of dehydration (e.g., lethargy, sunken eyeballs, dry mucus membranes, poor skin turgor, decreased urinary output, urine concentration), and electrolyte imbalance (e.g., hypokalemia)
- Assist the patient with diarrhea to cleanse the anal region with soap and water as often as necessary and apply a mild emollient cream to act as a skin barrier.
- Accurately record intake and output and monitor vital signs; listen for bowel sounds and record the exact number and character of the stools
- Assist in the collection of stool samples for lab testing.
- Educate the patient and family as to appropriate food and fluid items to consume. Gatorade, tea or broth, dry crackers or toast, plain gelatin, and bland foods such as pasta, rice, and cooked chicken are generally well tolerated in small amounts
- Administer antidiarrhea drugs as ordered

Do You UNDERSTAND?

DIRECTIONS: Fill in the blanks to complete the following statements.

1. Constipation is defined as _____

   _____

2. The fundamental mechanism of constipation involves the _____

   _____

3. What 2 groups of patients are at risk and need to be evaluated promptly when diarrhea occurs? _____ and

   _____

4. Acute diarrhea is usually of _____ or _____ _____ origin.

What IS Fecal Incontinence?

Pathogenesis

Normally, feces pass from the sigmoid colon into the rectum, causing distention. Stretch receptors in the rectal muscles provide the sensation of rectal filling. This causes a reflex relaxation of the internal anal sphincter and contraction of the external anal sphincter. Sensory receptors in the epithelium of the anal canal can usually distinguish among solid, liquid, and gas. The combination of contraction of abdominal muscles, relaxation of pelvic muscles, squatting (which straightens the anorectal angle), and voluntary relaxation of the external anal sphincter allows for elimination of feces. Motor (muscle contraction) or sensory (ability to perceive presence of stool or experience the urge to defecate) problems or a combination of both can result in fecal incontinence.

At-Risk Populations

Physiologic and psychologic conditions can be contributing factors to fecal incontinence.

Patients at risk for fecal incontinence include those with neurologically-based sensory and motor defects such as are seen with stroke or spinal cord injury; pathologic conditions that impair the integrity of the rectal sphincters such as tumors, lacerations, fistulas, and loss of sensory innervation; altered levels of consciousness; and severe diarrhea. Psychologic factors include anxiety, confusion, disorientation, depression, and despair. Fecal incontinence can also be secondary to fecal impaction, in which there is an accumulation of feces in the rectum or sigmoid colon that the patient is unable to move.

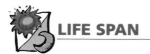

LIFE SPAN

Fecal incontinence caused by fecal impaction is a common problem in older adults.

What You NEED TO KNOW

Clinical Manifestations

Fecal incontinence is an inability to control bowel movements resulting in soiling of clothing, skin breakdown, and alterations in self-image.

Prognosis

The prognosis for fecal incontinence depends on the underlying cause. Stooling may not be correctable for patients with neurologic or motor deficits and for those with conditions of the anal sphincter, and thus may be life-long for some patients.

What You DO

Treatment

The goals for the patient with fecal incontinence is to return normal bowel control, maintain perianal skin integrity, and to minimize self-esteem problems related to issues with bowel control.

Nursing Responsibilities

For the patient with fecal incontinence, the nurse should do the following:

- Encourage regular bowel function by teaching adherence to healthful habits of diet and exercise.
- Help the patient develop an awareness of the need to establish a regular routine for elimination (adequate time for evacuation in a quiet, unhurried environment; thighs flexed toward abdomen).
- Establish a regular scheduled time for toileting; offer a bedpan, get the patient up to use a bedside commode, or assist the patient to the bathroom.

- Administer a rectal suppository (e.g., bisacodyl, glycerin) or a small phosphate enema before toileting time to stimulate the anorectal reflex (the lack of stool in the rectum reduces the likelihood of incontinence).
- Help the patient to make necessary dietary changes.
- Help the patient explore the use of biofeedback techniques to help maintain higher tone in the anal sphincter.

Do You UNDERSTAND?

DIRECTIONS: Unscramble the italicized letters to form terms associated with fecal incontinence.

1. _____ (*lasiboycd yrotssioppu*)
2. _____ (*nnnneeiiyoc*)
3. _____ (*latcerona xelfer*)
4. _____ (*atcerl hrspitnec*)

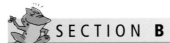

SECTION B

DISORDERS OF THE ESOPHAGUS

What IS Gastroesophageal Reflux Disease?

Pathogenesis

Normally, contents of the stomach are prevented from entering the esophagus because of the structural location of, and pressures within the LES. Gastroesophageal reflux disease (GERD) is a disorder in which the LES is relaxed or ineffective, permitting reflux (or upward movement) of gastric secretions from the stomach into the lower portion of the esophagus.

Answers: 1. bisacodyl suppository; 2. incontinence; 3. anorectal reflex; 4. rectal sphincter

At-Risk Populations

The populations at risk for GERD include Caucasian males who have a hiatal hernia and who smoke, since both factors contribute to acid trapping. Many of those afflicted with GERD have a body mass index over 30 mm². Foods that lower LES pressure contribute to GERD by forcing a relaxation of the sphincter muscles; these foods include yellow onions, chocolate, peppermint, and high fat foods. Drugs that tend to lower LES pressure include theophylline, anticholinergics, progesterone, calcium channel blockers (i.e., nifedipine, verapamil.), alpha adrenergic drugs, diazepam, and meperidine. NSAIDs used chronically are notorious for contributing to the irritation from GERD. Patients who have had chest trauma and those with a nasogastric tube are at risk for reflux, as well as patients with Down syndrome, mental retardation, cerebral palsy, or who have a repaired tracheoesophageal fistula.

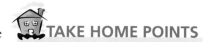

TAKE HOME POINTS

A strong relationship exists between reflux and reclining within 2 to 3 hours after eating.

What You NEED TO KNOW

Clinical Manifestations

The pain of GERD is described as a burning sensation radiating up and down the esophagus ("heartburn"). The pain is usually more severe when the patient is lying down or after eating a meal. In some situations, the pain may radiate to the jaw, the neck, or the back. Other symptoms of GERD include a bitter or sour liquid entering the esophagus or mouth (**regurgitation**), a feeling of a lump in the throat, and difficulty swallowing (**dysphagia**). The pain of GERD may mimic that of a MI.

Prognosis

The prognosis of GERD depends on early identification and treatment. When the underlying cause is not treated, the patient continues to have symptoms. Of patients with GERD, 50% have chronic symptoms but with no real progression of the disease. Patients with chronic GERD develop alterations of the distal esophageal mucosa, changing from the usual stratified squamous epithelium to a columnar epithelium (**Barrett's esophagus**). This mucosal change is also associated with esophageal ulcers, strictures, hemorrhage, and increased risk of adenocarcinoma. Five percent of patients progress to these severe stages of GERD and may require surgery.

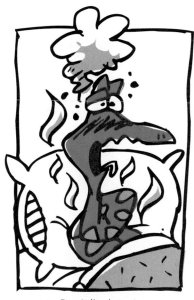

Don't lie down!

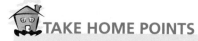

TAKE HOME POINTS

Heartburn is the hallmark symptom of GERD.

What You DO

Treatment

Conservative treatment of the patient with GERD includes weight reduction and avoidance of foods and drugs that increase acid secretion and decrease LES pressure. A high-protein, low-fat diet with small, frequent meals should be encouraged. Tobacco products should be avoided. The patient should avoid eating for at least 2 to 3 hours before going to bed, thus preventing a full stomach at bedtime, and the head of the bed should be elevated on 4- to 6-inch blocks to facilitate gastric emptying. Fluids should be taken between meals to decrease gastric distention. The patient should avoid lifting, straining, and bending. Tight-fitting clothing around the abdomen should also be avoided.

Drugs frequently used in the treatment of GERD include proton pump inhibitors, histamine 2 (H_2) antagonists, antacids, as well as cytoprotective agents and drugs that increase LES pressure. Surgical intervention is sometimes required. A Nissen fundoplication is an antireflux procedure that helps relieve reflux and its associated symptoms. Other surgical procedures strengthen the LES, thus preventing acid reflux. Either an open surgical approach or a laparoscopic approach may be used.

Nursing Responsibilities

For the patient who has surgery for GERD, the nurse should do the following:

- Provide the patient and the family with education regarding nutrition and drug management while assessing the effects of medications administered.
- Maintain IV fluids when required.
- Promote comfort, and manage the patient's pain (see Chapter 2).
- Maintain nasogastric tube patency, and monitor the amount, and color of drainage.
- Keep the head of the patient's bed elevated.
- Monitor respiratory status, and facilitate deep breathing and coughing while splinting the incision.
- Monitor the incision for redness or drainage; maintain a closed-chest drainage system, when needed.
- Provide discharge instructions regarding diet, medications, and symptom management.

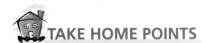

TAKE HOME POINTS

The patient with symptoms of GERD but who has not been diagnosed with the disorder is treated as though an MI has occurred until an accurate diagnosis is made. An electrocardiogram will help rule out an MI.

Do You UNDERSTAND?

DIRECTIONS: **Complete the following crossword puzzle.**

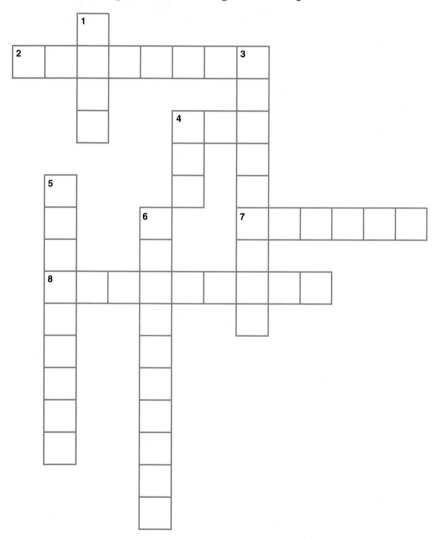

Down

1. Abbreviation given for gastroesophageal reflux disease
3. Term used for difficulty in swallowing
4. Individuals who do not smoke or use alcohol have a _____ risk for developing GERD.
5. Common symptom of GERD
6. The process of bitter liquid entering the mouth as a result of GERD

Across

2. To decrease the chances of a nighttime flare-up of GERD, the head of the patient's bed should be kept _____.
4. A relaxed _____ causes GERD. *(an abbreviation)*
7. _____ is a risk factor for GERD.
8. Weight _____ is recommended for patients suffering from GERD.

What IS a Hiatal Hernia?

Pathogenesis

A hiatal hernia is a protrusion of the upper part of the stomach through the gastroesophageal junction into the thoracic cavity. The actual cause of a hiatal hernia is unknown. Muscle weakness of the gastroesophageal junction and increased intraabdominal pressure contribute to the development of hiatal hernias.

Two major types of hiatal hernias have been identified: sliding hernias and rolling hernias. A sliding hiatal hernia is the most common type and involves protrusion of the gastroesophageal junction and the upper portion of the stomach through the diaphragm. In a rolling hernia, the LES stays below the level of the diaphragm, but the upper portion of the stomach protrudes through a second opening in the diaphragm and lies alongside the esophagus.

At-Risk Populations

Women are affected more frequently than men. Any factor that increases intraabdominal pressure (e.g., pregnancy, obesity, ascites, straining at stool) increases the risk for hiatal hernia. Research studies have refuted a close association between hiatal hernia and GERD.

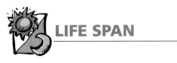

LIFE SPAN

Advancing age is a risk factor for hiatal hernia. Of those over the age of 60, 60% may have hiatal hernias.

Answers: *Down:* 1. GERD; 3. dysphagia; 4. low; 5. heartburn; 6. regurgitation. *Across:* 2. elevated; 4. LES; 7. asthma; 8. reduction.

What You NEED TO KNOW

Clinical Manifestations

The signs and symptoms of hiatal hernia vary, depending on the type of hernia. Most patients with hiatal hernias are asymptomatic. With a sliding hiatal hernia, heartburn related to reflux is common. However, the patient with a rolling hernia frequently complains of a feeling of fullness and pain that is frequently compared with anginal pain. In both cases, symptoms are worse when the patient is in a reclining position.

Prognosis

The prognosis for a patient with a hiatal hernia depends on the severity of the problem. A herniated gastric pouch can cause difficulty in swallowing and can be the site of gastritis and ulceration, the latter of which causes chronic blood loss.

What You DO

Treatment

Treatment of the patient with a hiatal hernia is the same as that for the patient with GERD. Patients are advised to lose weight. Treatment includes small, frequent meals of high-protein, low-fat foods, although eating is avoided within 2 to 3 hours of bedtime. The head of the bed is elevated on 4- to 6-inch blocks to facilitate gastric emptying. Patients should avoid alcohol, tobacco, and constrictive clothing around the abdomen.

Drugs frequently used in the treatment of hiatal hernias include the nonsystemic antacids, H_2 antagonists, and proton pump inhibitors. Surgical intervention is considered in patients with "rolling" paraesophageal hiatal hernias because of the increased incidence of strangulation. The surgical management of hiatal hernia is similar to that of the patient with GERD.

Nursing Responsibilities

For the patient with a hiatal hernia who is undergoing surgery, the nurse should do the following:

- Educate the patient and family about nutrition requirements and drug management.

- Assess the effects of medications administered.
- Maintain IV fluids for the patient who has had surgery.
- Promote comfort and manage the patient's pain.
- Assess the nasogastric tube for patency, amount, and color of drainage.
- Keep the head of the bed elevated to facilitate gastric emptying.
- Assess respiratory status and encourage deep breathing and coughing (despite any postoperative discomfort) and splinting the incision.
- Assess the incision for drainage and redness.
- Maintain closed-chest drainage when a thoracic approach was used for the surgery.
- Educate the patient and family regarding diet, medications, and symptom management.

Do You UNDERSTAND?

DIRECTIONS: **Fill in the blanks to complete the following statements.**

1. Muscle weakness and increased _____ pressure contributes to the formation of hiatal hernias.

2. In a hiatal hernia, part of the stomach extends through the diaphragm and into the _____ cavity.

3. The major symptom observed with a sliding hiatal hernia is _____ _____.

4. One medication that is frequently used for treatment of hiatal hernias is _____.

5. The most common type of hiatal hernia is termed a(n) _____ _____ hernia.

6. _____, _____, and _____ can increase abdominal pressure and predispose the individual to the development of a hiatal hernia.

7. In a(n) _____ hiatal hernia, the LES stays below the diaphragm, but the upper portion of the stomach protrudes through a second opening in the diaphragm.

Answers: 1. intraabdominal; 2. thoracic 3. heartburn; 4. antacids 5. sliding 6. pregnancy, obesity, ascites; 7. rolling.

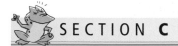

SECTION C

DISEASES OF THE STOMACH

What IS a Stress Ulcer?

Pathogenesis

Stress ulcers (also known as Curling's ulcers) are an acute form of peptic ulcers that may go along with events such as severe illness, systemic trauma, burns, or neural injury. Curling's ulcers develop within 72 hours of the patient's injury. Stress ulcers that occur in patients with severe head injuries are known as Cushing's ulcers. Excessive physiologic stress can lead to the development of stress ulcers. Severe injury or illness causes vasoconstriction, leading to a decreased gastric blood flow (related to sympathetic nervous system stimulation) as the body shunts blood to vital organs. This activity produces ischemia of gastric tissues, which in turn leads to a loss of the normal protective functions of the stomach lining and to GI bleeding.

At-Risk Populations

Individuals at risk for stress ulcers include those with a major illness or severe injury such as burns, shock, sepsis, head injuries, and spinal cord injury. Most people with burns over 35% or more of their body will develop stress ulcers. Other patients at risk include those receiving large dosages of drugs, particularly corticosteroids or NSAIDs.

What You NEED TO KNOW

Clinical Manifestations

The clinical manifestations of a stress ulcer include painless upper GI tract bleeding until complications such as hemorrhage develop, usually 2 to 3 days after the initial injury. Bleeding may manifest as blood in the stools (**melena**) or as bloody sputum (**hematemesis**).

Prognosis

Because a stress ulcer is a complication of a preexisting condition, the prognosis depends upon the treatment of the precipitating event. Early recognition and treatment contribute to a positive outcome.

What You DO

Treatment

Prevention is the key to management. Treatment of the patient with a hemorrhaging stress ulcer includes nasogastric intubation with suction. Endoscopic procedures may be needed to treat the bleeding.

Drugs used in the treatment of stress ulcers include proton-pump inhibitors, H_2 antagonists, mucosal protectants, and non–calcium-containing antacids. IV fluids are started to maintain and improve fluid and electrolyte balance. For severe hemorrhage or perforation, surgical procedures may be required.

Nursing Responsibilities

For the patient with a stress ulcer, the nurse should do the following:
- Identify patients who are at risk for the disorder while assessing for early signs and symptoms.
- Assess stools for hidden or occult blood and assessing vital signs for evidence of hemorrhage or shock.
- Palpate the abdomen. A board-like or rigid finding may indicate perforation of the viscera.

Do You UNDERSTAND?

Juan, a 55-year-old trauma victim, has been hospitalized for 3 days. The health care provider noticed symptoms of a developing stress ulcer.

DIRECTIONS: **Provide answers for the following questions.**

1. What is a stress ulcer? _____.

2. What occurs physiologically in a trauma situation that causes a stress ulcer to develop? _____
   _____

3. What factors place Juan at increased risk for developing a stress ulcer?
   _____

4. What symptoms might you notice if Juan develops a stress ulcer?
   _____
   _____

5. What measures might be taken to prevent the development of a stress ulcer? _____
   _____

What IS Peptic Ulcer Disease?

Pathogenesis

Peptic ulcer disease (PUD) is an acute or chronic inflammation from altered gastric secretions that produces erosions in the mucosal lining of the lower esophagus, the stomach, or the duodenum. Several factors are involved in the development of PUD. Chronic inflammation, imbalance between acid-pepsin and protective effects, damage to the protective mucosal barrier of the stomach by irritating substances, and infection from *Helicobacter pylori* (**H. pylori**) bacteria have all been implicated.

Answers: 1. a gastric ulcer that develops as a result of excessive physiologic stress; 2. a reduced blood flow to the GI tract is present as the body moves blood to more vital organs. This activity results in ischemia of gastric tissues, which, in turn, leads to a loss in the normal protective functions of the stomach lining, and ulcers form; 3. the patient was subjected to trauma that placed significant physiologic stress on his body; 4. most stress ulcers are painless until GI bleeding occurs; hematemesis or melena can occur; 5. prophylactic administration of proton-pump inhibitors, H$_2$ antagonists, mucosal protectants, and non–calcium-containing antacids.

An *H. pylori* infection is the most significant factor in the development of PUD and is associated with more than 90% of all duodenal peptic ulcers and 70% of all gastric ulcers. This organism releases mucolytic enzymes and toxins that breakdown the mucosal lining, causing cellular injury and inflammation. The process also alters gastric secretions and sustains inflammation, resulting in ulcerative lesions. Two different mechanisms for the disease, in addition to *H. pylori* infection, have been proposed as contributing to the development of ulcerations.

The tight, nonpermeable junctions between epithelial cells and the slightly alkaline layer of mucus that coats the surface of the gastric epithelium normally prevent the flow of hydrochloric acid from the lumen of the stomach. Gastric ulcers form when one or more of a number of injurious substances (e.g., aspirin, NSAIDs, glucocorticoids, caffeine, alcohol, phenylbutazone, adrenocorticotropin hormone) interrupts this diffusion barrier. These drugs stimulate acid production and cause local mucosal damage or suppress mucus secretion. The epithelial cell membranes degenerate with massive backward diffusion of acid into the gastric epithelial wall.

The pathogenesis of duodenal ulcers appears to be different. Vagus nerve activity is increased in patients with duodenal ulcers, particularly at night or when the patient is fasting. The vagus nerve stimulates the antrum cells in the pylorus to release gastrin. The gastrin travels through the circulation to act on the gastric parietal cells. The parietal cells stimulate the release of hydrochloric acid.

At-Risk Populations

Individuals with *H. pylori* infection are at high risk for developing PUD. Other individuals who are at risk include those who abuse alcohol, smoke, or use NSAIDs on a chronic basis, and those who have type O blood. The incidence of PUD is increased in individuals with Crohn's disease, Zollinger-Ellison syndrome, and hepatic or biliary disease. The older patient may present with vague description of discomfort, chest pain, dysphagia, weight loss, or anemia.

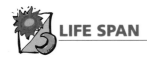

LIFE SPAN

Gastric ulcerations are likely to occur during the fifth and sixth decades of life. Duodenal ulcerations commonly occur during the fourth and fifth decades in men and in persons with type O blood. In women, the occurrence tends to be approximately 10 years later in life. Men are more likely to develop both gastric and duodenal ulcers than women.

What You NEED TO KNOW

Clinical Manifestations

The signs and symptoms of PUD include pain localized to the epigastric region. Gastric ulcer pain occurs in the upper epigastrium and is localized to the left of midline. The pain of gastric ulcers is variable and frequently described as aching, gnawing, burning, and cramplike, occurring from 1 to 3 hours after eating. The condition is made worse with eating but relieved with vomiting. Antacids fail to relieve the pain. Patients with duodenal ulcers have pain on an empty stomach and at night. Ingesting food or antacids frequently relieves the discomfort.

Patients with ulcers bleed when the ulcer erodes through a blood vessel. Massive bleeding can develop, or the bleeding can be occult from slow oozing. Approximately 25% of patients with gastric ulcers experience bleeding. Steady pain near the midline of the back can indicate perforation of the ulcer. The patient may also complain of nausea, regurgitation, constipation, or diarrhea, and may show evidence of blood in the stools.

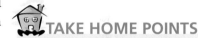

TAKE HOME POINTS

Of those with chronic gastric ulcers, 10% are at risk for gastric malignancy. Early treatment and preventive health measures are vital to prevent future disease.

Prognosis

The pain of both gastric and duodenal ulcers tends to recur daily for a time, and then it and all signs and symptoms disappear for months or years, to be followed eventually by another episode of pain. Reoccurrence of the disease is likely if risk factors are not reduced.

What You DO

Treatment

The treatment of PUD includes proton pump inhibitors, H_2 antagonists, mucosal protectants, and stress-modification strategies. In addition, antibiotics (e.g., clarithromycin, tetracycline, metronidazole, amoxicillin) in combination with the drugs just mentioned play a crucial role in the treatment and prevention of further disease.

Surgical intervention may be required in some cases. Possible surgical interventions include a vagotomy, pyloroplasty, antrectomy, subtotal gastrectomy, and total gastrectomy. A vagotomy is the partial or complete severance of the vagus nerve to reduce the acid-secreting stimulus to gastric cells. A pyloroplasty is a widening of the exit of the stomach to prevent stasis of stomach contents. This procedure is usually performed in connection with a vagotomy. An antrectomy is the removal of the antrum of the stomach. This portion of the stomach contains the cells that secrete gastrin. A subtotal gastrectomy (i.e., partial removal of the stomach) may be performed using a Billroth I or a Billroth II technique. A Billroth I procedure removes the distal portion of the stomach, including the antrum, with anastomosis to the duodenum. The Billroth II procedure removes the distal portion of the stomach, including the antrum and the duodenum, with anastomosis to the jejunum.

Nursing Responsibilities

For the patient with PUD, the nurse should do the following:

- Educate the patient and family regarding the disease and the treatment regimen (rest and stress reduction, diet modification to avoid oversecretion and hypermotility of the GI tract).
- Promote comfort, adequate hydration, and nutrition.
- Monitor drug therapy for effectiveness and adverse effects.
- Assess for signs and symptoms of complications, such as perforation (assess abdomen for pain, tenderness, and rigidity, and monitor vital signs), hemorrhage (assess vital signs, symptoms of shock, emesis of coffee-ground material), upper GI bleeding or blood in the stool, and obstruction (monitor for nocturnal pain, and assess type and amount of emesis).
- Assess for postoperative complications, such as the following:
  1. *Dumping syndrome.* May occur after a gastrectomy when food rapidly enters the jejunum. Symptoms include distention, feelings of fullness, cramping, nausea, and rumbling and gurgling in the bowel **(borborygmi).** To slow gastric emptying, the nurse should advise an increased fat and protein diet with avoidance of sugars. Patients should drink liquids between meals and rest after meals.
  2. *Anemia.* Loss of absorbing surface in the intestine predisposes the patient to anemia. Assess lab data for signs of anemia. Administer vitamin B_{12} and iron as appropriate.
- Promote postoperative wound healing.

Do You UNDERSTAND?

DIRECTIONS: Provide answers for the following questions.

1. What three factors predispose an individual to the development of gastric ulcers? _____

   _____

2. What factor has been identified as the most significant in the development of gastric ulcers? _____

   _____

3. What clinical manifestations are observed in the patient with a gastric ulcer? _____

   _____

4. What is the difference between the Billroth I and the Billroth II surgical procedures for the treatment of gastric ulcer disease?

   _____

   _____

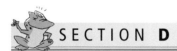

SECTION **D**

DISEASES OF THE PANCREAS

What IS Pancreatitis?

Pathogenesis

Pancreatitis is an acute or chronic inflammation of the pancreas that results in a release of pancreatic enzymes. This process leads to autodigestion of the pancreas by its own enzymes. Although the process is unclear, the causative factors activate enzymes in the pancreas rather than in the intestine, leading to autodigestion of the pancreas and surrounding tissues.

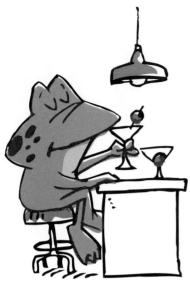

Drinking can cause acute pancreatitis.

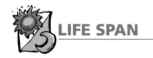

LIFE SPAN

Middle-aged men have the highest incidence of pancreatitis.

Of those patients with acute pancreatitis, 10% develop life-threatening complications.

The enzyme activity can be triggered by reflux of bile from the common bile duct into the pancreatic duct or by pancreatic duct obstruction. After pancreatic inflammation begins, a vicious cycle continues the process of further tissue damage and enzyme activation. As the process continues, destruction of the pancreas itself occurs. Severity of the disease varies from edema and pain to hemorrhage and necrosis of the pancreas.

At-Risk Populations

Long-term alcohol use is a common cause of acute pancreatitis. Of patients with acute pancreatitis, 90% have biliary disease or excessive alcohol intake. Other known causes of pancreatitis are pancreatic trauma, infection, drug reactions, and GI surgery on or near the pancreas. In addition, patients who are obese, those who have had pancreatic trauma or surgery, and those who have any condition that blocks the pancreatic ducts have an increased risk of developing pancreatitis. Other individuals at risk for pancreatitis include those who have hyperlipidemia, hypercalcemia, or pancreatic ischemia. Pancreatic ischemia occurs during periods of hypotension, cardiopulmonary bypass, and vasculitis. Visceral atheroembolism also raises the risk for pancreatitis.

What You NEED TO KNOW

Clinical Manifestations

The primary symptom of pancreatitis is pain. The pain is sudden in onset, constant, and severe, located in the midepigastrium and periumbilical region. The pain can also radiate to the back and is accompanied by nausea and vomiting, abdominal distension, and decreased bowel sounds. Pain is frequently more intense when the patient is supine. Relief from pain is obtained when the patient sits with trunk flexed and knees drawn up. Jaundice may become apparent.

When the pancreatitis is related to gallstones, the stools can be pale, frothy, and foul-smelling with high fat content (**steatorrhea**) as a consequence of impaired fat digestion. In patients with alcohol-related pancreatitis, the pain frequently begins 12 to 48 hours after an episode of drinking.

A low-grade fever, hypotension, tachycardia, and decreased breath sounds with crackles can also be present. The decreased breath sounds and crackles are related to irritation of the pleura from pancreatic enzyme action. Laboratory values are altered, with elevations in serum and urinary amylase, serum lipase, leukocytosis, hyperglycemia, hyperlipidemia, and hypocalcemia.

Other clinical manifestations include subcutaneous fat necrosis and alterations in consciousness, such as belligerence, confusion, psychosis, and coma. Transient hypoglycemia is evident in 50% of patients, most likely because of damage to the islets of Langerhans. Because all endocrine functions of the pancreas are disrupted, the patient can develop diabetes secondary to tissue damage.

Prognosis

Acute pancreatitis usually resolves when the cause has been eliminated. Patients with severe pancreatitis can experience circulatory complications such as hypotension, pallor, cool and clammy skin, hypovolemia, hypoperfusion, and obtundation. One third of the patients develop a left pleural effusion or an elevation of the left side of the diaphragm.

What You DO

Treatment

The primary goal for the patient with pancreatitis is rest for the GI tract. The rest decreases secretion of pancreatic enzymes. Withholding food and fluids, inserting a nasogastric tube, and giving pain drugs accomplish this goal. Oral intake is resumed after abdominal pain and tenderness have subsided.

IV fluids help maintain or improve fluid and electrolyte balance. Patients with moderate to severe pancreatitis will need total parenteral nutrition (TPN) and lipids to support nutritional status. IV therapy can also be used to administer pain drugs. Pancreatic enzymes, such as pancrelipase, are used for patients who have pancreatitis or for those who have had pancreatic surgery. Proton pump inhibitors, H_2 antagonists, anticholinergics, and antacids may be used. Antibiotics may be used prophylactically, particularly in patients with more severe pancreatitis.

Peritoneal lavage through a percutaneous dialysis catheter may be required to rid the peritoneum of the potentially toxic compounds commonly found in the exudate (e.g., histamine, vasoactive kinins, elastase, prostaglandins, phospholipase A, trypsin, and chymotrypsin). These toxins contribute to the hypotension, respiratory failure, hepatic

⚠ Premature return to oral intake has been associated with the development of pancreatic abscess and worsening inflammation. Morphine is contraindicated because it can cause spasm of the sphincter of Oddi, which can then cause ongoing pancreatic injury.

TAKE HOME POINTS

Advise the patient to eliminate alcohol, reduce dietary intake of fats, and avoid ingestion of drugs known to cause pancreatitis.

TAKE HOME POINTS

P— Pain control with meperidine (morphine causes contraction of the sphincter of Oddi)

A— Antacids to neutralize acidity

N— NPO and use of NG to rest GI tract and decrease pancreatic activity

C— Calcium replacement; check for tetany with possible hypocalcemia

R— Rest and replacement fluids

E— Electrolyte replacement

A— Antibiotics for acute pancreatitis

S— Surgery, usually Roux-en-Y procedure

failure, and altered vascular permeability that are present in pancreatitis. Peritoneal lavage is usually reserved for patients who show a worsening state, despite other interventions.

In severe cases of pancreatitis, surgery may be necessary to drain the pancreatic duct and remove injured and necrotic tissue. A Roux–en–Y procedure connects the pancreatic duct to the proximal jejunum. A subtotal pancreatectomy (removal of a portion of the pancreas) or a Whipple procedure (removal of the distal third of the stomach, duodenum, common bile duct, gallbladder, and the head of the pancreas) may be required in advanced disease states.

Nursing Responsibilities

For the patient with acute pancreatitis, the nurse should do the following:

- Maintain NG tube patency, and assess vital signs, while monitoring for evidence of hemorrhage, shock, and infection.
- Administer IV fluids to prevent fluid and electrolyte imbalance, monitor vital signs, weight, and lab values such as glucose, calcium, chloride, sodium, and potassium.
- Administer pancreatic enzyme drugs as ordered.
- Assess the patient's respiratory status.
- Educate the patient and family regarding restriction of alcohol intake, dietary restrictions, preventive measures, and follow-up care.

Do You UNDERSTAND?

DIRECTIONS: Fill in the blanks to complete the following statements.

1. Inflammation of the pancreas results in the release of _____ _____ that lead to _____ of the pancreas itself.
2. _____ have the highest incidence of pancreatitis.
3. The primary clinical manifestation of pancreatitis is _____.
4. When the pancreatitis is related to gallstones, the stools can be pale, bulky, and foul-smelling as a consequence of impaired fat digestion. This type of stool is referred to as _____.
5. The primary goal of treatment for the patient with pancreatitis is to decrease _____, thus resting the GI tract.

Answers: **1.** enzymes, autodigestion; **2.** middle-aged men; **3.** pain; **4.** steatorrhea; **5.** pancreatic enzyme function.

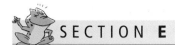

SECTION **E**

DISEASES OF THE INTESTINES

Inflammatory bowel disease (IBD) includes two chronic disorders: Crohn's disease and ulcerative colitis. Both disorders are characterized by periods when symptoms are worse (**exacerbations**) and periods when the diseases are less problematic (**remissions**). The recurrent diseases affect predominantly younger people. Treatment is symptomatic, and responses are frequently unpredictable.

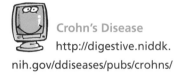

LIFE SPAN

The risk for Crohn's disease is highest among adolescent and young adult women ages 15 to 25.

What IS Crohn's Disease?

Pathogenesis

Crohn's disease is a recurring inflammation of the small intestine, usually occurring in the terminal ileum. Rectal involvement is common (in up to 95% of cases). Chronic, extensive inflammation results in ulcerations involving the entire thickness of the intestinal wall. As the disease progresses, the bowel mucosa thickens and shortens, decreasing the surface area available for absorption of water and nutrients.

Although the cause is unknown, Crohn's disease is believed to have a familial tendency, related in some way to an abnormal immune response to an unidentified etiologic agent. Extensive research continues the attempt to identify the cause of the disease. Possible causes include infection, autoimmune reaction, food allergies, and hereditary factors.

At-Risk Populations

Crohn's disease is more prevalent in urban, upper middle-class, and higher educated populations. The highest incidence of ulcerative colitis is among females ages 10 to 40. Stressful events frequently precipitate exacerbations.

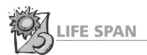

Crohn's Disease
http://digestive.niddk.nih.gov/ddiseases/pubs/crohns/

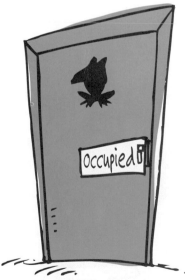

Bathroom trips are common for Crohn's patients.

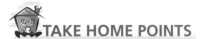

TAKE HOME POINTS

Absorption of fat-soluble vitamins is decreased in patients with Crohn's disease. Vitamin K deficiency predisposes the patient to bleeding disorders.

What You NEED TO KNOW

Clinical Manifestations

The signs and symptoms of Crohn's disease include nonbloody diarrhea up to 20 times a day. Steatorrhea is common, with the stools being pale, bulky, greasy, and foul-smelling. The stools are also the color and consistency of oatmeal. Rectal bleeding is not typically present in Crohn's disease. A cramping (colicky) abdominal pain is common. Systemic symptoms such as fever, malaise, anorexia, dehydration, fatigue, and weight loss are also noted. Weight loss and malnutrition are common. Coping behaviors are often inappropriate or ineffective.

Prognosis

The segmental nature of Crohn's disease results in reoccurrence in the majority of patients in a different area of the intestine.

What IS Ulcerative Colitis?

Pathogenesis

Ulcerative colitis is an inflammatory bowel disease that causes inflammation and ulceration of the mucosa and submucosa of the entire length of the colon. The cause of ulcerative colitis is unknown. Extensive research continues the attempt to identify the cause. Infection, autoimmune reactions, food allergies, and hereditary factors have been identified as possible causes of the disorder.

Beginning in the rectum, ulcerative colitis moves up the colon in a continuous pattern. Inflammation causes edema and an increase of blood flow (hyperemia) of the bowel mucosa. Multiple abscesses develop, leaving ulcerations, which bleed and cause increased peristalsis and diarrhea. As the disease progresses, the bowel mucosa thickens and shortens, decreasing the surface area available for absorption of water and nutrients.

At-Risk Populations

Ulcerative colitis is more prevalent in urban, upper middle-class, and higher educated populations. Ulcerative colitis affects women more than men, and usually in their productive years (between 20 and 40 years of age). Stressful events frequently precipitate exacerbations.

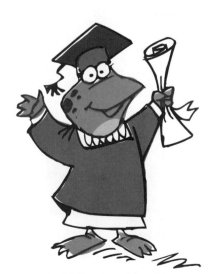

At risk for ulcerative colitis.

What You NEED TO KNOW

Clinical Manifestations

The signs and symptoms of ulcerative colitis include bloody diarrhea, occasionally up to 20 times a day. Abdominal pain can be cramplike in nature. Patients may develop systemic symptoms such as fever, malaise, and anorexia; they may also experience weight loss, anemia, and dehydration.

Prognosis

Ulcerative colitis progresses with periods of exacerbations and remissions. If the patient fails to respond to intense medical management the surgical removal of the colon (colectomy) may be necessary. Those who have had the disease more than 20 years have an increased incidence of cancer of the colon.

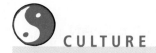

CULTURE

A genetic predisposition to inflammatory bowel disease may be present because ulcerative colitis and Crohn's disease are observed frequently in Caucasians and Jews.

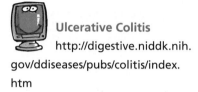

Ulcerative Colitis
http://digestive.niddk.nih.gov/ddiseases/pubs/colitis/index.htm

What You DO

Treatment of Inflammatory Bowel Diseases

The treatment for Crohn's disease and ulcerative colitis is symptomatic, with the goals of reducing inflammation, providing adequate nutrition, and preventing a secondary infection. Antibiotics such as sulfasalazine and mesalamine—a combination of sulfapyridine and 5-aminosalicyclic acid—are the mainstay of treatment because of their antimicrobial and antiinflammatory effects. Corticosteroids are also used for their antiinflammatory effect. Immunosuppressive drugs such as azathioprine or cyclosporine are used to reduce the immune response. Anticholinergics such as methantheline bromide and propantheline help slow gastric motility.

Providing the patient with a low-residue, high-protein diet with supplemental vitamins maintains nutritional balance. Providing the patient's GI tract with rest (NPO) and providing TPN may be necessary during acute exacerbations. TPN allows for total bowel rest and decreases gastric stimulation. Stress reduction techniques are helpful in assisting patients to deal with their reaction to conflicts (anxiety) and the distressing situation.

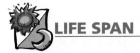

LIFE SPAN

Inflammatory bowel disease affects young people with many issues related to body image. Nurses advocate for both physical and psychosocial needs.

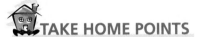

TAKE HOME POINTS

Inflammatory bowel disease affects a younger population in their productive years, focusing them on a disease process instead of building relationships with family and friends. An important aspect of nursing care is to educate the patient to help them maintain a more normal lifestyle.

Surgical intervention is used only to treat complications of Crohn's disease. The length of the small bowel is protected, when possible, to preserve the patient's ability to absorb nutrients.

When chronic ulcerative colitis fails to respond to drug therapy, four surgical procedures are used to treat this disease. A J-pouch (ileal pouch–anal anastomosis) prevents the need for an ostomy and preserves the rectal sphincter muscle. The colon is removed and the ileum attached to a reservoir created in the anal canal. This surgical procedure is frequently preferred for patients with ulcerative colitis.

The entire colon and rectum may be removed and the anus closed. The terminal ileum is brought out through the abdominal wall, and a permanent ileostomy is formed (total proctocolectomy with ileostomy). This procedure is the most extreme measure. An ileorectal anastomosis attaches the ileum to the rectum, and the remainder of the colon is removed, representing an early alternative to total proctocolectomy.

A procedure known as a continent ileostomy **(Koch's pouch)** creates a reservoir constructed from a loop of the ileum. Stool is stored in the ileum until it is drained through a nipple valve. This procedure is rarely performed as a first choice.

Nursing Responsibilities

For patients with ulcerative colitis or Crohn's disease, the nurse should do the following:

- Provide health teaching regarding medication therapy, diet, and stress-management strategies.
- Provide information about community resource groups available to support the patient and to help the patient cope with changes in body image and self-esteem.
- Monitor the effectiveness and adverse effects of drug therapy.
- Monitor intake, output, and daily weights.
- Assess the number, consistency and type of stools. Educate the patient about meeting his or her nutritional needs. Small, frequent meals that are low in residue and high in protein, carbohydrates, and calories are recommended after surgery, along with supplemental fat-soluble vitamins and vitamin B_{12}.
- Administer antidiarrheal drugs as needed.
- Encourage the patient to verbalize fears regarding changes in sexuality. The patient with an ileostomy has no physiologic reasons for sexual dysfunction; however, psychologic changes can occur.

In addition, for the patient with ulcerative colitis, the nurse should do the following:

- Educate the patient about the implications of a proposed surgical procedure.
- Involve an enterostomal therapist, and recommend a preoperative visit from a member of the ostomy association early in the treatment.
- Provide postoperative care and pain management as necessary.
- Educate the patient on how to manipulate ostomy equipment or supplies that will be needed postoperatively and how to monitor skin for breakdown.

Do You UNDERSTAND?

DIRECTIONS: **Indicate which statements are** *true* **(T) and which are** *false* **(F). If false, correct the statement in the margin space to make it true.**

_____ 1. Crohn's disease is a chronic, inflammatory disease that affects the terminal ileum.

_____ 2. Blood in the feces is a common finding in patients with Crohn's disease.

_____ 3. An expected outcome of Crohn's disease is increased absorption of the fat-soluble vitamins.

_____ 4. Rectal involvement is rare in Crohn's disease.

_____ 5. Steatorrhea is absent in Crohn's disease.

_____ 6. The lesions of Crohn's disease typically develop in several discontinuous segments of the bowel.

_____ 7. Anticholinergic drugs are given to the patient with Crohn's disease to relieve abdominal cramping and help control diarrhea.

_____ 8. Sulfasalazine is the most commonly prescribed drug used in the treatment of Crohn's disease.

_____ 9. Vitamin D deficiency predisposes the patient with Crohn's disease to bleeding disorders.

_____ 10. TNP provides total bowel rest and decreases gastric stimulation for the patient with Crohn's disease.

Answers: 1. T; 2. T; 3. F—an expected outcome of Crohn's disease is decreased absorption of the fat-soluble vitamins; 4. F—rectal involvement is common in Crohn's disease; up to 95% of patients have rectal involvement; 5. F—steatorrhea is seen with Crohn's disease; 6. T; 7. T; 8. T; 9. F—vitamin K deficiency predisposes the patient with Crohn's disease to increased bleeding; 10. T.

What IS Diverticular Disease?

Pathogenesis

Diverticuli are saclike outpouchings of mucosa through the muscle layers of the colon wall. Diverticuli develop most often in the sigmoid colon but can occur anywhere in the GI tract. Diverticulosis occurs when the large intestine, usually the descending and sigmoid portions, tries to move highly compacted fecal material. To accomplish this task, the longitudinal and circular muscles of those areas enlarge. The resulting increase in force on the nonmuscular tissues of the large intestine is similar to squeezing clay between the fingers as you clamp down on the soft clay. The clay between the fingers represents the diverticula, the outpouchings of soft tissue between the muscle fibers. Hypertrophy and contraction of the colonic muscles increase the pressure and can add to the degree of herniation.

Diverticulitis develops when small amounts of undigested foods (e.g., nuts, seeds, popcorn) or stool (**fecaliths**) become trapped. The area becomes irritated, and infection and inflammation result. The inflamed area may bleed as it becomes congested with blood. Diverticulitis can lead to perforation of the colon when the trapped mass in the diverticulum erodes through the colon wall. Chronic diverticulitis can result in scarring and narrowing of the lumen of the colon, potentially leading to colon obstruction. Extension of the inflammation to adjacent organs can lead to fistulas of the bladder or vagina.

At-Risk Populations

Diverticular disease is common in men and women over age 45 and in obese individuals. This disorder is present in approximately one third of the population over the age of 60 who do not have adequate fiber or roughage (cellulose) in their diets. The incidence appears to be increasing, particularly for persons who live in developing countries in which much of the diet consists of refined foods and little residue. Many older adults have lost their teeth or simply prefer a soft diet. As a result, these people do not ingest adequate cellulose to prevent diverticular disease.

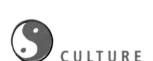

CULTURE

Diverticular disease is common in the United States, the United Kingdom, Australia, and France.

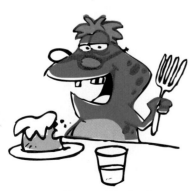

Avoid low-residue foods.

What You NEED TO KNOW

Clinical Manifestations

The signs and symptoms of diverticular disease can be vague or even absent in some patients. Anorexia, a change in bowel habits (constipation, diarrhea, or both), distention, cramping pain of the left lower abdomen, or the development of gas (**flatulence**) may be noted. When diverticula become inflamed or abscesses form, the patient develops fever, increased white blood cell count (**leukocytosis**), and tenderness of the left lower quadrant. Arterial bleeding (bright red blood) from the rectum is a serious sign of diverticular disease.

Prognosis

Habitual consumption of low-residue diet reduces fecal bulk, thus reducing the diameter of the colon. Pressure within the narrow lumen of the colon can thus increase sufficiently to rupture the diverticula. However, severe complications, such as hemorrhage, peritonitis, bowel obstruction, and fistula formation, are rare.

What You DO

Treatment

Diverticular disease is frequently discovered during diagnostic tests for other problems. Direct observation of the lesions is possible through examination of the rectal colon (**sigmoidoscopy** or **colonoscopy**). A barium enema may reveal muscle hypertrophy, but the barium can become trapped in the outpouchings and form hard masses.

Asymptomatic diverticular disease requires no specific treatment other than dietary modification. Mild disease is treated with a high-fiber diet and the use of bran and bulk laxatives.

Diverticulitis is treated conservatively by allowing the colon to rest. Food and fluids are withheld (NPO), antibiotics given to minimize the risk of infection, and pain drugs are used if needed. In more severe cases the patient is hospitalized, an NG tube is inserted, and IV fluids administered until pain, inflammation, and fever subside. When the acute episode has quieted, the patient can take in oral fluids and slowly advance the diet as tolerated.

A colon resection may be needed if the patient develops complications such as hemorrhage, obstruction, abscesses, or perforation. With abscess or obstruction, a colon resection with temporary colostomy may be performed until the patient's condition improves. A colostomy permits evacuation of the colon by creating an artificial opening (**stoma**) in the large intestine and bringing it to the surface of the abdomen (colostomy). For some patients, the temporary colostomy allows the colon to rest and heal.

Nursing Responsibilities

For the patient with diverticular disease, nursing responsibilities are aimed at controlling inflammation. The nurse should do the following:

- Educate the patient about the importance of consuming a high-fiber diet, bulk laxatives, and at least eight glasses of water every day to help prevent constipation.
- Encourage the obese patient to lose weight.
- Teach the patient to notify the health care provider of any changes in bowel pattern (constipation or diarrhea) or character of stools (presence of blood or mucus), or when fever, abdominal pain, or urinary symptoms develop.
- Educate the patient with acute diverticulitis to rest the colon by remaining NPO until the pain, fever, and inflammation subside.
- Administer IV fluids and antibiotics as prescribed.
- Insert and maintain the patency of an NG tube to rest the bowel.
- Provide postoperative care as needed for the patient who has had a colon resection with colostomy.
- Teach patients with chronic diverticulitis about the importance of avoiding indigestible fiber foods such as nuts, corn, popcorn, tomatoes, cucumbers, or strawberries, to help prevent further inflammation.

Do You UNDERSTAND?

DIRECTIONS: Provide answers for the following questions.

1. Diverticuli are defined as what? _____

   _____

2. When does diverticulitis develop? _____

3. At what age is diverticular disease found most frequently in patients? It is also becoming more common in what other age group?

   _____

4. What is the most common treatment for mild diverticular disease?

   _____

5. When surgery is required for the patient with diverticulitis, what is the procedure most commonly performed? _____

   _____

What IS Gluten-Sensitive Enteropathy?

Pathogenesis

Patients with gluten-sensitive enteropathy (**celiac sprue**) have intolerance to gluten—a protein found in wheat, barley, rye, malt, and possibly oats—which may trigger an autoimmune response in genetically predisposed individuals. The autoimmune responses damage the villi of the small intestines, resulting in flattening of the villi with a loss of surface area and decreased absorption. The damaged surface cells have a decreased ability to stimulate pancreatic secretions, which leads to further impaired digestion and absorption of nutrients.

Destruction of mucosal cells causes inflammation and the secretion of water and electrolytes, which leads to watery diarrhea. The loss of potassium leads to muscle weakness. Malabsorption of calcium and magnesium can cause seizures or tetany. Unabsorbed fatty acids combine with calcium, and the secondary hyperparathyroidism increases phosphorus

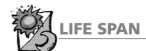

LIFE SPAN

Gluten-sensitive enteropathy affects primarily infants and children. As early as 3 to 4 months of age, growth failure, anorexia, and constipation can begin. In older children, constipation is observed occasionally despite steatorrhea. Vomiting and cramplike abdominal pain are prominent in infants but are unusual in older children. In older children, delayed puberty and infertility can develop.

excretion, resulting in bone mineral resorption. Fat malabsorption in the jejunum leads to steatorrhea.

At-Risk Populations

Of persons diagnosed with this disease, 70% are female. A strong genetic influence has been identified.

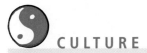

CULTURE

Gluten-sensitive enteropathy occurs largely in Caucasians but has been documented in persons from India and Pakistan. In native African, Japanese, and Chinese populations, gluten-sensitive enteropathy is nearly nonexistent. The incidence has been estimated to be 1 in 1000 in Europe, South America, and North Africa; however, it is diagnosed infrequently in the United States.

What You NEED TO KNOW

Clinical Manifestations

The signs and symptoms of this disorder include steatorrhea; three to five such movements occur daily. Malnutrition, anemia, weight loss, abdominal distention, and a symmetric skin rash (**dermatitis herpetiformis**) are also present. Low serum magnesium and calcium levels cause irritability, tremor, seizures, tetany, bone pain, osteomalacia, and dental deformities. Rickets and clubbing of the fingers are likely when vitamin D deficiency is prolonged.

Prognosis

The prognosis for the patient with gluten-sensitive enteropathy is good, as long as a gluten-free diet is maintained. Dietary management can prevent acute episodes of the disease. The incidence of non-Hodgkin's lymphoma is greatly increased in patients who fail to respond to gluten-free diets.

What You DO

Treatment

The treatment for gluten-sensitive enteropathy includes life-long, permanent attention to a gluten-free diet. A gluten-free diet means avoiding cereal grains such as wheat, rye, barley, oats, and malt. Milk-sugar (**lactose**) intolerance is presumed, thus these products are also excluded from the diet.

Corticosteroids may be used in acute episodes along with antidiarrheal and anticholinergic drugs. Infants are routinely given vitamin D, iron, and folic acid supplements to treat deficiencies.

Nursing Responsibilities

For the patient with gluten-sensitive enteropathy, the nusrse should do the following:

- Assess nutritional adequacy while the patient adheres to a gluten-free diet.
- Monitor daily weights, and periodically evaluate growth status.
- Monitor laboratory values, and assess for anemia and vitamin deficiency.
- Assess the frequency and consistency of stools while maintaining fluid and electrolyte balance.
- Provide health teaching for the patient or caregiver regarding the disease process, gluten-free diet, and medications.

Do You UNDERSTAND?

DIRECTIONS: **For each of the following diagnoses for gluten-sensitive enteropathy, identify the appropriate outcome statement and interventions.**

1. Alteration in nutrition (less than body requirements) related to an inability to tolerate gluten.
   a. Evaluation and outcome statement: _____
   _____

   b. Interventions: _____
   _____

2. Diarrhea related to intestinal response to gluten in the diet.
   a. Evaluation and outcome statement: _____
   _____

   b. Interventions: _____
   _____

3. Fluid volume deficit related to losses via excessive diarrhea.
   a. Evaluation and outcome statement: _____
      _____
   b. Interventions: _____
      _____

4. Knowledge deficit related to dietary restrictions.
   a. Evaluation and outcome statement: _____
      _____
   b. Interventions: _____
      _____

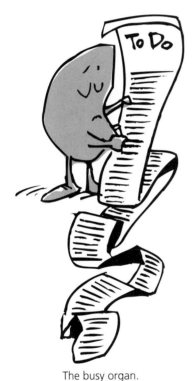

The busy organ.

SECTION F

DISEASES OF THE LIVER AND GALLBLADDER

The liver is responsible for over 1300 functions within the body. Included among these functions are the storing and filtering of blood, production of bile (bile is then stored in the gallbladder), conversion of glucose to glycogen, and the synthesis and breakdown of fats. The liver also temporarily stores fatty acids. As the chief supplier of glucose for the body, the liver is occasionally called on to convert glucose from protein and fats. This conversion may also work in reverse. The liver cells can convert excess sugar into fat and send it for storage in other parts of the body. The liver is also responsible for the synthesis of serum proteins, such as steroids, globulins, and albumin (which helps regulate blood volume), as well as fibrinogen and prothrombin (essential clotting factors). In addition to these functions, the liver stores many essential vitamins until they are needed by other parts of the body.

Answers: 1. a, the patient will experience no further weight loss; the patient will meet metabolic needs through adequate nutritional intake; b, maintain gluten-free diet high in calories, protein and vitamins; monitor daily weights; intake, and output 2. a, the patient will experience a normal number and consistency of stools; b, monitor frequency and consistency of stools; maintain gluten-free diet; administer antidiarrheal medications as ordered and needed; maintain good skin care to perianal area; 3. a, the patient will obtain and maintain a normal fluid and electrolyte balance; b, monitor intake and output; assess for symptoms of dehydration; monitor laboratory values for electrolyte imbalance; 4. a, the patient will develop a working understanding of the disease and treatment; b, provide health education to patient and family concerning the nature of the disease; establish dietary restrictions and allowances; monitor for complications and effects of noncompliance with diet; maintain medications and other treatments.

The liver protects the body by disposing of depleted blood cells and filtering and destroying bacteria. One of the most important protective functions of the liver is the detoxification of medications, alcohol, and environmental poisons by the endoplasmic reticulum. Kupffer cells are an important part of the mononuclear phagocyte system (known previously as the reticuloendothelial system). The liver also helps maintain the balance of sex hormones in the body. Finally, the liver monitors the proteins that pass through the digestive system. The body cannot use some of the amino acids that pass through the digestive tract. The liver rejects and neutralizes these acids and sends them to the kidneys for disposal. When the liver is affected by disease, any or all of these functions are affected.

What IS Hepatitis?

Pathogenesis

Hepatitis is an inflammation of the liver. Five strains of viruses cause various types of hepatitis (A, B, C, D, and E). Hepatitis G and F viruses have recently been identified. The pathogenesis of viral hepatitis is similar regardless of the virus. Cellular injury is promoted by cell-mediated immune mechanisms (i.e., cytotoxic T cells and natural killer cells). Liver cells become inflamed and die as a result of the body's antigen/antibody response to the virus. The endoplasmic reticulum (responsible for the synthesis of protein and steroids and the detoxification of drugs and poisons) is the first to be affected. The degree of impairment depends on the amount of cellular damage and the subsequent inflammatory process. The inflammatory process can damage and obstruct bile draining pathways, leading to cholestasis and obstructive jaundice. Damage tends to be most severe with hepatitis B and hepatitis C viruses. These viral infections may manifest acutely and, without treatment, may become chronic.

At-Risk Populations

Viral hepatitis occurs worldwide. The incubation period ranges from 30 to 180 days, depending on the specific type of virus.

Characteristic	Hepatitis A	Hepatitis B	Hepatitis C	Hepatitis D	Hepatitis E
Age group	Children, young adults	Any group	Any group	Any group	Children, young adults
Incubation	30 days	60-180 days	35-60 days	30-180 days	15-60 days
Transmission	Fecal-oral, parenteral, sexual	Parenteral, sexual	Parenteral	Parenteral, ? fecal-oral, sexual	Fecal-oral
Onset	Acute with fever	Insidious	Insidious	Insidious	Acute
Carrier state	No	Yes	Yes	Yes	No
Severity	Mild	Severe, prolonged, or chronic	Mild to severe	Severe	Severe in pregnant women
Chronic hepatitis	No	Yes	Yes	Yes	No

What You NEED TO KNOW

Clinical Manifestations

The clinical manifestations of the various types of hepatitis are very similar. The greatest chance for developing hepatitis is during the incubation period (about 2 weeks after exposure) and ends with the appearance of jaundice. Reduced energy metabolism by the liver causes fatigue and malaise. A low-grade fever results from the release of pyrogens during the inflammatory process. Changes in the stomach or bowel produce anorexia, nausea, and vomiting. Stretching of the liver capsule produces the right upper quadrant pain, and a weight loss of 5 to 10 pounds is not unusual. Hepatitis infection is highly transmissible during this prodromal phase.

The acute phase of illness (icteric phase) starts 1 to 2 weeks after the prodromal phase. Impaired excretion of conjugated bilirubin and the build-up of urobilinogen in the blood cause jaundice (noted first in the sclera), clay-colored stools, increased serum bilirubin levels, and dark urine. The dark urine and clay-colored stools appear before the onset of jaundice (icterus) which can last 2 to 6 weeks or longer. The GI and respiratory symptoms subside, but fatigue and abdominal pain persist or become severe. Itchy skin (pruritus) results from the accumulation of bile salts in the skin. Bleeding tendencies increase as a consequence of the reduced prothrombin synthesis by injured liver cells. Reduced bile in the intestines leads to reduced vitamin K absorption. Liver function test (LFTs) results are elevated.

The recovery phase (posticteric phase) begins when the jaundice disappears, about 6 to 8 weeks after exposure. Although the liver may still be enlarged and tender, symptoms diminish. Liver function test results return to normal 2 to 12 weeks after the onset of jaundice.

Chronic hepatitis may begin after the recovery phase. Chronic active hepatitis is the persistence of signs and symptoms and liver inflammation after acute hepatitis B, hepatitis C, or hepatitis D. Liver function tests remain abnormal for 6 months or longer, and the hepatitis B surface antigen (HbsAg) persists. The mortality rate for hepatitis is less than 1%.

> Life-threatening **(fulminant)** hepatitis resembles acute liver failure. This disorder may occur as a complication of hepatitis B or hepatitis C. Toxic reactions to drugs and congenital metabolic disorders also can cause fulminant hepatitis.

What You DO

Treatment

There is no specific treatment for hepatitis, but care generally centers on rest, drug therapy, dietary management, relief of pruritus, and postexposure prophylaxis. Small, frequent meals high in calories and low in fats, as well as abstinence from alcohol, is recommended for all patients.

Few drugs are available for treating hepatitis. Interferon can be useful in the treatment of chronic hepatitis B and hepatitis C. Antiemetics may be given to control nausea and vomiting. Parenteral vitamin K is given to patients who have prolonged INR times. Antihistamines are used to control pruritus. Certain antilipemic drugs (bile acid resins) may be used to treat pruritus because they bind bile acids which are then excreted in the stool. Hepatotoxic drugs, such as acetaminophen, phenobarbital, phenytoin (Dilantin), chlorpromazine, morphine, paraldehyde, codeine, and alcohol, should be avoided.

Vaccines and postexposure prophylaxis is used for primary and secondary prevention of hepatitis. Hygienic measures should be used by all persons. Hepatitis A vaccine and immune globulin provides protection from hepatitis A. Hepatitis B vaccines promote immunity to hepatitis B and D. No vaccines are available for hepatitis C or E.

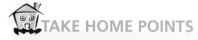

TAKE HOME POINTS

Health care workers must understand the importance of protecting themselves and others from this disease. Health care workers also need to understand the mode of transmission for the different types of viral hepatitis.

Nursing Responsibilities

For the patient with hepatitis, the nurse should do the following:

- Identify patients whose behaviors put them at risk for contracting viral hepatitis to determine the possible type and cause of disease.
- Educate the patient and family regarding the risk factors for transmitting the infection.
- Assess for jaundice (light-skinned patients), checking the sclera (dark-skinned patients), and checking the hard palate of the mouth and the inner canthus of the eye.
- Promote adequate nutritional intake and rest.
- Teach the patient to use tepid or emollient baths, to avoid alkaline soaps, and to apply lotion frequently to help with the pruritus. Encourage the patient to wear loose, soft clothing and to keep the room cool.
- Monitor the blood count, liver function (alanine aminotransferase [ALT], aspartate aminotransferase [AST], bilirubin, alkaline phosphatase), gamma globulin levels, and INR.
- Provide patient and family teaching regarding the risk for transmitting infection.
- Provide the patient and family education regarding jaundice being a temporary condition that will resolve as the patient's condition improves. Encourage the patient to discuss feelings about self-image.

Do You UNDERSTAND?

DIRECTIONS: **Unscramble the italicized words to complete the following statements.**

1. One cause of hepatitis is _____.
   (citxo stbusacsen)
2. The part of the liver that is responsible for protein and steroid synthesis is _____
   _____.*(mpedlnaicos cirultume)*
3. One way to contract hepatitis is coming in contact with _____
   _____
   _____.*(icnfetde yodb udifsl)*

What IS Cirrhosis?

Pathogenesis

Cirrhosis is an irreversible, progressive liver disease characterized by inflammation, cell death, scarring, and fibrosis. Cirrhosis is the final stage of many types of liver problems. Extensive destruction of liver cells occurs, which are then replaced by nodular scar tissue. The scarring alters the biliary and vascular flow within the liver, resulting in bile stasis and portal hypertension (the portal vein receives blood from the intestines and spleen). As a result of the pressure increase in the portal vein and altered protein synthesis by the liver, fluid accumulates in the peritoneum (ascites), varicose veins develop in the esophagus (esophageal varices), and protein metabolic wastes are not adequately cleared. This results in an increase in ammonia levels and deteriorating mental function (encephalopathy).

Four major types of cirrhosis have been identified: alcoholic cirrhosis, biliary cirrhosis, postnecrotic cirrhosis, and cardiac cirrhosis. Alcoholic cirrhosis (Laënnec's cirrhosis) is related to excessive alcohol intake, which results in an accumulation of fat in the liver. The fatty deposits are eventually replaced by scar tissue. Biliary cirrhosis is chronic, characterized by obstruction and infection of bile ducts that results in fibrosis scar formation. Postnecrotic cirrhosis is a complication of hepatitis, which results in replacement of necrotic tissue with scarred liver tissue. Cardiac cirrhosis is related to severe, right-sided heart failure, which ultimately causes liver scarring.

At-Risk Populations

Persons at primary risk for cirrhosis are those who abuse alcohol, particularly in the absence of proper nutrition. However, cirrhosis can also develop in patients with chronic obstructive biliary disease, long-standing heart failure, and chronic hepatitis.

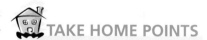

TAKE HOME POINTS

Countries with the highest incidence of cirrhosis also have the greatest per capita consumption of alcohol. However, do not be misled into believing that all patients who have cirrhosis are alcoholic. Many patients have the disease as a result of other GI problems.

What You NEED TO KNOW

Clinical Manifestations

The signs and symptoms of cirrhosis include abdominal pain, enlarged liver palpated as firm with a sharp edge, ascites, jaundice, dependent edema, bleeding tendencies, esophageal varices, hemorrhoids, anemia, and encephalopathy. An enlarged spleen (splenomegaly) indicates severe portal hypertension. Anemia, leukopenia, or thrombocytopenia can result from splenomegaly. Laboratory tests reveal elevated liver serum enzymes (AST, ALT, lactate dehydrogenase [LDH]), low serum albumin, anemia, and elevated prothrombin time. These abnormal lab results indicate impaired liver function.

Prognosis

The outcome of cirrhosis depends on the extent of liver damage and the degree to which the patient responds to treatment. Progression of the disease is characterized by liver failure, gram-negative bacterial infections, infection of the peritoneum (peritonitis), liver tumors, and death in a significant number of patients.

What You DO

Treatment

Liver damage is irreversible, although measures that halt the inflammation and destruction of liver cells prolong life. Treatment of cirrhosis includes abstaining from all alcohol, reducing dietary protein, restricting fluid, and preventing infection. Drug therapy with vitamins, particularly fat-soluble ones, B complex, and vitamin K, helps maintain an adequate nutritional state. Potassium-sparing diuretics are used to decrease ascites and edema. Neomycin and lactulose help decrease serum ammonia levels and reduce encephalopathy. Corticosteroids decrease inflammation. Vasopressin may be needed to control bleeding from esophageal varices. Proton pump inhibitors and H_2-receptor antagonists decrease gastric upset caused by ammonia buildup.

Some patients require the insertion of a portacaval shunt to reduce portal hypertension. A portacaval shunt involves the surgical anastomosis of the portal vein from the liver to the vena cava, which helps reduce the pressure in the portal circulation. Inserting a peritoneovenous shunt (LeVeen shunt) helps remove ascitic fluid from the peritoneal cavity. A peritoneovenous shunt consists of insertion of a peritoneal tube leading from the abdominal cavity to the superior vena cava or the jugular vein. For some patients, a liver transplant may be needed to sustain life.

Nursing Responsibilities

For the patient with cirrhosis, the nurse should do the following:

- Assist the patient to consume nutritional intake sufficient to meet metabolic needs—decreased protein and sodium and increased calories.
- Educate the patient to avoid drugs that are toxic to the liver while administering required drugs (e.g., diuretics, vitamins).
- Assess for skin integrity, and promote measures to maintain intact skin.
- Monitor daily weights, intake, and output.
- Assess for edema, ascites, and ineffective breathing patterns related to pressure on the diaphragm from ascites (by measuring abdominal girth and checking lower extremities).
- Assess for signs and symptoms of infection related to decreased white blood cell count.
- Assess for potential complications, such as encephalopathy (altered mental status, speech patterns, ammonia levels, and blood pH); bleeding (hemoglobin, hematocrit, and prothrombin times); nose-bleeds (epistaxis), bruising, blood in the urine (hematuria), and blood in the stool (melena).

Do You UNDERSTAND?

DIRECTIONS: **For the following symptoms of cirrhosis, explain why they occur in the patient and provide two nursing interventions appropriate when the patient experiences these symptoms.**

1. Ascites
   a. Occurs because: _____
   _____

   b. Appropriate nursing interventions: _____
   _____

2. Portal hypertension
   a. Occurs because: _____
   _____

   b. Appropriate nursing interventions: _____
   _____

3. Jaundice
   a. Occurs because: _____
   _____

   b. Appropriate nursing interventions: _____
   _____

What IS Cholecystitis?

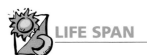

LIFE SPAN

Obese, Caucasian, multiparous women over the age of 40 are most at risk for cholecystitis.

Pathogenesis

Cholecystitis is an acute inflammation of the gallbladder and is associated most frequently with gallstones (cholelithiasis). In the absence of stones, bacteria that reach the gallbladder via the vascular or lymphatic system may be the cause of the inflammation. Inflammation of the gallbladder is

Answers: **1. a, pressure increase in the portal vein and altered protein synthesis by the liver fluid; b, semi-Fowler's to Fowler's position decreases pressure on diaphragm from ascites, daily abdominal girths; monitor daily intake and output and daily weights; administer diuretics as ordered to decrease edema; 2. a, destruction of hepatic tissue with resultant scarring leads to obstruction to blood flow and lymph; b, monitor vital signs frequently; maintain low-protein diet; monitor daily intake and output and daily weights; 3. a, inability of liver to clear normal amounts of bilirubin from the blood, which results in hyperbilirubinemia, leading to jaundice; b, assess for appearance and amount; assess urine and stool; provide skin care.**

accompanied by spasm within the biliary system, causing pain. When gallstones are present, distention of the gallbladder can occur, venous and lymphatic drainage becomes impaired, and proliferation of bacteria, localized irritation, and ischemia are present. This process can lead to pus (empyema) in the gallbladder. The inflamed gallbladder is edematous and thickened. Areas of gangrene or necrosis may also be present. Recurrent episodes of acute cholecystitis can cause fibrosis of the walls of the gallbladder.

Gallstones are of 2 types: cholesterol and pigmented. Pigmented gallstones are caused by cholesterol produced by the liver, calcium bilirubinate, or pigmented polymers. The formation of pigmented stones is related to biliary tract obstruction, bacterial breakdown, and the precipitation of biliary fats. This type of stone occurs later in life and is associated with cirrhosis. Cholesterol stones, by far the most common, form in bile that is supersaturated with cholesterol. Supersaturation sets the stage for cholesterol crystal formation and the development of stones. The more crystals that deposit, the larger the stone. Cholesterol stones are round and faceted and range in size from 0.5 to 3 cm. Gallstone formation can be such that the stones accumulate, filling the entire gallbladder.

At-Risk Populations

Cholecystitis is a prevalent disorder in developed countries. Obese, Caucasian, multiparous women over the age of 40 are most at risk for cholecystitis. Genetics appears to play a role in the development of gallstones for some patients and is evident in Pima and Chippewa Native Americans, Chinese, Jewish, and Italian populations, all of whom have an increased incidence of the disease. Patients with pancreatic or ileal disease are at risk for cholelithiasis.

TAKE HOME POINTS

A higher incidence of gallbladder disease is present in large women who have had multiple pregnancies. Symptoms related to intolerance of a fatty diet should alert the health care provider of the possibility of cholecystitis.

What You NEED TO KNOW

Clinical Manifestations

Assessment of the patient usually reveals a history of flatulence, bloating, dyspepsia, eructation, intolerance to fatty foods, and vague upper abdominal sensations. Nausea, pain in the upper right quadrant of the abdomen (biliary colic), fever, and leukocytosis are frequent. If gallstones are present and causing an obstruction, the patient may develop obstructive jaundice, dark amber urine, and clay-colored stools.

Prognosis

Approximately one third of complications are a result of perforation of the gallbladder. A gangrenous area becomes necrotic, and bile leaks into the peritoneal cavity. Peritonitis with systemic distribution of pepsin has a mortality rate of approximately 20%. Pericholecystic abscess accounts for 50% of the complications, although it is the least severe of the complications, having a mortality rate of approximately 15%. In some cases, a fistula develops when the gallbladder becomes attached to a portion of the gastrointestinal tract and perforates. The duodenum is the most common site for fistula formation, followed by the colon.

What You DO

Treatment

Removal of the gallbladder and obstructing gallstones is usually effective in reducing symptoms. Once the patient is symptomatic, intervening to prevent progression to more severe, occasionally fatal, complications of gallbladder disease is essential.

The treatment of cholecystitis includes promoting comfort and managing bacterial infection in severe cases. Meperidine is the drug of choice for pain control. Morphine and its derivatives are more likely to cause spasms in the biliary system and should be avoided.

A laparoscopic cholecystectomy is the preferred intervention for gallstones that cause obstruction or inflammation. This surgical procedure involves making four small incisions into the abdomen: one near the umbilicus to visualize the gallbladder, one for grasping the gallbladder, one for suction and irrigation, and the last one for the dissection instruments and applying clips. This procedure is performed under general anesthesia, and patients are usually discharged within 24 hours.

Extracorporal shock wave lithotripsy may be used when a handful of small stones are producing symptoms. This procedure requires general anesthesia. The patient is placed in a large tub of water and shock waves are directed to the stones. These waves are administered repeatedly until the stones are crushed. The patient is then able to pass the stones through the feces.

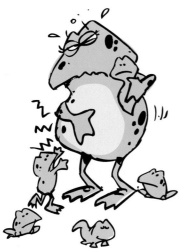

Removal of the gall bladder and the obstructing gallstones is usually effective in reducing symptoms.

Percutaneous cholecystolithotomy removes gallstones using endoscopy and stone baskets. General anesthesia is not required for this procedure.

Although less common, an open cholecystectomy removes the gallbladder through an upper right transverse incision on the abdomen. This procedure usually involves insertion of a T tube into the common duct to ensure adequate bile drainage after surgery. The procedure is performed under general anesthesia and usually requires up to a 6-week postoperative healing time.

Cholesterol-dissolving drugs such as chenodeoxycholic acid and ursodeoxycholic acid are especially useful in dissolving cholesterol gallstones.

Nursing Responsibilities

For the patient with cholecystitis, the nurse should do the following:

- Assess for pain, usually upper right quadrant pain that frequently radiates to the back. The pain may appear in "waves" (biliary colic), or it may be steady, consistent pain that is related to inflammation.
- Implement measures appropriate to treat nausea and vomiting. Distention of the bile ducts and fat intolerance trigger the vomiting center in the brain. Antiemetics, NPO status, and possible NG decompression may be used.
- Educate patients to modify their diet, such as limiting the amount of fat in the diet, which decreases the amount of bile released from the inflamed gallbladder and thus decreases symptoms.
- Assess for signs of infection; fever and leukocytosis are common in acute cholecystitis.
- Assess for jaundice, as a means of identifying biliary obstruction.
- Educate the patient and family regarding the disease and possible treatment options.
- Implement postoperative care, and monitor for postoperative complications.

Do You UNDERSTAND?

DIRECTIONS: **Fill in the blanks to complete the following statements.**

1. Postoperative symptoms to monitor that might indicate an infection are fever and _____.

2. _____ is the drug of choice for pain control in the patient with cholecystitis.

3. A surgical procedure that involves four small incisions into the abdomen for the treatment of cholecystitis is termed a _____ _____ cholecystectomy.

4. The pain frequently experienced by patients with acute cholecystitis is termed _____ colic.

5. The descriptive term for stones in the gallbladder is _____.

6. _____ is inflammation of the gallbladder.

7. A complication of a perforated gallbladder is _____, which is inflammation of the peritoneal cavity.

8. The population most at risk for developing cholecystitis is obese, _____ women over the age of 40.

9. Measures to treat nausea and vomiting during an acute attack of cholecystitis include antiemetics, _____ _____ decompression, and NPO status.

10. The pain of cholecystitis is usually found in the upper right _____ of the abdomen.

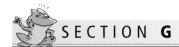

SECTION **G**

NUTRITIONAL DISORDERS

What IS Malnutrition?

Pathogenesis

Malnutrition is poor nourishment from improper intake or a defect in metabolism that prevents the body from using its food properly. Weight loss occurs when expended energy is greater than caloric intake and stored energy. Body proteins are used for energy, which causes a negative nitrogen balance. As malnutrition progresses to a state of starvation, fat cells become small, and accumulations of fat are depleted. The liver is reduced in size, the muscles shrivel **(atrophy),** and the lymphatic system, gonads, and blood deteriorate.

Vomiting and diarrhea cause nutrient loss from the GI tract. Infection, surgery, bowel obstruction, cancer, burns, draining wounds, and chronic illnesses also contribute to malnutrition. People with chronic obstructive pulmonary disease **(COPD)** can develop malnutrition when air hunger interferes with the ability to eat. The resulting malnutrition further complicates respiratory function and food consumption.

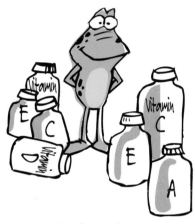

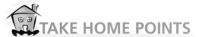

Get the nutrients.

At-Risk Populations

Although poverty remains the major cause of malnutrition, the condition is by no means confined to the underdeveloped areas of the world. Many risk factors for malnutrition exist.

Factors that increase the risk of malnutrition include inadequate nutrient intake resulting from poor availability of food, a knowledge deficit regarding the basic principles of nutrition, and substance abuse. Alcohol abuse frequently causes a person to rely on alcohol at the expense of food intake. Misplaced faith in vitamins as a substitute for food can cause malnourishment when carried to extremes. Overreliance on processed foods can occasionally result in a deficiency of valuable nutrients.

TAKE HOME POINTS

Persons at increased risk for malnutrition include infants and children, pregnant women, elderly adults, hospitalized patients, those who are cognitively impaired, substance abusers, minority populations, immigrants, and the homeless.

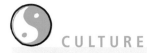

CULTURE

Patients with cultural differences who reside in long-term care facilities when the facility serves no ethnic food are also at risk for malnutrition.

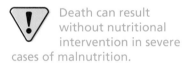

LIFE SPAN

High-fasting triglyceride and phospholipid concentrations are predictive of a poor prognosis for children with kwashiorkor.

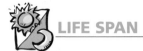

Death can result without nutritional intervention in severe cases of malnutrition.

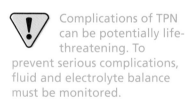

Complications of TPN can be potentially life-threatening. To prevent serious complications, fluid and electrolyte balance must be monitored.

What You NEED TO KNOW

Clinical Manifestations

The clinical manifestations of malnutrition are numerous. Each body system is affected by the lack of appropriate nutrients; however, in general the symptoms of malnutrition are physical weakness, lethargy, and an increasing sense of detachment from the world. In severe cases, the patient may appear starved (emaciated), have intolerance to cold, have an increased number of infections, and experience poor wound healing. Loss of muscle mass, reduced vital capacity as a result of respiratory muscle atrophy, diminished cardiac output, ankle edema, and dry flaking skin are common. Laboratory testing may reveal low hemoglobin, serum albumin, and transferrin levels. Serum triglyceride and phospholipid levels increase with increasing severity of malnutrition; however, other serum values, such as cholesterol, are normal or slightly reduced.

Prognosis

Malnutrition may be mild or severe to the extent that damage done to the body is irreversible.

What You DO

Treatment

High-calorie, high-protein foods are used most frequently to treat malnutrition. Oral feeding is the preferred method for nutritional intake. A fortified nutritional supplement (e.g., Ensure) may be added to the diet, and vitamin and mineral supplements may be given. When the patient is unable to eat, enteral feeding may be administered through a nasogastric, nasoduodenal, gastrostomy, or jejunostomy tube. TPN is a third option when the oral or enteral routes are inappropriate methods for feeding. TPN is a form of intravenous (IV) therapy that delivers all required nutrients to the patient.

Other treatment may be necessary, based on assessment findings. Some patients need financial help or assistance with eating. Lack of appetite, frequently related to depression or interaction of medications, may be identified and treated by the health care provider.

Nursing Responsibilities

For the patient who is malnourished, the nurse should do the following:

- Identify patients at risk for malnutrition.
- Obtain a dietary history with attention to protein and calorie intake, and availability and access to appropriate foods.
- Assess food preferences while ensuring a pleasant environment in which to eat.
- Administer oral, enteral, or parenteral nutrition, and vitamin and mineral supplements as ordered.
- Monitor electrolyte values and serum glucose and serum albumin levels.
- Record accurately intake and output.
- Obtain daily weight readings at the same time, on the same scale, and in the same type of clothing.
- Provide age-appropriate and culturally appropriate patient and family teaching regarding the disorder and required treatment.
- Arrange with social services for financial and transportation assistance, when appropriate.

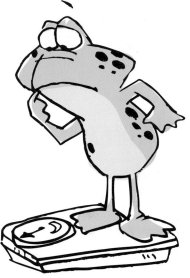

Same time, same place.

Do You UNDERSTAND?

DIRECTIONS: Fill in the blanks by unscrambling the italicized words.

1 A cause of increased loss of nutrients is _____.
   (heardria)

2. The _____ population is at increased risk of malnourishment. *(lydrele)*

3. _____ feeding is administered intravenously. *(rneaplarte)*

4. The nurse is responsible for obtaining _____ daily while the patient is receiving parenteral nutrition. *(htgiwe dasinreg)*

5. _____ is a condition of severe protein deficiency. *(oorwasikhkr)*

Answers: 1. diarrhea; 2. elderly; 3. parenteral; 4. weight readings; 5. kwashiorkor.

What IS Obesity?

Pathogenesis

Obesity is an imbalance between energy intake and expenditure that leads to an increase in weight beyond that considered desirable with regard to age, height, and bone structure. Obesity can be classified as occurring from the ingestion of excess calories (exogenous) or resulting from inherent metabolic problems (endogenous). Physiologically, obesity is classified according to the structure and distribution of fat (adipose) tissue.

Although numerous theories of obesity exist, the leading cause of obesity is consumption of excess calories. In addition, various neuroendocrine dysfunctions and some drugs, including corticosteroids, estrogens, and NSAIDs, are causes of obesity in some people.

Weight gained during certain periods in life leads to an increased number of fat cells. These periods are between 12 and 18 months, 12 and 16 years, and during pregnancy. Weight gain results from consuming foods, particularly calories and fat, in excess of body requirements. Furthermore, after a fat cell is formed, it is there to stay. When food intake equals metabolic needs, weight remains fairly constant throughout life.

At-Risk Populations

In the United States, 25% of adult women and 20% of adult men are obese.

Modifiable risk factors for obesity include a diet high in saturated fats, poor nutritional education, and minimal aerobic exercise. Nonmodifiable risk factors include heredity. When parents are overweight or obese as adults, particularly the biologic mother, a 75% chance exists that the children will be overweight or obese. Metabolism slows with advancing age, thus contributing to the risk of obesity. The metabolic rate decreases significantly after menopause, which places women at risk for being overweight or obese.

Numerous diseases and complications are associated with obesity, including depression, sleep apnea, pulmonary disease, stroke, gallbladder disease, liver disease, and degenerative arthritis. The altered metabolism of obesity can lead to atherosclerosis and related ischemic heart diseases. Hypertension and left-sided heart failure (left ventricular hypertrophy)

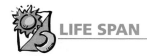

LIFE SPAN

Child-onset obesity is related to a greater-than-normal number of fat cells (hyperplastic obesity) and larger-than-normal fat cells (hypertrophic obesity). In children, the fat tissue is located over the entire body, and few metabolic abnormalities exist. In contrast, adult-onset obesity is hypertrophic. The fat tissues are centrally located, and metabolic abnormalities are more common. However, abnormalities of metabolism are believed to be the result, rather than the cause, of obesity.

LIFE SPAN

Non-Hispanic African American women, Mexican American women, and Native American men and women are at greater risk than is the general population for obesity.

occur because blood must be pumped through an enlarged vascular system. Diabetes mellitus is 4 times more common in the obese patient compared with the person with average weight. In addition, recent studies indicate a link between obesity and breast, endometrial, and ovarian cancer.

What You NEED TO KNOW

Clinical Manifestations

Height and weight tables, body mass indices (BMI), waist circumference, and a variety of other methods can be used to determine whether a person is overweight or obese. Generally, a person is considered as overweight when they weigh 10% more than optimal weight. Obese people are 15% above their optimal weight. Individuals who are 20% or more above their optimal weight are considered morbidly obese.

The BMI is used to predict problems associated with obesity. A BMI more than 30 is considered obese. The BMI is calculated as follows:

$$BMI = \text{Weight in kg} \div \text{height in meters}^2$$

Waist circumference is an indicator of obesity. Body fat that is distributed primarily in the abdominal area is of greater concern because of its association with other health problems **(morbidity).** Men with a waist circumference of 40 inches or more (102 cm) and women with a waist circumference of 35 inches or more (88 cm) are considered as obese.

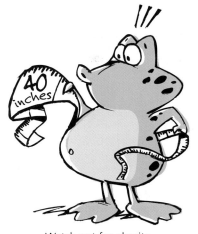

Watch out for obesity.

Prognosis

Obesity is considered as a serious disease and has been linked to a shortened life span.

 Obesity is the second leading cause of preventable death in the United States.

What You DO

Treatment

Treatment of obesity includes assisting the patient to establish a healthy meal plan. The dietary changes should be realistic for long-term success. A daily exercise routine should be incorporated with physical activity that is slowly increased and maintained. A support system for the obese patient is important to facilitate adherence to the meal and exercise plan.

Morbidly obese patients who do not respond to dietary management strategies to lose weight may require surgical procedures. Surgery is usually performed when patients are at high risk for complications associated with their obesity and/or once they have reached a weight 100 pounds over their ideal body weight. The procedures involve removal of adipose tissue, jaw wiring, stapling the stomach, or banding the esophagus. The jejunal bypass (intestinal bypass) has been abandoned because of complications, particularly hepatic failure. All of the surgical procedures have advantages and disadvantages but are designed to reduce the body's ability to ingest or absorb nutrients. The procedures do not always cause permanent weight reduction.

Nursing Responsibilities

For the obese patient, the nurse should do the following:

- Obtain a health and dietary history before implementing treatment.
- Evaluate the patient's body image. Recognize that obese patients frequently have low self-esteem and poor body image. Patients frequently view self-control of food intake as a way to improve self-esteem. The patient's family must help find other ways to improve the patient's body image that are unrelated to food.
- Provide information to the patient and family on community resources for support with weight loss, such as Weight Watchers, Take Off Pounds Sensibly (TOPS), or Overeaters Anonymous (OA). Many support groups offer nutrition and weight-loss programs.
- Encourage the patient and family to develop and use an exercise program that works for them and is maintained on at least a 3-times-per-week schedule.
- Manage the procedure-specific perioperative care of the patient who is undergoing a surgical procedure to treat obesity.

Do You UNDERSTAND?

DIRECTIONS: **Using the following illustrations, color in the box on the graph provided that most accurately depicts the definition of obesity for each of the measurements.**

1. Percentage over ideal body weight

5	10	15	20	25	30	35	40	45	50

2. BMI

5	10	15	20	25	30	35	40	45	50

3. Waist circumference in inches in men

5	10	15	20	25	30	35	40	45	50

4. Waist circumference in inches in women

5	10	15	20	25	30	35	40	45	50

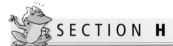

SECTION **H**

MALIGNANCIES OF THE GASTROINTESTINAL TRACT

Squamous (scaly or platelike) cell carcinomas involve the epidermis of the skin and linings of the mouth, the pharynx, the esophagus, the anus, and the vagina. Adenocarcinomas arise from glandular tissue or when the tumor cells form recognizable glandular structures.

Answers: 1. 15; 2. 30; 3. 40; 4. 35.

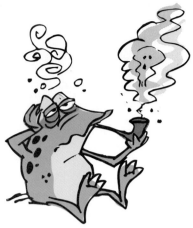

Cause & effect.

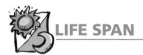

LIFE SPAN

In northern China, the rate of esophageal carcinoma is extremely high. The rate in men is twice that found in women and usually occurs after the fifth decade of life.

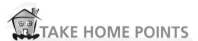

TAKE HOME POINTS

Esophageal cancer can be mistaken for GERD. Early identification and treatment is essential for a positive prognosis.

What IS Esophageal Carcinoma?

Pathogenesis

Squamous cell carcinoma is the most common form of esophageal cancer. Adenocarcinoma of the esophagus is far less common. The cause of cancer of the esophagus is unknown. Esophageal carcinoma usually begins as benign tissue changes associated with chronic esophagitis. Most squamous cell carcinomas are found in the middle third of the esophagus. Adenocarcinomas are usually found in the lower third of the esophagus. The malignancy may extend through the muscle layers of the lymphatics.

At-Risk Populations

GERD and chronic ingestion of hot food and beverages are risk factors. Alcohol abuse and nutritional deficiencies have also been implicated. Tobacco and opium smoking are known causative factors.

What You NEED TO KNOW

Clinical Manifestations

The first symptom of esophageal carcinoma is difficulty in swallowing (**dysphagia**), initially of solid food, or the sensation of burning or squeezing pain when swallowing (**odynophagia**). A sore throat, a feeling of choking, and hoarseness may also occur. Weight loss is common. As the disease progresses, dysphagia may develop to liquids also.

Prognosis

Unfortunately, by the time significant symptoms are apparent, esophageal cancer has usually invaded the deep layers of the esophagus and metastasized to adjacent tissues and lymph nodes. For this reason, the overall 5-year survival rate is 15%.

What You DO

Treatment

Treatment of esophageal carcinoma depends on the location of the tumor and the extent of growth and metastasis. Unfortunately, most tumors are discovered in the advanced stages, thus treatment is palliative and directed at relieving dysphagia and assisting the patient to obtain adequate nutrition. Radiation therapy is especially useful in treating tumors in the upper third of the esophagus. Radiation therapy is used to shrink the tumor, thus providing for a larger lumen in the esophagus. Radiation therapy may be used alone or in conjunction with surgical intervention. By dilating the esophagus with various dilators, or placing stents or prostheses that enlarge the lumen of the esophagus, the obstruction is lessened.

Surgical intervention may be needed for some patients. Laser therapy may be used to vaporize the tumor through endoscopy. An esophagectomy involves removal of all or part of the esophagus followed by insertion of a graft to replace the resected esophagus. An esophagogastrostomy removes all or part of the esophagus, with anastomosis to the stomach. An esophagoenterostomy removes all or part of the esophagus, with anastomosis to the intestine.

Nursing Responsibilities

For the patient with esophageal carcinoma, the nurse should do the following:

- Assess and promote nutritional status, including small frequent feedings of soft foods. Placing a feeding tube may be necessary. Keep the head of bed elevated at least 30 degrees.
- Monitor intake and output, and record daily weights.
- Promote effective respiratory function while assessing for potential aspiration.
- Promote effective coping through the use of stress-management techniques.
- Monitor the patient for postoperative complications.

Do You UNDERSTAND?

DIRECTIONS: **Study the following set of orders. Identify the order from the health care provider that you would question for the patient diagnosed with esophageal cancer. Provide the rationale for your answer.**

1. Nutritional status is a priority for clients with esophageal cancer. Your patient has lost 5 pounds this week.

_____ a. Order 1: Elevate the head of the bed no more than 15 degrees. Insert NG tube. Initiate tube feeding at 300 cc per hour.

_____ b. Order 2: Check swallowing reflex each shift. Provide soft, bland diet. Eat 6 small meals per day.

Rationale: _____

_____

_____

_____

What IS Gastric Carcinoma?

Pathogenesis

Gastric carcinoma is characterized by malignant neoplasm in the stomach. No single causative agent has been identified for gastric carcinoma. Adenocarcinomas comprise the majority (90%) of gastric carcinomas. The pyloric and antral areas of the stomach are most frequently involved. Metastasis occurs early, frequently to the pancreas.

At-Risk Populations

Gastric carcinoma is found twice as often in men as it is in women. Chronic gastritis, presence of *H. pylori,* environmental factors including a diet with large amount of added salt, food additives (nitrates) found in smoked fish and meat, and exposure to radiation and trace metals have been identified in the etiology of gastric cancer. Genetic predisposition appears evident for patients who have type A blood.

What You NEED TO KNOW

Clinical Manifestations

Early detection of gastric carcinoma is difficult because of its vague symptoms. There are no early physical signs of the disease, and generally the disease is not diagnosed until metastasis has occurred and symptoms become more pronounced. The symptoms in many cases are identical to PUD, with heartburn, a feeling of fullness, and mild discomfort. Anemia related to chronic blood loss is common, although bleeding into the stool is usually occult. Weight loss is also common.

Prognosis

The prognosis for gastric carcinoma depends on the stage of the disease at diagnosis. Most tumors are identified late in the course of the disease. The 5-year survival rate is approximately 15%.

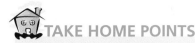**TAKE HOME POINTS**

Gastric cancer is diagnosed late in the course of the disease because the symptoms frequently mimic PUD.

What You DO

Treatment

The only effective treatment for gastric carcinoma is surgery. The invasiveness of the tumor determines the extent of surgery. When significant metastasis is present, the surgery may be palliative. A Billroth I or Billroth II procedure removes lesions in the atrium and pylorus. A total gastrectomy with esophagojejunostomy is used to treat lesions in the cardia or high in the fundus. Radiation and chemotherapy are adjunctive therapies, along with blood transfusions, to treat anemia. Gastric decompression is required.

Nursing Responsibilities

For the patient undergoing surgery for the removal of gastric carcinoma, the nurse should do the following:

- Assess and promote adequate nutritional status, including monitoring daily weights, intake, and output.
- Implement TPN or jejunostomy feedings while assessing for complications.

- Maintain the patient's comfort level, assessing level of pain and administering analgesics before they are needed and implementing adjunctive measures when possible.
- Monitor the patient's activity level, implementing a safe environment while providing for rest and activity.
- Educate the patient and family regarding the diagnosis, treatment, and home care.
- Provide support related to diagnosis and condition.

Do You UNDERSTAND?

DIRECTIONS: **Indicate which statements are *true* (T) and which are *false* (F). If false, correct the statement in the margin space to make it true.**

_____ 1. No single causative agent has been identified for gastric carcinoma.

_____ 2. Squamous cell carcinomas comprise the majority of gastric cancers.

_____ 3. A risk factor for gastric cancer of which most people may be unaware is consumption of smoked fish.

_____ 4. The symptoms of gastric cancer are frequently confused with gallbladder disease.

_____ 5. Anemia is a frequent finding in patients who have gastric cancer.

_____ 6. A Billroth I surgical procedure involves a subtotal gastrectomy.

_____ 7. The prognosis for gastric cancer is excellent because few tumors metastasize.

What IS Colorectal Carcinoma?

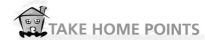

Pathogenesis

The term colorectal carcinoma refers to a malignant neoplasm found in the lower intestinal tract. The causes of colorectal cancer remain unclear, although several risk factors have been identified.

Adenocarcinomas are the most common type of colorectal cancers. These malignancies usually arise from colon polyps. The vast majority of tumors are found in the rectal and sigmoid areas of the colon. Metastasis is common because of the vascularity and the lymphatic system surrounding the intestines.

At-Risk Populations

Risk factors for colorectal cancer include advancing age, familial polyposis, colorectal polyps, chronic inflammatory bowel disease (i.e., Crohn's disease and ulcerative colitis), and a family history of colorectal cancer. A low-residue, high-fat diet has also been identified as a risk factor.

What You NEED TO KNOW

Clinical Manifestations

Symptoms are generally vague until the disease is advanced; they also differ depending on the location of the tumor. Bright red blood on the surface of the stool is the most common symptom of left-sided colorectal cancer. In addition, alternating constipation, diarrhea, and a change in stool (ribbonlike and narrow) are common. Symptoms of obstruction occur as the tumor grows. Right-sided lesions are usually asymptomatic. Nonspecific abdominal pain, anemia, and occult bleeding may be present. Arterial bleeding (bright red) from the rectum is most frequently a result of one of two causes: colorectal cancer or diverticular disease. In both cases, the sign is grim.

Prognosis

The prognosis of colorectal cancer depends on the degree of cancer involvement at the time of diagnosis. Unfortunately, most colorectal cancer remains unrecognized until it is in the advanced stages. The overall 5-year survival rate is 50%.

What You DO

Treatment

Surgery is the only curative treatment available for colorectal cancer. The type of surgery depends on the location and extent of cancer growth. The tumor and a section of colon on either side of the tumor are removed. This procedure is known as a colon resection. When the tumor is located within the intestine, a colostomy may be created during the surgical procedure. A colostomy is a connection between the bowel and an opening on the abdominal wall through which bowel contents can be eliminated. A colostomy can be either temporary or permanent, depending on the reason for the procedure.

A temporary colostomy allows the bowel to rest and repair when attachment of the proximal bowel to the remaining segment of distal bowel (**reanastomosis**) is anticipated. A permanent colostomy provides fecal diversion for the rest of the patient's life. An abdominal perineal resection is performed when invasive rectal tumors require removal of surrounding tissue and the development of a permanent colostomy. Radiation and chemotherapy are used as adjuncts to decrease tumor size and prevent further metastasis.

Nursing Responsibilities

For the patient with colorectal carcinoma, the nurse should do the following:

- Assess for and promote adequate nutritional status while monitoring intake, output, and daily weights.
- Monitor for postoperative complications, such as infection, deep vein thrombosis, hemorrhage, and altered wound healing.
- Educate the patient and family about the diagnosis and treatment regimen.
- Educate the patient and family regarding the care and maintenance of a colostomy.
- Offer support to the patient and family during diagnosis and treatment of disease.
- Educate the patient and family regarding the development and implementation of effective coping mechanisms.
- Provide support to the patient and family regarding changes in body image.

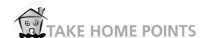

TAKE HOME POINTS

Patients with colorectal cancer require a great deal of support and education to deal with both the diagnosis and the treatment.

Do You UNDERSTAND?

DIRECTIONS: **Complete the following crossword puzzle.**

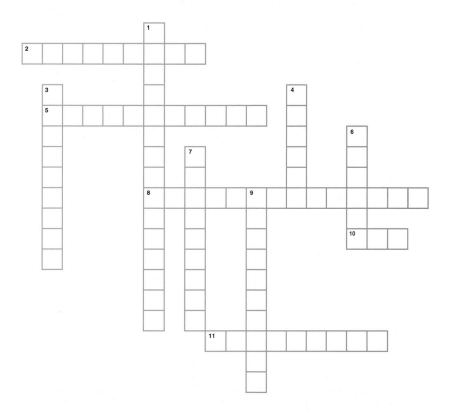

Down

1. _____ arise from glandular tissues or polyps in which the tumor cells form recognizable glandular structures.
3. Gastric carcinoma is characterized by _____ neoplasm in the stomach.
4. Adenocarcinomas usually arise from colon _____.
6. The vast majority of colorectal cancer tumors are found in the _____ and sigmoid areas of the colon.
7. A _____ is a connection between the bowel and an opening on the abdominal wall through which bowel contents can be excreted.
9. _____ colorectal cancer lesions are usually asymptomatic.

Across

2. Rectal bleeding is the most common symptom of _____ _____ colorectal cancer.

5. An esophagogastrostomy removes all or part of the esophagus, with _____ to the stomach.

8. The procedure during which a tumor and a section of colon on either side of the tumor are removed is known as a _____ _____.

10. _____-residue, high-fat diets have also been indicated as a risk factor for colon cancer.

11. One nursing intervention in colorectal cancer is to provide support to the patient and family regarding changes in _____.

References

Arcangelo V: *Pharmacotherapeutics for advanced practice: a practical approach,* Philadelphia, 2001, Lippincott.

Black J, Matassarin-Jacobs E: *Medical-surgical nursing: clinical management for positive outcomes,* ed 6, Philadelphia, 1997, WB Saunders.

Gutierrez K, Queener S: *Pharmacology for nursing practice,* Philadelphia, 2004, Mosby.

Huether S, McCance K: *Understanding pathophysiology,* St Louis, 1999, Mosby.

Lehne R: Pharmacology for nursing care, ed 5, Philadelphia, 2004, WB Saunders.

Lewis SM, Heitkemper MM, Dirksen SR: *Medical-surgical nursing: assessment and management of clinical problems,* ed 6, St Louis, 2004, Mosby.

Lilley L, Harrington S, Snyder J: *Pharmacology and the nursing process,* ed 4, St Louis, 2005, Mosby.

McCance K, Huether S: *Pathophysiology: the biologic basis for disease in adults and children,* ed 4, St Louis, 2002, Mosby.

Answers: *Down:* 1. adenocarcinomas; 3. malignant; 4. polyps; 6. rectal; 7. colostomy; 9. right-sided. *Across:* 2. left-sided; 5. anastomosis; 8. colon resection; 10. low; 11. body image.

NCLEX® Review

Section A

1. Older patients and young children are at particular risk for _____ when nauseated and vomiting develop.
   1 Nutritional deficits
   2 Aspiration
   3 Electrolyte imbalance
   4 Fever

2. Fecal incontinence caused by fecal impaction is a common problem in older adults: True or false?
   1 True
   2 False

3. Which of the following statements is incorrect in describing the causes of diarrhea?
   1 Decreased fluid reabsorption in the small or large intestine or alters bowel motility
   2 Increased fluid secretion (e.g., deranged electrolyte transport)
   3 Is associated with mucosal injury
   4 Increased fluid uptake from the gut

Section B

4. Risk factors for GERD do *not* include which of the following?
   1 Asthma
   2 Smoking
   3 Alcohol
   4 Genetics

5. The treatment for hiatal hernia does *not* include advising the patient to
   1 Avoid alcohol.
   2 Avoid restrictive clothing.
   3 Elevate the head of the bed.
   4 Eat three large meals each day.

Section C

6. Curling's ulcers are stress ulcers that occur in patients
   1 With burns.
   2 With preexisting ulcers.
   3 With severe head injuries.
   4 Who are bedridden.

7. Peptic ulcer disease caused by *H. pylori* is often treated with antibiotics and
   1 Proton pump inhibitors.
   2 H_2-receptor antagonists.
   3 Sucralfate.
   4 Anticholinergics.

Section D

8. The major clinical manifestation of acute pancreatitis is which of the following?
   1 Cardiovascular hypotension
   2 Disseminated intravascular coagulation
   3 Mild to severe abdominal pain
   4 Serum amylase of 100 units

9. The major therapy for acute pancreatitis is
   1 Control of alcohol intake.
   2 Meperidine for pain management.
   3 Peritoneal lavage.
   4 Placement of an NG tube and keeping the patient NPO.

10. For which condition should the patient with pancreatitis be monitored?
    1 Hypercalcemia
    2 Hyperkalemia
    3 Hypocalcemia
    4 Hypoglycemia

11. Following recovery from acute pancreatitis, the pancreas should do which of the following?
    1 Cease to produce insulin
    2 Appear normal, except for alcohol-induced pancreatitis
    3 Continue to be inflamed and become necrotic
    4 Atrophy when the inflammatory process is gone

Section E

12. Which of the following characteristics is common to both ulcerative colitis and Crohn's disease?
    1 Involves mucosal layer of intestinal wall
    2 Frequent fatty stools
    3 Malabsorption of small intestine
    4 Nutritional deficit

13. You are caring for a 21-year-old female college student who was admitted to your unit with severe abdominal pain. She states she has had 25 episodes of bloody diarrhea today and has lost 15 pounds in the last 2 weeks. She has not been able to eat and feels extremely weak and tired. What outcomes would you assess to indicate a positive outcome in treatment for the patient?

    _____

    _____

14. What nursing interventions would you initiate to detect or prevent complications for the patient described in question 13? _____

    _____

Section F

15. The primary clinical manifestation of cholecystitis is which of the following?
    1 Jaundice
    2 Decreased bilirubin levels
    3 Constipation
    4 Intolerance to fatty foods

16. Hepatic encephalopathy is manifested by which of the following?
    1 Ascites
    2 Cerebral dysfunction
    3 Dark urine
    4 Splenomegaly

17. Medical management of the patient with cirrhosis is primarily directed toward _____.

Section G

18. The nurse is preparing to administer a feeding to the patient receiving enteral nutrition through a nasogastric tube. What is the priority nursing action?
    1 Measuring intake and output
    2 Weighing the patient
    3 Assessing the patient for diarrhea
    4 Determining tube placement

19. The nurse is caring for a 2-year-old patient who is diagnosed with a form of malnutrition known as kwashiorkor. The nurse knows this patient is deficient in which nutrient?
    1 Carbohydrates
    2 Proteins
    3 Fats
    4 Vitamins and minerals

Section H

20. Which of the following is not considered a predisposing factor in the development of colon cancer?
    1 Low-fiber, high-fat diet
    2 High-fiber diet
    3 High–refined carbohydrate diet
    4 Ulcerative colitis

21. Which of the following is a predisposing factor in the development of Barrett's esophagus?
    1 Crohn's disease
    2 Duodenal ulcers
    3 Uncontrolled GERD
    4 Repeated episodes of constipation

22. Patients at risk for gastric carcinoma include those who consume a diet containing
    1 Large amounts of added salt and food additives
    2 Inadequate amounts of calcium
    3 Excessive amounts of fiber
    4 Large amounts of fruits and vegetables

NCLEX® Review Answers

Section A

1. **2** Aspiration is the greatest risk with nausea and vomiting in the very young and older adults. Nutritional deficits, electrolyte imbalances, and fever are all possible but usually not the greatest risk.

2. **1** True

3. **4** Options 1, 2, and 3 are all basic causes of diarrhea. Option 4 is incorrect, because it is essentially the same as saying the patient is resorbing fluid from the gut and thus is at risk for constipation.

Section B

4. **4** Genetics has not been shown to be a risk factor for GERD. Asthma, tobacco use, and alcohol use are all risk factors for GERD.

5. **4** The patient should be advised to eat small, frequent meals high in protein and low in fat and also to avoid eating within 2 to 3 hours of bedtime to lower pressure on the LES. The patient should avoid alcohol and restrictive clothing and also elevate the head of the bed to decrease pressure on the LES.

Section C

6. **1** Patients with burns experience stress ulcers known as Curling's ulcers. A preexisting ulcer does not progress to become a stress ulcer. The patient with severe head injuries may experience stress ulcers known as Cushing's ulcers. Pressure ulcers frequently occur in patients who are bedridden when their positions are not changed on a regular basis and care of skin integrity is not maintained.

7. **1** Proton pump inhibitors in combination with antibiotics are used to treat PUD. The other options are possible but are not usually first-line drugs.

Section D

8. **3** Abdominal pain is the major clinical manifestation of acute pancreatitis. Cardiovascular hypotension, disseminated intravascular coagulation, and a serum amylase of 100 units are not the major clinical manifestations of acute pancreatitis.

9. **4** Resting the GI tract is the major treatment in helping to resolve acute pancreatitis. This approach is accomplished by placement of an NG tube and keeping the patient NPO. Controlling alcohol intake reduces the likelihood of reoccurrence of acute pancreatitis. Meperidine treats the pain associated with acute pancreatitis but does not cure the underlying disorder. Peritoneal lavage does nothing to treat the acute pancreatitis.

10. **3** The patient with pancreatitis should be monitored for hypocalcemia. Pancreatitis reduces, not increases, calcium levels, thus hypercalcemia is unlikely. Hypoglycemia is unusual; hyperglycemia is more likely. Hyperkalemia requires increased intake of potassium or decreased elimination.

11. **2** After recovery from acute pancreatitis, the pancreas should function normally, but the patient may experience future bouts of alcohol-induced pancreatitis. The pancreas will continue to produce insulin following recovery from acute pancreatitis. The pancreas will continue to be inflamed and can become necrotic only when the patient continues to ingest alcohol. Atrophy is not associated with resolution of the inflammatory response.

Section E

12. **4** Nutritional deficit is common in both Crohn's disease and ulcerative colitis because of the quick transit of materials through the large intestine. Ulcerative colitis involves the mucosal layer of the intestinal wall and has characteristic fatty stools. Small intestine malabsorption is common in Crohn's disease only because this disease frequently affects the small intestine.

13.   The patient will experience a decrease in the number of stools; increase intake to meet metabolic needs; provide relief from abdominal pain and effective coping with the disease.

14.   Administering antidiarrheal medications as ordered and needed; monitoring the skin for breakdown, keeping it clean and dry; monitoring intake, output, and daily weights; consuming small, frequent easily digestible meals; monitoring IV fluids and TPN as indicated; assessing the patient's pain level frequently; administering pain medication as needed and assessing the adequacy of pain management; and educating the patient and family about disease and course of treatment.

Section F

15.   **4** Cholecystitis is associated with increased bilirubin levels. Intolerance to fatty foods is more common than jaundice and constipation in cholecystitis.

16.   **2** Hepatic encephalopathy is a cerebral dysfunction. Ascites, dark urine, and splenomegaly are gastrointestinal and urinary manifestations of liver disease.

17.   **1** Helping the patient stop drinking alcohol.

Section G

18.   **4** Determining placement of the feeding tube is the priority nursing action. Not taking this action can lead to aspiration. Measuring intake and output, weighing the patient, and assessing the patient for diarrhea are not directly related to the tube-feeding procedure.

19.   **1** Kwashiorkor is associated with protein deficiency. Marasmus is a severe deficiency of all nutrients.

Section H

20.   **2** Low-fiber, high-fat, high–refined carbohydrate diets and ulcerative colitis are associated with colon cancer. A high-fiber diet is not a predisposing factor to development of colon cancer.

21.   **3** Uncontrolled GERD is a major contributing factor in the development of Barrett's esophagus and possible esophageal cancer. The other factors involve the lower gastrointestinal tract and are not directly involved in reflux.

22.   **1** Patients at risk for gastric carcinoma are those who consume large amounts of foods containing salt or additives. The other options are unrelated to gastric carcinoma.

Notes

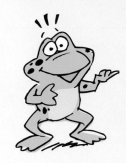

Alterations in Urinary Tract Function

What You WILL LEARN

After reading this chapter, you will know how to do the following:

- ✔ Define what is meant by the term urinary incontinence.
- ✔ List the organisms commonly associated with cystitis and pyelonephritis.
- ✔ Identify the population that is at most risk for renal calculi.
- ✔ Compare and contrast the 5 types of neurogenic bladder in terms of causes, clinical manifestations, and treatment.
- ✔ Explain the primary cause of acute glomerulonephritis, the population at most risk, and the sequelae of this infection on other body systems as well as its relationship to IgA nephropathy.
- ✔ Identify the most common cause of nephrotic syndrome.
- ✔ Compare and contrast acute renal failure with chronic renal failure in terms of mechanisms, clinical manifestations, and treatment modalities.
- ✔ Discuss the pathogenesis of polycystic kidney disease.
- ✔ Identify the population at most risk for bladder and renal cell carcinomas.

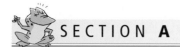

SECTION **A**

FUNCTIONAL DISORDERS OF THE GENITOURINARY TRACT

What IS Urinary Incontinence?

Urinary incontinence is the involuntary loss of urine from the bladder. It can occur while asleep or awake. The amount of urine lost can vary greatly. The condition comes to medical attention when it is perceived to be a social and/or hygiene problem by the patient or caregiver.

Pathogenesis

The pathogenesis of urinary incontinence relates to the primary cause of the incontinence. Urinary tract infections are often a primary cause of incontinence, but there may be an intrinsic urinary sphincter disorder, prostatic hypertrophy, a neurogenic bladder, or a bladder tumor.

At-Risk Populations

Women are more likely to have urinary incontinence than men; less than 10% of women under age 65 are affected and more than 35% of women over 65. Men under age 65 have a 1.5% incidence of urinary incontinence, and 22% of men over age 65 are affected. In patients over 65 who are institutionalized the incidence increases 30% to 50%.

Risk factors for urinary incontinence include increasing age, estrogen deficiency, women who have had a hysterectomy or multiple vaginal births, and men with prostatic hypertrophy. Urinary incontinence is also found in patients with dementia, stroke, diabetes, spinal cord injury, multiple sclerosis, and obesity.

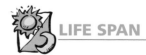

LIFE SPAN

Neurogenic, congenital, and idiopathic overactive bladder also occurs in children.

What You NEED TO KNOW

Clinical Manifestations

The primary sign of urinary incontinence is an involuntary loss of urine. The loss may be accompanied by urinary urgency, frequency, and nocturia. It is sometimes helpful when assessing the patient to ask the patient to reproduce the activities (e.g., coughing, sneezing, laughing) which result in loss of urine.

Prognosis

The prognosis for the patient with urinary incontinence is generally good. Most patients can achieve an increase in bladder control with appropriate medical and behavioral management. Some health care providers feel sphincter incompetence is best treated surgically.

There are several complications of urinary incontinence, the most common of which are skin irritation or infection and an increased incidence of falls and fractures in the older adult with an overactive bladder.

What You DO

Treatment

The least invasive and least dangerous procedure that is appropriate for the patient should be the first choice when treating urinary incontinence. All primary conditions relating to the incontinence should be identified and treated specifically (e.g., urinary tract infection, bladder tumors, prostatic hypertrophy, and diabetes). Regular pelvic floor exercises (Kegel exercises) are helpful in most patients. Biofeedback and behavioral training have been used for some patients with success. For selected patients, intermittent catheterization may be needed. Indwelling catheterization is rarely used. Condom catheters and incontinence pads may be helpful. Vaginal cones and electrical stimulation are also treatment options for select patients.

Drug therapy for urinary incontinence is based on the cause of the incontinence. If the incontinence is from an overactive bladder, antispasmodic anticholinergic drugs such as oxybutynin, tolterodine, and trospium may help by antagonizing acetylcholine at parasympathetic receptors and thereby relaxing bladder smooth muscle and inhibiting involuntary detrusor muscle contractions. Imipramine inhibits norepinephrine and serotonin reuptake and may be helpful for nocturnal enuresis. When the cause is sphincter incompetency, pseudoephedrine or imipramine can be used. A number of different drugs can be used when the cause of urinary incontinence is prostatic enlargement. These drugs include doxazosin, terazosin, tamsulosin, which antagonize alpha-1 adrenergic receptors, thus relaxing bladder smooth muscle. Finasteride and dutasteride are type II 5 alpha–reductase inhibitors, which help in some male patients. Alternative drugs may include oral or topical estrogens for stress incontinence associated with atrophic vaginitis, prostaglandin inhibitors, calcium channel blockers, and desmopressin (DDAVP) nasal spray for nocturnal enuresis.

Male patients with overflow incontinence secondary to prostatic hypertrophy may benefit from a surgical procedure known as a transurethral resection of the prostate (TURP). Men who have had a removal of their prostate (prostatectomy) and those having had a TURP may be candidates for bulking agents, artificial sphincters, or other surgical procedures. Female patients with stress incontinence may benefit from bladder suspension or sling procedures. Women with poor urethral tone may benefit from periurethral bulking agents or sphincter implants.

Nursing Responsibilities

For the patient with urinary incontinence, the nurse should do the following:

- Encourage the patient to maintain full activity.
- Have the patient keep a voiding diary over a period of 2 to 3 days so that a pattern to the incontinence may be identified.
- Advise the patient to avoid high-volume fluid intake when in situations where access to bathroom facilities is limited.
- Know that caffeine may aggravate overactive bladder symptoms by increasing urine volume and by causing an irritant effect on the bladder.
- Encourage the patient to gain an understanding of the disorder as well as an understanding of good nutrition and exercise.

- Encourage the patient to maintain a rational toileting schedule based on the pattern of incontinence.
- Instruct women in the routine use of pelvic floor exercises (Kegel exercises) after childbirth.
- Ask about the side effects of drugs used to treat incontinence but they also may cause incontinence.

Do You UNDERSTAND?

DIRECTIONS: **Fill in the blanks to complete the following statements.**

1. Pelvic floor exercises are also known as _____ exercises.
2. _____ intake may aggravate overactive bladder symptoms by _____ urine volume and causing a(n) _____ effect on the bladder.
3. Antispasmodic anticholinergic drugs such as _____ may help by antagonizing acetylcholine at parasympathetic receptors, thereby relaxing bladder smooth muscle and inhibiting involuntary detrusor muscle contractions.
4. The most common cause of urinary incontinence in the older adult is _____.

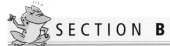

SECTION **B**

INFECTIOUS DISEASES OF THE GENITOURINARY TRACT

Urinary tract infections (UTIs) are commonly occurring disorders that result from pathogenic microorganisms. UTIs are classified according to the site of the infection. The two UTIs that are important to understand are cystitis (bladder infection) and pyelonephritis (kidney infection).

Answers: 1. **Kegel;** 2. **Caffeine,** irritant; 3. oxybutynin tolterodine, or trospium; 4. urinary tract infection.

What IS Cystitis?

Pathogenesis

The bladder is the second most common infection site in the body, second only to the respiratory tract. Cystitis is an inflammation of the bladder wall, usually resulting from ascending bacteria. Although *Enterobacter, Klebsiella, Proteus, Serratia,* and *Pseudomonas* are common offending organisms, the most common organism is *Escherichia coli*. Gram-positive organisms, fungi, or tubercular bacilli are less common causes of infection. However, fungal infections of the bladder are on the rise because of the overuse of antibiotics that alter the normal flora and fauna of the urinary tract.

The bladder and urine are normally resistant to infection because the lining of the bladder is composed of mucin-producing cells. These cells maintain the integrity of the bladder lining, which prevents inflammation and damage. However, the presence of pathogenic organisms in the bladder acts as an irritant. The irritation triggers the inflammatory response with an inappropriate need to void.

At-Risk Populations

The female urethra is short and close to the anus and vaginal opening, thus increasing the possibility of bacterial contamination and cystitis. Cystitis is uncommon in adult men, except for those with a sexually transmitted disease, prostate enlargement, or those with structural deformity of the genitourinary (GU) tract that contributes to urinary stasis. The length of the urethra and perhaps the antibacterial properties of prostatic fluid reduce the risk of cystitis in men.

Individuals also at risk for cystitis include patients with urinary stasis and alkaline urine because these factors provide a favorable environment for microorganisms to grow. Anything that breaks down the integrity of the bladder lining leads to possible infection, such as an indwelling catheter, urinary tract instrumentation, and frequent or traumatic sexual intercourse. People with diabetes mellitus, a neurogenic bladder, poor hygiene, or a history of recurrent bladder infections are at risk.

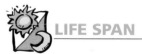

LIFE SPAN

Cystitis is more common in women; 30% of women develop cystitis sometime in their lives. Cystitis is uncommon in adult men.

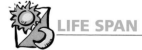

LIFE SPAN

Asymptomatic cystitis occurs commonly in older adults, with the only clinical manifestation being a change in their mental status. Of those with positive urine cultures, 10% are asymptomatic.

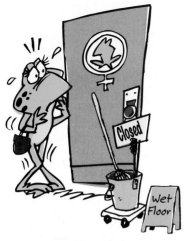

Urgent!

What You NEED TO KNOW

Clinical Manifestations

The cardinal signs and symptoms of infection are frequency, urgency, burning pain on urination (dysuria), voiding in small amounts, incomplete emptying of the bladder, and low back or suprapubic pain. The patient may also have malaise, chills, fever, and nausea; vomiting can occur when the ureters are also inflamed. Assessment may reveal cloudy urine, blood in the urine (hematuria), and abdominal or flank pain, which may indicate pyelonephritis.

Bacterial counts of 10,000/mL (for freshly voided specimens) may indicate cystitis, particularly when the patient has the cardinal signs and symptoms of infection. In contrast, one third of patients with symptoms of cystitis have no bacteria in the urine. This finding is then known as urethral syndrome and is not considered as an infectious disease of the urinary tract. The persistent, chronic form of nonbacterial cystitis occurring primarily in women is known as interstitial cystitis.

Prognosis

The prognosis for cystitis depends on whether it is an uncomplicated or complicated case of cystitis, as well as the patient's clinical manifestations, immune status, and the presence of risk factors. The prognosis is good in a patient who exhibits mild symptoms of uncomplicated cystitis. Complicated cystitis is characterized by the presence of more serious clinical manifestations. Prolonged, advanced cases of cystitis can lead to bladder ulceration or necrosis.

What You DO

Treatment

The treatment for cystitis depends on its severity. Ordinarily, no treatment is required for the patient who has asymptomatic bacteruria. In patients with acute, but uncomplicated, cystitis who are symptomatic, urinary tract antimicrobial or antiseptic drugs (e.g., sulfamethoxazole-trimethoprim, nitrofurantoin) are prescribed. Patients with asymptomatic bacteruria who are scheduled to undergo urologic surgery may also receive an antimicrobial drug. Urinary tract analgesics (e.g., phenazopyridine) may be used for symptom relief.

An additional intervention includes minimizing the use of indwelling catheters. Acidifying the urine and optimizing hydration are also important measures in treating the underlying causes of the cystitis. Surgical intervention may be required for the patient who has a structural defect of the GU tract that predisposes the patient to cystitis.

Nursing Responsibilities

For the patient with cystitis, the nurse should do the following:

* Identify patients who are at risk for cystitis and assess for signs and symptoms of the infection.
* Maintain optimal hydration (at least 3 L daily) while monitoring intake and output.
* Teach the patient about the importance of an acid-ash diet (e.g., cranberry juice, meats, eggs, cheese, prunes, cranberries, plums, whole grains, vitamin C) to help acidify the urine.
* Administer antimicrobial and urinary analgesic drugs as ordered.
* Obtain the results of urinalysis, urine culture, and sensitivity tests when able before starting antimicrobial therapy.
* Provide patient and family teaching regarding primary prevention strategies, such as wiping front to back after toileting; showering rather than bathing in a tub; voiding and drinking a glass of water after intercourse; wearing cotton underwear and avoiding wearing pantyhose with slacks or tight jeans; not sitting around in a wet bathing suit; avoiding feminine hygiene sprays and other irritants, such as perfumed toilet paper or sanitary pads; voiding every 2 hours; and using a water-soluble lubricant for coitus, especially after menopause.
* Practice preventive techniques when providing care, for example, inserting urinary catheters using strict aseptic techniques, and maintaining closed urinary drainage systems for patients who require indwelling catheters.

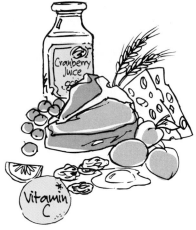

An acid-ash diet helps to acidify the urine.

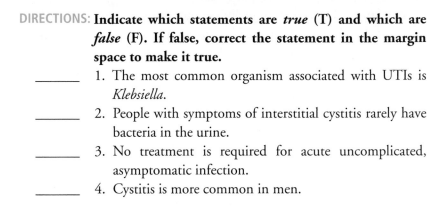

Do You UNDERSTAND?

DIRECTIONS: **Indicate which statements are *true* (T) and which are *false* (F). If false, correct the statement in the margin space to make it true.**

_____ 1. The most common organism associated with UTIs is *Klebsiella*.

_____ 2. People with symptoms of interstitial cystitis rarely have bacteria in the urine.

_____ 3. No treatment is required for acute uncomplicated, asymptomatic infection.

_____ 4. Cystitis is more common in men.

What IS Pyelonephritis?

Pathogenesis

Pyelonephritis is an inflammation of the kidney pelvis and parenchyma from a bacterial infection. Pyelonephritis can occur as an acute episode or progress into a chronic, persistent, or recurrent disorder. The two forms differ, primarily in their clinical manifestations and long-term effects. One or both kidneys can be affected.

The most common cause of pyelonephritis is *E. coli,* although viruses or fungi can also cause the infection. *Proteus* or *Pseudomonas* may also be isolated in a urine culture. Causative organisms spread to the kidney through the bloodstream, or they ascend through the urinary tract. The presence of pathogenic organisms in the kidney acts as an irritant. The irritation triggers the inflammatory response with an increase in the number of white blood cells. The inflammation leads to edema and swelling of the involved tissues. The inflammatory response is usually focal and irregular, affecting the kidney pelvis, calyces, and medulla. After the acute phase, healing occurs with scar tissue formation and atrophy of affected tubules. If the infection recurs, more and more scar tissue develops, which leads to altered tubular resorption and secretion.

At-Risk Populations

Pyelonephritis is most common in women, and the risk increases with age. Other individuals at risk for pyelonephritis include those who have alkaline urine. Alkaline urine, particularly when associated with a kidney stone or neurogenic bladder, provides a favorable environment for organisms to grow.

Risk factors for acute pyelonephritis include urinary tract instrumentation and female sexual trauma. People with a history of recurrent bladder infections or chronic urinary tract obstruction with reflux are at an increased risk.

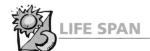

LIFE SPAN

Bacteruria is more common among pregnant women compared to nonpregnant women in the same age group. Pregnancy is also associated with increased risk for pyelonephritis because of urinary stasis from mechanical obstruction and ureteral relaxation.

What You NEED TO KNOW

Clinical Manifestations

The signs and symptoms of acute pyelonephritis are related to the degree of infection and include frequency, dysuria, costovertebral angle (CVA) tenderness, flank or groin pain, headache, muscular pain, and general prostration. The pain is described as colicky, radiating down the ureter or toward the epigastric region in the abdomen. The patient typically appears to be in acute distress and may appear intoxicated. The patient frequently experiences symptoms of cystitis for several days. Urine may be cloudy or bloody, foul-smelling, and contain a large number of white blood cell casts and white blood cells. Older adults with pyelonephritis may experience gastrointestinal (GI) and respiratory symptoms but no fever.

The signs and symptoms of chronic pyelonephritis are similar to those present in the acute phase of pyelonephritis, although early symptoms are frequently minimal or vague. Chronic pyelonephritis is frequently diagnosed incidentally when the patient is examined for hypertension or its complications. Hypertension is the most common sign of the disease. Chronic pyelonephritis gradually progresses to diffuse scarring, atrophy of functional units in the kidney, and renal failure.

Prognosis

Acute pyelonephritis rarely leads to renal failure but is associated with the development of perinephric abscesses, renal abscesses, emphysematous pyelonephritis, and chronic pyelonephritis. Chronic pyelonephritis can lead to renal failure.

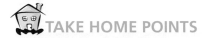

TAKE HOME POINTS

A urine culture is needed to differentiate pyelonephritis from cystitis. The presence of antibody-coated bacteria is associated more closely with pyelonephritis.

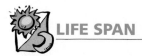

What You DO

Treatment

Treatment of pyelonephritis includes attention to the underlying cause. The use of urinary tract antimicrobial drugs is based on the results of urine culture and sensitivity. Uncomplicated pyelonephritis usually responds well to organism-specific antibiotics administered for 2 weeks or until the patient has been without a fever for 24 to 48 hours. Urinary tract analgesics are used as needed for symptom relief. Acidifying the urine and optimizing hydration aids recovery. Most importantly, hypertension must be controlled. Additional drug therapy may be required to correct any predisposing factors.

Surgical intervention may be needed for patients who have structural defects that predispose them to pyelonephritis. Intravenous (IV) pyelography and cystoscopy procedures are used to identify structural defects amenable to surgical correction.

Nursing Responsibilities

For the patient with pyelonephritis, the nurse should do the following:
- Identify patients who are at risk for the disorder, and assess them for signs and symptoms of the kidney infection.
- Monitor the results of urinalysis and urine culture and sensitivity.
- Maintain optimal hydration, minimize nausea and vomiting, and monitor intake and output.
- Provide an acid-ash diet (e.g., cranberry juice, meats, eggs, cheese, prunes, cranberries, plums, whole grains, vitamin C) to acidify urine.
- Administer antibiotics and analgesic drugs as ordered.
- Provide patient and family teaching about ways to prevent recurrent infections and the importance of follow-up care after the infection has been resolved.

Do You UNDERSTAND?

DIRECTIONS: **Indicate which statements are *true* (T) and which are *false* (F). If false, correct the statement in the margin space to make it true.**

_____ 1. Pyelonephritis is defined as an inflammation of the urethra.

_____ 2. Pyelonephritis can occur as an acute episode or progress into a chronic disorder that is persistent or recurrent.

_____ 3. The primary cause of pyelonephritis is fungal.

_____ 4. One or both kidneys can be affected in pyelonephritis.

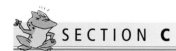

SECTION C

OBSTRUCTIVE DISORDERS OF THE GENITOURINARY TRACT

What IS a Renal Calculus?

Pathogenesis

Kidney stones (**renal calculi**) are hardened clusters of organic crystals. Although kidney stones can form anywhere in the urinary tract, the most frequent site of stone formation is in the kidneys.

Three factors must be present for a kidney stone to form: saturated urine, organic material to serve as the basis for stone formation, and deficiency of substances that hinder stone formation. Individuals born with abnormally high production of mucoproteins and a deficiency in substances that bind stone-forming material are at an increased risk for forming kidney stones. Extremely high concentrations of stone-forming crystals also promote stone formation. Urine pH, temperature, ionic strength, and concentration of urine can increase the concentration of stone-forming substrates.

Calcium is the most common stone-forming substance, although stones can also form as a result of high concentrations of other substances,

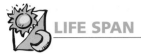 A patient with an infection above the level of the kidney stone needs urgent care to protect the kidney from further damage.

LIFE SPAN

Caucasian men between the ages of 20 and 40 are 3 times more likely to form kidney stones than women.

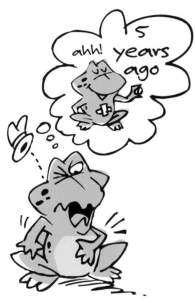

Should have had treatment.

such as uric acid, cystine, and struvite. Struvite kidney stones are also called infective stones.

Urinary organic matter (mostly mucoproteins) provides a structure for the deposition of crystals. As crystals become trapped in the organic matter, a stone is formed. Stones that are sufficiently small to pass through the urinary tract have no medical consequences. However, larger stones may be unable to pass, causing the patient severe, colic-like pain as these stones stretch the ureters. Kidney stones increase the risk of urinary obstruction and infection.

At-Risk Populations

Stone formation is more frequent in the patient who has a family history of kidney stones or metabolic disorders (e.g., overactive parathyroid gland) that increases serum calcium levels. A previous kidney stone places the patient at an increased risk for another kidney stone. When no medical treatment is provided, 50% of patients will form another stone within 5 years. Anything that increases the concentration of the urine (e.g., dehydration) or that causes urinary stasis (e.g., immobility) places the patient at risk for stone formation. Certain drugs facilitate the formation of kidney stones. For example, a patient with human immunodeficiency virus (HIV) who is taking indinavir, a protease inhibitor drug, is prone to forming kidney stones unless he or she can be properly hydrated.

The incidence of stone formation is greatest in the summer months and in areas of high humidity and high temperatures (southeastern United States). Massive doses of vitamin C and certain other drugs also contribute to high concentrations of stone-forming substances.

What You NEED TO KNOW

Clinical Manifestations

The signs and symptoms of kidney stones are related to obstruction of the urinary tract. The manifestations include a sudden, severe pain in the back flank that radiates to the abdomen and into the testis or labium. The pain may be described as colicky, cramping, dull, achy, or as having a heavy feeling. The patient may be restless and unable to find a position of comfort. Urinary urgency and frequency is noted when the stone is lodged where the ureter joins the bladder. Blood is frequently present in the urine (hematuria). Nausea, vomiting, pallor, and sweating (diaphoresis) may be present with severe pain. Fever and chills indicate that an infection is present.

Prognosis

Most kidney stones pass spontaneously. Of those patients with kidney stones, 20% require medical intervention. The greatest dangers are obstruction and kidney infection; either could lead to the loss of a kidney.

What You DO

Treatment

The goal of therapy is to prevent kidney damage from obstruction or infection and to prevent further stone formation. Treatment of acute episodes of kidney stones is based on the size of the stone. Stones less than 6 mm in diameter usually pass spontaneously. However, appropriate pain management is important. Because pain is thought to be related to prostaglandin-E_2, nonsteroidal antiinflammatory drugs (NSAIDs) give as much or better pain relief as opioid analgesics. Antiemetic drugs may be used if pain relief does not eliminate the nausea and vomiting. When required, IV drugs may be given. The urine should be strained for stones with each voiding.

Stones greater than 6 mm in diameter are frequently removed using an instrument placed through the skin and into the kidney. The stones are broken down and the pieces removed. Kidney stones can also be removed through a procedure known as extracorporeal shockwave lithotripsy (ESWL), during which the stones are broken down using sound waves and then allowed to pass through the urinary system. Stone removal from the ureters may also be accomplished using a special instrument (ureteroscope). The ureteroscope is passed through the urethra and bladder and into the ureter for stone removal. Surgical removal of the stones may be needed if all other strategies for removal have failed.

When the kidney stones are infected, immediate drainage of the infected kidney is required. A special instrument is inserted through the skin and into the kidney. The kidney is then drained of the infectious materials. This procedure includes the use of IV antibiotics and the

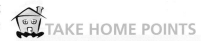

TAKE HOME POINTS

- A history of kidney stones, dehydration, and immobility increases the patient's risk of forming kidney stones.
- The severity of signs and symptoms do not directly correlate with the size of the stone.
- Kidney stones can be life-threatening when associated with kidney infection; however, death related to kidney stones is rare.

placement of a special drainage apparatus **(ureteral stent)** that allows infected material and urine to drain.

Modalities used to prevent further stone formation include developing a life-long habit of increased fluid intake (10 to 12 large glasses of water per 24 hours). Daily consumption of coffee, tea, beer, or wine may decrease the risk of stone formation; intake of apple or grapefruit juice increases the risk of stone formation.

The patient may be given drugs that control the acid or alkali nature of the urine. Allopurinol reduces the risk of forming kidney stones in patients with high urinary calcium or uric acid levels. Thiazide diuretics (e.g., hydrochlorothiazide) increase the elimination of calcium. Sodium cellulose phosphate helps bind calcium in the intestines for elimination in the stool. A number of other drugs can be used to reduce the quantity of cystine or struvite in the body, thus reducing the risk of stone formation.

Nursing Responsibilities

For the patient with kidney stones, the nurse should do the following:

- Obtain the patient's history, including drug history, dietary habits, and risk factors such as immobility, history of urinary tract infections, or gout.
- Monitor the patient for signs and symptoms of obstruction or infections, such as fever and chills, pain, nausea, vomiting, and irritative voiding behaviors (e.g., frequency, urgency, incontinence).
- Monitor laboratory results of white blood cell counts and urinalysis for evidence of infection or the presence of blood.
- Provide adequate pain management before pain is out of control.
- Encourage a high normal fluid intake (10 to 12 glasses of water per 24 hours).
- Strain all urine, and save any stones that are captured for laboratory analysis.

Do You UNDERSTAND?

DIRECTIONS: **Provide short answers for the following questions.**

1. Based on what you know about the formation of kidney stones, what do you think should be areas of research to prevent kidney stone formation? _____
   _____
   _____
   _____

2. What would you include in a teaching plan for a patient who has a kidney stone? _____
   _____
   _____
   _____

What IS a Neurogenic Bladder?

Pathogenesis

A neurogenic bladder is one that has lost its response to nervous system stimulation. When all nerve response is lost, the bladder does not receive the impulses that cause muscle relaxation or contraction. Additionally, the brain does not receive the message that the bladder is filling. The interruption causes loss of voluntary bladder control or loss of bladder sensation and results in urinary retention and, eventually, overflow incontinence. The patient is at risk for infection and backup of urine into the kidney.

Five classifications of a neurogenic bladder have been identified and further broken down into those caused by upper motor neuron

Answers: 1. studies that examine how we predict or screen those at risk for getting stones; genetic studies to determine whether there are genes that increase the risk of stone formation; studies that examine the substances that inhibit stone formation and whether they should be given to patients who are at risk for stone formation; 2. drinking at least 10 to 12 large glasses of water every day; monitoring for signs and symptoms of infection; teaching the importance of exercise, purpose of medications, and role of calcium and uric acid in stone formation.

involvement and those caused by lower motor neuron involvement. The causes, mechanisms, clinical manifestations, and treatment for neurogenic bladder are displayed in the accompanying table.

Neurogenic Bladder: Mechanisms, Causes, Clinical Manifestations, and Treatment

Type: Mechanism	Causes	Clinical Manifestation	Treatment
Upper Motor Neuron Disorders			
Uninhibited: (loss of cortical inhibition)	Lack of voluntary control in infancy Multiple sclerosis	Small urine volume Frequency, urgency, incontinence, enuresis	Anticholinergic drugs
Reflex or automatic: (reflex arc maintained below the level of the lesion with spontaneous voiding)	Spinal cord transection Spinal cord tumors Multiple sclerosis above T_{12}	Involuntary voiding Incomplete emptying of bladder Urinary retention and infection	Catheter or condom drainage Bladder training
Autonomous: (loss of cortical inhibition and interruption of spinal reflexes)	Sacral cord trauma Herniated disk Surgery with damage to pelvic para-sympathetic nerves	Overflow incontinence	Catheter Urinary diversion surgery
Lower Motor Neuron Disorders			
Motor paralysis (intact sensory function)	Spinal cord lesions at S_2 to S_4 Poliomyelitis Trauma Tumors	Overflow incontinence	Manual compression of bladder (Credé's maneuver)
Sensory paralysis (intact motor function)	Damage to lumbar nerve roots Diabetes mellitus Degeneration of dorsal column of spinal cord and sensory nerve trunks	Dribbling Overflow incontinence Loss of sensation of bladder fullness	Bladder training

At-Risk Populations

Individuals with trauma to the brain or spinal cord and those who have a neurologic condition such as Parkinson's disease, multiple sclerosis, stroke, or damage to the nerves from tumors are at risk for a neurogenic bladder. Patients who have poorly controlled diabetes and those with UTIs are also at risk.

What You NEED TO KNOW

Clinical Manifestations

The signs and symptoms of a neurogenic bladder include incontinence or urinary retention, loss of sensation to void, and loss of the ability to void spontaneously.

Prognosis

The prognosis for a patient with neurogenic bladder depends on the cause of the nerve damage. Currently, no method is available to repair nerves that are damaged within the central nervous system.

What You DO

Treatment

Treatment depends on the type of neurogenic bladder. The foregoing table identifies possible treatment modalities.

For some patients, surgical intervention is indicated. An artificial sphincter can be created if the urinary sphincter is not working. Interrupting the nerve innervation to the bladder reflex may help the patient with an uninhibited bladder. Electrodes that interfere with reflex bladder contractions can be implanted.

Drug therapy can also be used for some patients. The use of baclofen, a skeletal muscle–relaxant, may help some patients. The drug decreases the frequency and amplitude of bladder muscle spasms through an action in the spinal cord.

Nursing Responsibilities

For the patient with a neurogenic bladder, the nurse should do the following:
- Teach the patient ways to recognize a UTI and to perform self-catheterization if needed; educate the patient about a bladder training program and ways to protect the skin from breakdown.
- Link the patient with effective support systems.
- Assess for signs and symptoms of urinary retention and infection.
- Assess for skin breakdown caused by urine leakage.

- Assess for signs of excessive autonomic response (e.g., hypertension, bradycardia, headache, blurred vision).
- Monitor the patient for adverse drug effects.

Do You UNDERSTAND?

DIRECTIONS: Provide short answers for the following questions.

1. A patient has had a stroke that results in the loss of the regulatory tracts for bladder control. What type of neurogenic bladder will this patient have? _____

   _____

   _____

2. Why does a patient with paralyzed bladder muscles have incontinence? _____

   _____

   _____

3. What are the risks associated with a neurogenic bladder? _____

   _____

   _____

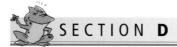

SECTION D

GLOMERULAR DISORDERS OF THE GENITOURINARY TRACT

What IS Glomerulonephritis?

Pathogenesis

Glomerulonephritis is an autoimmune response that results in inflammation of the glomeruli. Acute glomerulonephritis comes on rapidly and is self-limiting 95% of the time. For the remaining 5%, the disorder becomes

Answers: 1. uninhibited neurogenic bladder; 2. the bladder is unable to empty on command and eventually becomes full to the extent that urine leaks out of the bladder; 3. possible infection from urinary retention; skin breakdown from urine leakage; kidney disease from backed-up urine.

chronic, and glomeruli damage is more gradual. Insulin-dependent diabetes mellitus and lupus erythematosus are secondary causes of chronic glomerulonephritis.

The most common cause of acute glomerulonephritis in the United States is immunoglobin A (IgA) nephropathy (a deposit of IgA antibodies in the glomeruli)—see following discussion. However, anything that causes inflammation of the glomeruli can cause glomerulonephritis, including drugs, toxins, vascular disorders, and systemic diseases (e.g., lupus erythematosus). One rare form of the disease progresses rapidly (rapidly progressive glomerulonephritis), resulting in end-stage renal disease (ESRD) within a few weeks.

Two types of acute glomerulonephritis have been identified: infectious glomerulonephritis and postinfectious glomerulonephritis. Infectious glomerulonephritis develops within a few days of an infection. Bacterial, viral, or parasitic infections are the primary causes. Postinfectious glomerulonephritis occurs 14 to 21 days after the infection that caused the damaging antigen-antibody complexes to be formed. It is frequently the result of a type A beta-hemolytic strep infection, although other organisms and diseases can also cause the immune response (e.g., pneumococcus, staphylococcus, meningococcus, chicken pox, and hepatitis).

In glomerulonephritis, antigen-antibody complexes from an infection somewhere in the body are sent through the bloodstream to the kidneys for elimination. Most of the antigen-antibody complexes are filtered from the blood to become part of the urine. Occasionally, antigen-antibody complexes are simply the wrong size. Rather than passing into the urine, these complexes become lodged in the tiny openings of the glomerulus, and their presence excites the immune system and initiates an inflammatory response. The immune-mediated inflammatory response with cellular infiltration decreases the glomerular filtration rate, which leads to fluid retention.

The cells and chemicals that are part of the inflammatory response injure the glomerulus. The damaged cells allow large molecules such as proteins and red blood cells to move from the circulation into the filtrate of the kidneys. The kidneys' tubule cells cannot move these large molecules back into the capillaries that surround the tubules and are thus lost to the urine.

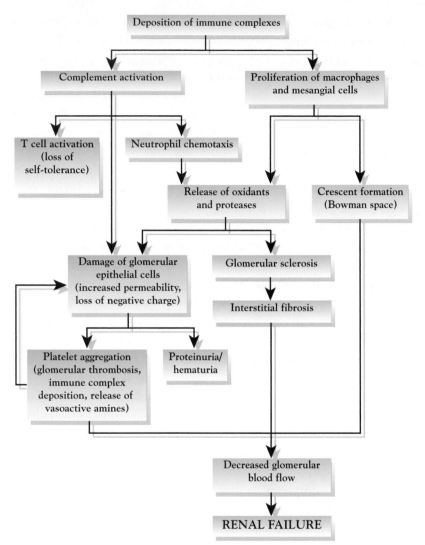

Pathophysiology of renal failure. *(Redrawn from Causer WG: Am J Kidney Dis 11:449, 1998.)*

At-Risk Populations

Patients who have had a streptococcal infection (e.g., scarlet fever or erysipelas) are at risk for glomerulonephritis, as well as people with autoimmune diseases such as systemic lupus erythematosus. The long-term prognosis of a child with glomerulonephritis is excellent; almost all patients recover completely without sequelae. Immediate mortality rate is less than 0.5%.

The incidence of acute glomerulonephritis decreases with age, although adults between the ages of 40 and 60 and those with preexisting renal lesions are at the greatest risk for the rapidly progressing form of glomerulonephritis.

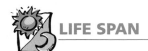

LIFE SPAN

Children between the ages of 2 and 16 years have the highest risk for acute glomerulonephritis, although any individual with an untreated type A beta-hemolytic strep infection is susceptible. The incidence of acute glomerulonephritis decreases with age.

What You NEED TO KNOW

Clinical Manifestations

A streptococcal infection (e.g., pharyngitis, impetigo) precedes renal lesions by 1 to 3 weeks. The patient with acute disease experiences a sudden onset of symptoms, including protein in the urine (**proteinuria**), blood in the urine (**hematuria**), tea-colored urine, and hypertension. The patient may have decreased or no urine output (**oliguria** or **anuria**) for several days. Edema of the face and eyes in the morning and of the feet and ankles in the afternoons and evenings is seen. Signs of infection such as a sore throat, upper respiratory infection, scarlet fever, fever, chill, and nausea and vomiting may also be noted.

Chronic glomerulonephritis encompasses several glomerular diseases with a progressive course leading to chronic renal failure. It develops slowly and may not be recognized for several years. Symptoms of chronic glomerulonephritis include the signs and symptoms of renal insufficiency or failure, such as fatigue, mental sluggishness, edema, and dizziness. Excessive urine output (**polyuria**) develops as a result of the kidney's inability to concentrate urine. High blood pressure, severe anemia, hematuria, proteinuria, and casts of white blood cells and kidney tubular cells in the urine may also be present.

Prognosis

In acute glomerulonephritis, symptoms are usually self-limiting to 2 to 3 weeks, although full recovery may take from weeks to months. Generally, the damaged cells are repaired and normal kidney function returns. Of those patients with acute, self-limiting glomerulonephritis, 95% experience a full recovery.

With chronic glomerulonephritis, the damaged cells fail to heal and are gradually replaced with scar tissue. As more and more scar tissue forms, normal kidney function is lost. Although chronic glomerulonephritis progresses at variable rates, in some patients it can progress to ESRD.

What You DO

Treatment

No specific treatment is available that will repair damaged kidneys. The goal is to prevent further damage and allow the kidneys to heal. Most patients can be safely followed as outpatients.

Treatment of acute glomerulonephritis includes a no-added-salt diet and diuretics until edema and hypertension improve; antibiotics and steroid therapy to decrease immune system damage (although they do not change the course of the disease); and removal of antibodies from the circulation (plasmapheresis) to decrease immune response. Dialysis or kidney transplant may be required in some patients for symptomatic azotemia, intractable acidosis, or diuretic-resistant pulmonary edema.

Nursing Responsibilities

For the patient with acute glomerulonephritis, the nurse should do the following:
- Obtain a complete history of recent infections or invasive procedures.
- Monitor and recognize complications.
- Monitor the patient's vital signs (particularly blood pressure), intake and output, daily weights, and the severity and pattern of edema.
- Advise the patient that urine will have to be evaluated for color, amount, and abnormal substances at 2, 4, and 8 weeks and again at 4, 6, and 12 months to check for resolution of hematuria and proteinuria.
- Teach the patient and family about the disorder and the need to limit sodium and potassium intake, as appropriate. Restrict protein in the presence of azotemia and metabolic acidosis.
- Remind patients that they can return to full activity after clinical improvement but that they may have increased hematuria after exercise for up to 2 years.

For the patient with chronic glomerulonephritis, the nurse should do the following:
- Monitor the patient for signs of renal failure (see Section E).
- Provide symptomatic relief.
- Assist the patient and family in developing support systems for coping with a chronic illness.
- Provide supportive therapy if the glomerulonephritis leads to kidney failure.

Do You UNDERSTAND?

DIRECTIONS: **Provide short answers for the following questions.**

1. Why is it important to treat strep infections early? _____
   _____
   _____

2. Why is protein found in the urine of patients with glomerulone-phritis? _____
   _____
   _____

3. How would greater knowledge of the immune system help in treat-ing this disease? _____
   _____
   _____

What IS Nephrotic Syndrome?

Pathogenesis

Nephrotic syndrome is not a disease at all but rather a manifestation of protein wasting that occurs with glomerular damage. In a normal kidney, protein molecules are too large to enter the filtrate and remain in the body. However, with glomerular damage from disease, "holes" in the glomeruli allow the large protein molecules to become part of the filtrate and, eventually, part of the urine. This protein loss is difficult to replace with dietary measures.

The result of nephrotic syndrome is a loss of plasma proteins, particularly albumin, to the urine. As much as 30 g of protein may be lost in a single day. The protein is lost because the glomeruli have been damaged from drugs, toxins, or disease, which causes them to be abnormally permeable. The most common cause of nephrotic syndrome is glomerulonephritis. However, systemic disorders such as diabetes mellitus,

Answers: **1.** antigen-antibody complexes that build up can cause an inflammatory response and damage the kidneys; **2.** the inflammation and subsequent damage to the kidney by glomerulonephritis allows large molecules through the glomeruli that would ordinarily not be lost to the urine; **3.** if ways to stop the inflammation from occurring could be found, the damage to the kidneys would not occur.

systemic lupus erythematosus, hepatitis B, leukemia, infectious disease, or preeclampsia can also cause nephrotic syndrome.

When protein is lost from the plasma, the pressure that draws fluid from the spaces between cells (**interstitial spaces**) back into the circulation is greatly reduced. As the concentration of protein decreases, the pressure for water to move to the higher concentration of proteins increases. This causes loss of fluid in the circulation and leads to decreased fluid volume (**hypovolemia**) and low blood pressure. The excess fluid in the tissues results in edema.

A satisfactory blood pressure reading and adequate renal perfusion is required for the kidneys to filter blood. When blood pressure decreases, the kidneys release renin, which raises blood pressure and causes the release of aldosterone. Aldosterone increases the amount of sodium and water retained by the kidneys. This extra fluid also leaks out of the capillaries, which further contributes to the developing edema.

Complications of nephrotic syndrome include severe deficit of circulating fluids, blood clot formation in the renal vein, abnormal thyroid function, and softening of the bones (**osteomalacia**). The patient also has an increased susceptibility to infections.

At-Risk Populations

No specific age group is at higher risk than any other group. Anyone with a disorder that permits the kidneys to filter plasma proteins into the urine is at risk for nephrotic syndrome. Predisposing risk factors to nephrotic syndrome include allergic drug reactions. Drugs associated with nephrotic syndrome include anticonvulsants, probenecid, captopril, gold salts, NSAIDs, penicillamine, and heroin.

What You NEED TO KNOW

Clinical Manifestations

The signs and symptoms of nephrotic syndrome are the result of protein loss and the accumulation of extracellular fluid. The classical signs include proteinuria, a decrease in the amount of protein (particularly albumin) in the plasma, and edema. Edema is usually the patient's primary complaint.

High levels of fats in the blood are thought to result from the liver's increased synthesis of lipoproteins. The elevated lipid levels are primarily

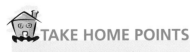

TAKE HOME POINTS

Nephrotic syndrome is the combination of signs and symptoms that occur with protein wasting from kidney disease. The major outcomes are hypovolemia and edema.

related to increased synthesis, decreased lipoprotein catabolism, reduced plasma oncotic pressure from low serum albumin levels, and increased delivery of precursors of cholesterol.

Depending on the severity of kidney involvement, patients have some degree of anemia. Other manifestations of nephrotic syndrome include loss of appetite, fatigue and malaise, irritability, abnormal menses or stoppage of menstrual periods (amenorrhea), and depression.

Serum albumin concentrations may drop as low as 1 to 2.5 g/dL. Some hematuria may be present. Large amounts of protein are present in the urine. The amount of protein lost in the urine may reflect losses of 4 to 30 g/day. If vitamin D_3 is lost in the urine, there will be decreased absorption of intestinal calcium. Hypocalcemia, osteomalacia, and secondary hypoparathyroidism result, along with the signs and symptoms of vitamin D deficiency.

Prognosis

The prognosis for the patient with nephrotic syndrome depends on the extent of kidney damage, the degree of protein wasting, and the extent of edema. Complete remission is expected if the basic underlying cause is treatable, otherwise the disease may progress to dialysis dependence.

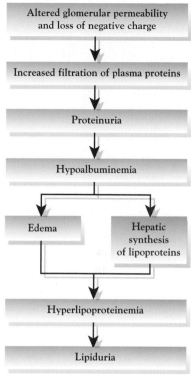

Mechanisms of lipiduria. *(Redrawn from McCance KL, Huether SE: Pathophysiology: the biologic basis for disease in adults and children, ed 3, St. Louis, 1998, Mosby.)*

What You DO

Treatment

The goal of treatment is to heal the glomerulus and stop the loss of protein in the urine. Through attention to these two goals, the cycle of edema is broken. Treatment includes mild dietary restrictions of fats, sodium, and potassium, with a daily intake of 1 to 1.5 g of high–biologic-value protein per kilogram of body weight. The protein requirement is designed to prevent further protein breakdown. A liberal potassium intake and supplemental multivitamins and minerals, especially vitamin D and iron, are important. Fluids should be restricted if the patient is hyponatremic. Infections should be treated vigorously (especially bacteruria, endocarditis, and peritonitis).

Drug therapy includes angiotensin converting enzyme (ACE) inhibitors to reduce proteinuria and to control hypertension, if present. Judicious use of thiazide and loop diuretics such as furosemide, along with salt restriction, helps with the edema. IV administration of protein-based plasma-volume expanders such as albumin may also be used to treat edema. Depending on the cause of the disorder, glucocorticosteroids such as prednisone may be used to reduce inflammation. Anticoagulants may be needed to prevent further clot formation if a renal vein thrombosis is present. Cholesterol-lowering drugs and a low-fat diet should be used as appropriate.

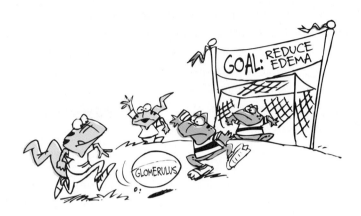

Nursing Responsibilities

For the patient with nephrotic syndrome, the nurse should do the following:

- Teach the patient and family about the underlying cause or causes of the disorder, the importance of dietary therapy, and the prevention of infection.
- Monitor vital signs for fluid volume deficit. Assess breath sounds for pulmonary edema as fluid moves into interstitial spaces in the lungs.
- Assess for signs and symptoms of electrolyte imbalance and infection.
- Monitor intake, output, and daily weights.
- Promote adequate dietary intake by monitoring the patient's degree of anorexia, depression, and malaise and making interventions as appropriate.
- Assist the patient and family in developing adequate coping skills for a chronic illness.

Do You UNDERSTAND?

DIRECTIONS: **Select the correct option from the italicized words that makes each statement correct.**

1. Nephrotic syndrome is the result of _____ *(glomerular/tubular)* damage and is manifested as the loss of ____ _____ *(albumin/red blood cells)* to the urine.

2. The most common cause of nephrotic syndrome is _____ _____ *(pyelonephritis/glomerulonephritis)*.

3. The loss of albumin from the circulation leads to _____ _____ *(hypervolemia/hypovolemia)* and a subsequent drop in _____ *(blood pressure/heart rate)*.

4. When blood pressure _____ *(increases/decreases)*, the kidneys release _____ *(renin/aldosterone)*, which in turn causes the release of _____ *(renin/aldosterone)*. There is a subsequent increase in the amount of _____ *(sodium/potassium)* retained by the kidneys. The extra fluid leaks out of the capillaries into the _____ *(interstitial/intravascular)* spaces, contributing to the edema seen in nephrotic syndrome.

5. The high levels of fats in the blood are thought to be the result of the liver's _____ *(increased/decreased)* synthesis of lipoproteins.

Fill in the blanks to complete the following sentences.

6. Serum albumin concentrations in the patient with nephrotic syndrome may drop as low as _____.

7. The prognosis for the patient with nephrotic syndrome depends on the extent of _____, the degree of _____ _____, and the extent of the _____.

8. Drug therapy for the patient with nephrotic syndrome may include the use of _____, _____, _____, and _____.

9. Assess the patient's _____ for evidence of pulmonary edema.

10. Monitor the patient's vital signs for evidence of _____.

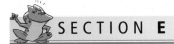

SECTION E

RENAL FAILURE

What IS Acute Renal Failure?

Pathogenesis

Acute renal failure (ARF) is the sudden inability of the kidneys to maintain normal function. This inability affects most of the body's systems because of the kidneys' important role in maintaining fluid balance, regulating electrolytes, providing constant protection against acid-base imbalances, and controlling blood pressure.

The causes of ARF are generally classified into three major areas: prerenal (associated with decreased renal blood flow), intrarenal (associated with renal ischemia or toxins), or postrenal (associated with the obstruction of urine flow out of the kidneys).

Prerenal disorders include factors that decrease the amount of blood going to the kidneys. Severe blood loss, burns, septic shock, or massive trauma are major causes of prerenal failure. Prerenal failure may also be related to the systemic inflammation present with burns, septic shock, or massive trauma. Decreased blood volume from dehydration, fluid shifts from the vascular tree to interstitial tissues, and heart failure are also prerenal sources of acute kidney failure.

Intrarenal causes of ARF include factors that damage the kidneys themselves. Intrarenal failure can occur as a result of ischemia, physical trauma, infection, inflammation, or exposure to toxic chemicals. Nephrotoxic drugs include the penicillins, sulfonamides, aminoglycosides, tetracyclines, radiographic iodine contrast materials, and heavy metals.

Death of the renal tubule cells (**acute tubular necrosis**) from decreased renal perfusion and ischemia or from nephrotoxins accounts for the majority of ARF. Glomerulonephritis, pyelonephritis, diabetic sclerosis, thrombus, or narrowing of the renal arteries can also be responsible for acute renal failure.

A postrenal cause of ARF is usually a result of an obstruction in the urinary tract below the level of the kidneys. The obstruction leads to a backup of urine and kidney damage. Obstructions can be from prostatic disease, tumors, narrowing of the ureters or urethra, kidney stones, or neurogenic bladder.

The exact pathogenesis of ARF is unclear. Acute tubular necrosis is a major contributing factor to ARF. The renal tubular cells are injured and are no longer able to effectively excrete waste products into the urine or resorb needed electrolytes and other molecules from the filtrate. The damaged tubular cells allow leakage of tubular fluid back into the interstitial area. Tubular cells may be obstructed by dead cells from tubular cell damage, or they may be damaged from a lack of sufficient blood flow (excessive vasoconstriction or extreme hypovolemia, usually secondary to severe blood or fluid loss). A buildup of waste products in the blood and a loss of important electrolytes to the urine result.

 Any episode of severe hypovolemia increases the risk for acute renal failure.

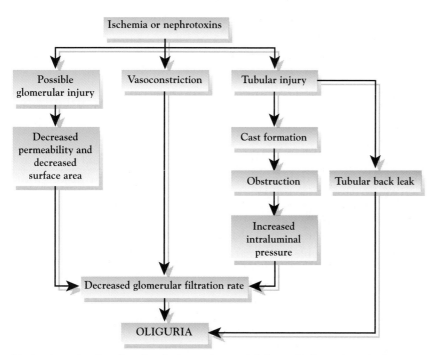

Mechanisms leading to oliguria in acute renal failure. *(Redrawn from McCance KL, Huether SE: Pathophysiology: the biologic basis for disease in adults and children, ed 3, St. Louis, 1998, Mosby.)*

At-Risk Populations

The very young and the very old are at highest risk for acute renal failure. Any patient who suffers decreased perfusion to the kidneys or who is exposed to kidney toxins is at risk. Patients experiencing trauma, sepsis, or acute blood loss are at the greatest risk for acute renal failure.

What You NEED TO KNOW

Clinical Manifestations

The progression of ARF with recovery of renal function occurs in 3 phases: oliguria, diuresis, and recovery. The *oliguric phase* begins within 24 hours of a hypotensive event and lasts for 1 to 3 weeks. The signs and symptoms of ARF include decreased urinary output (less than 30 mL/hr or less than 400 to 600 mL/day for 8 to 15 days). Edema, weight gain, anemia, and hypertension develop. Proteinuria develops, particularly when the cause is glomerulonephritis. The urine is mud-colored when the cause of renal failure is acute tubular necrosis. Elevated blood urea nitrogen (BUN) and creatinine levels and changes in electrolytes are present. Patients are prone to elevated serum levels of potassium and phosphates from cellular breakdown. Nausea and vomiting accompany the electrolyte imbalances. Fluid retention causes edema, weight gain, and elevated blood pressure.

A *diuresis phase* develops at a later point in this disorder; the urinary output increases with fluid losses of 3 to 4 L/day, and the BUN and creatinine levels begin to fall. This stage lasts from 7 to 10 days. The inability to concentrate urine can lead to excessive fluid and electrolyte loss, which in turn leads to hypovolemia and hypoperfusion of the kidneys.

Serial measurements of creatinine and BUN provide an index of renal function during the recovery phase. The *recovery phase* of ARF starts the day the BUN is stable and may take from 3 to 12 months.

Prognosis

The prognosis for the patient with acute renal failure depends on the cause and extent of renal damage. Most types of ARF are reversible if diagnosed and treated early. Patients who have decreased urinary output for longer than 15 days may never regain normal kidney function. Approximately 30% of patients do not have a full recovery of a normal glomerular filtration rate or tubular function. When renal function has deteriorated to a point that it is considered irreversible and no longer adequate to sustain life, the patient has ESRD.

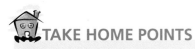

TAKE HOME POINTS

Always be aware of decreased fluid volume, and take precautions to prevent prolonged fluid volume deficit. Assess for urinary obstruction and kidney disease. Early assessment and early intervention can save lives.

What You DO

Treatment

Prevention of ARF is the primary goal; however, when prevention is not possible, the treatment goal for ARF is to prevent further renal damage and support the kidneys as they heal. Treating reversible problems such as urinary obstruction, replacing fluid volume, and correcting anemia with the use of packed red blood cells (when anemia is severe) provide the means to accomplish this goal. A high-calorie, low-protein diet helps decrease waste products, although protein replacement is used when protein wasting is also present. Electrolyte imbalances are corrected with restrictions in sodium and potassium. Hemodialysis may be necessary to correct fluid volume, electrolyte level, and acid-base imbalances.

Nursing Responsibilities

Nurses can have a significant effect on preventing ARF by closely monitoring patients at risk and by understanding the potential toxicity of drugs. The nurse should do the following:

- Assess patient's fluid balance by accurately monitoring intake, output, daily weights, and edema.
- Check vital signs, particularly blood pressure.
- Evaluate mucous membranes and skin turgor for signs of dehydration.
- Teach the patient and family about protein intake and dietary restrictions of sodium and potassium.
- Provide or offer frequent oral hygiene to reduce the effects of renal waste products on taste and smell sensations, and integrity of mucous membranes.
- Treat any associated nausea, vomiting, and anorexia.
- Assess for complications of ARF (e.g., pleural effusion, pericarditis, acidosis, uremia); monitor the patient's level of consciousness; assess breathing and heart sounds.
- Prevent secondary infection through good hand washing practices, providing meticulous skin, respiratory, and central IV line care; assess for signs and symptoms of infection.
- Teach the patient basic hygiene skills, when necessary.
- Avoid the use of nephrotoxic drugs; use protocols to provide appropriate, adequate dosages.
- Provide psychologic support to help the patient cope with the disorder and required therapy.

Do You UNDERSTAND?

Healthy People 2010:
Chronic Renal Failure

http://www.
healthypeople.gov/document/
html/volume1/04ckd.htm

DIRECTIONS: **Match the type of renal failure in Column A with the cause in Column B.**

Column A

_____ 1. Prerenal
_____ 2. Intrarenal
_____ 3. Postrenal

Column B

a. Obstruction of urine flow out of the kidneys
b. Renal ischemia or toxins
c. Decreased renal blood flow

DIRECTIONS: **Indicate which statements are *true* (T) and which are *false* (F). If false, correct the statement in the margin space to make it true.**

_____ 4. Urine is red when the cause of renal failure is acute tubular necrosis.

_____ 5. The very young and the very old are at highest risk for ARF.

_____ 6. Clinical manifestations of ARF include a urine output of less than 400 to 600 mL/day for 8 to 15 days.

What IS Chronic Renal Failure?

Pathogenesis

Chronic renal failure (CRF) is a slow, progressive, and irreversible loss of kidney function. Chronic renal failure may follow an episode of ARF, depending on the extent of nephron loss. The causes of chronic renal failure are many but can generally be divided into three groups: (1) those that directly affect the kidney by infection, inflammation, and upper urinary tract obstruction; (2) those in which an obstruction of the lower urinary tract is present; and (3) those associated with systemic diseases and toxicities, such as elevated serum calcium levels, hypertension, disseminated lupus erythematosus, atheroma, and diabetes mellitus.

Whatever the cause, the result of renal failure is destruction of the functional units of the kidneys. The patient has no clinical manifestation of renal failure until 75% or more nephrons no longer function. When the nephrons are lost, body wastes accumulate and fluids and electrolytes become out of balance.

The clinical course of CRF is described in four stages. A glomerular filtration rate (GFR) between 30 and 75 mL/min suggests chronic renal insufficiency. (A normal GFR is between 100 and 150 mL/min.) In early chronic renal failure, the GFR declines to between 10 and 30 mL/min. The GFR in late renal failure is between 5 and 10 mL/min. In the terminal stages of renal failure, the GFR is less than 5 mL/min. Because all of the creatinine (a by-product of muscle energy metabolism) that is filtered by the kidneys in a given period appears in the urine, the serum creatinine level is equivalent to the GFR.

A decreased production of erythropoietin—a hormone produced by the kidneys to increase red blood cell formation—is present, thus anemia develops. In addition, a decrease in the activation of vitamin D is present, which leads to decreased absorption of calcium.

The BUN and serum creatinine levels rise. Sodium, calcium, phosphate, and potassium imbalances lead to hypertension, pulmonary edema, altered metabolism, a loss of calcium from the bones (osteoporosis), changes in mental status, and peripheral nerve conduction delays. Decreased platelet factor III, decreased fat metabolism, and decreased white blood cell activity contribute to dermatologic problems.

At-Risk Populations

Patients who have diabetes mellitus are at a significant risk for chronic renal failure, particularly when blood sugar levels are not well controlled. Patients with long-standing, untreated hypertension are also at risk.

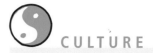

CULTURE

African Americans and Native Americans with diabetes mellitus or long-standing, untreated hypertension are especially at increased risk for developing chronic renal failure and ESRD.

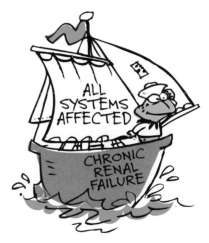

What You NEED TO KNOW

Clinical Manifestations

All body systems are affected by CRF. The signs and symptoms include the following:

Cardiovascular: Hypertension, arrhythmias, heart failure, pericarditis, atherosclerosis, anemia-clotting factor disorders

Genitourinary: Decreased creatinine clearance, oliguria, anuria

Chronic renal failure affects every system in the body and, without treatment, will end in death within a short time.

Musculoskeletal: Soft tissue calcifications; osteodystrophy related to phosphate and calcium imbalance; decreased absorption of calcium, which leads to increased stimulation of parathyroid glands; increased loss of calcium from bones; joint swelling and pain

Perceptual: Retinal changes related to hypertension, conjunctival calcification, blurred vision

Reproductive: Decreased libido, infertility, impotence, enlarged mammary glands (gynecomastia)

Dermatologic: Pallor, bruising, pruritus, edema, dry skin, dry hair, altered pigmentation

Gastrointestinal: Decreased appetite, nausea, vomiting, changes in taste and smell), stomatitis, an offensive breath odor (uremic fetor), bloody emesis, blood in the stools, diarrhea, and constipation

Respiratory: Pleural effusions, pulmonary edema, deep rapid respirations (Kussmaul respirations), lack of respirations (apnea).

Neurologic: Numbness, burning, tingling feet, jumpy feeling (peripheral neuropathy), insomnia, irritability, altered level of consciousness, changes in motor function, changes in cognition or behavior

Prognosis

The clinical manifestations of nephron loss are prominent in late renal failure and life-threatening in ESRD. The mortality rate exceeds 20% despite careful attention to fluid and electrolyte balance or other treatments.

What You DO

Treatment

The care of the patient with CRF must emphasize interventions to conserve residual renal function, such as controlling blood pressure and blood sugar and avoiding nephrotoxins. Relieving symptoms and maintaining ideal body weight and fluid and electrolyte balance are important as the kidneys fail.

Dietary restrictions are aimed at minimizing urea toxicity, controlling various metabolic upsets, and providing optimal nutrition. Modifications involve adjustments to protein, carbohydrate, fat, sodium, potassium, and phosphate intake.

Drug therapies includes cation exchange resins, such as sodium polystyrene to lower serum potassium levels, anticonvulsants to control seizures caused by elevated BUN levels (when necessary), antihypertensive drugs to control blood pressure, diuretics to manage excessive circulating fluid volume **(hypervolemia)**, antimicrobial drugs to treat infection, phosphate-binding drugs to prevent absorption of phosphorus from the intestinal tract, H_2-receptor antagonists and antiemetics to control gastrointestinal upset, erythropoietin to manage anemia, inotropic drugs to manage heart failure, antipruritics to relieve pruritus caused by buildup of urea on the skin, laxatives or stool softeners to manage diarrhea and constipation, and vitamins and minerals to enhance nutritional status.

Nursing Responsibilities

The nursing responsibilities of caring for the patient with CRF includes recognizing changes in renal function; electrolyte balances; cardiovascular, skin, electrolytes, gastrointestinal, metabolic, neurologic, perceptual, reproductive, respiratory, and musculoskeletal systems; and to provide supportive care.

Medical and nursing interventions are aimed at providing the highest quality of life. To do so, the nurse should do the following:

- Collaborate with the patient and health care team to provide optimal quality of life within the limitations of the disease.
- Accurately record intake and output with consideration to fluid and dietary restrictions.
- Obtain weights at the same time daily, on the same scale, and in the same type of clothing.
- Provide age-appropriate and culturally appropriate patient and family teaching regarding the disorder and the treatment regimen.
- Assess the extent of the patient's anorexia, nausea, vomiting, diarrhea, and constipation, taking measures to relieve symptoms.
- Assist in obtaining laboratory specimens.
- Administer drugs as ordered with consideration to declining renal function and monitor for adverse effects.
- Monitor for clinical manifestations of infection, dehydration, overhydration, pruritus, petechiae, purpura, edema, and changing neurologic status.
- Maintain patient safety precautions reorienting the patient to reality, when necessary.
- Assess the patient's fatigue and activity tolerance and adjust care to permit rest periods.
- Assess sexual dysfunction and effect on patient-spouse relationship.
- Offer emotional support; arrange for family counseling, teach coping strategies, and provide information about available support groups.

TAKE HOME POINTS

The only treatment for ESRD is dialysis or kidney transplantation.

Do You UNDERSTAND?

DIRECTIONS: Using the numbers provided below, fill in the blanks to complete the following statements.

5   5 to 10   10 to 30   30 to 75   50   100 to 150

1. A patient usually has no clinical manifestations of renal failure until _____% or more nephrons no longer function.
2. A normal GFR is _____ mL/min.
3. A GFR of _____ ml/min suggests chronic renal failure.
4. In early chronic renal failure, the GFR declines to _____ mL/min.
5. The GFR in late renal failure is _____ mL/min.
6. In terminal stages of chronic renal failure, the GFR is less than _____ mL/min.

SECTION F

HEREDITARY DISEASES OF THE GENITOURINARY TRACT

What IS Immunoglobulin A Nephropathy?

National Institute of Diabetes and Diseases of the Kidneys
(IgA Nephropathy)
http://kidney.niddk.nih.gov/kudiseases/pubs/iganephropathy/

Pathogenesis

Immunoglobulin A (IgA) nephropathy (IgA glomerulonephritis) is one of the many types of acute glomerulonephritis. IgA, and also some IgM and complement proteins, deposit in the mesangium of glomerular capillaries, even though there is no evidence of systemic immunologic disease. IgA nephropathy is rare, affecting 2% to 4% of the population. A renal biopsy may be required for a diagnosis.

Evidence suggests that the disorder is a result of either increased production or reduced clearance of IgA and immune complexes that are ultimately deposited in the kidneys. IgA nephropathy is frequently associated with an upper respiratory infection or influenza-like illness with high serum IgA levels, although normal IgA may be present.

The glomeruli normally filter wastes and excess water from the blood, sending them to the bladder as urine. IgA causes "holes" in the glomeruli, which leads to blood and protein in the urine. Patients with IgA nephropathy have a marked deposit of IgA (and, occasionally, IgG with complement) in the glomeruli.

At-Risk Populations

IgA nephropathy is the most common form of glomerulonephritis in developing countries, especially Asia. Men are twice as susceptible as women to this disease.

What You NEED TO KNOW

Clinical Manifestations

The symptoms of IgA nephropathy occur 24 to 48 hours after an upper respiratory or gastrointestinal viral infection. Gross or microscopic hematuria occurs in 30% to 40% of patients. The urine is foamy and tea-colored for 2 to 6 days. Proteinuria, edema, and hypertension are less common. Puffiness develops around the eyes, hands, or feet. Patients may complain of a pain in the small of the back immediately below the ribs that is not aggravated by motion. The urge to urinate becomes frequent, particularly at night, and a reduced amount of urine is produced.

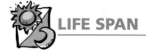

LIFE SPAN

Adults with IgA nephropathy progress to loss of renal function more frequently than children.

Prognosis

IgA nephropathy is a self-limiting, single-occurrence disorder for over 50% of patients. The remaining patients have a gradual progression of glomerular disease over a period of 10 to 20 years with recurrent episodes of hematuria and mild proteinuria. Of affected children, 20% develop the progressive form of the disease. Patients with early hypertension and proteinuria that exceeds 3 g/day tend to progress to renal failure. Hypertriglyceridemia and hyperuricemia are predictors of poor outcomes.

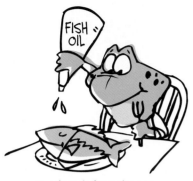

Our friends from the sea.

What You DO

Treatment

No widely accepted medical treatment for IgA nephropathy is available. The treatment is primarily supportive. ACE inhibitor drugs help control blood pressure and delay the deterioration of kidney function. Some evidence suggests that daily consumption of fish oil slows the progression of the disease. Reducing cholesterol through diet and drugs or both appears to help slow the progression of the disease.

Nursing Responsibilities

The nursing responsibilities for patients with IgA nephropathy are similar to the care of the patient with glomerulonephritis. The nurse should do the following:

- Obtain a complete history of recent infections or invasive procedures.
- Monitor for and recognize complications.
- Assess the severity of the patient's edema, vital signs (particularly blood pressure), and intake and output.
- Examine urine for color, amount, protein, and blood.
- Obtain weight readings at the same time daily, on the same scale, and in the same type of clothing.
- Provide age-appropriate and culturally appropriate patient and family teaching regarding the disorder.
- Provide relief of symptoms.
- Assist the patient and family in developing support systems and coping skills when the disease becomes progressive.

Do You UNDERSTAND?

DIRECTIONS: **Indicate which statements are *true* (T) and which are *false* (F). If false, correct the statement in the margin space to make it true.**

_____ 1. Patients with early hypertension and proteinuria that exceeds 3 g/day tend to progress to renal failure.

_____ 2. Hypertension is a common finding of IgA nephropathy.

_____ 3. ACE inhibitors delay deterioration of renal function in IgA nephropathy.

_____ 4. Urine is nonfoamy and greenish in the patient with IgA nephropathy.

What IS Polycystic Kidney Disease?

Pathogenesis

Polycystic kidney disease (PKD) is a genetic disorder characterized by multiple dilations of the collection ducts, which appear as if they are fluid-filled cysts. The proportion of dilated collecting ducts varies from less than 10% to greater than 90%. The grapelike cysts replace normal kidney tissue. People with PKD live decades without developing symptoms.

Normal kidney cells are crowded out by groups of cysts filled with fluid, blood, or even urine. The kidneys enlarge along with the cysts, which can number in the thousands, while roughly retaining their kidney shape. In fully developed PKD, a cyst-filled kidney can weigh as much as 22 pounds.

High blood pressure occurs early in the disease, frequently before the cysts appear. Kidney stones usually develop, and kidney infection is common because of the compression and obstruction of the urinary tract. Cysts may also form in other areas, such as the lung, the liver, and the pancreas.

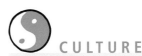

CULTURE

PKD is thought to occur more frequently in Caucasians than in African Americans, and more frequently in females than in males.

At-Risk Populations

Patients at risk for PKD are those who carry the defective gene. Both adults and children are affected. Approximately 90% of all PKD is a genetic, autosomal dominant disorder. When one parent has the disease, the chances are 50% that the disease will pass to a child. In some rare cases, the cause of the autosomal dominant disease occurs spontaneously in the child soon after conception. In these cases, the parents are not the source of the disease. A genetic flaw different from that causing autosomal dominant PKD causes autosomal recessive PKD. Parents who do not have the disease can have a child with the disease if both parents carry the abnormal gene and both pass the gene to their child. The chance of this happening, when both parents carry the abnormal gene, is one in four. When only one parent carries the abnormal gene, the child does not get the disease.

What You NEED TO KNOW

Clinical Manifestations

The symptoms of the autosomal dominant form of the disease usually develop between the ages of 30 to 40, but they can begin earlier, even in childhood. The most common clinical manifestations of PKD are pain in the back and sides and headaches. The dull pain can be temporary or persistent, mild or severe. Additionally, patients with autosomal dominant PKD can have urinary tract infections, blood in the urine, liver and pancreatic cysts, abnormal heart valves, high blood pressure, kidney stones, bulges in the walls of blood vessels (aneurysms) in the brain, and small outpocketings of the wall of the colon (diverticulosis).

Symptoms of the autosomal recessive form of the disease begin in the earliest months of life, even in utero. Children with PKD experience high blood pressure, urinary tract infections, and frequent urination. The disease usually affects the liver, the spleen, and the pancreas, resulting in low blood cell counts, varicose veins, and hemorrhoids.

Prognosis

Many people with autosomal dominant form of PKD live for decades without developing symptoms. Adults show signs of hypertension and kidney failure 5 to 15 years after the onset of symptoms.

Children with autosomal recessive PKD usually develop kidney failure within a few years. Babies with the worst cases die hours or days

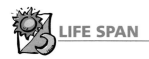

LIFE SPAN

Because kidney function is crucial for early physical development, children with autosomal recessive PKD are usually smaller compared with the average child.

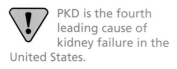

PKD is the fourth leading cause of kidney failure in the United States.

after birth. Children with an infantile version may have sufficient renal function for normal activities for a few years. People with the juvenile version may live into their teens and twenties but usually have liver problems as well.

What You DO

Treatment

Currently, the course of PKD cannot be genetically altered. Treatment is aimed at preserving kidney function for as long as possible. Interventions include prompt treatment of UTIs, prompt recognition and treatment of urinary tract obstruction, and maintenance of fluid and electrolyte balance. Genetic counseling is vital to reduce the likelihood of transmission of the disease.

Nursing Responsibilities

For the patient with PKD, the nurse should do the following:

- Accurately record intake and output, and monitor laboratory tests that assess kidney function.
- Assess for and teach the patient to recognize the signs and symptoms of UTIs (e.g., urgency, frequency, dysuria).
- Assess vital signs, particularly blood pressure for hypertension.
- Avoid invasive procedures of the urinary tract.
- Evaluate the patient's level of pain related to compression of internal structures.
- Administer analgesics as ordered, and monitor the patient's response to the drugs.
- Assist the patient and family in obtaining genetic counseling.
- Help the patient and family understand and cope with effects of the disease.
- Provide information about renal dialysis and transplantation when appropriate.

Do You UNDERSTAND?

DIRECTIONS: **Fill in the blanks to complete the following statements.**

1. PKD leads to renal failure because nonfunctioning _____ gradually replace _____.
2. Patients at risk for PKD are those who carry the defective _____.
3. _____ counseling is important in reducing the transmission of PKD.

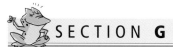

SECTION **G**

MALIGNANCIES OF THE GENITOURINARY TRACT

What IS Bladder Carcinoma?

Pathogenesis

Bladder carcinoma is a cancer of the cells that line the bladder. Of all bladder cancers, 90% are transitional cell carcinomas, approximately 8% arise from squamous cells, and 1% to 2% are adenocarcinomas. Transitional cell carcinomas develop from the epithelial lining of the urinary tract, thus they may occur in the ureters, the renal pelvis, and the urethra. The carcinomas frequently grow as stalks. Growths that are not papillary are more aggressive.

Damage to a cell irreversibly changes the structure of the cell, thus it no longer sends or receives normal cell messages; it does not know when to stop dividing. The abnormal cell undergoes uninhibited growth, which crowds out normal cells. Without treatment, the cancer cells invade nearby organs and spread to lymph nodes, bones, the liver, and the lungs.

At-Risk Populations

Individuals over age 55 are at an increased risk for bladder cancer, as well as those who have a long history of chronic bladder stones or chronic bladder irritation. Cigarette smoking is associated with the development of bladder cancer. Industrial exposure to chemicals such as textile chemicals, petroleum products, leather finishes, and benzidine have also been linked to bladder cancer. Genetic changes (i.e., mutations in gene p53—a tumor-suppressor gene—may also be a precursor for the development of bladder cancer.

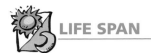

LIFE SPAN

Men are twice as likely to develop bladder cancer as women, and the risk increases with age. Caucasian men are at greater risk for bladder carcinoma than are African American men.

What You NEED TO KNOW

Clinical Manifestations

The signs and symptoms of bladder cancer are subtle in onset. Twenty or more years may elapse between contact with a carcinogen and the clinical appearance of a tumor.

Hematuria is the initial symptom of bladder cancer in 80% of the cases, although in the early stages it is often intermittent. Frequency and urgency appear late in the disease, but these symptoms are nearly always accompanied by either gross or microscopic hematuria. Pelvic pain develops in patients with advanced bladder cancer.

TAKE HOME POINTS

Bladder cancer is a "silent cancer," meaning that it is usually asymptomatic until it invades nearby tissues. Blood in the urine, particularly when produced painlessly, always warrants further evaluation.

Prognosis

The prognosis for patients with bladder cancer depends on the extent to which the cancer has advanced at the time of diagnosis. Patients with localized bladder cancer have a 95% survival rate. Patients with tumors that extend beyond the bladder wall have a poorer prognosis (46% to 49%, 5-year survival rate).

What You DO

Treatment

Choices of treatment for bladder cancer are limited. Surgical removal of the cancer cells can be performed using a procedure called transurethral resection of the bladder tumor (TURBT). In some cases, the entire bladder may need to be removed (cystectomy). Radiation is not extremely effective but may be used in combination with antineoplastic therapy.

Nursing Responsibilities

The nursing responsibilities for the patient with bladder cancer are aimed at helping the patient cope with the diagnosis and treatment plan. Postoperative nursing care will be needed if the patient has had a surgical procedure; however, generally, the nurse should do the following:

- Elicit a history of exposure to known cancer-causing chemicals (carcinogens).
- Encourage the patient to stop smoking; provide smoking cessation materials to patients.
- Assess the urine for quantity, color, and characteristics.
- Encourage the patient to increase fluid intake after a cystoscopy and to report any signs of infection (e.g., blood in the urine, burning, pain, increased frequency with urination).
- Teach about the importance of follow-up care.
- Teach the patient and family about care of the skin after radiation therapy.
- Provide age- and culture-supportive, symptomatic care for the patient who is receiving antineoplastic therapy.
- Provide perioperative care based on the surgical procedure performed.
- Evaluate the patient's and the family's support systems, and assist with learning effective coping strategies.

Do You UNDERSTAND?

DIRECTIONS: **Fill in the blanks to complete the following statements.**

1. Eighty percent of patients with bladder cancer are seen with _____ _____.

2. Ninety-five percent of patients with _____ bladder cancer survive.

3. _____ or a TURBT are the surgical options for bladder cancer.

Answers: 1. painless hematuria; 2. localized; 3. cystectomy

What IS Renal Cell Carcinoma?

Pathogenesis

Renal cell carcinoma, also known as renal adenocarcinoma, is a cancer of cells lining the tubules of the kidneys and is the most common renal cancer. The right and left kidneys are at equal risk for development of cancerous tumors. At least 85% of all renal tumors are malignant.

Cancerous cells usually begin in the outer layer of the kidney. Tumor growth is slow, usually developing in one kidney and spreading through lymph nodes and blood vessels to other lymph nodes, the liver, bones, the lungs, the thyroid gland, and the central nervous system. Tumor growth places pressure on blood vessels and surrounding tissues, which contributes to tissue death and interruption of kidney function. Metastasis can occur even after the diseased kidney is removed.

At-Risk Populations

Renal cell carcinoma occurs 2 to 3 times as often in men as in women. A genetic predisposition to renal cell carcinoma may exist. Tobacco use doubles the risk of renal cancer, although the exact mechanism of cell damage is unclear. Occupational exposure to petroleum products, heavy metals, or asbestos increases the risk for renal cell carcinoma. Other risk factors include high-protein diets, obesity, cigarette smoking, hypertension, the use of antihypertensive drugs and diuretics, and autosomal dominant polycystic kidney disease. Long-term use of dialysis also places the patient at greater risk.

LIFE SPAN

Renal cell carcinoma may be diagnosed at any age but is most common in adults aged 50 to 70 years.

What You NEED TO KNOW

Clinical Manifestations

Because one kidney can maintain fluid and electrolyte balance, the signs and symptoms of renal cell carcinoma are usually not apparent until tumor growth is extensive. Hematuria is the most common symptom, occurring in 40% to 60% of patients. Flank pain is described as dull and aching. Other findings may include a palpable flank or abdominal mass, although tumor palpation is difficult in all but the thinnest people. The patient may note weight loss and develop an intermittent fever.

Hypertension develops as a result of increased renin production. Liver function tests are altered with an elevated serum alkaline phosphatase, prothrombin, and bilirubin.

Prognosis

A patient with clinical symptoms nearly always has advanced disease, although the prognosis for the patient with renal cell carcinoma depends highly on the tumor grade, tumor cell type, and the extent of metastasis at the time of diagnosis (staging). A stage I tumor is contained within the renal capsule. The 5-year survival rate for stage I disease (after a partial nephrectomy) has ranged from 73% to 92%. Unfortunately, 20% to 30% of patients with localized tumors eventually relapse, with the lung the most common site of metastasis.

Stage II carcinoma is evidenced by spread of the cancer through the renal capsule but within the surrounding fascia. Stage III carcinoma involves regional lymph nodes, the renal vein, or the vena cava. Stage IV carcinoma involves the spread of the cancer to distant sites. Survival beyond 5 years is rare for patients with carcinomas of stages III and IV.

What You DO

Treatment

Treatment of renal cell carcinoma is usually surgical removal of the affected kidney (partial or radical nephrectomy). The combination of antineoplastic drugs and biologic response–modifying drugs is frequently used. Interleukins and interferons (IL-2, INF-α) show promise in treating this cancer. Radiation therapy may be used preoperatively to shrink the tumors or postoperatively to destroy remaining tumor cells.

Nursing Responsibilities

For the patient with renal cell carcinoma, the nurse should do the following:

- Increase fluid intake, when indicated, to ensure adequate excretion of waste products before surgery.
- Assure the patient that the remaining kidney will function sufficiently to meet the body's needs.

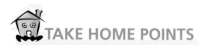

TAKE HOME POINTS

Kidney tumors are nearly always malignant and difficult to find in the early stages, which makes early intervention particularly challenging.

- Advise the patient of the importance of postoperative deep breathing and coughing. Coughing is difficult because the incision is near the diaphragm.
- Evaluate and manage the patient's pain with patient-controlled analgesia (PCA).
- Accurately record intake and output.
- Provide meticulous catheter care, which is necessary to prevent postoperative UTI.
- Listen to bowels sounds for the development of failure of the forward movement of intestinal contents (**paralytic ileus**) during the postoperative period.
- Provide age-appropriate and culturally appropriate patient and family teaching regarding the disorder, surgery, antineoplastic therapy, and radiation therapy.
- Assist the patient and family with the grieving process and the development of coping skills.

Do You UNDERSTAND?

DIRECTIONS: **Fill in the blanks to complete the following statements.**

1. The most common cancer that arises in the kidney is _____ _____.
2. Tobacco use _____ the risk of renal cell carcinoma.
3. The survival rate for renal carcinoma is lower than for many other cancers because: _____ _____

References

Black J, Hawks J, Keene A: *Medical-surgical nursing: clinical management for positive outcomes,* ed 6, Philadelphia, 2001, WB Saunders.

Gutierrez K, Queener S: *Pharmacology in nursing,* Philadelphia, 2004, WB Saunders.

Huether S, McCance, K: *Understanding pathophysiology,* ed 3, St Louis, 2005, Mosby.

Answers: 1. cell carcinoma; 2. doubles; 3. it has frequently reached the advanced stages before diagnosis.

Lewis S, Heitkemper M, Dirksen S: *Medical-surgical nursing: assessment and management of clinical problems,* ed 6, St Louis, 2004, Mosby.

McCance K, Huether S: *Pathophysiology: the biologic basis for disease in adults and children,* ed 4, St Louis, 2002, Mosby.

National Institute of Diabetes and Diseases of the Kidneys: *Polycystic kidney disease,* 2005. URL http://www.niddk.nih.gov/health/kidney/pubs/polycyst/polycyst/htm.

National Institute of Diabetes and Kidney Disease: *Kidney disease,* 2005, URL http://www.niddk.nih.gov.

National Library of Medicine: *Bladder diseases,* 2005, URL http://www.nlm.nih.gov/medlineplus/bladderdiseases.html.

NCLEX® Review

Section A

1. The primary cause of urinary incontinence is
   1 Bladder tumor.
   2 Neurogenic bladder.
   3 Sphincter disorder.
   4 Urinary tract infection.

2. The primary sign of urinary incontinence is
   1 Involuntary loss of urine.
   2 Frequency.
   3 Nocturia.
   4 Urgency.

3. The primary treatment modality for urinary incontinence is
   1 Treat the underlying cause.
   2 Urinary catheters.
   3 Drugs.
   4 Kegel exercises.

Section B

4. The health care provider teaches a patient with cystitis about proper fluid intake. What is the recommended fluid intake per 24 hours?
   1 1000 mL
   2 1500 mL
   3 2000 mL
   4 3000 mL

5. Hypertension may be a sign of which of the following UTIs?
   1 Acute cystitis
   2 Chronic cystitis
   3 Acute pyelonephritis
   4 Chronic pyelonephritis

6. The most common organism causing cystitis or pyelonephritis is
   1 *Escherichia coli.*
   2 *Klebsiella pneumoniae.*
   3 *Proteus.*
   4 *Staphylococcus aureus.*

7. Which of the following menus would *not* be most appropriate for the patient with chronic cystitis?
   1 Tossed vegetable salad, milk, apple
   2 Grilled cheese, prunes, tea
   3 Egg salad, ham, milk
   4 Hamburger on whole wheat bread, milk, tea

8. Your 15-year-old patient has been diagnosed with cystitis. To prevent recurrence of the infection, you would teach her which of the following behavior modifications?
   1 Increasing her fluid intake
   2 Wiping front to back after a bowel movement
   3 Adhering to an alkaline-ash diet
   4 Taking showers rather than baths

9. Which of the following findings on a urinalysis most likely indicates a UTI?
   1 Four to five red blood cells; high power field
   2 Bacteria count of over 100,000/mL
   3 Glucose level of 3+
   4 4+ ketones

Section C

10. Which of the following is a risk factor in calculi formation?
    1 Excessive calcium intake
    2 Family history of renal calculi
    3 High concentrations of struvite
    4 Reduced production of inhibitors

Section D

11. Which renal condition usually has a history of recent infection with beta-hemolytic streptococcus?
    1 Chronic renal failure
    2 Glomerulonephritis
    3 Nephrosis
    4 Pyelonephritis

Section E

12. An individual has an elevated blood level of urea and creatinine as a result of blockage of one ureter by calculi. This condition is referred to as
    1 Prerenal disease.
    2 Intrarenal disease.
    3 Postrenal disease.
    4 Hypercalcemia.

13. What is the earliest symptom of chronic renal failure?
    1 Increased BUN
    2 Oliguria
    3 Polyuria
    4 Pruritus

Section F

14. What is the most common cause of IgA nephropathy?
    1 Increased production or reduced clearance of IgA in the kidneys
    2 Poststreptococcal glomerulonephritis
    3 Decreased production or increased clearance of IgA in the kidneys
    4 Genetic, autosomal dominant disorder

Section G

15. Cigarette smoking is associated with the development of
    1 Bladder cancer.
    2 Cystitis.
    3 Glomerulonephritis.
    4 Polycystic kidney disease.

16. Stage I renal cell carcinoma is usually
    1 Contained within the renal capsule.
    2 Located in the renal capsule but within the surrounding fascia.
    3 Found in the regional lymph nodes, renal vein, or vena cava.
    4 Spread to distant sites such as the lungs.

NCLEX® Review Answers

Section A

1. **4** Urinary tract infections are a primary cause of incontinence. Intrinsic causes of incontinence include urinary sphincter disorder, prostatic hypertrophy, a neurogenic bladder, or a bladder tumor.

2. **1** The primary sign of urinary incontinence is an involuntary loss of urine. The loss may be accompanied by urinary urgency, frequency, and nocturia.

3. **1** The primary treatment modality for urinary incontinence is to treat the underlying cause of the incontinence, although the other options are also used.

Section B

4. **4** A minimum of 3000 mL of fluid is required per 24 hours to treat cystitis adequately. 1000 mL, 1500 mL, and 2000 mL are insufficient.

5. **4** Because blood pressure is, in part, regulated by kidney function, chronically altered renal function (e.g., chronic pyelonephritis) may contribute to hypertension. Cystitis is a bladder problem unrelated to blood pressure. Acute pyelonephritis is a temporary, not a chronic condition.

6. **1** *S. aureus, K. pneumoniae,* and *Proteus* may be found in the urine, but *E. coli* is the most common cause of cystitis or pyelonephritis.

7. **1** An acid-ash diet (e.g., cranberry juice, meats, eggs, cheese, prunes, cranberries, plums, whole grains, vitamin C) acidifies the urine and thus reduces symptoms and the risk of chronic cystitis. Tossed vegetable salad, milk, and apple may cause alkaline urine, which can increase symptoms and the chronic nature of the cystitis.

8. **2** Wiping front to back is the most important behavior to teach. Increasing fluid intake and taking showers rather than baths reduces the risk. An alkaline-ash diet may increase the risk of cystitis.

9. **2** A UTI is identified by bacteria in the urine and, occasionally, by red blood cells; however, the cell count is normal. Glucose and ketones in the urine are not associated with infection.

Section C

10. **4** Reduced production of inhibitors is a risk factor for calculi formation since the inhibitors prevent kidney stone formation. Calcium is the most common stone-forming substance. Mucoproteins provide the structure for the deposition of crystals, which become trapped and form stones. Struvite is a common stone-forming substance for infective stones.

Section D

11. **2** Glomerulonephritis may develop after an untreated beta-hemolytic streptococcal infection. Chronic renal failure and nephrosis are not commonly related to streptococcal infection. Pyelonephritis is most commonly associated with *E. coli* infection.

Section E

12. **3** Postrenal disease is anything that causes obstructions to urinary outflow, which in turn elevates BUN and creatinine levels. Prerenal disease is caused by obstruction to blood flow to the kidney. Bacteriuria is the presence of bacteria in the urine. Hypercalcemia is elevated serum calcium levels in the blood.

13. **1** BUN levels are increased in chronic renal failure. Oliguria and pruritus are later signs of chronic renal failure. Polyuria is not associated with chronic renal failure.

Section F

14. **1** Increased production or reduced clearance IgA in the kidneys is a common cause of IgA nephropathy. IgE is an immunoglobulin found in patients with allergies and is unrelated to IgA nephropathy. IgA nephropathy is an immune disorder unrelated to infection. No known genetic influence on IgA nephropathy exists.

Section G

15. **1** Cigarette smoking is associated with the development of bladder cancer. *E. coli* is the most common cause of cystitis. The most common cause of glomerulonephritis in the United States is IgA nephropathy. IgA nephropathy is a type of acute glomerulonephritis. Polycystic kidney disease is a genetic disorder.

16. **1** A stage I tumor is contained within the renal capsule. Stage II carcinoma spreads through the renal capsule but remains within the surrounding fascia. Stage III carcinoma involves regional lymph nodes, the renal vein, or the vena cava. Stage IV carcinoma involves the spread of the cancer to distant sites.

Notes

Alterations in Genital and Reproductive Function

What You WILL LEARN

After reading this chapter, you will know how to do the following:

- ✔ Describe infectious processes that may affect the male reproductive tract.
- ✔ Compare and contrast the differences between benign prostatic hyperplasia and prostate cancer.
- ✔ Explain the various benign disorders that affect the endometrium and uterus.
- ✔ List the major risk factors for the development of reproductive malignancies.
- ✔ Describe the signs and symptoms of malignancies of the male and female reproductive organs.
- ✔ Identify treatment modalities for the various reproductive disorders.

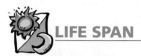

LIFE SPAN

Of male newborns, 2% have a congenital anomaly of the reproductive system.

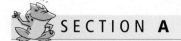

SECTION A

MALE REPRODUCTIVE DISEASES

The male reproductive system produces, sustains, and transports sperm; introduces sperm into the female vagina; and produces hormones. The male gonads (testes) develop within the abdominal cavity and descend into the scrotum before birth. Their position within the scrotum is necessary for the production of viable sperm. Sperm production begins at puberty and continues throughout life.

The male urethra, which is composed of the prostatic urethra, membranous urethra, and penile urethra, is the passageway for sperm, fluids from the reproductive tract, and urine. The seminal vesicles, prostate, and bulbourethral glands secrete fluids that nourish sperm and enhance the motility and viability of the sperm. These structures also help neutralize the acidity of the urethra and vagina, providing lubrication during intercourse.

Three hormones are the primary regulators of male reproductive functioning. Follicle-stimulating hormone (FSH) stimulates the development of sperm (spermatogenesis). Luteinizing hormone (LH) stimulates the production of testosterone. Testosterone, in turn, stimulates the development of male secondary sexual characteristics and sperm production.

What IS Cryptorchidism?

Pathogenesis

Failure of one or both of the testes to descend into the scrotum is known as cryptorchidism. As the male fetus grows, the testes develop in the abdomen. At approximately 7 months' gestation, the testes descend to the upper part of the groin, from which they move into the inguinal canal and then normally descend into the scrotum. However, the descent of the testes may be halted in the abdomen or within the canal. In most cases, only one testis is involved. Testes that remain in the abdomen may not produce the hormones that induce secondary sexual characteristics. A testis lodged in the inguinal canal can induce secondary sex characters but cannot produce spermatozoa. Most testes that have not descended spontaneously at birth do so during the first 6 to 9 months of life. After the first year, spontaneous descent is unlikely to occur.

Most undescended testes are a result of a short spermatic cord, fibrous bands, adhesions in the normal pathway of the testes, or a narrowed inguinal canal. Failure of the testes to descend can also be the result of a congenital gonadal defect that makes the testis insensitive to gonadotropins (the likely explanation for unilateral nondescent), or of a lack of maternal gonadotropins (the likely explanation for bilateral nondescent of prematurity). Research also indicates this condition may be due to abnormalities of the epididymis. Chromosomal studies do not support a genetic cause.

At-Risk Populations

Cryptorchidism is found in 3% of full-term and 30% of premature male infants. The incidence of cryptorchidism in adults is less than 1%.

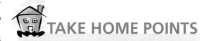

TAKE HOME POINTS

Patients with cryptorchidism or a history of undescended testes have a 35 to 50 times greater risk for testicular cancer in later life compared with the general male population.

What You NEED TO KNOW

Clinical Manifestations

Cryptorchidism may be unilateral or bilateral. Examination of the male genitalia reveals an absence of one or both of the testes in the scrotal sac. The male adult with cryptorchidism may complain of infertility.

Prognosis

The prognosis for the child with cryptorchidism is good. Early repair decreases the risk of infertility, malignancy, and testicular torsion.

What You DO

Treatment

Because cell changes occur in the cryptorchid testis by 1 year of age, the most favorable age for treatment is 9 to 12 months. Treatment usually begins with the administration of human chorionic gonadotropin (HCG), a hormone that may initiate descent and make surgery unnecessary. If hormone therapy is unsuccessful, the testis is located and surgically moved in young children **(orchiopexy).** The surgery is best performed before the patient is 5 to 7 years of age, because operating at a later age can involve more risk to the cells that produce spermatozoa. The testes may be removed entirely (orchiectomy) in children over age 10 and in adults who fail hormone therapy. Testes that are properly placed in the scrotal sac provide adequate hormone function and give the scrotum a normal appearance. A testicular prosthesis is available for patients who have an orchiectomy.

Nursing Responsibilities

For the patient with cryptorchidism, the nurse should do the following:

- Teach the caregivers of young patients how to care for the surgical incision and to watch for the clinical manifestations of infection.
- Advise adult patients on ways to care for the scrotal incision and to notify the health care provider should signs and symptoms of infection appear.
- Elevate the scrotum with a scrotal support to reduce edema and discomfort caused by the surgical incision. Keep the wound clean and dry.

Do You UNDERSTAND?

DIRECTIONS: **Indicate which statements are *true* (T) and which are *false* (F). If false, correct the statement in the margin space to make it true.**

_____ 1. Cryptorchidism is caused by a genetic abnormality.

_____ 2. The treatment for cryptorchidism in a child under age 10 is referred to as an orchiectomy.

_____ 3. Surgical repair of cryptorchidism must be performed after puberty to preserve testicular function.

_____ 4. The risk of testicular cancer in the patient with a history of cryptorchidism is low compared with that of the general male population.

_____ 5. The most favorable age for treatment of cryptorchidism is 9 to 10 months.

Answers: 1. F—cryptorchidism is the result of a short spermatic cord, fibrous bands, or adhesions in the pathway of the testes, or a narrowed inguinal canal; 2. F—treatment of cryptorchidism in a child under age 10 is known as an orchiopexy; 3. F—surgical repair is performed at age 9 to 10 months; 4. F—the risk of testicular cancer is 35 to 50 times greater than that of the general population; 5. T.

What IS Orchitis?

Pathogenesis

Orchitis is a rare, acute inflammation of one or both testes and may be associated with trauma or infection elsewhere in the body. Mumps is the most common cause of orchitis. Infectious organisms can reach the testis through the blood or lymphatics but most commonly by ascent through the urethra, vas deferens, and epididymis. Other disorders that cause orchitis include fungal infections, mycobacterial infections, and syphilis. Occasionally, in middle-aged men, a nonspecific, apparently noninfectious inflammatory process can occur. The inflammation may contribute to the development of a painless collection of fluid along the spermatic cord **(hydrocele).**

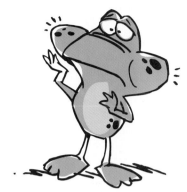

Orchitis occurs in approximately 25% to 38% of postpubertal men, but sterility is rare.

At-Risk Populations

Orchitis is uncommon except as a complication of systemic infection or as an extension of an associated epididymitis.

What You NEED TO KNOW

Clinical Manifestations

Orchitis is unilateral in 75% of cases. Orchitis presents with sudden onset of severe pain and a red, warm, and tender testis, usually occurring 3 to 4 days after the onset of the infection. Other signs and symptoms include high fever, marked prostration, bilateral or unilateral erythema, edema, and tenderness of the scrotum and leukocytosis. The acute phase lasts approximately 1 week. An acute hydrocele may develop. Orchitis is frequently difficult to diagnose because the inflammatory edema and pain of palpation prevent accurate evaluation.

Prognosis

In patients with orchitis secondary to mumps, atrophy with irreversible damage to spermatogenesis may result. Bilateral orchitis does not affect androgenic function but may cause permanent sterility.

What You DO

Treatment

Therapy for orchitis involves administration of the appropriate antimicrobial drugs based on culture and sensitivity reports. Severe infections may require parenteral antimicrobials. Supportive measures include suspending the scrotum in a suspensory or toweling and using hot or cold compresses. Opioids and antiinflammatory drugs are used to reduce pain and inflammation. When an acute hydrocele develops, it is aspirated. Testicular abscess usually requires surgical removal of the testis. Corticosteroids may be necessary in cases of nonspecific, noninfectious inflammatory orchitis.

Nursing Interventions

Because male patients may be reluctant to ask for help, skillful communication techniques are essential to help them express concerns. Be sensitive and give the patient permission to talk about the problem. The nurse should do the following:

- Teach the patient about using hot and cold compresses to control swelling.
- Be aware of the patient's discomfort, administering analgesic and other drugs as ordered.
- Reassure the patient that orchitis is not a threat to androgenic function.

Do You UNDERSTAND?

DIRECTIONS: **Indicate in the space provided which statements are** *true* **(T) and which are** *false* **(F). If false, correct the statement in the margin space to make it true.**

_____ 1. Orchitis is a common disorder in men.

_____ 2. The most common disorder associated with orchitis is mumps.

_____ 3. In all cases, orchitis occurs in both testes.

_____ 4. Bilateral orchitis does not affect androgenic function.

_____ 5. A hydrocele associated with the development of orchitis is treated by aspiration.

Answers: 1. F—orchitis is an uncommon disorder of men; 2. T; 3. F—orchitis can occur unilaterally; 4. T; 5. T.

What IS Epididymitis?

Pathogenesis

Epididymitis is an inflammation of the epididymis that may be chronic or acute in nature. Infection causes most cases of epididymitis. Pathogens reach the epididymis through the vas deferens from infected urine, the distal urethra, or seminal vesicles. In rare cases, heavy lifting or straining can result in reflux of urine from the bladder into the vas deferens and epididymis, with the subsequent development of epididymitis. Urine is also irritating to the epididymis and may initiate an inflammatory response.

At-Risk Populations

Epididymitis generally occurs in sexually active young men under the age of 35 but is uncommon before puberty. When it does occur in prepubescent males, it is often a consequence of genitourinary anomalies. In patients over the age of 35, it may occur as a result of underlying obstructive urinary disease.

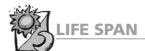

LIFE SPAN

In young men, the cause of epididymitis is usually a sexually transmitted organism such as *Neisseria gonorrhoeae* or *Chlamydia trachomatis* (see Section C in this chapter). Non–sexually transmitted forms typically occur in older men and are associated with intestinal bacteria and *Pseudomonas aeruginosa* from urinary tract infections and prostatitis. Although uncommon, tuberculosis epididymitis can occur in regions in which the incidence of pulmonary tuberculosis is high.

What You NEED TO KNOW

Clinical Manifestations

The main symptoms of epididymitis are scrotal pain and swelling. Acute, severe pain develops in the scrotum and can radiate to the spermatic cord. The spermatic cord may be swollen and tender to palpation. Lower abdominal pain can occur as the urethra passes over the spermatic cord. Pain relief when the inflamed testis and epididymis are elevated is a diagnostic sign of epididymitis **(Phren sign).**

Swelling of the spermatic cord obstructs the urethra. The patient may have pyuria and bacteruria and a history of urinary symptoms, including urethral discharge. The scrotum on the involved side is red and edematous as a result of the inflammatory changes and is tender during palpation. The tail of the epididymis near the lower pole of the testis usually swells first, followed by the head of the epididymis. Fever occurs in approximately 50% of patients, with accompanying nausea and vomiting. A hydrocele may accompany epididymitis.

Prognosis

Complete resolution of swelling and the pain of epididymitis can take from several weeks to months. Complications of epididymitis include abscess formation, testicular necrosis, recurrent infection, and infertility.

What You DO

Treatment

Treatment of epididymitis is directed toward the identified pathogen. Appropriate antimicrobial therapy, bed rest, and scrotal elevation are integral parts of treatment. Scrotal elevation facilitates maximal lymphatic and venous drainage. The patient's sexual partner should be treated with an antimicrobial drug if the causative organism is a sexually transmitted pathogen. Although rare, when an abscess develops it is drained surgically. An orchiectomy may be necessary in some cases, but is usually a treatment of last resort.

Nursing Responsibilities

For the patient with epididymitis, the nurse should do the following:
- Advise the patient to avoid straining while voiding.
- Offer the patient comfort measures such as scrotal elevation and an ice pack.
- Counsel patients with epididymitis from sexually transmitted organisms to contact their partner and advise them of the necessity for treatment.

Do You UNDERSTAND?

DIRECTIONS: **Fill in the blanks to complete the following statements.**
1. Sexually transmitted organisms such as _____ _____ and _____ _____ cause epididymitis.
2. Epididymitis usually occurs in sexually active men under the age of _____.

3. The main symptom of epididymitis is _____.

4. Epididymitis unresponsive to antibiotic therapy may require a surgical procedure known as _____.

What IS Prostatitis?

Pathogenesis

Prostatitis is an inflammation or infection of the prostate gland and occurs in four common forms: acute bacterial, chronic bacterial, nonbacterial, and prostatodynia (pain in the prostate). Prostatitis can result from an ascending urethral infection, reflux of infected urine, extension of a rectal infection, or from hematogenous spread. Pathogens associated with acute and chronic bacterial prostatitis include gram-negative bacilli, *Enterobacter, Klebsiella, Pseudomonas,* and *Proteus.* Gardnerella, chlamydia, and mycoplasma are organisms associated with nonbacterial prostatitis. In nonbacterial prostatitis, the cause may be unknown, or it may be associated with an autoimmune process, an allergic reaction, neuromuscular dysfunction, or a psychologic factor. Prostadynia is not caused by a pathologic condition but by spasms in the genitourinary tract, a disorder of the bladder outlet, or tension in the muscles of the pelvic floor.

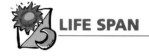

LIFE SPAN

Approximately 50% of older adult men have prostatic inflammation.

At-Risk Populations

Some degree of prostatic inflammation is present in 4% to 36% of the male population. It is the most common urologic disorder in men over the age of 50.

What You NEED TO KNOW

Clinical Manifestations

The signs and symptoms of acute bacterial prostatitis are those of urinary tract infection. Symptoms include painful or difficult urination (**dysuria**) and excessive urinary frequency. The patient may also have a slow, small urinary stream, an inability to empty the bladder, and the

Answers: 1. *Chlamydia trachomatis; Neisseria gonorrhoeae;* 2. 35; 3. pain; 4. orchiectomy.

need to void frequently during the night **(nocturia).** An acute inflammation can cause a urinary obstruction that compresses the urethra. Systemic signs of infection include high fever, fatigue, and joint and muscle pain. Prostatic pain may be present when the patient is in an upright position. Some patients experience low back pain, painful ejaculation, and rectal or perineal pain. Digital rectal examination reveals an extremely tender, swollen, firm, indurated, warm prostate.

Chronic bacterial prostatitis is characterized by recurrent urinary tract infections and persistence of pathogenic bacteria. This form is the most common recurrent urinary tract infection in men. The clinical manifestations are variable and similar to that of acute bladder infection: frequency, urgency, dysuria, perineal discomfort, low back pain, and muscle and joint pain. Physical examination reveals the prostate to be only slightly enlarged or boggy, but fibrosis can cause it to be firm and irregular in shape.

Men with nonbacterial prostatitis may complain of a continuous or sporadic dull ache in the suprapubic, infrapubic, scrotal, penile, or inguinal areas. Other clinical manifestations include pain during ejaculation and urinary symptoms. The prostate gland feels normal during palpation.

Prognosis

Complications associated with acute bacterial prostatitis include urinary retention requiring bladder drainage with a suprapubic catheter, prostatic abscess, epididymitis, bacteremia, and septic shock.

What You DO

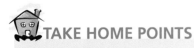

TAKE HOME POINTS

A fluoroquinolone or trimethoprim-sulfamethoxazole antibiotic is used for at least 30 to 42 days to treat patients with acute prostatitis. Men with chronic prostatitis may require continuous, low-dose suppressive therapy, or they may benefit from a radical transurethral prostatectomy.

Treatment

The treatment for prostatitis is based on the cause; thus management of the disease begins with making an accurate diagnosis. In severe cases, the patient is hospitalized and treated with aminoglycoside antibiotics and ampicillin. Analgesics, antipyretics, bed rest, and adequate hydration are also therapeutic. An indwelling, urethral catheter is contraindicated in patients with acute bacterial prostatitis and urinary retention, thus a suprapubic catheter may be required.

No generally accepted treatment for nonbacterial prostatitis is available. Alpha-blockers or anticholinergic drugs may be helpful in some patients.

Other treatments include muscle relaxants, nonsteroidal antiinflammatory drugs (NSAIDs), low-dose anxiolytic drugs, biofeedback, diathermy, exercise, and sitz baths. Evidence of obstruction, an elevated creatinine level, and recurrent infection are clear indications for referral to an urologist.

With the exception of acute bacterial prostatitis, prostatic massage can be helpful for most types of prostatitis. By squeezing out excess secretions, swelling of the gland decreases and thus decreases the patient's pain. Sexual intercourse will also help to drain secretions and should be encouraged.

Nursing Responsibilities

Generally, patients with prostatitis are treated on an outpatient basis. For those patients hospitalized with the condition, the nurse should do the following:

- Monitor creatinine levels. An increase in creatinine levels should be reported to the urologist.
- Encourage the patient to drink plenty of fluids.
- Administer medications as ordered.

Do You UNDERSTAND?

DIRECTIONS: **Indicate which statements are *true* (T) and which are *false* (F). If false, correct the statement in the margin space to make it true.**

_____ 1. Pathogens associated with acute and chronic bacterial prostatitis include gram-negative bacilli, *Enterobacter, Klebsiella, Pseudomonas*, and *Proteus*.

_____ 2. Gardnerella, chlamydia, and mycoplasma are organisms associated with nonbacterial prostatitis.

_____ 3. The clinical manifestations of acute bacterial prostatitis are those of urinary tract infection.

_____ 4. The pain of prostatitis may be present when the patient is supine.

_____ 5. An indwelling, urethral catheter is contraindicated in patients with acute bacterial prostatitis and urinary retention.

Answers: 1. T; 2. T; 3. T; 4. F—the pain of prostatitis is present when the patient is in an upright position; 5. T.

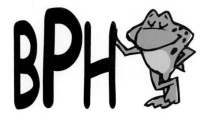

What IS Benign Prostatic Hyperplasia?

Pathogenesis

Benign prostatic hyperplasia (BPH) is an enlargement of the prostate gland. BPH begins in the periurethral glands, the inner portion of the prostate. The prostate enlarges as nodules form and grow, and glandular cells enlarge. The resulting hyperplasia leads to hypertrophy of the gland. Because hyperplasia, not hypertrophy, causes the major prostatic changes, the term *benign prostatic hyperplasia* is preferred. The hyperplastic process results in mechanical obstruction of the urethra as it passes through the prostate. The obstruction of the urethra leads to clinical symptoms of the disease.

During the early stages of BPH, the detrusor muscle hypertrophies to help the bladder force urine out against increasing resistance. As obstruction progresses, the detrusor muscle decompensates, and the bladder is unable to empty all of the urine. Increasing volumes of urine are retained until urinary retention becomes a chronic problem. The amount of urine that is retained can be large to the extent that it produces uncontrollable overflow incontinence with any increase in abdominal pressure.

Progressive bladder distension causes outpouchings in the bladder wall, and some neural degeneration of smooth muscle cells occurs. The ureters may become obstructed, with subsequent development of hydroureters, hydronephrosis, bladder calculi, and bladder or kidney infections.

The causes of BPH are uncertain, but several factors appear to play a role. Changes in hormones associated with the aging process appear to be a contributing factor to this disease. Increased testosterone, increased estrogen, stimulation of alpha-adrenergic nerve endings that interfere with opening of the bladder sphincter, and smoking may all have effects on the gland. Although dihydrotestosterone (DHT) is necessary for normal prostate development, its role in BPH remains unclear.

At-Risk Populations

BPH is the most common benign tumor in men, and its incidence is age-related. The main risk factors are age and the presence of androgens. Other risk factors include a family history of the disease, environment, and diet. Men who consume a diet high in animal fats are more likely to develop this problem.

What You NEED TO KNOW

Clinical Manifestations

Because the disease develops slowly, symptoms are gradual in onset. The symptoms of BPH include reduced or interrupted urinary flow, an inability to empty the bladder, and increased frequency of urination. Most patients have a gradual worsening of obstructive symptoms, including a weak urinary stream, abdominal straining to void, hesitancy, intermittency, incomplete bladder emptying, terminal dribbling, frequency, nocturia, and urgency.

Urinary obstruction can occur in patients who have a small prostate; and conversely, large prostates do not necessarily cause obstruction, which makes diagnosis and treatment difficult. The palpated prostate does not always reveal the degree of BPH because a substantial portion of the enlargement is within the gland itself.

Prognosis

The development of BPH occurs over a prolonged period. Changes within the urinary tract are slow. Reversing progressive BPH is impossible.

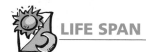

LIFE SPAN

Symptoms of BPH usually begin after age 55, with approximately 25% of men reporting obstructive voiding. At age 75, 50% of men report a decrease in the force of the urinary stream.

What You DO

Treatment

Because BPH is not always progressive, the timing of intervention is variable and depends on the severity of symptoms and the presence of complications. The treatment of BPH ranges from watchful waiting to drug therapy or surgery. BPH is treated with alpha-blocking drugs (**prazosin** and **terazosin**) to relax the smooth muscle of the bladder and prostate. Antiandrogen drugs such as finasteride selectively block androgens at the prostate cellular level and cause the prostate gland to shrink. Hormonal therapy may also be used for less severe symptoms. The 5-α reductase inhibitors such as finasteride block the conversion of hormones to androgen, which causes regression of hyperplastic tissue. In some cases plant extracts can be helpful. Saw palmetto has been shown to improve urinary flow.

Patients with prostate glands weighing over 60 grams are treated with transurethral resections of the prostate (TURP) or laser therapy. Even larger glands are surgically removed **(prostatectomy).** A urinary catheter may be used. The length of time the catheter remains in use depends on the type of surgery, the patient's recovery, and the health care provider's preference. A permanent, indwelling urinary catheter may be inserted for the patient who cannot undergo surgery.

Nursing Responsibilities

Conservative measures for the patient with BPH include advising patients with this problem to avoid alcohol and caffeine, since both of these agents have a diuretic effect and may increase bladder distention. The patient should also follow a planned voiding schedule (usually every 2 to 3 hours) to decrease urinary stasis and acute urinary retention. Teach the patient that over-the-counter cold remedies containing pseudoephedrine and phenylephrine may worsen urinary symptoms. Patients often restrict their fluid intake, believing that this will decrease urinary symptoms; they should be instructed to drink an adequate amount in order to decrease the risk for urinary stasis and infection. Preoperatively, the nurse should do the following:

- Assess the patient's ability to urinate.
- Assess both physical and psychosocial aspects.
- Assess the patient's knowledge base regarding treatment options. The patient may not understand the implications of the many treatment options.
- Encourage the patient and significant other to discuss concerns about sexuality while providing empathic listening, accurate information, and ongoing support. Referral for sexual counseling may be helpful.

Post-operatively, the nurse should do the following:

- Monitor intake and output to evaluate fluid balance. Advise the patient to drink at least 2 liters of fluid daily and to urinate at least every 2 to 3 hours to avoid urinary stasis.
- Maintain patency of the catheter at all times.
- Encourage patients to manage rather than treat postoperative pain.
- Instruct the patient on the proper way to manage urinary irrigation devices and collection bags.
- Teach the patient the proper way to care for the urinary or suprapubic catheter postoperatively. Increase fluid intake while the catheter is in place to promote free flow of urine and minimize clot formation.

- Advise the patient to avoid straining for defecation for 6 weeks after surgery, which can lead to bleeding from the operative site. Administer stool softeners or laxatives as ordered.
- Advise the patient to avoid strenuous activity, heavy lifting, or prolonged periods of travel for 4 to 6 weeks after discharge.

Do You UNDERSTAND?

DIRECTIONS: Fill in the blanks to complete the following statements.

1. Benign prostatic hypertrophy is defined as _____.
2. Benign prostatic hypertrophy is the most common _____ tumor in men.
3. Treatment of BPH includes conservative treatment with _____ _____, _____, or _____.
4. TURP is used for patients whose prostate gland weighs over _____ grams.

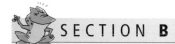

SECTION B

FEMALE REPRODUCTIVE DISEASES

The uterus is a pear-shaped organ consisting of two parts: the body and the cervix. The uterus secures and protects the fertilized ovum, provides an optimal environment while the ovum develops, and pushes the fetus out during delivery. The inner lining of the uterus (**endometrium**) thickens and becomes rich with blood vessels to prepare for the implantation of the fertilized egg. When fertilization does not occur, the endometrium sloughs off as part of the menstrual flow.

The cervix is located at the lower one third of the uterus. The cervix acts as a barrier to microorganisms that may be present in the vagina. The cervical os, through which the child will be born, dilates during labor. It also opens into the vagina to allow menstrual blood to flow out of the uterus during menstruation.

Answers: 1. enlargement of the prostate gland; 2. benign; 3. watchful waiting, medication, surgery; 4. 60.

The fallopian tubes serve as a pathway for the ova from the ovaries to the uterus. Near the end of each fallopian tube is an ovary. The ovaries contain the materials needed to produce ripened eggs (ova). Because hormones regulate ovarian function, any disorder that disrupts hormone secretion or reception by target cells can result in ovarian dysfunction and infertility.

For the menstrual cycle to remain normal and consistent, there must be synchronized interaction between the brain and reproductive organs. The interaction of six hormones produced by the hypothalamus, the anterior pituitary gland, and the ovaries controls menstruation. It is important to understand the effect of hormones on the endometrium and ovaries to implement diagnostic testing correctly and to identify the appropriate treatment when disorders arise.

What IS Dysfunctional Uterine Bleeding?

Pathogenesis

Dysfunctional uterine bleeding (DUB) is excessive, prolonged, irregular bleeding unrelated to structural or systemic disease. This disease may originate as a primary disorder of the ovaries or as a secondary defect in ovarian function related to hypothalamic-pituitary stimulation. Most cases of DUB are the result of anovulatory menstrual cycles that cause high levels of estrogen without the counter-balance of progesterone. The latter can be initiated by emotional stress, marked variation in weight, or nonspecific endocrine or metabolic disturbances. Organic causes of DUB include reproductive tumors, infection, pregnancy complications, endometrial polyps, polycystic ovary syndrome, and pregnancy. Blood dyscrasias (e.g., thrombocytopenia, aplastic anemia, von Willebrand's syndrome) and systemic diseases such as hepatic, adrenal, or pituitary disorders and hyperthyroidism, diabetes, and colorectal cancers can also alter menstrual patterns. Iatrogenic causes of DUB include contraceptives, androgens, anabolic drugs, and hypothalamic depressants.

At-Risk Populations

Dysfunctional bleeding patterns occur in any woman of childbearing age, but tend to occur during the beginning or end of a woman's reproductive life.

What You NEED TO KNOW

Clinical Manifestations

DUB can occur in the following patterns:

- Absence of menses for 6 months, or longer than three of the patient's normal menstrual cycles (amenorrhea)
- Bleeding in which the interval varies from 36 days to 6 months (oligomenorrhea)
- Profuse or prolonged bleeding occurring at regular intervals, lasting more than 7 days and resulting in a blood loss of more than 80 ml in volume (menorrhagia)
- Excessive uterine bleeding that occurs at irregular intervals (menometrorrhagia)
- Bleeding that occurs at regular intervals of less than 21 days (polymenorrhea)

Prognosis

The prognosis for DUB is generally good but is relative to the severity of the disorder. Most patients respond well to pharmacologic therapy.

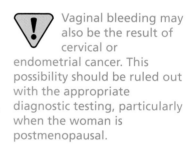

Vaginal bleeding may also be the result of cervical or endometrial cancer. This possibility should be ruled out with the appropriate diagnostic testing, particularly when the woman is postmenopausal.

What You DO

Treatment

When no organic pathologic factor is found for the abnormal bleeding pattern, medical therapy is preferred over surgery. The treatment of choice for DUB is drug therapy. Treatment is based on the need to interrupt the growth of the endometrium and create a hormonal environment that is not conducive to endometrial thickening. The drug regimens may include progestins, estrogens, and NSAIDs. Progestins (e.g., medroxyprogesterone), not only stop endometrial growth, but also support and organize the endometrium, thus sloughing occurs in an organized fashion. When contraception is required, an oral contraceptive accomplishes the same purpose.

When tissue for progestational action is insufficient, or when prolonged intractable bleeding has occurred, estrogen therapy is warranted. Estrogen causes rapid growth of the endometrium and also stimulates clotting at the capillary level. Medroxyprogesterone should be given following the estrogen therapy or concomitantly.

NSAIDs alter the balance between the platelet aggregating substance thromboxane A2 and the antiplatelet substance prostacyclin. Blood loss has been shown to be reduced by as much as 50%.

Other methods used to treat DUB include antifibrinolytic drugs, androgenic steroids, ergot derivatives, desmopressin, and gonadotropin-releasing hormone (GnRH) analogues. The choice of drug therapy is based on factors such as the patient's desire for fertility, extent of bleeding, accompanying symptoms, other medical conditions, side effects, cost, and patient preference.

Patients who don't respond to drug therapy may require a dilation and curettage (D and C) to remove the overgrown endometrial tissues; however, repeated procedures may cause uterine adhesions. Lasers and thermal balloons may also be used to ablate the endometrium and control bleeding. In refractory cases, the woman may ultimately require a hysterectomy.

Nursing Responsibilities

For the patient with DUB, the nurse should do the following:

- Obtain a thorough history that includes the woman's age; age at menarche; a thorough history of menses, including flow, pattern, frequency, duration; sexual history; pregnancies, contraception, and medications (including over-the-counter medications); any type of violence; surgical history; family history; and all lifestyle patterns. The number of pads or tampons used during each period should be estimated. The patient should also be questioned about other symptoms experienced during menses or any abnormal bleeding, premenstrual syndrome, premenstrual breast tenderness, bloating, or cramping.
- Evaluate the patient for anemia, particularly if she has had heavy menstrual cycles for a prolonged period.
- Assess the meaning of menses to the patient and the way in which it affects her view of body image.
- Encourage the patient to achieve a balance between diet and exercise and to keep a chart of each menstrual cycle.
- Instruct the patient on the relationship of emotional stress to the menstrual cycle.

Do You UNDERSTAND?

DIRECTIONS: **Indicate which statements are *true* (T) and which are *false* (F). If false, correct the statement in the margin space to make it true.**

_____   1. The most common treatment for DUB is surgical removal of the ovaries and uterus.

_____   2. DUB occurs only in postmenopausal women.

What IS Amenorrhea?

Pathogenesis

Amenorrhea is the absence of menses. Primary amenorrhea is the failure to menstruate by age 16, or by age 14 when accompanied by the absence of secondary sex characteristics. Faulty gonadal development, congenital agenesis, testicular feminization, or a hypothalamic-pituitary-ovarian axis disorder are usually the causes of primary amenorrhea.

Secondary amenorrhea is the cessation of menses for at least 6 months in a woman who has established normal menstrual cycles. The leading cause of secondary amenorrhea is pregnancy. Other causes of secondary amenorrhea include ovarian, pituitary, or hypothalamic dysfunction, intrauterine adhesions, infections, pituitary tumor, anorexia nervosa, and strenuous physical exercise. When abnormalities in the hormonal function or the structure of the reproductive organs are present, amenorrhea can occur.

At-Risk Populations

The majority of women experience amenorrhea at some time in life.

What You NEED TO KNOW

Clinical Manifestations

The major manifestation of primary and secondary amenorrhea is the absence of menses for 6 months, or longer than three of the patient's normal menstrual cycles.

Prognosis

Successful treatment of amenorrhea depends on the underlying pathologic factors. Amenorrhea may require long-term therapy. Without treatment, infertility can result.

What You DO

Treatment

Treatment for primary amenorrhea involves the correction of any underlying disorder and hormonal replacement to induce the development of secondary sexual characteristics. Depending on the cause of the amenorrhea, treatment may involve hormonal replacement or surgical removal of any adenoma. Surgical alteration of the genitalia may be required to correct abnormalities. Before treatment for secondary amenorrhea can be implemented, pregnancy must be ruled out.

Nursing Responsibilities

For the patient with amenorrhea, the nurse should do the following:
- Educate the patient on the importance of following all treatment plans.
- Teach the patient about the causes and treatment for amenorrhea and the importance of an adequate diet and exercise.
- Instruct the patient to take hormonal replacement therapy as prescribed.

Do You UNDERSTAND?

DIRECTIONS: **Indicate which statements are *true* (T) and which are *false* (F). If false, correct the statement in the margin space to make it true.**

_____   1. Amenorrhea is the occurrence of irregular periods.

_____   2. The leading cause of amenorrhea is menopause.

What IS Dysmenorrhea?

Pathogenesis

Dysmenorrhea is painful menses or severe menstrual cramps. Prostaglandin synthesis at the time of menses produces strong uterine contractions. Contractions constrict blood vessels supplying the uterus, causing ischemia and pain. Excess prostaglandins in smooth muscle also contribute to the gastrointestinal manifestations of dysmenorrhea, such as nausea, vomiting, or diarrhea. Headache is also common.

Primary dysmenorrhea is pain associated with ovulation but not a result of any disease process. Regardless of the cause, the outcome is the same: dysmenorrhea. The most common cause of secondary dysmenorrhea is endometriosis. Other causes include pelvic inflammatory disease, uterine prolapse, fibroids, polyps, invasion of the uterine tissue by endometrial tissue, or the use of an intrauterine device (IUD).

At-Risk Populations

The true incidence and prevalence of dysmenorrhea are unknown, although most women are affected to some degree at one time or another during their lifetime. Risk factors for primary dysmenorrhea include nulliparity, obesity, cigarette smoking, and a positive family history for this disorder. Secondary dysmenorrhea is associated with infections of the pelvis, sexually transmitted diseases, and endometritis.

Answers: 1. F—amenorrhea is the lack of periods; 2. F—the leading cause of amenorrhea is pregnancy.

What You NEED TO KNOW

Clinical Manifestations

Primary dysmenorrhea begins with the onset of ovulatory cycles, increases in severity until the woman is in her mid-20s, and then begins to decline. The symptoms appear within a few hours of the onset of menses and can last from 1 to 2 days. Most discomfort is ordinarily experienced during the first 24 hours of flow. The pain is usually located in the lower abdomen and may radiate to the lower back, labia majora, or inner thighs. Headache, fatigue, nausea, vomiting, or diarrhea may accompany the discomfort. The pain of secondary dysmenorrhea may begin after many years of relatively pain-free menstruation.

Prognosis

Dysmenorrhea may ultimately affect women's productivity and increase absenteeism.

What You DO

Treatment

The treatment of primary dysmenorrhea emphasizes prevention and education. Women who wish to avoid medications use non–drug therapies such as biofeedback, therapeutic touch, or acupuncture. Exercise has been used as a remedy for dysmenorrhea because it increases blood flow of beta-endorphins, thus making them available for pain relief. NSAIDs such as ibuprofen, indomethacin, and naproxen are commonly used to provide relief because they decrease prostaglandin activity. Oral contraceptives may be helpful because they reduce menstrual flow and prevent ovulation. Patients who fail to obtain relief from standard pharmacologic measures may benefit from calcium channel blockers and tocolytic drugs.

Treatment of secondary dysmenorrhea is directed toward the underlying cause. When pelvic inflammatory disease causes dysmenorrhea, identifying the causative organism and selecting the appropriate antimicrobial drug is important. When dysmenorrhea results from the use of an IUD, removal may be warranted.

Nursing Responsibilities

Assessment, education, and the use of supportive measures are important nursing responsibilities in the care for women with primary dysmenorrhea. The nurse should do the following:

- Determine the relationship between pain and bleeding, including the frequency, amount, and duration of menses, and the effect on the patient's activities of daily living.
- Encourage regular exercise, a diet low in fat, and appropriate rest and sleep.
- Advise the patient that local application of heat, massage, relaxation techniques, and orgasm are common comfort measures.
- Educate the patient about the mechanisms involved in dysmenorrhea and the actions and adverse effects of drugs used for therapy.
- Explain the importance of taking all drugs as prescribed and to report any increase in physical discomfort.
- Assess the patient's need for sex education, including the mode of disease transmission, pathologic factors, and consequences of acquiring a sexually transmitted disease.

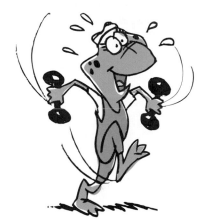

Keep active.

Do You UNDERSTAND?

DIRECTIONS: Fill in the blanks to complete the following statements.

1. Prostaglandin synthesis at the time of menstruation produces strong _____ _____.
2. The most discomfort associated with dysmenorrhea is ordinarily experienced during the first _____ of flow.
3. The primary treatment for dysmenorrhea emphasizes _____ and _____.
4. Advise the patient that local application of _____, _____, _____ _____, and _____ are common comfort measures.

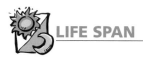

What IS Endometriosis?

Pathogenesis

Endometriosis is a condition in which the tissue that normally lines the uterus (**endometrium**) escapes the uterus and migrates to other area of the body, where it grows. The abnormal tissue growth can develop outside the uterus in the pelvic area, on the ovaries, the fallopian tubes, the bowel, the rectum, and the bladder. Endometriosis frequently occurs in other areas of the body as well.

Endometrial cells implant outside the uterus, where they respond to menses in a manner similar to that of uterine endometrium. At the end of every cycle, when hormones cause the uterus to shed the endometrial lining, endometrial tissue outside the uterus breaks apart, migrates to other areas, and bleeds. The blood has no place to go, thus the surrounding tissues become inflamed or swollen. The continuous cycle of bleeding and healing causes scar tissue to form. Endometrial cells can also penetrate the ovary and multiply, causing ovarian cysts. Repeated episodes of bleeding by ectopic endometrial tissue causes blood to collect in cystlike nodules that are typically bluish-black in color. When these cysts rupture, severe pain may occur. The irritation that results from constant bleeding can cause pelvic adhesions.

At-Risk Populations

Endometriosis is a major cause of dysmenorrhea and infertility, affecting 7% of women, regardless of socioeconomic class, age, or race, during the reproductive years. Endometriosis appears to be hereditary, occurring more commonly in women whose mothers had the disorder.

Factors that increase the risk for endometriosis include heredity, higher estrogen levels, prolonged heavy menses, low weight, and smoking. Oral contraceptive use and pregnancy may reduce the risk of developing endometriosis.

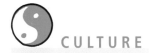

What You NEED TO KNOW

Clinical Manifestations

Many women are unaware that they have endometriosis, although many experience significant symptoms. Over the years, symptoms tend to gradually increase as endometriosis increases in size. Pain is the most common symptom in 50% of patients. The pain occurs as cramping before and during menses, pain after sexual activity, and heavy or irregular bleeding.

Other symptoms include fatigue, painful bowel movements, low back pain with menses, diarrhea or constipation with menses, and intestinal upset. When the bladder is affected, pain during urination and blood in the urine may be present.

Prognosis

Endometriosis is a progressive disease, but the rate of progression and the nature of the lesions vary from patient to patient. The disease can be life-long when symptoms are untreated. Infertility occurs in approximately 25% of patients.

TAKE HOME POINTS

Pain does not correlate with the severity of the endometriosis.

What You DO

Treatment

The objectives of treatment are to remove or destroy the ectopic tissue, relieve symptoms, maintain or restore fertility, and avoid or delay recurrence of the disease. The treatment chosen depends on the manifestations, age, parity, and extent of the disease. In determining the treatment option for endometriosis, the woman's reproductive goals should also be evaluated.

When endometriosis is mild, the woman is provided support, information about the disease, and suggestions for coping with the disorder. Analgesics and NSAIDs can be helpful for those with mild discomfort associated with endometriosis. Drug treatment can last from 2 to 6 months. When a woman is infertile or wishes not to become pregnant, a progesterone-containing oral contraceptive may be used. Progesterone causes the ectopic endometrium to slough off. This drug controls the endometriosis and works as long as the hormone is taken. In some instances, endometriosis can be forced into remission for months or years after this hormone medication is discontinued.

When progesterone therapy is ineffective, danazol may be used. Danazol is a synthetic androgen that suppresses the ovarian-pituitary axis by inhibiting the release of gonadotropins from the pituitary gland.

When severe symptoms are present, removal of the uterus and ovaries may be recommended, which stops menses and therefore stops the symptoms. Although this procedure is considered by some to be an absolute cure, some women experience a recurrence of the disease nonetheless.

Nursing Responsibilities

Nursing responsibilities in the care for the woman with endometriosis are individualized, based on the severity of the patient's manifestations, the severity of the disease, the patient's age, and her childbearing status. The nurse should do the following:

- Discuss the nature of endometriosis, its treatment, and ways to cope with the manifestations.
- Provide information and support in decision making when infertility is present.
- Help the patient find positive ways to cope with the disease and its symptoms.

Do You UNDERSTAND?

DIRECTIONS: **Indicate which statements are *true* (T) and which are *false* (F). If false, correct the statement in the margin space to make it true.**

_____ 1. Mild endometriosis is treated with support and mild analgesics.

_____ 2. Danazol, a synthetic androgen used to treat endometriosis, suppresses the ovarian-pituitary axis by inhibiting the release of gonadotropins from the pituitary gland.

_____ 3. The prognosis for endometriosis has no relationship to the rate of progression and the extent of the lesions.

_____ 4. Pain is the most common symptom of endometriosis.

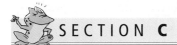

SECTION C

INFECTIOUS DISEASES

Sexually transmitted diseases (STDs) present a major public health problem. STDs include over 25 infectious organisms that are transmitted through sexual activity (vaginal, oral, and anal intercourse). The pathogens that cause STDs may be bacterial or viral. The illnesses they cause may also be due to contact with blood, blood products, or autoinoculation. Most infections begin with lesions on the genitals and other mucous membranes, and from there spread to other parts of the body. All STDs are characterized by a latent or asymptomatic phase.

What IS Chlamydia?

Pathogenesis

Chlamydia is the most common STD in the United States and is caused by the organism *Chlamydia trachomati*. A bacterium with at least 15 variations, chlamydia spreads through lymph channels and lymph nodes. Typically, the site of infection in women is the genital tract in the transition zone of the endocervix. In men, the urethra is the most common site of infection. Incubation is variable but is usually at least 1 week.

Coinfection with gonococci and chlamydiae is common, and postgonococcal urethritis may persist following successful treatment of the gonococcal component. For this reason, the Centers for Disease Control and Prevention (CDC) recommend treating for both chlamydia and gonorrhea when either STD is present.

At-Risk Populations

Chlamydia is common in the United States, particularly among adolescents and young adults. Newborns are at risk for gonococcal ophthalmia from contact with infected vaginal discharge during vaginal birth. This disease is underreported because most people who have it are asymptomatic.

What You NEED TO KNOW

Clinical Manifestations

When they occur, symptoms in men include urethral discharge, swelling and tenderness of the scrotum, fever, rectal discharge, and pain during defecation. Women may experience cervicitis, urethritis, abnormal vaginal bleeding, nausea, and vomiting.

Prognosis

This disease is easily cured with antibiotics. Untreated, this disease may cause pelvic inflammatory disease (PID), chronic pelvic pain, ectopic pregnancy, premature deliveries, and infertility. Reiter's syndrome (reactive arthritis, conjunctivitis, and urethritis) is a complication of untreated chlamydial infection that occurs primarily in men.

What You DO

Treatment

Treatment for uncomplicated urethral, endocervical, or rectal chlamydia infections includes administration of doxycycline or azithromycin. Erythromycin administration is the treatment of choice in pregnant patients.

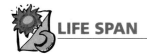

LIFE SPAN

The CDC recommends that all pregnant women be screened for gonorrhea.

What IS Gonorrhea?

Pathogenesis

Gonorrhea is transmitted almost exclusively sexually, because the organism, *Neisseria gonorrhoeae,* cannot survive outside the body. Columnar epithelial tissues in the mucosa are prone to gonococcal infection. The incubation period is 3 to 4 days. The infection may also spread into the uterus and fallopian tubes, which can cause PID. Gonorrhea is the major cause of PID, tubal infertility, ectopic pregnancy, and chronic pelvic pain.

At-Risk Populations

The infection rate is highest in sexually active young adults. The transmission risk from an infected man to a woman is 70% after one exposure.

What You NEED TO KNOW

Clinical Manifestations

Initially, symptoms of gonorrhea may be mild, and a small number of people with the infection are asymptomatic. As the infection progresses, women will experience pain and bleeding with vaginal intercourse, pain and burning with urination, and yellow or bloody vaginal discharge. Men are more likely to be symptomatic than women. Their symptoms will include white, yellow or green-tinged discharge from the penis with pain, severe dysuria, and painful, swollen testicles. Symptoms of rectal infection include pruritus, discharge, painful bowel movements, and stools with frank blood. Symptoms of widespread disease include inflammation of the tendon sheath (tenosynovitis), skin lesions, fever, and multiple joint pains. Widespread disease usually occurs when the infection is acquired during menses or pregnancy. Less common manifestations include endocarditis and perihepatic involvement. Conjunctivitis and progressive corneal ulceration can occur as a result of inoculation into the conjunctiva.

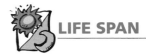

LIFE SPAN

The eyes of newborns may become infected with gonorrhea during a vaginal delivery from an infected mother. For this reason most state health departments mandate newborns be treated with a one-time prophylactic dose of an ophthalmic antibiotic ointment or an aqueous solution of silver nitrate.

Treatment

Gonorrhea in the early stages can be successfully treated with antibiotics. Treatment of adults with uncomplicated gonococcal infections of the cervix, urethra, and rectum include regimens of ceftriaxone, cefixime, ciprofloxacin, or ofloxacin. Retesting following treatment is usually unnecessary.

All sexual contacts made in the 30 days prior to the onset of symptoms should be evaluated and treated. With asymptomatic patients, all sexual contacts made within 60 days should be evaluated and treated. The CDC recommends screening for and treating chlamydia for all persons diagnosed with gonorrhea because the two infections are commonly found together.

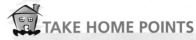

TAKE HOME POINTS

Advise the patient with gonorrhea to refrain from oral sexual activity when a pharyngeal infection is present. A primary measure for controlling gonorrhea is the screening of high-risk women for both chlamydia and gonorrhea.

Prognosis

Without treatment, women will develop PID and infertility. In men, the disease may cause epididymitis, prostatitis, and scarring of the urethra. Occasionally, the infection will spread via the blood to joints, heart valves, and the brain.

What IS Syphilis?

Pathogenesis

Syphilis is a systemic disease caused by the spirochete *Treponema palladium*. The organism penetrates intact skin or mucous membranes during sexual contact, multiplies, and rapidly spreads to regional lymph nodes. The spirochete enters the bloodstream within hours and is transported to other tissues. It is capable of infecting almost any organ or tissue in the body. The incubation period for primary syphilis is approximately 3 weeks but ranges from 10 to 90 days after exposure. Syphilis can be transferred via the placenta from mother to fetus after the tenth week of pregnancy **(congenital syphilis).**

At-Risk Populations

Factors such as limited access to health care, decreases in health department clinical services, increased use of illicit drugs, and contact with multiple sexual partners increase the risk of contracting syphilis. Women of childbearing age, sexually active teens, drug users, inmates of penal institutions, and persons with multiple sex partners are most at risk. Early congenital syphilis occurs from birth to age 2.

What You NEED TO KNOW

Clinical Manifestations

Primary syphilis produces a painless **chancre** at the site of inoculation. The chancre is a solitary macule with a well-defined, indurated border and a clear, red base that becomes encrusted. The chancre frequently goes unnoticed and heals spontaneously. Chancres outside the genitals, such as on the breasts and lips, are usually painful. If treatment is not initiated the disease will progress to the second stage.

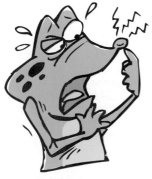

Painful chancre.

Secondary syphilis develops 6 to 8 weeks after exposure and is characterized by enlarged lymph nodes, generalized rash, and influenza-like symptoms. The rash may be macular, maculopapular, or papular, extending to palmar and plantar surfaces. Fever, headache, malaise, fatigue, and muscle or joint pain usually accompanies the rash.

The latent phase begins with healing of the lesions from the secondary stage and may last a few years or a lifetime. After a variable period, approximately 33% of untreated cases develop into tertiary syphilis. Neurologic and cardiovascular disease, soft tumors, auditory or ophthalmic involvement, and cutaneous lesions are characteristics of tertiary syphilis. During the tertiary stage neurologic effects include degeneration of brain tissue, mental deterioration, and progressive locomotor ataxia.

Congenital syphilis is characterized by mucocutaneous lesions, runny nose, and other symptoms. Congenital syphilis can be asymptomatic, particularly in the first weeks of life. Late congenital syphilis is characterized by bone and joint disorders, cardiovascular disease, cranial neuropathies, soft tumors of the liver and respiratory system, and interstitial iritis, which can cause blindness if untreated.

Prognosis

Although syphilis is treatable, reinfection is possible with continued exposure. An infection does not provide lasting immunity to the disease. Blindness is possible in late congenital syphilis, and approximately 28% of patients will die. *T. palladium* may be eradicated with antibiotics even in the late stage of the disease, but unfortunately treatment at this point will not reverse organ and tissue damage that has already occurred.

What You DO

Treatment

The most commonly used tests for syphilis are provided by the Venereal Disease Research Laboratory (VDRL) and rapid plasma reagin (RPR). The fluorescent treponemal antibody absorption (FTA-ABS) test is most widely used. All patients with syphilis should have a human immunodeficiency virus (HIV) test at the time of diagnosis.

Treatment of syphilis is parenterally administered penicillin G. Sexual contacts of patients who are being treated should be evaluated and treated presumptively if their exposure to the patient was within the previous

90 days. Patients with syphilis must abstain from sexual activity until they are found to be uninfected.

Nursing Responsibilities

For the patient with a syphilis, chlamydia, or gonorrhea infection, the nurse should do the following:

- Provide the patient with accurate information about transmission, early detection, treatment, follow-up, reinfection, sequelae, proper hygiene, and safe sexual practices.
- Individualize teaching to meet the patient's needs and psychosocial situation.
- Encourage the patient to complete the entire course of drug therapy and to return for follow-up evaluation.
- Advise the patient to abstain from all sexual contact (intercourse, oral-genital contact, oral-anal contact, or anal penetration) until after the treatment period is completed. All sexual contacts identified within the previous 60 days of exposure should be examined, cultured, and treated.

Do You UNDERSTAND?

DIRECTIONS: Fill in the blanks to complete the following statements.

1. Syphilis is caused by the spirochete known as _____.

2. Persons at high risk for syphilis include the following groups:

   _____

   _____

   _____

   _____

   _____

3. Primary syphilis is characterized by a painless _____ at the site of inoculation.

4. Secondary syphilis occurs approximately 6 to 8 weeks after sexual exposure and is characterized by _____, _____, and _____.

DIRECTIONS: **Write the letter in the space provided that accurately completes each of the following statements.**

_____ 5. Most persons infected with chlamydia are _____.
   a. Symptomatic
   b. Asymptomatic

_____ 6. The site of infection in women typically is the genital tract in the transition zone of the _____.
   a. Endocervix
   b. Ovaries

_____ 7. Anyone with whom the patient has had ongoing sexual exposure within _____ days of a positive test result should be treated.
   a. 60
   b. 120

Fill in the blanks to complete the following statements.

8. Treatment for uncomplicated urethral, endocervical, or rectal chlamydia infections is _____ or _____ administration.

9. The causative organism of gonorrhea is _____ _____.

10. Common sites of infection with the gonococcal organism are the following: _____, _____, _____, _____, and _____ _____.

11. Treatment of adults with uncomplicated gonococcal infections of the cervix, urethra, and rectum include regimens of the following: _____, _____, _____ and _____ _____.

12. All sexual contacts identified within the previous _____ days of exposure should be examined, cultured, and treated presumptively.

What IS Genital Herpes?

Pathogenesis

Genital herpes is the result of the type II herpes simplex virus (HSV2). Two types of herpes simplex viruses exist, both of which cause painful, blisterlike lesions. Type I HSV ordinarily affects the oral cavity but can affect other body areas; type II HSV most often affects the genitalia. Contact with an infected person allows the virus to enter via the mucous membranes or via breaks in the skin. The virus then moves to the peripheral or autonomic nerves and ascends to the ganglia, where it may become dormant. In most cases, the virus persists for life. The presence of the virus predisposes the patient to recurrent outbreaks.

At-Risk Populations

The incidence of active genital herpes is difficult to determine. The difficulty arises because many patients have mild symptoms that are self-limiting and thus are not called to the attention of the health care provider. However, genital herpes affects both genders, is highly contagious, and is transmitted by direct person-to-person contact. Transmission is not limited to sexual contact. Transmission from one person to another via the hands is possible; for example, from a lip ulcer to the genital area or from the lip or genitals to the eye.

Factors that contribute to recurrent herpes outbreaks are not well understood, but exposure to sunlight, local trauma, fever, or emotional stress may precipitate an outbreak. Hormonal changes that precede menses have been associated with recurrences in women.

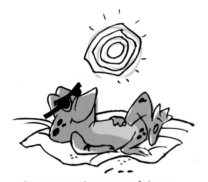

Be smart and stay out of the sun.

What You NEED TO KNOW

Clinical Manifestations

A genital rash and mild itching are usually the earliest signs of genital HSV infection. Eventually, blisters form on the skin surface, enlarge, break open, and ulcerate. The lesions are painful, particularly during intercourse, and can cause intense itching. When the urethra is involved, painful urination can result. In men, the blisters are found on the glans, the shaft of the penis, the prepuce, the scrotum, and the inner thighs. In women, the blisters usually involve the vulva, the vagina, the cervix,

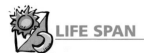

LIFE SPAN

An infant can become infected with genital herpes as the newborn passes through the birth canal. Genital herpes have also been implicated as a cause of cervical cancer.

the perineum, the inner thighs, and the buttocks. The blisters may or may not be present with first exposure to the virus. The blisters usually last from 1 to 3 weeks, with recurrent episodes becoming milder and less frequent. However, some patients may have weekly or monthly outbreaks that are quite painful and severe. Other symptoms include anorexia, malaise, myalgia, lymphadenopathy, and fever.

Because the virus lives in the blisters and nerve cells and not in the blood, antibody titers and cultures taken from the lesions are helpful in identifying the stage of the disease. A culture of the blisters is sensitive and specific for HSV. The presence of HSV antibodies at the time of an initial episode indicates a previous HSV infection. High antibody titers are usually found in patients with recurrent HSV.

Prognosis

Primary genital herpes is usually self-limiting, and immediate complications are rare, barring secondary infection and neurologic damage. Occasionally lower motor neuron damage may cause atonic bladder, impotence, and constipation. Women with genital herpes are 8 times more likely to develop carcinoma in situ than are those who lack HSV2 antibodies in their serum.

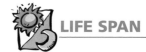
LIFE SPAN

Pregnant women who are having their first episode of HSV infection and have open lesions on their genitals may transmit the virus to the fetus during vaginal delivery. In this case, a cesarean section delivery is indicated.

What You DO

Treatment

Drugs currently used for genital herpes include topical, oral, or intravenous (IV) acyclovir, famciclovir, or valacyclovir. These drugs help shorten the outbreak but do not provide a cure. Treatment goals include keeping the blisters clean and dry, controlling pain with analgesics, promoting healing with frequent sitz baths, and preventing secondary bacterial infections.

Mothers with HSV who have had two negative cervical smears for the virus within 1 week of delivery and those who have no active lesions at the time they go into labor can safely deliver their child vaginally.

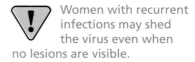
Women with recurrent infections may shed the virus even when no lesions are visible.

Nursing Responsibilities

For the patient with genital herpes, the nurse should do the following:
* Provide accurate information, support, and counseling to help the patient cope with the disease and its effects, including the usual

frequency of recurrence, asymptomatic shedding, and mode of transmission. Inform the patient that the attacks are less frequent and severe as time passes. Recommend abstention from sexual activity while symptoms or lesions are present. Advise patient to inform all sexual partners from time of suspected exposure. Encourage the use of condoms during sexual activity with any new or uninfected partners. Note, however, that condom use does not always prevent viral transmission. Recommend that all sexual partners be evaluated for mild or atypical signs of infection and treated appropriately.

- Instruct the patient to wear loose, cotton clothing to avoid trapping moisture in the genital area. Help the patient find effective coping mechanisms to help control outbreaks.
- Advise the patient to avoid the use of perfumed soaps, feminine deodorant sprays, and douches.
- Assist patients in finding support groups that allow them to express anger and talk about their guilt. The American Social Health Association sponsors self-help groups and provides educational materials.
- Encourage female patients to have a Papanicolaou (Pap) smear every 6 months.
- Instruct the pregnant patient to abstain from intercourse during the last trimester when there is a history of genital herpes in either partner.

Do You UNDERSTAND?

DIRECTIONS: **Circle the correct answer.**

1. Which of the following are symptoms of herpes?

blisters	painless chancre	enlarged lymph nodes
fever	vaginal discharge	pelvic pain
genital rash	dysuria	abnormal vaginal bleeding

Answers: **blisters, genital rash.**

What IS Genital Human Papilloma Virus Infection?

Pathogenesis

Over 100 different strains of the human papillomavirus (HPV) have been identified, and approximately 30 of them may be transmitted by sexual contact. The virus can infect the genital regions of both men and women, as well as the cervix, the vagina, and the rectum. Some of the viral strains carry a high risk of severe disease and have been identified as a causative agent in the development of cancer of the vagina, the vulva, the cervix, the anus and the penis. Other strains may cause mildly abnormal Pap smears and genital warts. Lesions that are characteristic of HPV infection are thought to be the result of growth and replication of infected basal keratinocytes.

At-Risk Populations

Any individual who engages in unprotected sexual intercourse is at risk for becoming infected by this virus.

What You NEED TO KNOW

Clinical Manifestations

In most cases, HPV infections are asymptomatic. Some individuals will develop genital warts, which may be located anywhere within the genital area. The warts are soft, pink, flesh-colored swellings, and may be raised or flat, single lesions or in a group, and are sometimes shaped like a cauliflower.

Prognosis

Genital warts may subside spontaneously, or may be treated with topical drugs. Occasionally surgical excision is necessary, particularly if the warts are blocking the birth canal. Persistent infection with high-risk strains of the virus has been identified as one of the most important risk factors for cervical cancer.

What You DO

Treatment

HPV has no known cure. When genital warts are so large, numerous, or growing in such a location that they require removal, various measures can be used. Topical therapies that may be helpful include 5-fluorouracil cream and a podophyllin solution. Smaller warts may be treated with cryotherapy or electrocautery, and lasers may be used to remove them. If these measures fail, or if the warts are very large, surgery may be needed.

Nursing Responsibilities

For the patient with an HPV infection, the nurse should do the following:
- Advise patients that they may spread the virus to sexual partners and that a condom may help to avoid infection but is by no means fool-proof.
- Teach patients how to apply topical medications. Warn them that some burning and stinging may result, and that relief may be obtained with sitz baths and cold compresses.
- Identify patients who fall into a high-risk category for the development of cancer, and explain the necessity for life-long screening.
- Refer patients to a support group when indicated, since many people will have feelings of fear, shame, and guilt after having contracted a sexually transmitted disease.
- Advise the patient to obtain the HPV vaccine for prevention of HPV as appropriate.

Do You UNDERSTAND?

Directions: **Indicate which statements are *true* (T), and which are *false* (F). If false, correct the statement in the margin space to make it true.**

1. All patients who have HPV infection have genital warts. _____
2. Signs and symptoms of HPV infection include fever, myalgia, nausea, and lower abdominal pain. _____
3. HPV may be cured by taking antiviral medications. _____
4. Many different treatments are available for genital warts. _____

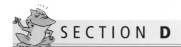

SECTION D

REPRODUCTIVE MALIGNANCIES

What IS Testicular Carcinoma?

Pathogenesis

Germ cells are responsible for sperm production and are the site of almost 98% of testicular tumors. This is the most common solid tumor in men between the ages of 15 to 35. Metastasis occurs primarily through lymphatic spread. Drainage from the right testis is to the interaortic lymphatic system, whereas the left testis drains to the preaortic lymph nodes. Retroperitoneal lymph nodes are commonly affected. The lungs are common sites for distant metastases. The cause of testicular carcinoma is unknown, but congenital and acquired factors have been associated with tumor development. It is more likely to occur in individuals with certain genetic disorders such as Down syndrome. Environmental exposures to chemical agents may also contribute to this disease.

At-Risk Populations

Lack of descent of the testicles and damage to the testicles appear to be common risk factors for testicular carcinoma. The incidence is approximately 2 to 3 cases per 100,000 men in the United States each year.

What You NEED TO KNOW

Clinical Manifestations

Men with testicular tumors experience a painless enlargement in the testis. Some men describe the sensation as a dragging sensation. Pain is rare unless the tumor is found during an examination after injury. A hydrocele or hematocele may develop. Back pain, vague abdominal pain, nausea and vomiting, changes in bowel or bladder patterns, anorexia, and weight loss are common and suggest metastasis to the retroperitoneal lymph nodes. When the lungs are involved, manifestations may include cough, dyspnea, and hemoptysis. Testicular cancer is slightly more common on the right side than it is on the left side.

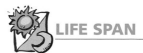

LIFE SPAN

Testicular carcinoma seldom occurs in men younger than age 15 or older than age 40. Men who were extremely physically active in their youth may have an increased risk. Men who have breast development (**gynecomastia**) should also be screened for this disease.

CULTURE

- Caucasians are more likely to develop testicular cancer than African American men. The overall survival rate from all types of testicular cancer is approximately 89% in Caucasians and 78% in African Americans.
- Factors that appear to increase the risk of testicular carcinoma are Caucasian heritage, high socioeconomic status, family history, gonadal dysgenesis, fetal exposure to DES, a synthetic estrogen or oral contraceptives, and a history of orchitis.

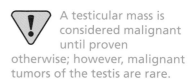

A testicular mass is considered malignant until proven otherwise; however, malignant tumors of the testis are rare.

Prognosis

The cure rate is nearly 100% when this disease is detected in early stages. Tumors of the sexually undifferentiated embryonic gonads (**seminomas**) generally have a favorable prognosis with a 90%, 5-year survival rate, because they are usually localized and metastasize late.

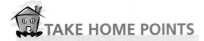

TAKE HOME POINTS

TSE is the most effective strategy for early detection of testicular carcinoma.

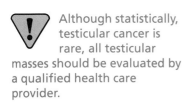

Although statistically, testicular cancer is rare, all testicular masses should be evaluated by a qualified health care provider.

What You DO

Treatment

A removal of the entire testis is the major intervention for testicular carcinoma. Surgery is used because a needle or open biopsy would lead to rapid spread and because after a tumor has been shown to be a solid mass (through ultrasound imaging), the chance of it being malignant is nearly 100%. A decision must be made as to whether to do a lymph node dissection in addition to testicular removal. Antineoplastic or radiation therapy is required for advanced disease.

Nursing Responsibilities

Teach all male patients how to perform a testicular self-examination (TSE) on a monthly basis. For the patient with a diagnosis of testicular cancer, the nurse should do the following:

- Carefully assess the patient's understanding of and readiness for surgery, because the time between diagnosis and surgery may be a few days at most.
- Discuss sperm banking with the patient, because fertility may be impaired postoperatively or as a consequence of antineoplastic or radiation therapy.
- Teach the postoperative patient to monitor for complications (e.g., hematoma, infection) and self-care strategies.
- Recommend the use of ice bags to control scrotal edema. Analgesics are ordered for pain management, usually through the use of a PCA pump or epidural infusion.
- Encourage ambulation as soon as possible to help prevent postoperative phlebitis.

Do You UNDERSTAND?

DIRECTIONS: **Fill in the blanks to complete the following statements.**

1. Metastasis secondary to testicular carcinoma occurs primarily through _____ spread.
2. Factors increasing the risk of testicular carcinoma are _____ heritage, _____ socioeconomic status, family history, gonadal dysgenesis, _____ exposure to DES or oral contraceptives, and a history of _____.
3. Men with testicular tumors experience a _____ enlargement in the testis.
4. The overall survival rate from all types of testicular cancer is about _____% in Caucasians and _____% in African Americans.
5. A radical _____ is the major treatment for testicular carcinoma.

What IS Prostatic Carcinoma?

Pathogenesis

The majority of prostatic cancers are adenocarcinomas. The prostatic tumor begins in the periphery of the posterior lobe of the gland in contrast to BPH, in which the disorder occurs centrally. The lesions are confined to the prostatic capsule and grow slowly. Occasionally, the tumor grows rapidly, with metastasis occurring through direct extension to the bladder neck and seminal vesicles. Other spread occurs through lymphatic and circulatory routes. With advanced disease, metastasis to the bone, the lungs, and the liver is common. The most common sites of bony metastasis are the lumbar spine, the pelvis, the femur, and the skull.

Answers: 1. lymphatic; 2. Caucasian, low, fetal, orchitis; 3. painless; 4. 89, 78; 5. orchiectomy.

CULTURE

African Americans, men with a family history of prostate cancer, those with a history of high dietary fat intake, and perhaps men who have undergone vasectomy are at an increased risk for developing prostatic cancer. Japanese men have low rates of prostate cancer until they migrate to the United States, which suggests dietary habits are a possible risk factor for the disease. A higher incidence is found in urban areas, which suggests an environmental consideration. Occupations linked to higher rates of prostate cancer include employment in fertilizer, textile, and rubber industries, as well as working with cadmium-containing batteries. Gonorrhea is also associated with an increased incidence of prostate cancer.

At-Risk Populations

Prostatic cancer is the most common male cancer and the third leading cause of death among men in the United States. On a global basis, African American males have the highest incidence of prostate cancer, with a much poorer survival rate than is found in Caucasians. Even when there is equal access to health care, African American men tend to have more aggressive disease than their Caucasian counterparts. Other risk factors relate to lifestyle, age, and heredity. Diets high in animal fat and obesity are thought to contribute to the increased incidence of prostate cancer among African American men. Certain carcinogens such as pesticides, smoking, and heavy alcohol abuse are also thought to contribute to the development of this disease. Before the age of 50, prostate cancer is uncommon. When it does occur in younger individuals, the disease is often more aggressive and tends to have a poorer prognosis. Patients who have a first-degree relative (brother or father) with prostate cancer have a greater risk for developing the disease.

What You NEED TO KNOW

Clinical Manifestations

Unless BPH is present at the same time, prostate cancer does not manifest itself on digital examination. The presenting findings are those of prostatitis. Urinary obstruction is rare unless BPH is present. Rectal pressure or obstruction from local tumor growth can produce stool changes and painful bowel movements. Painful ejaculation may also be noted. Many men arrive to be seen at a late stage in their disease, complaining of hip or back pain and possible sensory or motor changes from spinal cord pressure. Lymphatic metastases are usually identified in the obturator lymph node chain. Late in the disease, thrombophlebitis and lower extremity lymphedema may develop.

Prostate-specific antigen (PSA) is a glycoprotein produced in the cytoplasm of benign and malignant prostate cells. PSA measurements can be useful in detecting and staging prostate cancer, monitoring response to treatment, and detecting recurrence before it becomes clinically evident. Approximately 24% of men with moderate elevations of PSA are found to have prostate cancer. Patients with urinary retention or ureteral obstruction from local or regionally advanced prostatic cancers may show elevations in blood urea nitrogen (BUN) or creatinine levels.

Patients with bony metastases may have elevations in alkaline phosphatase or hypercalcemia. Prostatic biopsy and imaging are also used to evaluate and detect prostatic cancer. Metastatic prostate cancer may cause hydronephrosis (due to obstruction of the ureter), bone pain, rectal obstruction, weight loss, defects in coagulation, and suppression of hematopoiesis if the disease invades the bone marrow.

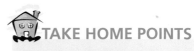

TAKE HOME POINTS

Few forms of prostate cancer become metastatic.

Prognosis

Prostate cancer tends to be diagnosed in men over the age of 50, many of whom will die of other causes before they become symptomatic from prostate cancer.

What You DO

Treatment

Treatment of prostatic cancer remains controversial. The adverse effects of treatment combined with the relatively long life expectancy of many patients with prostate carcinoma makes aggressive treatment an option for only certain patients. Some untreated patients may have a life expectancy equal to or better than that of patients who are treated.

Treatment decisions are based on staging and grading of the tumor and the patient's age. Most patients with an anticipated survival in excess of 10 years should be considered for treatment with irradiation or surgery. Radiation therapy and radical prostatectomy allow for acceptable levels of local control. Radiation therapy may be curative for men with early stage disease. Patients who are candidates for radical prostatectomy are those who have no other serious medical problems, those who have a discrete tumor involving less than one lobe of the prostate, and those who have an expected survival of at least 10 to 15 years.

Certain tumors are sensitive to hormonal manipulation, and may respond well to antiandrogen drugs. For patients with hormone-refractory disease, antineoplastic drugs given singly or in combination have been used to treat or occasionally stabilize the disease. Palliative therapy with oral androgen blockers (e.g., flutamide) and gonadotropin-releasing hormone analogs (e.g., leuprolide) are used in symptomatic patients with advanced disease. Antineoplastic therapy and radiation can also provide additional symptomatic disease relief to patients with advanced disease.

Nursing Responsibilities

Nursing responsibilities for the patient with prostate carcinoma is essentially the same as that for the patient with BPH. However, the psychosocial and emotional care of these patients is different because the issues of cancer must be addressed. Some patients may refuse treatment because of the fear of impotence. These patients need a great deal of emotional support to understand the options available to them. Patients who are on hormonal therapy may experience distressing adverse effects, including gynecomastia, loss of facial hair, vasomotor instability (hot flashes) and impotence, and should be warned of the possibility that they may occur. In addition, the nurse should do the following:

- Advise the patient who is undergoing radiation therapy about the possibility of radiation cystitis, impotence, or proctitis. These adverse effects may not occur until several years after treatment. The patient must learn about the need to control diarrhea and ways to protect the perianal skin surfaces, which can become excoriated. Antidiarrheal drugs may help control diarrhea.
- Teach the patient who is undergoing antineoplastic therapy about the adverse effects of the drugs. Make suggestions about ways to cope with and manage the adverse effects.
- Encourage patients who are receiving antineoplastic therapy to have their blood counts assessed as recommended.
- Provide preoperative and postoperative care as needed. The specifics of care will depend on the procedure used. Generally, care involves close monitoring of surgical wounds, fluid intake, urinary output, and vital signs.
- Teach patients who are going home with a urinary catheter how to care for the device. Urinary incontinence usually occurs after removal of the catheter, but leakage subsides within approximately 6 months in the majority of patients.
- Provide bladder retraining, which may be required for the patient who undergoes laser or cryosurgery of the prostate.
- Instruct patients to prevent strain on the perineal incision. Recommend the use of a scrotal support, T-binder, or mesh pants to prevent wound trauma and to hold the dressing in place.

Do You UNDERSTAND?

DIRECTIONS: **Indicate which statements are** *true* **(T) and which are** *false* **(F). If false, correct the statement in the margin space to make it true.**

_____ 1. The majority of prostatic cancers are seminomas.

_____ 2. With advanced prostate carcinoma, metastasis to the bone, the lungs, and the liver is common.

_____ 3. The PSA can be useful in detecting and staging prostate cancer, monitoring response to treatment, and detecting recurrence before it becomes clinically evident.

_____ 4. The adverse effects of treatment combined with the relatively long life expectancy of many patients with prostate carcinoma make aggressive treatment an option for only certain patients.

_____ 5. Nursing responsibilities for the patient with prostate carcinoma is essentially the same as that for the patient with BPH.

What IS Breast Cancer?

Pathogenesis

Breast cancer is the most commonly occurring solid tumor in women who do not smoke. Like most malignancies, breast cancers are identified based on the characteristics of the breast tissue in which they first started growing, as well as growth patterns of the malignant cells. Usually breast cancer begins in the epithelial lining of the ducts of the breast, or in the epithelium of the lobules. Breast cancer may spread to almost any organ in the body, but it is most likely to metastasize to the bone, the lungs, the lymph nodes, the brain, and the liver. Breast cancer must be treated as a systemic rather than a localized disease because of its ability to spread to other parts of the body very early in the process. Over the last 40 years, the lifetime risk of breast cancer has increased from 1 in every 18 women to 1 in every 8 women. In some cases, breast cancer clusters in families as

Answers: 1. F—the majority of cancers are adenomas; 2. T; 3. T; 4. T; 5. T.

a result of genetic mutations that predispose the individual to the development of cancer.

At-Risk Populations

Many different factors are thought to contribute to the development of breast cancer. No single causative factor for this disease has been identified. Rather, this disease is thought to be the result of a combination of genetics, environment, and lifestyle. Women are much more likely to develop this disease than men, although it does occur in men occasionally, particularly if they have a positive family history of the disease or are obese. Research indicates that there is a strong hormonal connection as well. Women who have early menarche, are nulliparous, or delay their childbearing until after the age of 30 or have late menopause are considered to have a higher risk for the disease. Women who live in developed countries have a higher risk for this disease than those in developing countries. People who emigrate from countries of low risk to regions of higher risk exhibit the higher risk by the third generation, which is a strong argument for an environmental cause.

Obesity is also a contributing factor, particularly in women who have gained 25 kg or more since their teen years. Both high and low doses of ionizing radiation have a carcinogenic effect on breast tissue. This has been well demonstrated in studies of survivors of the atom bomb, as well as patients who have received therapeutic doses of radiation for the treatment of other malignancies.

What You NEED TO KNOW

Clinical Manifestations

In most cases breast cancer is detected as either a palpable mass or radiologic abnormality that shows up on a mammogram. Some breast cancers may cause nipple discharge from one breast that may be clear or bloody. The nipple may become retracted, and the texture of the skin on the breast may begin to look like an orange peel *(peau d'orange)*. Induration and dimpling of the skin over the tumor may also be noted.

Prognosis

Survival rates for breast cancer depend upon many factors, including the stage at the time of diagnosis, the type of breast cancer, growth characteristics of the malignant cells, and the presence of other comorbidities that may affect the patient's ability to undergo treatment. In the year 2000, African American women had a 32% higher death rate from this disease than their Caucasian counterparts. Breast cancer patients under the age of 35 have a worse prognosis than older individuals.

What You DO

Treatment

Therapy depends upon the stage of the disease at the time it was diagnosed, as well as the general health of the patient. Small tumors may be treated with local excision and a course of external radiation. Larger tumors will require wide excision or mastectomy, as well as antineoplastic therapy and radiation to maximize survival.

Nursing Responsibilities

Patient education is an extremely important part of the care of any cancer patient. Help patients facing a cancer diagnosis make an informed decision about their treatment plan. Provide them with the opportunity to ask questions and seek clarification. Because the breasts form an aspect of body image and sexuality, explore possible concerns with the patient and their partner. If the patient has had a mastectomy, allow them to grieve over the change in their body image.

After surgery, monitor incisions for drainage or evidence of infection, and help the patient do range of motion exercises on the affected side if approved by the physician. Teach patients about the risk of lymphedema on the operative side, and instruct them on how to care for the operative arm.

For patients receiving radiation therapy, monitor their skin over the radiated area for evidence of radiation damage. Teach the patient to use only lotions and creams that are approved by the radiation oncologist in order to avoid further damage from topical agents. Monitor lab values, particularly the complete blood count (CBC), for evidence of myelosuppression associated with the radiation therapy. Severe skin reactions or myelosuppression may indicate the patient needs a treatment holiday so that normal tissue can recover.

Patients who are receiving antineoplastic therapy will require monitoring for evidence of myelosuppression, as well as adverse effects associated with antineoplastic therapy. These adverse effects include myocardial damage, photosensitivity, nausea, vomiting, diarrhea, and mouth ulcers, hair loss, and weight gain.

Do You UNDERSTAND?

Directions: Indicate the correct answer.

1. Breast cancer is classified according to all of the following characteristics *except*
   a. The size of the tumor.
   b. Cellular growth rate.
   c. Encapsulation of the tumor.
   d. The presence of metastatic disease.
2. _____ is/are a risk factor for breast cancer.
   a. Multiparity
   b. Nulliparity
   c. Low body mass
   d. Low-fat diets
3. Patients who are receiving chemotherapy should be monitored for
   a. Excessive weight gain.
   b. Hyperkalemia.
   c. Myelosuppression.
   d. All of the above.

What IS Cervical Cancer?

Pathogenesis

Cancer may develop in that portion of the uterus that attaches to the cervix. Malignant transformation of this area is gradual and begins with dysplasia, a precursor to cancer, in which the tissue cells begin to show some abnormalities. These dysplastic cells may evolve into an actual cancer. If the cancer has not spread and is localized, it is called carcinoma in situ. If it has spread only a few millimeters into surrounding tissue, it is described as microinvasive. After this process occurs the cancer may

Answers: 1. *c*; 2. *b*; 3. *c*

spread into close surrounding tissues or may go to distant sites such as the liver, the lungs, the bladder and the intestines. The disease spreads by penetrating the basement membrane to invade the stromal layers of the cervix. The lesion then enlarges and spreads in any direction by direct extension. This tumor is capable of invading the bloodstream and the lymphatic system, which facilitates its ability to invade remote parts of the body. Invasive cervical cancer is classified according to the tissue type of the malignant cells involved. The three main classifications are squamous cell carcinoma, adenocarcinoma, and glassy cell carcinoma.

At-Risk Populations

Infection with the HPV virus is the most significant risk factor for the development of cervical cancer. Genital herpes and chronic chlamydial infections increase risk for this disease. Other contributing factors include immunosuppression (cervical cancer is one of the indicator diseases for acquired immunodeficiency syndrome [AIDS]), age, smoking, exposure to tobacco products, vitamin deficiencies, multiple sexual partners, and sexual activity beginning at an early age. Cervical cancer is almost never found in women who have practiced lifelong celibacy. Women whose mothers took diethylstilbestrol (DES) during pregnancy are at increased risk for clear cell carcinoma of the cervix and the vagina.

What You NEED TO KNOW

Clinical Manifestations

In its earliest and most treatable stage, cervical cancer is asymptomatic. As the disease progresses, the woman may have a watery or mucoid vaginal discharge. Later symptoms of disease progression include postcoital or intramenstrual bleeding and heavy menstrual flow. Symptoms indicative of late-stage disease include pain in the lower abdomen, the lower back, the buttocks, the legs and the pelvis. Foul-smelling mucopurulent vaginal discharge may also occur. Urinary structures may be invaded or compressed by tumor, which will then result in dysuria. With end-stage disease, swelling of the legs may occur, along with massive vaginal hemorrhage and renal failure.

Prognosis

Early-stage cervical cancer has an excellent prognosis for most individuals if appropriate treatment and monitoring is provided. It is a curable disease if it is diagnosed in the early stages. The prognosis is influenced by the stage of the disease at the time of diagnosis, the size and volume of the tumor, the presence of lymphatic and endometrial involvement, and the presence or absence of epidermal growth factors in the tumor.

What You DO

Treatment

Treatment options depend upon the stage of the disease. Very–early stage disease can be treated with a surgical procedure called conization if the woman wishes to preserve fertility. Patients in this circumstance must be followed closely by their health care provider because there is a risk for recurrence. Other treatment modalities include surgery, radiation, and antineoplastic therapy.

Nursing Responsibilities

Early detection and screening with a Pap test can significantly decrease mortality and morbidity associated with this disease. Nurses should encourage women to do the following:

- Begin having Pap tests 3 years after the start of sexual activity or at the age of 21, whichever is earlier.
- Screening should be done on a yearly basis until the age of 30. After that time, women who have had 3 consecutive normal smears may be screened every 2 to 3 years.
- Women with risk factors such as exposure to DES in utero will need more frequent screening.
- Women who have had a total hysterectomy may stop screening unless the surgery was done to treat cervical cancer.

Patients undergoing treatment for cervical cancer require extensive information and education so that they may actively participate in their care. Patient education should include the following:

- Explanation and clarification of the various treatment options in conjunction with the health care provider.

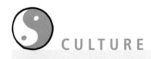

CULTURE

Allow patients to express their fears and concerns regarding their cancer diagnosis. Help them explore alternate ways of expressing sexuality with their partner when necessary.

- Complications and adverse effects associated with treatment, and how to manage and minimize these issues after discharge. Adverse effects of treatment include but are not limited to:
  - Infertility.
  - Sexual dysfunction.
  - Urinary dysfunction.
  - Radiation cystitis.
  - Intestinal malabsorption.

Patients who have undergone a hysterectomy should be monitored postoperatively for bleeding, infection, and urinary dysfunction. If the patient had an exploratory surgery to look for possible metastatic disease in the abdomen, anticipate a possible delay in the return of bowel function. When dissecting out peritoneal lymph nodes, occasionally nerves that innervate the bladder and colon may be traumatized, which in turn can cause problems with urination and bowel elimination.

Mobilize the patient as soon as possible to minimize complications associated with prolonged bed rest and inactivity. When the patient is ready for discharge, instruct her on signs and symptoms of infection, the importance of medical follow-up visits, and activity restrictions. These patients should not drive, engage in strenuous physical activity, or have sexual intercourse until they have the health care provider's approval.

Monitor the CBC of patients receiving radiation therapy for evidence of decreased platelets and white cells. Advise these patients of possible long-term effects of radiation therapy due to scatter beams that affect normal tissue outside of the radiation field. Radiated mucosal tissue may become thinner, more fragile, or fibrotic. Patients who are receiving radiation therapy via an implant may experience vaginal stenosis. These individuals should be instructed to engage in sexual intercourse using a water-based lubricant. Patients who do not have a sexual partner should obtain a vaginal dilator and use it on a daily basis to avoid stenosis of the vagina.

Patients who are receiving antineoplastic drugs may experience pancytopenia, renal damage, and further changes in body image. Monitor them carefully for evidence of bleeding, anemia, infection, and renal compromise.

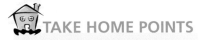

TAKE HOME POINTS

Maintaining patency of the vagina is important in order to preserve the possibility of having a bimanual pelvic exam, which is helpful in the detection of recurrent disease.

Do You Understand?

Directions: **Indicate the correct answer.**

1. The _____ _____ virus may contribute to the development of cervical cancer.

2. Cervical cancer, particularly in young women, is an indicator disease for _____.

3. Annual Pap smears should begin no later than _____ years of age.

4. A patient who had a hysterectomy yesterday now has declining urinary output. The nurse is aware that this may be _____.
   a. A normal finding
   b. Evidence of hypervolemia
   c. A complication of the surgery
   d. None of the above

References

Abeloff MD et al: *Clinical oncology,* Philadelphia, 2004, Churchill Livingstone/ Elsevier.

American Cancer Society: *Cancer facts and figures: 2004,* Atlanta, 2004, Author.

Applegate E: *The anatomy and physiology learning system,* Philadelphia, 2000, WB Saunders.

Centers for Disease Control and Prevention: 1998 guidelines for treatment of sexually transmitted disease, *Morb Mortal Wkly Rep* 47, 1-116: 1998.

Edmunds M, Mayhew M: *Pharmacology for the primary care provider,* St Louis, 2000, Mosby.

Itano JK, Taoka KN: *Core curriculum for oncology nursing,* St Louis, 2005, Saunders/ Elsevier.

McConnell JD: Benign prostatic hyperplasia. In Rake RE: *Conn's current therapy,* Philadelphia, 2000, WB Saunders.

McMillan JA et al: *Oski's pediatrics: principles and practice,* ed 3, Philadelphia, 1998, Lippincott–Williams & Wilkins.

Meredith P, Horan N: *Adult primary care,* Philadelphia, 2000, WB Saunders.

Porth CM: *Pathophysiology: concepts of altered health states,* ed 7, Philadelphia, 2004, Lippincott.

Rakel RE: *Conn's current therapy,* Philadelphia, 1999, WB Saunders.

Schwartz MW: *Clinical handbook of pediatrics,* ed 2, Baltimore, 1999, Williams & Wilkins.

Sherwood L: *Human physiology,* ed 3, Belmont, CA, 1999, West.

Singleton JK et al: *Primary care,* Philadelphia, 1999, Lippincott–Williams & Wilkins.

Answers: **1. human papilloma;** 2. AIDS; 3. 21; 4. c.

NCLEX® Review

Section A

1. The most common symptom of cryptorchidism is
   1 Swelling of the scrotal sac.
   2 Perianal pain.
   3 Undescended testis.
   4 Infertility.

2. Signs of orchitis do *not* include
   1 Severe pain.
   2 High fever.
   3 Infertility.
   4 Edema.

3. Patients at risk for epididymitis include
   1 Men over the age of 50.
   2 Prepubescent males.
   3 Newborn males.
   4 Males between the ages of 12 and 35.

4. The four common forms of prostatitis are
   1 Acute bacterial, chronic bacterial, bacterial, and prostatodynia.
   2 Chronic bacterial, nonbacterial, prostatodynia, and viral.
   3 Acute bacterial, chronic bacterial, nonbacterial, and prostatodynia.
   4 Acute bacterial, chronic viral, nonbacterial, and prostatodynia.

5. The pathophysiologic factors of benign prostatic hyperplasia include
   1 Hypertrophy of the prostatic cells.
   2 Atrophy of prostatic cells.
   3 Stricture of the vas deferens.
   4 Inflammation of the epididymis.

6. The risk of developing benign prostatic hyperplasia _____ as men age.
   1 Decreases
   2 Increases
   3 Stays the same
   4 Increases tenfold

7. The cause of BPH is *not* related to which of the following factors?
   1 Increased testosterone and estrogen levels
   2 Stimulation of alpha-adrenergic nerve endings interfering with opening of the bladder sphincter
   3 Smoking
   4 Alcohol consumption

8. Testicular carcinoma metastasizes most frequently to which organ?
   1 Lung
   2 Brain
   3 Bladder
   4 Liver

9. Risk factors for prostatic carcinoma do *not* include
   1 African American men.
   2 Men who have undergone vasectomy.
   3 Men who work with fertilizer.
   4 Alcoholic men.

Section B

10. Primary dysmenorrhea is defined as
    1 Increased menstruation.
    2 The absence of menstruation.
    3 Painful menstruation.
    4 A symptom of pregnancy.

11. Secondary dysmenorrhea is *not* a result of
    1 Pelvic inflammatory disease.
    2 Adhesions or fibroids.
    3 Endometriosis.
    4 Urinary tract infections.

Section C

12. Recurrent genital herpes infections result from
    1 Reactivation of the virus from sacral dorsal root ganglia.
    2 Activation of virus from genital tissues.
    3 An immune response arising from repeated exposure to the virus.
    4 Reinfection with herpes simplex type I virus.

13. A patient with syphilis who complains of a maculopapular rash on the trunk, palms of the hands, and soles of the feet is most likely in which stage of the disease?
    1 Primary
    2 Secondary
    3 Latent
    4 Tertiary

14. The typical site of chlamydia infection in women is the
    1 Transition zone of the endocervix.
    2 Intrauterine tissue.
    3 Ovaries.
    4 Vulva region.

Section D

15. _____ is a risk factor for the development of testicular cancer.
    1 Prostatitis
    2 Gonorrhea
    3 Cryptorchidism
    4 Excessive testosterone

16. Symptoms of prostate cancer include all of the following *except*
    1 Changes in bowel habits.
    2 Burning urination.
    3 Rectal pressure.
    4 Painful defecation.

17. Obesity is a risk factor for which of the following malignancies?
    1 Breast cancer
    2 Prostate cancer
    3 Bladder cancer
    4 1 and 2 only

18. Patients who have undergone a hysterectomy should be monitored carefully for
    1 Problems with urination.
    2 Abdominal distention due to a paralyzed bowel.
    3 Bleeding.
    4 All of the above.

NCLEX® Review Answers

Section A

1. **3** The most common symptom of cryptorchidism is an undescended testis. The patient with epididymitis is more apt to experience swelling of the scrotal sac. The patient with an enlarged prostate experiences perianal pain. Infertility is a complaint among adult patients of cryptorchidism but is not the most common.

2. **3** Infertility is not a sign of orchitis. Male infertility can be the result of many causes. Severe pain, high fever, and edema are characteristics of orchitis.

3. **4** Epididymitis generally occurs in sexually active young men under the age of 35. To find epididymitis in males before they have experienced puberty is rare.

4. **3** The four common forms of prostatitis are acute bacterial, chronic bacterial, nonbacterial, and prostatodynia.

5. **1** Hypertrophy of prostatic cells is one of the pathophysiologic factors of benign prostatic hyperplasia. Atrophy of prostatic cells does not occur in benign hyperplasia. Stricture of the vas deferens and inflammation of the epididymis are not commonly observed in BPH.

6. **2** The risk of developing BPH increases, does not decrease, with age.

7. **4** The cause of BPH is not related to alcohol consumption, but rather is related to increased testosterone and estrogen levels, stimulation of the alpha-adrenergic nerve endings, which interferes with the bladder sphincter, and smoking.

8. **1** Testicular carcinoma spreads most frequently to the lung. Drainage from the testis enters the interaortic or preaortic lymph nodes. The brain, the bladder, and the liver are rarely affected by testicular carcinoma metastasis.

9. **4** Alcoholics do not appear to be at higher risk for developing prostatic carcinoma than the general population. African American men, men who have undergone a vasectomy, and men who work with fertilizer are at risk for developing prostatic carcinoma.

Section B

10. **3** Primary dysmenorrhea is pain associated with ovulation but is not caused by any disease process. Increased menstruation is known as either menorrhagia or menometrorrhagia. Absence of menstruation is known as amenorrhea. Dysmenorrhea is not a symptom of pregnancy.

11. **4** Urinary tract infections do not cause secondary dysmenorrhea. Secondary dysmenorrhea may be a result of pelvic inflammatory disease, adhesions or fibroids, or endometriosis.

Section C

12. **1** Recurrent genital herpes infections result from reactivation of the virus from sacral dorsal root ganglia. Herpes virus does not reside in the genital tissues. Reinfection does not contribute to recurrent infection. The patient already has the virus. Repeated exposure does not produce the immune response. The immune response is already present.

13. **2** A maculopapular rash on the trunk, the palms of hands, and the soles of feet characterizes the secondary stage of syphilis. Primary syphilis produces a painless chancre at the site of inoculation. Healing of the lesions is characteristic of latent syphilis. Neurologic and cardiovascular disease, soft tumors, auditory or ophthalmic involvement, and cutaneous lesions characterize tertiary syphilis.

14. **1** The transition zone of the endocervix is the typical site of chlamydia infection in women. The other structures (intrauterine tissue, ovaries, vulva region) are not typically associated with chlamydia.

Section D

15. **3** Cryptorchidism and damage to the testicles are the only known risk factors for the development of testicular cancer.

16. **2** Burning urination is indicative of infection, and is not ordinarily a symptom of prostate cancer. The other factors mentioned are due to obstruction that is typically caused by a tumor.

17. **4** Obesity is a risk factor for reproductive organs with glandular tissue, including the breast, the prostate, and the endometrial lining of the uterus.

18. **4** Dissection of the lymph nodes during the surgical procedure may lead to damage or trauma to the nerves that control micturition and defecation. Manipulation of the intestinal contents during surgery and anesthesia may lead to a paralytic ileus. Any surgical patient should be monitored for possible bleeding.

Notes

Alterations in Musculoskeletal Function

What You WILL LEARN

After reading this chapter, you will know how to do the following:

- ✔ Identify the clinical manifestations of a fracture.
- ✔ Compare and contrast a sprain with strains, and bursitis with tendonitis, in terms of their treatment.
- ✔ Relate the common treatment modalities for low back pain.
- ✔ Explain the causes and mechanism associated with the development of gout.
- ✔ Compare and contrast the pathogenesis of osteomalacia with that of osteoporosis, as well as the populations at most risk for the disorders.
- ✔ Compare and contrast osteoarthritis with rheumatoid arthritis in terms of clinical manifestations and treatment modalities.
- ✔ Correlate the treatment modalities for Paget's disease with the pathogenesis of the disorder.
- ✔ Explain the clinical significance of osteomyelitis and its prognosis.

The musculoskeletal system is composed of muscles and bones, together with associated structures such as joints, ligaments, cartilage, and tendons. The function of the musculoskeletal system is to protect internal organs, provide structure and motion, store minerals, and form blood cells. Bone is composed of collagen fibers and mineral salts, such as calcium and phosphorus, making bone the hardest tissue in the body and providing great strength. Bone cells include fibroblasts, fibrocytes, osteocytes, osteoblasts, and osteoclast cells. Fibroblasts and fibrocytes are used for collagen formation. Osteocytes maintain bone matrix. Osteoblasts form new bone tissue, and osteoclasts break down bone tissue. Bone tissue is quite vascular and has the ability for self-repair.

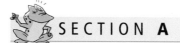

SECTION **A**

SKELETAL AND SOFT TISSUE DISORDERS

What IS a Fracture?

Pathogenesis

A fracture is a break or alteration in the normal contour of a bone. Fractures typically occur as a result of trauma but may also occur from muscle spasm or bone disease. Direct force is the most common cause of fractures.

Several terms are used to describe the type of break in the bone. A *transverse* fracture line is at a 90-degree angle to the longitudinal bone axis. *Spiral* fractures encircle the bone and are usually due to a twisting motion. An *oblique* fracture is diagonal or at a 45-degree angle to the longitudinal bone axis. A *comminuted* fracture involves multiple bone fragments, is most often due to a crushing injury, and is usually accompanied by extensive soft tissue damage of the skin, muscle, nerve tissue, and blood vessels.

Fractures are also classified according to the amount of soft tissue damage. A closed (or **simple**) fracture involves a break in the bone while the skin remains intact. Open (or **compound**) fractures are associated with the protrusion of a bone fragment through the skin.

Open fractures are further classified according to the extent of injury. The least severe injury is known as grade I, which has minimal skin and soft tissue damage associated with the fracture. If a wound is present, it is less than 1 cm in size with minimal contamination. Grade I fractures may be transverse or oblique or may be compound. A grade II fracture is more severe and is accompanied by moderate soft tissue damage and contamination. Grade II fractures are associated with crushing injury, comminuted fracture, and an open wound 1 to 2.4 cm in size. A grade III fracture, the most severe, is usually comminuted and markedly unstable. It is usually associated with extensive soft tissue damage and a large amount of wound contamination.

Bone healing is a five-stage process. The first stage (**hematoma stage**) begins immediately after the injury and lasts approximately 1 day. Bleeding into tissues surrounding the fracture site occurs from ruptured vessels in the bone, torn connective tissue that covers the bone (**periosteum**), and soft tissues. A hematoma forms around the injured site. The body's normal inflammatory response to injury results in vasodilation and edema.

The second stage (**cellular proliferation stage**) occurs 2 to 6 days after the fracture. Fibroblasts from the periosteum and nearby connective tissues enter the injured site and change the hematoma into fibrous connective or granulation tissue. A fibrin mesh is formed that protects the damaged bone and provides structure for capillaries, fibroblast activity, and new bone growth. White blood cells migrate into the injured area to contain the inflammation caused by phagocytosis of the red blood cells and tissue debris.

The third stage (**callus formation stage**) lasts 6 to 10 days. Osteoblasts, which emerge from fibroblasts, invade the clot and granulation tissue to form a soft tissue around the injured site. The granulation tissue changes into newly formed cartilage (**callus**) and bone matrix. The newly formed callus is sufficiently strong to hold bones together but not strong enough for weight-bearing activities.

The fourth stage (**callus ossification stage**) occurs in the period from 2 to 10 weeks after the injury. Calcium salts and cartilage are deposited in the soft-tissue callus, leading to rigid calcification and permanent callus formation.

The fifth stage (**consolidation and remodeling stage**) lasts 2 months to 1 year. Through osteoclastic activity (associated with resorption of bone), bone tissue overgrowth and excess calcium are remolded to the normal bone contour.

At-Risk Populations

Fractures occur in all age groups. The highest incidence of fractures occurs in men ages 15 to 24 and in older adults, particularly women over age 65.

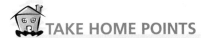

TAKE HOME POINTS

Patients with osteoporosis have a bone density that is inadequate for mechanical support and are at risk for fractures.

What You NEED TO KNOW

Clinical Manifestations

There are many signs and symptoms of a fracture. Fracture pain is usually immediate, continuous, and severe during movement. The major symptom is pain or tenderness on palpation of the site and is related to the rubbing, stretching, and swelling of the periosteum. Pain severity generally increases until the fracture site is splinted and protected. There may be abnormal sensations (paresthesia) as a result of injury from a pinched or severed nerve.

A grating-sound or sensation (crepitus) may be noted as jagged bone ends rub together. Muscle spasms are common and related to sudden involuntary contractions resulting from nerve irritation. Edema is usually present because of the leakage of blood into the tissues (extravasation) and an accumulation of serous fluid at the injury site, both of which contribute to a bruised appearance. When the break involves an arm or leg, the extremity may be in external or internal rotation. The extremity may appear shorter because of an overlapping of bone fragments.

An avulsion fracture occurs when a sudden pull on the tendon occurs. The bone to which the tendon is attached will break (tendons are stronger than bones). Common places for avulsion fractures include the lateral and medial malleolus (from twisted ankles) and the phalanges of the hand (from sports objects being thrown and hitting the ends of the fingers).

Prognosis

The prognosis for the patient with a fracture is usually good. Factors that affect healing are many and include the amount of trauma to surrounding soft tissue, the type of fracture, size of the broken bone, and adequacy of immobilization. Infection, underlying pathologic conditions, bone death (avascular necrosis), patient age, fracture location, stress level, accurate fracture reduction, early remobilization, the amount of circulation and nutrition to injured site, and the general condition of the patient all affect healing. When any of these factors are present, the prognosis is diminished.

LIFE SPAN

- Women over the age of 65 are the group most at risk for osteoporosis, which weakens bone and leaves this group more prone to fractures.
- Fractures in an older adult take longer to heal. Corticosteroid use and the lack of estrogen after menopause tend to decrease the body's ability to form new bone tissue and to heal injured bone.

What You DO

Treatment

Treatment of a fracture includes realignment (**reduction**) of the fractured bone, stabilization during the healing process, and pain management. A fracture should be reduced as soon as possible because soft-tissue swelling tends to increase for 6 to 12 hours after injury and the tissue becomes inelastic with time, making reduction more difficult.

Realignment of bone can be achieved with open or closed reduction or with traction. Closed reduction is accomplished through manual manipulation or reduction traction, which allows for realignment of the broken bones without direct visualization. Closed reduction is indicated when patients are unable to tolerate open reduction. Open reduction involves surgery with direct visualization of the injury and is usually performed within 24 to 48 hours in medically stable patients. Some patients may be unable to undergo open reduction because of the dangers associated with surgical anesthesia.

Reduction traction

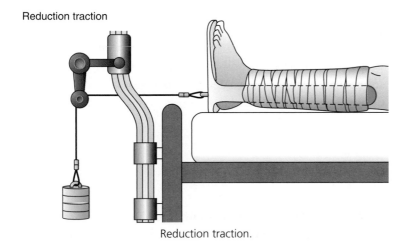

Reduction traction.

Traction may also be used to realign a broken bone. After the fracture is in a normal anatomic position, alignment is maintained by immobilizing the extremity with a cast or splint. Initially, a splint is applied after reduction to allow the injured soft tissue to swell and expand. After the danger period for swelling has passed, a rigid cast that completely encircles the injured part is applied for stabilization.

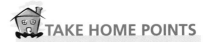

TAKE HOME POINTS

Adequate amounts of exercise stimulate healing. Healthy patients who have adequate nutrition and an exercise regimen heal more quickly than malnourished patients.

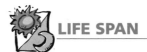

LIFE SPAN

In an older adult who has a fractured femur and fragile bones, and who is a poor surgical candidate, realignment may be achieved by Buck's traction.

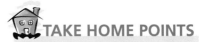

TAKE HOME POINTS

Although used less often today, a wet plaster cast should be handled with the palms rather than with the fingertips and placed on a soft surface to minimize the risk for pressure areas forming inside the cast.

Nursing Responsibilities

The nursing responsibilities for a patient with a fracture begin with initial assessment at the scene of injury or in the emergency department. In addition, the nurse should do the following:

- Evaluate the patient's ABCs (airway, bleeding, and circulation) and the presence of potentially life-threatening injuries.
- Assess the fracture site for deformity, shortening of the extremity, limited or abnormal movement, pain, swelling, diminished neurovascular status, discoloration, soft-tissue damage, or crepitus.
- Immediately immobilize the extremity above and below the fracture site before moving the patient, to prevent further injury.
- Carefully handle the fractured part, because movement and palpation aggravate pain and cause further damage.
- Avoid improper handling of a newly applied plaster cast to avoid leaving indentations in the cast and creating pressure areas under the cast.
- Instruct the patient to keep a plaster cast dry. When a plaster cast becomes wet, strength and integrity are lost, thus the function of support and immobilization is lost.
- Closely monitor and preserve neurovascular status, which prevents complications and restores independent function.
- Control the patient's pain to ensure that exercise and the activities of daily living can be accomplished with ease. Mobilize the patient with an adequate exercise regimen designed to increase circulation, promote healing, and assist in restoring function.

Do You UNDERSTAND?

DIRECTIONS: **Number the five stages of bone healing in order.**

_____   a. Callus ossification
_____   b. Consolidation with remodeling
_____   c. Cellular proliferation
_____   d. Hematoma formation
_____   e. Callus formation

Answers: a. 4; b. 5; c. 2; d. 1; e. 3.

What ARE Sprains and Strains?

Pathogenesis

A sprain is a tear in a ligament at any joint. This injury is usually caused by an abnormal joint movement. Sprains occur most often in the ankle joint with frequent involvement of the wrist, the elbow, and the knee.

In contrast, a strain involves excessive stretching of a muscle beyond normal capacity and the subsequent damage. Areas of the body prone to strains are the shoulder, the elbow, the cervical and lumbar vertebrae, and the feet.

At-Risk Populations

Sprains and strains can occur in any individual. Those at most risk are individuals who engage in vigorous exercise or repetitive muscle overuse. Adolescent athletes who are involved in gymnastics, diving, wrestling, and track are at a high risk for frequent hyperextension sprains.

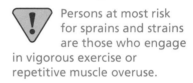

Persons at most risk for sprains and strains are those who engage in vigorous exercise or repetitive muscle overuse.

What You NEED TO KNOW

Clinical Manifestations

The clinical manifestations of a sprain are pain, swelling, discoloration, limited movement, and decreased function. A strain is primarily accompanied by pain, abnormal movement, instability, muscle spasm, and crepitus.

Prognosis

The prognosis of sprains and strains are good. With appropriate treatment and rest, 6 to 8 weeks or longer recovery time is required, depending on the severity of the injury. Collagen bundles begin to form within 4 to 5 days, with strength becoming adequate in approximately 4 to 6 weeks.

What You DO

Treatment

The treatment for sprains and strains is similar. Management of sprains can be remembered by using the acronym RICE (*Rest*, *Ice*, *Compression*, and *Elevation*). Cold packs and elevation are used for 24 to 48 hours after a strain to reduce swelling, with splints to provide support and immobilization. Initially, activity limitations are beneficial. Later, exercise is necessary to increase strength and mobility. Antiinflammatory drugs, skeletal muscle relaxants, and surgical repair are used when needed.

Nursing Responsibilities

For a patient with sprains and strains, the nurse should do the following:

- Advise the patient to elevate and apply ice to the affected area for 24 to 48 hours after the injury to decrease swelling and reduce pain.
- Apply heat after 72 hours for a strain to promote healing and hasten blood resorption.
- Instruct the patient to immobilize the injured part for approximately 2 weeks. Later, partial weight-bearing and rehabilitation exercises are usually begun to regain normal functions.
- Teach the patient how to wrap the affected extremity with an elastic bandage or the proper application of and care of an air-cast.
- Teach the patient how to take nonsteroidal antiinflammatory drugs (NSAIDs) correctly to reduce risk of gastric upset.
- Instruct the patient on the correct use of crutches while non–weight-bearing.

Do You UNDERSTAND?

DIRECTIONS: **Indicate which statements are *true* (T) and which are *false* (F). If false, correct the statement in the margin space to make it true.**

_____ 1. A sprain is extensive stretching of a muscle beyond normal capacity.

_____ 2. A sprain is primarily accompanied by pain, abnormal movement, instability, muscle spasm, and crepitus.

_____ 3. A sprain is primarily accompanied by pain, swelling, discoloration, limited movement, and decreased function.

_____ 4. Treatment of a sprain and strain is to apply ice to the affected area for 24 to 48 hours after injury to decrease swelling and reduce pain.

_____ 5. The prognosis for a strain or sprain remains poor.

What ARE Bursitis and Tendonitis?

Pathogenesis

Bursae are fluid-filled sacs near tendons and ligaments, and over bony prominences. Bursitis is an inflammation of the bursae, which become thickened. The joint most often affected by bursitis is the shoulder, but the elbow, the knee, and the hip are also frequently involved. Bursitis may be due to repeated trauma, overuse, excessive pressure, and various diseases such as gout and rheumatoid arthritis.

Tendonitis is painful inflammation of tendons. Usually tendonitis is caused by misalignment, hypermobility, and crystal deposits in a joint. The most common site of tendonitis is the Achilles tendon.

At-Risk Populations

Individuals between the ages of 40 to 50 are the most affected by bursitis. Risk factors for bursitis and tendonitis include trauma, repetitive activities, joint degeneration, gout, rheumatoid arthritis, and tumors.

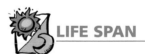 **LIFE SPAN**

Individuals between the ages of 40 to 50 are those most affected by bursitis.

What You NEED TO KNOW

Clinical Manifestations

The clinical manifestations of bursitis and tendonitis include evidence of inflammation, such as localized redness, swelling, warmth, and pain. Interrupted sleep and difficulty with ambulation may also occur.

Prognosis

Most bouts of bursitis heal without sequelae. Repetitive acute bouts may lead to chronic bursitis and necessitate repeated joint/bursal aspirations

Answers: 1. F—extensive stretching of a muscle beyond normal capacity is a strain; 2. F—not a *sprain* but a *strain* is primarily accompanied by pain, abnormal movement, instability, muscle spasm, and crepitus; 3. T; 4. T; 5. F—the prognosis for a strain or sprain is good.

or eventually surgical intervention to remove the involved bursa. The great majority of tendonitis subsides without complications.

What You DO

Treatment

The treatment for bursitis and tendonitis is consistent with the management of inflammation. Appropriate treatment includes rest, immobilization (i.e., sling, splint), elevation, ice packs, NSAIDs, mild analgesics, and corticosteroids (as required). Later, moist heat and range of motion exercises may be used for healing and remobilization.

Nursing Responsibilities

For a patient with bursitis and tendonitis, the nurse should do the following:

- Instruct the patient to reduce undesirable movement, such as repetitive activities.
- Teach the patient to wear oversize clothing and easy closures (i.e., shirts that button in front) to minimize discomfort when dressing.
- Teach the patient to put clothing on affected part first and take it off the affected part last.
- Teach the patient how to take NSAIDs correctly to reduce risk of gastric upset.
- Advise patients to apply ice or moist heat for no more than 20 minutes at a time to minimize the risk of increased pain rather than pain relief.

Do You UNDERSTAND?

DIRECTIONS: Circle predisposing factors of bursitis and tendonitis.

Repetitive activity	Poor eating habits	Dehydration	Trauma	Genetics
Emotional stress	Excess alcohol intake	Living in the tropics	Allergies	Gout

Answers: **Trauma, repetitive activity, gout.**

What IS Low Back Pain?

Pathogenesis

Low back pain is typically described as mild to severe discomfort in the lumbar vertebral area. This condition is usually due to injury from stretching tissues beyond normal capacity. Tissue injury to spinal structures includes bone, joints, ligaments, subcutaneous tissue, muscles, nerves, and blood vessels.

At-Risk Populations

Those who engage in heavy physical labor, strenuous exercise, and repeated stress are at risk for developing low back pain. Repeated stress may be due to improper body mechanics when lifting heavy objects (i.e., leaning forward to lift heavy objects without a strong base of support rather than squatting down with knees to pick it up). A vertebral disk rupture, or herniated nucleus pulposus, after strenuous labor may impinge on spinal nerves or nerve roots, causing pain.

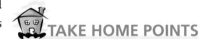

TAKE HOME POINTS

Individuals with weak abdominal and back muscles or who are overweight place added stress on the back and are at risk for low back pain.

What You NEED TO KNOW

Clinical Manifestations

Lower back pain often radiates from the back and buttock area down the sciatic nerve into the posterior thigh to the ankle. Disk herniation may also lead to groin pain. Numbness and tingling **(paresthesia),** muscle spasms, and decreased deep tendon reflexes frequently accompany low back pain. Aching pain upon standing and walking often occur with spinal stenosis.

Prognosis

The prognosis of lower back pain is good. There is a resumption of normal activity without residual symptoms in most cases; however, recovery may be hindered by secondary gain issues. Surgery typically relieves lower back pain faster than medical management.

What You DO

Treatment

The treatment for lower back pain includes cold and heat applications, ultrasonic heat treatments, massage, back brace, exercises to strengthen back and abdominal muscles, stretching exercises, and progressive muscle relaxation exercises. Bed rest on a firm mattress is no longer used in the treatment of low back pain. However, in some cases low back pain may be relieved by placing the patient in a side-lying position with knees flexed, a semi-sitting position, or supine with a pillow under the knees or legs. NSAIDs, short-term opioids, and muscle relaxants may be beneficial to relieve the pain. A transcutaneous electrical nerve stimulator (TENS) may also help to reduce the pain.

Surgical management may include removal of a herniated disk (percutaneous diskectomy), removal of a herniated disk with microsurgical instruments (microdiskectomy), removal of the posterior arch of vertebrae (decompressive laminectomy), spinal fusion, and an artificial disk replacement.

Nursing Responsibilities

For the patient with low back pain, the nurse should do the following:
- Help the patient adjust current lifestyle to reduce the risk of further back injury.
- Teach the patient safe methods to lift and bend.
- Teach the patient how to take NSAIDs correctly to reduce risk of gastric upset.
- Instruct the patient how to logroll after surgery and in the correct use of body mechanics.
- Inform the patient to increase fiber in the diet to reduce constipation when taking opioids.
- Reevaluate the patient who is not recovering for secondary gain issues.
- Encourage the patient to engage in a weight-loss and exercise program.

Do You UNDERSTAND?

DIRECTIONS: Indicate which of the following statements are *true* (T) and which are *false* (F). If false, correct the statement in the margin space to make it true.

_____ 1. A herniated vertebral disk typically causes low back pain.

_____ 2. Tight abdominal muscles place added stress on the back, leading to low back pain.

_____ 3. Medical treatment leads to a faster relief of low back pain than surgery.

What IS Gout?

Pathogenesis

Gout is defined as a metabolic disorder resulting from an overproduction or underexcretion of uric acid. Gout moves through progressive stages. Initially, uric acid levels exceed 7 to 10 mg/dL without other significant signs and symptoms. The asymptomatic stage can last years, with only 20% to 25% of patients progressing to the second stage.

The next stage is called acute gouty arthritis, during which the serum uric acid level exceeds 10 mg/dL. The supersaturation of uric acid in plasma and body fluids leads to urate crystal deposition in joints and surrounding tissue. Urate crystals tend to deposit in cooler body parts, such as fingers or toes. The metatarsophalangeal joint, also known as the great toe, is usually affected.

In the second stage of gout, the body's immune system attacks and treats the crystals as foreign substances. Polymorphonuclear leukocytes (PMNs) permeate the joint and phagocytize the urate crystals. Phagocytosis results in the death of PMNs and the release of lysosomal enzymes, as well as other inflammatory mediators, into surrounding tissues. Ordinarily, at least a 1-year lull exists between the first and second gouty attack. Recurrent attacks increase in frequency over a period of years.

The third stage of gout is the intercritical stage. With appropriate treatment, patients may be asymptomatic for months and up to 10 years.

Answer: 1. T; 2. F—weak abdominal and back muscles cause added stress; 3. F—surgery provides faster relief.

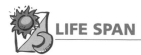

LIFE SPAN

Uric acid elevations usually occur in male adolescents; however, the male population at highest risk is over age 40. In women, gout is delayed until after menopause because estrogens tend to increase the renal excretion of uric acid.

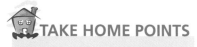

TAKE HOME POINTS

The great toe joint is most commonly affected, causing the patient to awaken at night with excruciating pain. The weight of the bed linens on the great toe is frequently intolerable.

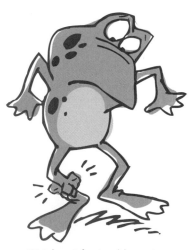

Watch out for trouble spots.

However, when the patient is not treated, the interval between attacks is usually less than 1 year.

The last phase is identified as chronic gout (**chronic tophaceous gout**) and may develop 10 years or more after the first attack. During this stage, chronic inflammation from urate crystals leads to the development of insoluble monosodium urate crystals (**tophi**). Tophi are commonly deposited in synovial membranes, cartilage, soft tissues, tendons, and other tissues that surround joints. Tophaceous gout attacks tend to have a rapid onset, developing over a period of a few hours. Without effective drug treatment, acute attacks may be observed every few weeks.

At-Risk Populations

Predisposing factors that lead to individual attacks of gout include genetics, poor dietary habits, dehydration, trauma, emotional stress, increased alcohol intake, and even several drugs. A diet high in purines can lead to a gout attack if the patient has an inborn faulty metabolism; otherwise, no direct relationship exists.

What You NEED TO KNOW

Clinical Manifestations

The clinical manifestations of gout include a localized inflammatory response that triggers excruciating pain, joint edema, warmth, redness, extreme sensitivity to the slightest touch, and limitation of joint movement. Fatigue, chills, fever, and an increased white blood cell count also accompany gout.

The first attack usually affects only one joint, but as the attacks occur more frequently, the attacks involve other joints and last longer. In later stages, tophi may be present in the helices of the ears and in the hands, the feet, the olecranon bursa, the infrapatellar bursa, and the Achilles tendon. Tophi are generally not painful but may restrict joint movement and cause deformities.

Prognosis

The prognosis for gout is good when successfully managed with a reduction of precipitating factors and drug therapy. If the patient has recurrent gout attacks, a successful adjustment of uric acid levels using antigout or uricosuric drugs is usually effective. Early diagnosis and drug treatment can prevent tophi.

What You DO

Treatment

The treatment for gout includes rest, joint immobilization, elevation of the affected part, cold applications, a low-purine diet, and increased fluid intake. Corticosteroids, the antimitotic drug colchicine, and the NSAID indomethacin are typically used for an acute attack. Colchicine usually resolves symptoms in 48 hours after initiation of oral tablets and 12 hours after intravenous treatment. Xanthine oxidase inhibitors or uricosuric drugs help reduce uric acid levels and are used in chronic gout and prophylaxis. Surgery is usually performed only to remove tophi deposits that have become extremely large and interfere with daily functioning or joint movement.

Nursing Responsibilities

For the patient with gout, the nurse should do the following:
- Emphasize the importance of reducing precipitating factors, such as stress and alcohol use.
- Instruct the patient about resting the affected joint until the acute phase of gout is controlled.
- Advise the patient to avoid sardines, anchovies, liver, and sweetbreads.
- Assist the patient to remain as comfortable as possible during an acute attack.
- Encourage weight reduction, because uric acid levels are higher in overweight people.
- Teach about the importance of diligent drug therapy.
- Monitor uric acid levels and kidney function tests.

Do You UNDERSTAND?

DIRECTIONS: Circle predisposing factors of individual gout attacks.

Genetics	Poor eating habits	Dehydration	Trauma
Emotional stress	Excess alcohol intake	Living in the tropics	Allergies

Answers: **Dehydration, emotional stress, excess alcohol intake, genetics, poor eating habits, trauma.**

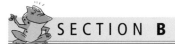

SECTION B

ALTERATIONS IN BONE MASS AND STRUCTURE

What IS Osteoporosis?

Pathogenesis

Osteoporosis is the most common bone disease and is defined as a reduction in bone density. Osteopenia is a decrease in bone mass that is greater than expected for the age, race, or gender of an individual. The primary etiology of osteopenia includes osteoporosis, osteomalacia, neoplasm, and endocrine disorders (i.e., hyperthyroidism). Estrogen stimulates bone growth activity and limits bone breakdown. In osteoporosis, the bone density is below the level required for mechanical support and can lead to fragile bones and fractures. Osteoporosis results from bone breakdown that exceeds the rate of bone formation. The bones are left porous and weaker than normal. The natural drop of estrogen in postmenopausal women is primarily responsible for osteoporosis.

At-Risk Populations

A positive family history of osteoporosis is a major risk factor. Women who have small, thin-framed bodies and who smoke are especially prone to osteoporosis. Men who work underground in large cities and who lead a sedentary life style are also at risk for osteoporosis. These people have limited exposure to sunlight and frequently have significant osteoporosis.

Additional factors predisposing a person to osteoporosis include genetics, the natural aging process, vitamin D and calcium deficiency, high intake of caffeine or alcohol, and hyperthyroidism. More than two cups' worth of caffeine per day in the form of coffee or soft drinks and daily alcoholic beverages cause calcium loss. Excessive corticosteroid therapy also contributes to bone demineralization and breakdown.

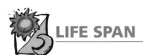

LIFE SPAN

The population at highest risk for osteoporosis is postmenopausal Caucasian women over age 65 although Asian women are also at high risk for osteoporosis.

What You NEED TO KNOW

Clinical Manifestations

The reduction in bone mass associated with osteoporosis is asymptomatic. Frequently though, the first manifestation of osteoporosis is a fracture of the wrist, the forearm, the hip, or vertebrae. Pain is a common complaint, as well as difficulty in bending over. When the rib cage is affected, the patient may have impaired breathing.

Bone density testing and x-rays will show reduced skeletal mass, with trabecular bone more often affected than cortical bone. There is a loss of trabecular connections. Bone marrow is minimal or atrophic.

Prognosis

The prognosis of an individual with osteoporosis is poor because the associated fractures lead to significant morbidity and mortality. Approximately 25% of patients over age 65 die within 1 year of a hip fracture. Of those who survive, 20% require institutional care with an average length of stay of 7 years.

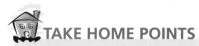

TAKE HOME POINTS

As osteoporosis progresses, the vertebrae become weak and collapse, resulting in a decrease in height, hump back **(kyphosis)**, and pathologic fractures.

What You DO

Treatment

The treatment for osteoporosis includes bisphosphonates, such as alendronate or risedronate, calcitonin, slow-release sodium fluoride, and teriparatide. Biphosphonates bind to calcium-phosphate crystals and inhibit osteoclastic activity. Calcitonin inhibits bone breakdown, and sodium fluoride stimulates bone formation. Teriparatide regulates bone metabolism, intestinal calcium absorption, and renal tubular calcium and phosphate resorption. Estrogen replacement therapy may be used in postmenopausal women to prevent further breakdown of bone mass.

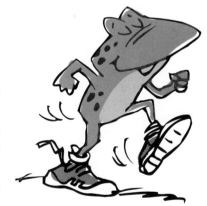

Walking for good posture.

Nursing Responsibilities

For the patient with osteoporosis, the nurse should do the following:

- Teach the patient about risk factors, the importance of weight-bearing exercise (walking or low-impact aerobics), adequate dietary calcium, vitamin D supplements, smoking cessation, and avoiding excess caffeine, alcohol, and soft drinks.

- Help the patient find a balance between rest and activity, while maintaining functional independence.
- Tell the patient to report pain and muscle spasms, which may be managed with analgesics and muscle relaxants.
- Instruct the patient to self-administer teriparatide, when ordered as a subcutaneous injection, to stimulate new bone formation.

Do You UNDERSTAND?

DIRECTIONS: **Circle the bone that most likely would be affected by osteoporosis.**

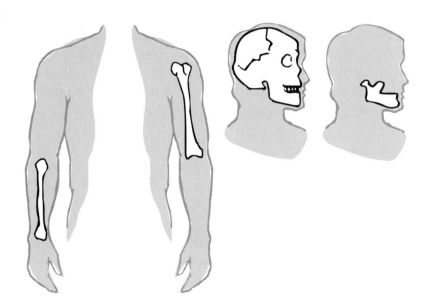

DIRECTIONS: **Circle the beverages that are most likely to predispose an individual to osteoporosis.**

Wine   Orange juice   Coffee   Milk   Pineapple juice

Answers: 1. radius; 2. wine, coffee.

What IS Osteomalacia?

Pathogenesis

The pathogenesis of osteomalacia includes inadequate mineralization of bone matrix by calcium and phosphorous, leading to disorganized bone formation that lacks density. In essence, the bones are softened, but there is no loss of bone matrix. Osteomalacia results from impaired absorption of vitamin D, impaired renal or hepatic activation of vitamin D to an active hormone, dietary deficiency, lack of exposure to sunlight, and malabsorption of fat. Osteomalacia usually affects the ribs, the spine, the pelvis, and the legs. When this disease is present in adults, it is called osteomalacia, and it is called rickets when occurring in children.

At-Risk Populations

Individuals in the northern hemisphere who endure long winters with inadequate exposure to sunlight are at risk. Other high-risk individuals include those with malabsorption syndromes and renal or hepatic disease.

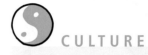

CULTURE

The population at the highest risk for osteomalacia includes people in developing countries. In the United States, osteomalacia is most common in children, pregnant women, or older adults with dietary vitamin D deficiency.

What You NEED TO KNOW

Clinical Manifestations

The clinical manifestations of osteomalacia include bone pain, tenderness on palpation, muscle weakness, and skeletal abnormalities such as short stature, pigeon-breast deformity of the chest, squaring of the head, and swayback (**lumbar lordosis**). Pain usually increases with activity. Bone cysts and fractures of the wrists, ribs, vertebrae, and hips are common.

Prognosis

The prognosis of osteomalacia is fairly good when treatment is begun early. Skeletal deformities may improve or disappear. When osteomalacia is the result of malabsorption or renal or hepatic failure, the prognosis is poor.

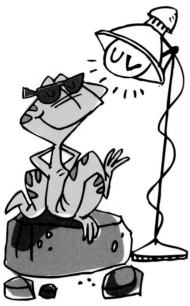

Soaking up the rays.

What You DO

Treatment

The treatment for osteomalacia involves correction of the underlying cause. Exposure to ultraviolet light, calcium and vitamin D supplements, and the replacement of pancreatic enzymes are used in managing rickets and osteomalacia.

Nursing Responsibilities

For the patient with osteomalacia, the nurse should do the following:

- Provide effective pain management.
- Prevent injury.
- Assess the home environment for safety and fall risks.
- Teach the patient and family about a diet that is adequate in calcium and vitamin D.
- Inform the patient of available ambulatory devices.

Do You UNDERSTAND?

DIRECTIONS: **Indicate which statements are *true* (T) and which are *false* (F). If false, correct the statement in the margin space to make it true.**

_____ 1. Osteomalacia is a result of a deficiency of vitamin C.

_____ 2. Bowed legs are the most common skeletal abnormality of osteomalacia.

What IS Osteoarthritis?

Pathogenesis

Osteoarthritis (OA), a degenerative joint disease (DJD), is a progressive, chronic, localized, noninflammatory deterioration that includes loss of

Answers: 1. F—vitamin D and calcium, lack of sunlight exposure, and malabsorption of fat cause osteomalacia; 2. F—short stature, squaring of the head, pigeon-breast, and lumbar lordosis or swayback are characteristics of osteomalacia.

articular cartilage with a proliferation of new bone and soft-tissue growth in and around joints. OA involves the articular cartilage at the end of weight-bearing joints and results from a breakdown of the articular cartilage, which ordinarily cushions bone ends. The most frequently affected joints are the proximal and distal joints of the fingers, lumbar and cervical vertebrae, hips, and knees.

The pathogenesis of OA initially involves enzymatic destruction of articular cartilage. The surface layers of articular cartilage flake off and develop deep cracks. Later in the disease process the articular cartilage erodes entirely, causing the ends of the bone to become thin and unprotected. When eroded bone ends make contact unprotected by cartilage, they rub against each other. This stress on the bone leads to further density, hardness, and proliferation of new bone and soft-tissue growth. The new, but disorganized, bone growth leads to the formation of bone spurs (osteophytes), which alter the contour of the bone and joint. Osteophytes project outward from the bone. Microscopic fractures of the osteophytes result in free-floating fragments within the joint.

> The population most at risk for osteoarthritis includes individuals over the age of 65.

At-Risk Populations

Younger people, athletes, or those with repeated joint trauma are at risk. Repetitive or congenital anomalies, instability, obesity, aging, or disease of the joint are risk factors contributing to OA.

What You NEED TO KNOW

Clinical Manifestations

The signs and symptoms of OA include brief morning stiffness that lasts 15 to 30 minutes, joint pain and swelling that worsens late in the day, limited movement, and crepitus. The symptoms vary from mild to severe, depending on the amount of degeneration that has taken place. When severe OA involves the hand, Heberden's nodes (found on the distal interphalangeal joints) or Bouchard's nodes (found on the proximal interphalangeal joints) develop. As OA progresses, a loss of muscle strength and size occurs, along with an increase of muscle spasms.

Prognosis

The prognosis for OA is good. This disease is chronically progressive, but the treatment is usually well tolerated and significantly improves mobility and the quality of life. Osteoarthritis is less crippling compared with rheumatoid arthritis, which may cause two bone surfaces to fuse, completely immobilizing the joint.

What You DO

Treatment

The treatment for OA involves weight loss, rest, positioning, and reduction of repetitive joint trauma. Surgical interventions include surgical fusion of the joint **(arthrodesis),** transection of the bone **(osteotomy),** and joint replacement. OA is the most common reason for total hip and knee replacement surgeries. Heat applications provide comfort, and cold applications help to reduce pain. Range of motion and isometric exercises are used to strengthen muscles around the affected joints. Oral drug therapy includes NSAIDs and analgesics; in addition, intraarticular glucocorticoid and hyaluronate injections may help some patients. In some cases, glucosamine and chondroitin have been helpful in reducing discomfort.

Nursing Responsibilities

For the patient with OA, the nurse should do the following:
- Provide pain management and maintain joint function and mobility.
- Help the patient find a balance between rest and activity, while maintaining functional independence.
- Monitor the patient for depression, and facilitate a referral as needed.

Do You UNDERSTAND?

DIRECTIONS: **Draw a figure with Bouchard's and Heberden's nodes at the site where they are most commonly found.**

Answers: Bouchard's nodes would be on the proximal interphalangeal joints; Heberden's nodes would be on the distal interphalangeal joints.

What IS Rheumatoid Arthritis?

Pathogenesis

Rheumatoid arthritis (RA) is a chronic, progressive, systemic, inflammatory disorder of connective tissue that affects symmetrical joints. The cause is unknown but is thought to be an autoimmune attack of the patient's own body tissue, a genetic predisposition, or a dormant infection.

RA is a progressive disease in which the immune system mistakes normal tissues for foreign tissues and tries to neutralize and rid the body of the perceived threat. Initially, the synovial membrane becomes inflamed. T cells activate macrophages and B cell–derived antibodies. These autoantibodies produce immune complexes that lead to inflammation. Inflammation of the synovium (synovitis) causes edema and excessive growth of the inflamed membrane. Exudate produced from the inflammatory process oozes into the articular cartilage, forming a fibrous pannus layer. Harder bone tissue replaces the fibrous material that eventually becomes completely immobile (ankylosis).

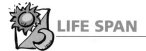
LIFE SPAN

RA that occurs before age 16 is known as juvenile arthritis. Juvenile arthritis usually resolves by adulthood.

At-Risk Populations

The population at the highest risk for RA includes middle-age women, but all age groups and races may be affected.

What You NEED TO KNOW

Clinical Manifestations

The initial manifestations of RA include low-grade fever, fatigue, malaise, anorexia, weight loss, and musculoskeletal pain. Morning stiffness usually lasts 30 minutes to 1 hour. As the disease progresses, joint inflammation occurs with accompanying redness, swelling, warmth, pain, limitation of movement, gait abnormalities, and the development of subcutaneous nodules over bony prominences.

Unlike DJD, which involves asymmetrical joints, in RA symmetrical joints are affected. Usually the hands and feet are affected first, with later involvement of the wrist, elbow, knee, and ankle joints. Joint deformities, such as ulnar deviation, hyperextension of the proximal interphalangeal joint (swan-neck deformity), and flexion of the proximal interphalangeal joint (boutonniere deformity) are characteristic findings of RA.

Prognosis

The prognosis of RA is rather poor because of the progressive joint destruction. Patients with severe RA have a survival rate of less than 50%. Death from RA is usually a result of cardiac, pulmonary, or vascular complications. In addition, deaths from RA may be related to the adverse effects of drug therapy, such as reduced resistance to infection or gastrointestinal (GI) bleeding. Progressive joint destruction can be disrupted with aggressive drug therapy begun early in the disease process.

What You DO

Treatment

Treatment includes rest, heat and cold applications, braces, devices to help with the activities of daily living, and physical therapy. Drug therapy includes NSAIDs, corticosteroids, immunosuppressives, antimalarial drugs, disease-modifying antirheumatic drugs (DMARDs) such as methotrexate, and biologic response modifiers.

Surgical techniques are also performed. A surgical synovectomy to remove the pannus layer and disrupt the inflammatory process is effective for some patients. Surgical total joint replacement is also successful in most patients.

Nursing Responsibilities

For the patient with RA, the nurse should do the following:
- Provide effective pain management and maintain joint function.
- Help with frequent position changes to prevent muscle spasms and contractures, and to minimize stress on joints.
- Help the patient find a proper balance between rest and activity.
- Teach about the disease, weight reduction, proper nutrition, and appropriate exercises.
- When appropriate, provide postoperative care, with attention to maintaining existing system functioning.
- Monitor the patient's complete blood count (CBC) for a decreased white blood cell (WBC) and platelet count from the bone marrow suppression that is an adverse effect of methotrexate.
- Instruct the patient to report oral ulcers and acute dyspnea.

Do You UNDERSTAND?

DIRECTIONS: **Place a check mark next to each sign or symptom of RA.**

_____   1. Low-grade fever
_____   2. Bad breath
_____   3. Swelling of joints
_____   4. Fatigue
_____   5. Tongue thickening
_____   6. Night blindness
_____   7. Joint deformities

What IS Ankylosing Spondylitis?

Pathogenesis

Ankylosing spondylitis is a chronic, progressive disorder involving inflammatory erosions where tendons and ligaments attach to bone. Usually the shoulders, the spine, the hips, the sacroiliac joints, and stabilizing ligaments are involved. The cause of this disease is unknown, but it is thought to have a strong genetic predisposition. *Klebsiella* infection or environmental triggers likely perpetuate the inflammatory response as well.

In ankylosing spondylitis, sacroiliac joint inflammation (sacroiliitis) occurs initially, followed by spinal joint involvement. The sacroiliitis and overgrowth of synovial tissues associated with the accumulation of lymphoid cells following inflammation leads to cartilage destruction and bony erosions. The inflammatory process destroys the articular cartilage on the ends of bones, replacing it with new bone formation. Later in the disease process, the entire spine becomes fused. The sacroiliitis progresses to fibrosis, calcification, and ossification of joints until ligaments are replaced by bone that becomes fixed.

At-Risk Population

The population at risk for ankylosing spondylitis is usually Caucasian men between the ages of 20 and 40.

Answers: **1, 3, 4, and 7.**

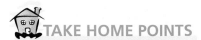

TAKE HOME POINTS

The pain of ankylosing spondylitis improves with exercise and is not relieved by rest.

What You NEED TO KNOW

Clinical Manifestations

Initially, the clinical manifestations of ankylosing spondylitis include early morning stiffness and chronic hip or low back pain. Later in the disease process, the low back pain progresses upward in the spine with a loss of spinal movement. Leg or buttock pain and leg weakness may also develop.

Systemic inflammatory effects, such as fatigue, malaise, low-grade fever, and weight loss occur. Patients may experience chest pain resulting from thoracic compression. With spinal fusion, increased forward curvature of the spine (kyphosis), and thoracic compression, cardiac, pulmonary, and GI involvement usually occur.

Prognosis

The prognosis for the patient with ankylosing spondylitis is poor. Over a 10- to 20-year period, the patient begins to flex the knees and hips in an effort to hold the head upright.

What You DO

Treatment

The treatment for ankylosing spondylitis includes the application of heat, resting joints, proper posture and positioning, and physical therapy. An exercise program that includes breathing exercises and mobility exercises is appropriate. Weight loss may help to reduce joint stress. Drug therapy includes NSAIDs and other analgesics, sulfasalazine, corticosteroids, DMARDs, and biologic response modifiers. Reconstructive surgery includes osteotomy, cervical spinal fusion, or total joint replacement.

Nursing Responsibilities

For the patient with ankylosing spondylitis, the nurse should do the following:
- Assist the patient in obtaining physical therapy services to help maintain proper posture.
- Encourage the patient and family to maintain an exercise regimen within the patient's abilities to maintain existing systems' functioning.

- Encourage the patient to stop smoking to decrease pulmonary complications.
- Monitor the patient's heart rate, rhythm, and respiratory status.
- Monitor the functioning of the patient's GI tract for evidence of worsening compression.
- Instruct the patient to sleep on a firm mattress in a supine position, using a small pillow, to promote sleep and control pain.
- Inform the patient that swimming is an exercise option to enhance muscle tone without creating joint stress.

Do You UNDERSTAND?

DIRECTIONS: **Write the letter in the space provided that accurately completes each of the following statements.**

_____ 1. In ankylosing spondylitis, pain is _____ at rest.
   a. Better
   b. Worse

_____ 2. Ankylosing spondylitis has _____.
   a. Local effects
   b. Systemic effects

_____ 3. After 20 years of ankylosing spondylitis, the patient has a _____.
   a. Bowed-leg position
   b. Stooped position

What IS Paget's Disease?

Pathogenesis

Paget's disease is the second most common bone disorder in the United States and usually affects the skull, the spine, the pelvis, and the long bones. The cause of Paget's disease is unknown. Theories suggest that genetic predisposition leads to a dormant skeletal infection.

Answers: **1. b; 2. b; 3. b.**

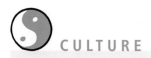

In the initial stages of the disease, rapid breakdown of bone occurs, followed by short periods of abnormal excessive bone formation. The rapid breakdown produces cavities in the bone that lead to frail bones. Newly formed bone is high in minerals but poorly constructed, resulting in bone that is thick but soft, hypertrophic, structurally weak, and deformed. The affected bone develops a greater blood supply to support its high metabolic demands. The risk of pathologic fracture is increased.

At-Risk Populations

The population at highest risk for Paget's disease is men over the age of 50.

What You NEED TO KNOW

Clinical Manifestations

The majority of patients with Paget's disease are asymptomatic (approximately 80%). Typically, the patient is diagnosed incidentally during routine laboratory or x-ray tests. When present, the clinical manifestations of Paget's disease include severe, persistent bone pain, stiffness, and pathologic fractures. Bowed-leg deformities lead to gait disturbances, such as a waddling gait. A thickening of cranial bones leads to skull enlargement, a change in the shape of the skull, and compression of cranial nerves. When the skull thickens and enlarges, the patient may complain that hats no longer fit properly. Cranial nerve compression can cause dizziness, headaches, blindness, facial paralysis, tinnitus, hearing loss, and mental deterioration. Bone deformity contributes to the complication of arthritis. Increased vascularity and high metabolic demands lead to complications of hypertension and cardiac failure.

Prognosis

The prognosis of a patient with Paget's disease depends on the degree of involvement. Because Paget's disease is gradual, most patients are unaware they have the disorder. Some patients have skeletal deformities but are asymptomatic and without pain. In the majority of patients, the deformities involve the skull or the long bones, contributing to cranial damage or bowed legs.

What You DO

Treatment

The treatment of Paget's disease includes preventing and treating fractures, pain, and deformities. Analgesics are used for the pain and NSAIDs are used to decrease the inflammation associated with bone breakdown. Bisphosphonates (i.e., alendronate, risedronate, etidronate, and tiludronate) prevent bone breakdown, thus decreasing the fracture risk. Etidronate produces rapid reduction in bone turnover and pain relief, thereby promoting disease remission. Calcitonin is used to slow the rate of bone breakdown. Mithramycin (Plicamycin) is a cytotoxic antineoplastic drug used in severe cases to control the disease and gives remission for months after the drug is discontinued.

Nursing Responsibilities

For the patient with Paget's disease, the nurse should do the following:
- Assess for and manage pain. Heat and gentle massage may be indicated.
- Teach patient strengthening exercises.
- Monitor drug levels, CBC, and liver enzymes' levels for early detection of toxicities.
- Assess for fatigue; specific skeletal alterations, such as shortened stature, enlarged skull, and bowed legs; and pathologic fractures.
- Counsel the patient and family safety about precautions to prevent falls and fractures.
- Teach the basic first-aid measures as necessary should fractures or injuries occur.
- Monitor for complications of Paget's disease such as cranial or spinal cord compression, hypertension, and cardiac failure.
- Instruct the patient as to the proper technique for taking the bisphosphonate drugs to reduce the risk of esophageal erosions and gastritis.

Do You UNDERSTAND?

DIRECTIONS: Select the outcome(s) from the following list and fill in the blanks.

Waddling gait disturbances	Hypertension	Cardiac failure
Diabetes	Sarcoidosis	Sore throat

1. Bowed-leg deformity of Paget's disease leads to _____

   _____.

2. Increased vascularity of bone affected by Paget's disease leads to

   _____ and _____.

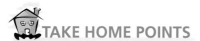

SECTION C

INFECTIOUS PROCESSES

What IS Osteomyelitis?

Pathogenesis

Osteomyelitis is an infection of the bone with progressive inflammatory bone destruction, which results most frequently from *Staphylococcus aureus* invading bone tissue. The second most common invading bacteria are gram-negative bacteria. Fungi have also been implicated as a causative microorganism in osteomyelitis.

Bacteria may also travel through the blood from a distant body site, such as an abscessed tooth, the sinuses or the upper respiratory tract, the middle ear, the gastrointestinal or the urinary tract, soft-tissue trauma, pressure sores, or burns.

Osteomyelitis begins with the introduction and adherence of bacteria to bone matrix. In the adherent state, bacteria are highly resistant to antibiotics. When bacteria invade the skeletal blood supply, an inflammatory response is triggered in the confined space. Drainage that results from the inflammation process enters the bone marrow, which forms abscess pockets. Because of the disruption in blood supply, the bone tissue

TAKE HOME POINTS

In osteomyelitis, bacteria may enter the bone directly from a fracture or wound or as a result of surgery, or they may travel through blood from another infection in the body.

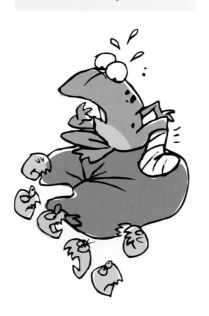

Answers: **1. waddling gait disturbances; 2. hypertension, cardiac failure.**

becomes necrotic. Ordinarily, the rapidly growing long bones of the tibia, the femur, and the humerus are affected.

At-Risk Populations

Males are at greater risk than females for osteomyelitis. Other risk factors include renal or hepatic dysfunction, alcoholism, malnutrition, and immunosuppression.

What You NEED TO KNOW

Clinical Manifestations

The clinical manifestations of osteomyelitis initially include vague pain in the affected extremity or back for 1 to 3 months. Later in the infection process, fever, chills, malaise, irritability, localized tenderness, redness, warmth in affected area, swelling, enlarged proximal lymph nodes, muscle spasm, and bone pain develop.

Prognosis

The prognosis for osteomyelitis is usually good. In severe cases, bone and joint deformity or a halt of bone growth can occur. Amputation is occasionally required to prevent the spread of bacteria throughout the body.

What You DO

Treatment

The treatments for osteomyelitis include long-term antibiotic therapy, surgical drainage and debridement of necrotic bone and, in some cases, bone grafting. The antibiotics used to treat *S. aureus* infections include nafcillin and cefazolin. Antibiotics that treat gram-negative bacteria include the third-generation cephalosporins, the aminoglycosides, and ciprofloxacin, a fluoroquinolone. Hyperbaric oxygen therapy may be used to increase tissue perfusion and treat anaerobic infections. The debridement of bone tissue may create cavities, which may be corrected with bone grafts or bone segment transfers. Donor sites usually include the patient's posterior ileum and fibula. Amputation may be required if necrosis of the bone is extensive.

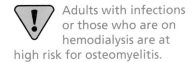

LIFE SPAN

The population at highest risk for osteomyelitis is children under 12 years of age and adults over 50 years of age.

Adults with infections or those who are on hemodialysis are at high risk for osteomyelitis.

Nursing Responsibilities

For patients with osteomyelitis, the nurse should do the following:

- Encourage good hand-washing practices and contact precautions to prevent transferring the bacteria to others.
- Administer antibiotic therapy as prescribed.
- Assist with dressing changes as needed.
- Provide effective pain management and assistance with avoiding immobility complications.
- Teach the patient to perform exercises that help maintain strength and joint flexibility.

Do You UNDERSTAND?

DIRECTIONS: **Indicate which statements are *true* (T) and which are *false* (F). If false, correct the statement in the margin space to make it true.**

_____ 1. Osteomyelitis is usually found in elderly adults.

_____ 2. Osteomyelitis can be the result of bacteria entering an abscessed tooth.

_____ 3. Osteomyelitis is an infection of the bone resulting from food poisoning.

_____ 4. Vague pain is usually the initial symptom of osteomyelitis.

References

Chen S et al: Pain and rheumatoid arthritis: an update, *Drug Topics* 144(7):47, 2000.

Copstead L, Banasik J: *Pathophysiology,* ed 3, Philadelphia, 2005, Saunders.

Fauci A et al: *Harrison's principles of internal medicine,* ed 14, St Louis, 1998, McGraw-Hill.

Ignatavicius D, Workman M: *Medical-surgical nursing across the health care continuum,* ed 3, Philadelphia, 1999, Saunders.

McCance K, Huether S: *Pathophysiology: the biologic basis for disease in adults and children,* ed 4, St Louis, 2002, Mosby.

Maher A, Salmond S, Pellino T: *Orthopedic nursing,* ed 2, Philadelphia, 1998, WB Saunders.

Answers: 1. F, 2. T, 3. F, 4. T.

Phipps W et al: *Medical-surgical nursing: health and illness perspectives,* ed 7, St Louis, 2003, Mosby.

Porth C: *Pathophysiology: concepts of altered health states,* ed 7, Philadelphia, 2005, Lippincott Williams & Wilkins.

Price S, Wilson L: *Pathophysiology: clinical concepts of disease processes,* ed 6, St Louis, 2003, Mosby.

Reeves C, Roux G, Lockhart R: *Medical-surgical nursing,* St Louis, 1999, McGraw-Hill.

Smeltzer S, Bare B: *Brunner and Suddarth's textbook of medical-surgical nursing,* ed 10, Philadelphia, 2004, Lippincott Williams & Wilkins.

NCLEX® Review

Section A

1. The stage of bone healing when the hematoma becomes strong granulation tissue is in the
   1 Callus ossification stage.
   2 Cellular proliferation stage.
   3 Callus formation stage.
   4 Cellular consolidation stage.

2. Match the terms in Column A to their definitions in Column B.

Column A	Column B
_____ 1. Spiral	a. Involves multiple bone fragments
_____ 2. Transverse	b. Usually due to a twisting motion
_____ 3. Comminuted	c. Fracture line is at 90-degree angle
_____ 4. Oblique	d. Fracture is diagonal to longitudinal axis of bone

3. Circle those of the following statements regarding sprain types of injury that are true. (More than one statement may be correct.)
   1 A sprain is a tear in a ligament at any joint.
   2 A sprain involves excessive stretching of a muscle beyond normal capacity.
   3 The clinical manifestations of a sprain include pain, swelling, discoloration, limited movement, and decreased function.
   4 Sprains most often involve the shoulder, the elbow, the lumbar vertebrae, and the feet.

4. Risk factors for bursitis and tendonitis include which of the following? (More than one answer may be correct.)
   1 Trauma
   2 Repetitive activities
   3 Joint degeneration
   4 Tumors
   5 Rheumatoid arthritis
   6 Gout
   7 Alcohol intake
   8 Diabetes mellitus

5. The pathophysiologic factors of gout involve
   1 Autoimmune lesions of collagen tissue.
   2 Increase of uric acid level in the blood.
   3 Inflammation of the synovial membrane in a joint.
   4 Cartilage and bone eroding the narrow joint spaces.

Section B

6. Which of the following populations has the highest risk for osteoporosis?
   1 Postmenopausal Asian women over age 65
   2 Postmenopausal Black women over age 65
   3 Postmenopausal Caucasian women over age 65
   4 Postmenopausal Native American women over age 65

7. Circle the description or descriptions of the underlying cause(s) of osteomalacia. (More than one answer may be correct.)
   1 Impaired absorption of vitamin D
   2 Impaired renal or hepatic activation of vitamin D
   3 Dietary deficiency of vitamin D
   4 Exposure to natural sunlight
   5 Malabsorption of fat in the diet

8. In rheumatoid arthritis, the changes in joints begins in the
   1 Tophi.
   2 Bursae.
   3 Cartilage.
   4 Synovium.

9. The pathophysiologic changes in osteoarthritis involve
   1 Faulty purine metabolism.
   2 Uric acid crystals that trigger a phagocytic response by leukocytes.
   3 A thick layer of granulation pannus tissue that covers and invades articular cartilage.
   4 Joint ends repeatedly hitting together, leading to a loss of joint matrix and erosion of cartilage.

10. Which of the following statements is true regarding the clinical manifestations of ankylosing spondylitis?
    1 Stiffness occurs late in the afternoon at the hip and low back.
    2 The back pain progresses downward with increased flexibility of thoracic vertebrae.
    3 Patients may experience chest pain resulting from thoracic compression.
    4 GI involvement does not usually occur.

11. Although patients with Paget's disease are often asymptomatic, the clinical manifestations of the disorder include which of the following? (More than one answer may be correct.)
    1 Severe, persistent bone pain and stiffness
    2 Pathologic fractures and a change in hat size
    3 Bowed-leg deformities with waddling gait
    4 Dizziness, headaches, facial paralysis
    5 Hearing loss and tinnitus

Section C

12. Osteomyelitis is an infection of the bone with progressive inflammatory bone destruction. The infection is most often caused by
    1 *Klebsiella pneumoniae.*
    2 *Staphylococcus aureus.*
    3 *Staphylococcus epidermis.*
    4 *Vibrio cholerae.*s

NCLEX® Review Answers

Section A

1. **2** Strong granulation tissue forms from the hematoma in the cellular proliferation stage of bone healing. No callus ossification stage exists in bone healing. The granulation tissue changes into newly formed cartilage during the callus formation stage. The calcium salts and cartilage are deposited in the soft-tissue callus, leading to rigid calcification and permanent callus formation in the cellular consolidation stage.

2. **1.** b

2. **2.** c

2. **3.** a

2. **4.** d

3. **1, 3, 4** Number 2 is incorrect because a sprain does not involve stretching of a muscle beyond normal capacity.

4. **1-6** These are risk factors for the development of bursitis and tendonitis. Alcohol intake is a risk factor in the development of gout. Diabetes mellitus is not related to bursitis and tendonitis.

5. **2** The pathophysiologic factors of gout involve an increase of uric acid level in the blood. Autoimmune lesions of collagen tissue are found in a variety of connective tissue disorders but not gout. Inflammation of the synovial membrane is associated with rheumatoid arthritis. Cartilage and bone erosion is associated with osteoarthritis.

Section B

6. **3** Postmenopausal Caucasian women over age 65 are at highest risk for osteoporosis as are Asian women. There is no evidence that Native American women are at a higher risk because of their ethnic background.

7. **1-5** All correct; all of these factors contribute to the development of osteomalacia.

8. **4** Changes for rheumatoid arthritis begin in the joint synovium. Tophi formation is related to elevated uric acid levels, not rheumatoid arthritis. The bursae and cartilage are not initially involved in rheumatoid arthritis.

9. **4** The pathophysiologic changes in osteoarthritis involve joint ends repeatedly rubbing together, leading to a loss of joint matrix and erosion of cartilage. Faulty purine metabolism and uric acid crystals triggering a phagocytic response by leukocytes are found in the patient with gout. A thick layer of granulation pannus tissue, which covers and invades articular cartilage, is associated with rheumatoid arthritis, not osteoarthritis.

10. **3** Patients may experience chest pain from thoracic compression. The back pain of ankylosing spondylitis progresses upward, with decreased flexibility of the lumbar vertebrae. Patients have stiffness in the morning at the hip and lower back. GI involvement usually occurs.

11. **1-6** All are correct; patients with Paget's disease may complain of all of these changes.

Section C

12. **3** *S. aureus* is the most common organism associated with osteomyelitis. *K. pneumoniae* is associated with asymptomatic bacteruria, pyelonephritis, and urinary tract infections in men and women. *S. epidermis* has been associated with osteomyelitis but is not the most common organism. *V. cholerae* is associated with acute gastroenteritis.

Notes

Alterations in Visual and Auditory Function

What You WILL LEARN

After reading this chapter, you will know how to do the following:

- ✔ Identify the risk factors for macular degeneration and possible steps to reduce those risks.
- ✔ Identify the population at most risk for retinal detachment and the significance of early intervention.
- ✔ Compare and contrast cataracts with glaucoma in terms of pathogenesis, clinical manifestations, and treatment modalities.
- ✔ Compare the eye structures commonly associated with dacryocystitis, hordeolum, conjunctivitis, keratitis, and blepharitis.
- ✔ Correlate the treatment of otosclerosis with the pathogenesis of the disorder.
- ✔ Discuss the prognosis and treatment of the patient who has Ménière's disease.
- ✔ Compare and contrast acute otitis externa with that of acute otitis media in terms of onset, offending organism, location of pain, discharge, swelling, and complications.

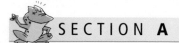

SECTION A

DISORDERS OF THE EYE

What IS Macular Degeneration?

Most cases of macular degeneration appear in people 50 to 60 years of age (**age-related macular degeneration**). Age-related macular degeneration is one of the most common causes of vision loss in older adults and is the leading cause of irreversible, severe visual loss in persons over 65 years of age. Stargardt's macular degeneration is present at the time of birth (**congenital**).

Pathogenesis

Macular degeneration is a breakdown of cells in the macula and surrounding tissues of the eye. The result of the degeneration is loss of central vision in the affected eye. The exact cause of macular degeneration is unknown in approximately 75% of cases.

Two stages of macular degeneration have been identified: "dry" and "wet." Both stages are bilateral and progressive. The "dry," atrophic stage of macular degeneration is characterized by a decrease in the size of normally developed eye tissues with degeneration of the outer retina and underlying structures. Deposits of material from the pigmented epithelial cells produce yellowish-white spots on the retina. Eventually, these spots increase, enlarge, and may calcify.

The "wet," exudative stage of macular degeneration involves the choroid, the layer immediately beneath the pigmented epithelial cell layer of the retina. When this layer is involved, a serous fluid leak with accompanying growth of choroidal blood vessels is noted. When the fovea is involved, central vision is lost.

At-Risk Populations

Exposure to sunlight without wearing sunglasses is a risk factor for macular degeneration. Other risk factors for the development of macular degeneration include a diet low in antioxidant nutrients, cigarette smoking, a blue or light iris color, and hyperopia, hypertension, or other circulatory problems. Macular degeneration may be hereditary.

What You NEED TO KNOW

Clinical Manifestations

The clinical manifestation of macular degeneration is a loss of central vision. The patient may also note a blurred spot in the central field of vision and scotomas. Scotomas are areas of vision loss or depressed vision within the visual field that are surrounded by other areas of less depressed or normal vision. The leakage of serous fluid from the choroid produces a blurred, wavy distortion of vision. On Amsler grid testing, the horizontal or vertical lines may become broken, distorted, or missing.

Yellowish round spots (drusen) may be observed on the retina and macula using an ophthalmoscope. A dome-shaped deposit of retinal pigment epithelium may also be present.

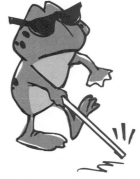

Macular degeneration can lead to blindness.

Prognosis

Currently, nothing can be done to prevent, stop, or reverse the process of macular degeneration. However, the condition does not progress to total blindness and is usually self-limiting.

What You DO

Treatment

Because the majority of cases of macular degeneration cannot be stopped or treated, care involves making the most of the vision that the patient has. A diet high in vitamins A, E, C, and beta-carotene along with zinc may be of benefit. Eating dark green, leafy vegetables (spinach or collard greens) that are rich in carotinoids may decrease the risk of developing the exudative stage of macular degeneration. Consumption of omega-3 fatty acids found in fish decreases the risk of macular degeneration when the patient's intake of linoleic acid is low. Occasionally, damage from "wet" macular degeneration can be stopped with the use of argon lasers, although laser treatment in this area results in a blind spot. The only helpful treatment when the fovea is involved is low-vision aids.

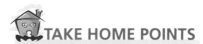

TAKE HOME POINTS

Macular degeneration is a progressive disorder resulting in loss of central vision. Patient safety becomes a primary consideration.

Nursing Responsibilities

For the patient with macular degeneration, the nurse should do the following:

- Identify yourself to the patient with each contact.
- Assess the patient for visual changes in both eyes. Explain to the patient that an extremely bright light may be noted when the eye is dilated for examination.
- Assist the patient in coping with the fears and reality of vision loss and adapting to changes in vision.
- Teach the patient the proper way to use Amsler's grid at home for evaluating the progression of macular degeneration.
- Assist the patient in maximizing remaining vision by using low-vision aids (e.g., large-print books and newspapers, magnifying television screens, programmable telephone equipment).
- Provide the patient with information about community resources and low-vision support groups (e.g., American Association for the Blind, National Industries for the Blind).
- Provide the patient and family with information about the disorder and strategies to promote safety measures in the home (e.g., avoiding throw rugs; keeping furniture and belongings in the same place; removing unnecessary furniture; installing handrails in hallways and bathrooms and on steps; obtaining pill organizers; "marking off" dials on stoves and microwaves with special tape or colors; obtaining special lighting).
- Avoid raising your voice to the patient; vision-impaired patients are not hearing-impaired.

Do You UNDERSTAND?

DIRECTIONS: **Identify five nursing measures that should be implemented to increase a visually impaired patient's safety and comfort.**

1. _____
2. _____
3. _____
4. _____
5. _____

TAKE HOME POINTS

Ophthamologist: a physician who specializes in the diagnosis and treatment of eye diseases and conditions.
Optometrist: a person qualified to carry out eye examinations and to prescribe and supply glasses and contact lenses.
Optician: a person who fits and supplies glasses and contact lenses but who does not examine eyes or prescribe corrective lenses.
Oculist: a person who makes and prepares lens for placement in glass frames.

Answers: 1. *Identify yourself to the patient with each contact*; 2. teach the patient the correct way to use a chart at home for evaluating macular degeneration (Amsler's grid); 3. help the patient maximize remaining vision with low-vision aids; 4. advise patient and family to examine the home for possible unsafe situations; 5. *avoid raising your voice to the patient.*

What IS Retinal Detachment?

Pathogenesis

Retinal detachment is characterized by a separation of the sensory retina from the underlying retinal pigment epithelium. In the most common type, vitreous fluid gains access to the space beneath the retina. Retinal holes and tears usually occur from spontaneous vitreous traction, but abnormal adhesions may be present between the retina and vitreous body secondary to diabetic retinopathy, injury, or other ocular disorders. Atrophy of the vitreous body may also result in a retinal tear.

The liquid seeps through the hole and separates the retina from its choroidal blood supply. Without intervention, the detachment continues to spread, and the detached retina loses the ability to function. The retina may become increasingly detached over a period of hours to years.

At-Risk Populations

Males develop retinal detachment more often than females, with the most common cause being diabetic retinopathy. Other predisposing factors to retinal detachment include aging, cataract extraction, degeneration of the retina, trauma, severe myopia, and a previous retinal detachment in the other eye. A family history of retinal detachment may also be a risk factor. One person in 10,000 develops retinal detachment each year. In patients who have had cataract surgery, one in three patients will develop a retinal detachment. Of patients with retinal detachment 4% to 7% have chronic open-angle glaucoma.

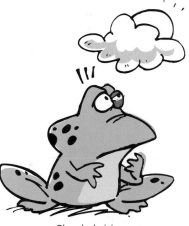

Clouded vision.

What You NEED TO KNOW

Clinical Manifestations

The clinical manifestations of retinal detachment are characteristic. Patients describe a shadow or curtain falling across the field of vision. No pain is present. The onset is usually sudden and may be accompanied by a burst of black spots or floaters, indicating that bleeding has occurred as a result of the detachment. The patient may also see flashes of light resulting from separation of the retina. Examination of the inner eye reveals the portion of the retina involved and the extent of the detachment.

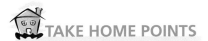

TAKE HOME POINTS

A detached retina requires urgent care. A permanent loss of vision is possible without timely intervention.

Without urgent care, the detachment may extend to involve the macula with subsequent loss of vision.

Prognosis

Involvement of the macula greatly compromises visual acuity. Visual acuity after treatment depends primarily on the status of the macula preoperatively. The length of time between the detachment and the repair also influences future visual acuity after treatment.

What You DO

Treatment

Ninety percent of retinal detachments can be reattached successfully with one or more surgical procedures. A freezing probe or cold laser is used to seal the hole (cryotherapy) if the damage has not progressed to detachment. Both freezing and laser treatments cause an inflammatory response around the affected area that scars over and seals the hole.

A procedure known as scleral buckling may be used when a detachment has occurred. The sclera is depressed from the outside of the eye using special bands to position the choroid next to the retina. An air or gas bubble is then injected into the eye to create pressure on the retina from the inside. The gas bubble holds the retina in place next to the choroid during the healing phase.

Nursing Responsibilities

For the patient with a detached retina the nurse should do the following:
- Assess the patient for visual changes in both eyes. Explain to the patient that an extremely bright light may be noted when the eye is dilated for examination.
- Teach the patient about the clinical manifestations of further loss of vision and to avoid any activities that increase intraocular pressure (IOP) (e.g., Valsalva maneuvers such as straining at stool, coughing, sneezing, lifting).
- Observe the eye patch postoperatively for any drainage. Only serous drainage is expected.

- During the immediate postoperative period, position the patient to maximize the benefits of pressure produced by the introduction of the gas or air bubble. The head of the bed is down, and the patient's head is turned to one side for a period lasting several days.
- Administer drugs as ordered to reduce IOP and to reduce discomfort, nausea, and vomiting.
- Instruct the patient about the correct use of mydriatic and postoperative eye drugs that help prevent infection and reduce inflammation.
- Apply warm or cold compresses to the affected eye several times daily for comfort.
- Advise the patient to clean the eye with warm tap water using a clean washcloth.
- Instruct the patient to avoid vigorous activities and heavy lifting during the immediate postoperative period.
- Advise the patient to avoid air travel during the postoperative period because the air or gas bubble expands at high altitudes.
- Assess the home environment for safety hazards, such as throw rugs, electrical cords, stairs, and poor lighting.
- Advise the patient to contact the health care provider as soon as possible should severe pain develop.

Do You UNDERSTAND?

DIRECTIONS: **Define the following terms.**

1. Scleral buckling: _____
2. Macula: _____
3. Cryotherapy: _____

Answers: 1. a surgical technique used to repair a retinal detachment; 2. an irregular, yellowish depression on the retina, lateral to and slightly below the optic disc that receives and analyzes light only from the center of the visual field; 3. freezing of tissues to close the hole associated with retinal detachment; 4. any movement that increases pressure within the chest; occurs when the patient strains with bowel movement or urination, uses the arms and upper trunk muscles to move up in bed, or strains during coughing, sneezing, gagging, or vomiting; the maneuver increases not only pressure within the chest and the skull, but also IOP.

What IS a Cataract?

Pathogenesis

A cataract is a clouding (opacity) of the lens of the eye. It can be either localized or generalized. The most common cataract is related to aging, although cataracts can have a variety of other causes.

Cataracts develop because of alterations in the metabolism and transport of nutrients within the lens. Both a reduction in oxygen uptake and an initial increase in water content occur. Dehydration of the lens follows these two processes. Sodium and calcium content of the lens are increased. Potassium, ascorbic acid, and protein are decreased. The protein in the lens undergoes numerous age-related changes, including yellowing from formation of fluorescent compounds and molecular changes.

Cataracts progress through four stages. In the early stage, the cataract is not completely cloudy. Some light is transmitted through the lens, which allows for useful vision. In the second stage, the cataract is completely opaque, and vision is significantly reduced. Third-stage cataract lenses absorb water and increase in size, resulting in IOP. In the last stage of cataract formation, the proteins in the lens break down and leak out through the lens capsule. Macrophages swallow up the proteins, which in turn may obstruct the trabecular meshwork, causing additional increases in IOP.

At-Risk Populations

Cataracts are the single largest cause of blindness in the world, affecting an estimated 17 million people. Patients who work in bright sunlight (e.g., lifeguards, commercial fisherman, construction workers, ski patrollers) and those who live at high altitudes develop cataracts earlier in life.

Cataracts may develop as a result of other eye disorders, such as retinal detachment, inflammation of the retina (retinitis), or an inflammation of the iris and ciliary body (iridocyclitis). Blunt trauma, lacerations, foreign bodies, radiation, exposure to infrared light, and chronic use of glucocorticosteroid drugs may also result in cataract formation. Cataracts may be congenital and are found in patients who have systemic disorders such as diabetes mellitus or Down syndrome.

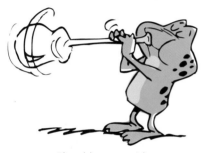

Glass blower at risk.

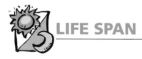

LIFE SPAN

Cumulative exposure to ultraviolet light over the life span is the single most important risk factor in the development of cataracts. Some degree of cataract formation is to be expected in most persons over the age of 70.

What You NEED TO KNOW

Clinical Manifestations

The clinical manifestations of cataracts include decreased visual acuity, blurred vision, occasionally, one-sided double vision, abnormal sensitivity to light **(photophobia),** and glare. Decreased color perception may also be present. Patients usually see "better" in low light when the pupil is dilated. The patient has no complaints of pain. A cloudy lens can be observed during examination of the eye. A cataract is suspected when the red reflex, which is normally observed with an ophthalmoscope, is distorted or absent.

Prognosis

In most cases of cataract, vision can be restored or improved by surgical intervention.

> ⚠️ Cataracts cause decreased visual acuity, blurred vision, double vision, and sensitivity to light and glare. Decreased color perception may also be present. Patient safety becomes a primary consideration.

What You DO

Treatment

Use of ultraviolet-protective glasses in sunny climates may slow progression of cataracts. Surgical removal of the cataract is the most common intervention. Antioxidants (e.g., vitamins C, E) are thought to be beneficial. There are no treatments or drugs at present that prevent or slow the progression of cataracts. Use of strong bifocals, magnification, appropriate lighting, and visual aids may be used as the cataract progresses. When these activities are no longer practical or successful, surgery is recommended.

Surgical removal of the cataract is indicated if visual impairment is producing symptoms distressing to the patient or interfering with lifestyle or occupation, or posing a risk of fall or injury. The most common surgical procedure, an extracapsular cataract extraction (ECCE), consists of removing the lens and the anterior portion of the lens capsule. The posterior portion of the lens capsule is left intact. In some cases, the lens material can be broken down using ultrasonic vibration **(phacoemulsification),** and pieces of the anterior lens capsule can be removed by suction. This technique requires a much smaller incision in the eye.

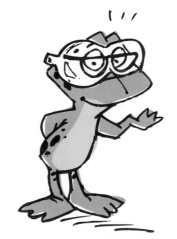

Treatment for retinal detachment.

Intracapsular cataract extraction (ICCE) is performed less frequently. This procedure consists of removing the lens and the lens capsule.

After the removal of a cataract, the patient's lens may be removed (**aphakia**) or a new lens inserted in the posterior chamber of the eye. The newest implants fold during insertion, which allows for a small incision and does not require postoperative eye-patching (except during sleep). Lens implants are permanent. Glasses may be needed after a lens implant.

Contact lens can be used for patients who have aphakia. The simplest and least expensive way to help the patient see after the lens has been removed is to use eyeglasses with extremely thick lenses. The thick lenses magnify objects, but vertical lines appear curved, and distances can be difficult for the patient to judge. Contact lenses help correct vision with significantly less distortion compared with the thick eyeglasses.

Nursing Responsibilities

Pain following cataract surgery should be minimal. Acute pain, which is a symptom of IOP, should be reported immediately. For the patient who has a cataract extraction, the nurse should do the following:

- Document visual acuity in each eye.
- Evaluate the patient's lifestyle, environment, and ability to perform the activities of daily living before and after surgery.
- Advise the patient who has had surgery to leave the eye patch in place, wear glasses, take the prescribed eye drops, and avoid rubbing the eye. Instruct the patient to wear a metal or plastic eye shield at night to protect the eye from accidental injury.
- Advise the patient to avoid lifting more than 5 pounds (the weight of a gallon of milk), avoid straining or bearing down, and sleep on the side of the body on which the operation was performed.
- Use acetaminophen for discomfort. Aspirin or drugs that contain aspirin should be avoided to reduce the risk of bleeding.
- Advise the patient to report any pain that is unrelieved, redness around the eye, nausea, or vomiting.
- Assess the patient and family's ability to properly administer eye drops. Review the rationale and schedule for the administration of eye drugs with the patient and family.
- Arrange for a home care referral, depending on the patient's age, ability, and support systems.
- Provide age-appropriate and culturally appropriate patient and family teaching regarding the disorder and postoperative care.

- Provide to the patient and family information on the disorder and strategies to promote safety measures in the home.
- Advise the patient who has a permanent implant to carry identification regarding the implant at all times.

Do You UNDERSTAND?

DIRECTIONS: **Match the terms in Column A with the definitions in Column B.**

Column A

_____ 1. Cataract
_____ 2. Visual acuity
_____ 3. Diplopia
_____ 4. Photophobia
_____ 5. Extracapsular cataract extraction
_____ 6. Intracapsular cataract extraction
_____ 7. Aphakia

Column B

a. Abnormal intolerance to light
b. Removal of the lens and the anterior portion of the lens capsule
c. Clouding of the lens
d. Clearness of visual perception of an image
e. Double vision
f. Removal of the lens including the entire lens capsule
g. Absence of the lens of the eye, occurring congenitally or as a result of surgery

What IS Glaucoma?

Pathogenesis

Glaucoma is a group of disorders characterized by IOP within the anterior chamber of the eye. IOP is controlled by the rate of aqueous humor production in the ciliary body and the resistance to outflow of aqueous humor from the eye. Normal pressure variations within the anterior

Answers: 1. c; 2. d; 3. e; 4. a; 5. b; 6. f; 7. g.

chamber usually do not exceed 2 to 3 mm Hg. However, as aqueous fluid increases in the eye, the increased pressure interferes with blood supply to the optic nerve and the retina. It should be noted that optic nerve damage can also occur in the setting of normal IOP and as a secondary manifestation of other disorders. The eye structures become ischemic and gradually lose function. IOP and arterial blood pressure are independent of each other, although changes in blood pressure can affect IOP.

The extent of pressure changes that cause ocular damage is not the same for each eye or in every patient. Some sustain damage with a relatively low pressure, while others sustain no damage from higher pressures. Glaucoma may be acute or chronic.

The angle between the cornea and the iris is used to describe glaucoma. Open-angle glaucoma (also known as wide-angle glaucoma) is chronic, resulting from degenerative changes in the trabecular meshwork of the eye. Open-angle glaucoma results from multiple factors that are genetically determined; it is usually bilateral, insidious in onset, and slow to progress. The angle between the cornea and the iris is wide, but the trabecular meshwork impairs drainage of aqueous humor. In closed-angle glaucoma (also known as acute-angle glaucoma), the angle is narrow, acute obstruction to the outflow of aqueous humor is present, and a markedly elevated IOP occurs.

At-Risk Populations

Ninety percent of primary glaucoma occurs in people who have open angles. Persons with a narrow anterior chamber angle are predisposed to an acute onset of closed-angle glaucoma. Congenital glaucoma is rare and is the result of developmental abnormalities of eye structures.

Risk factors for the development of glaucoma include hypertension, cardiovascular disease, diabetes mellitus, and obesity. Smoking, caffeine or alcohol intake, use of illicit drugs or glucocorticosteroids, and altered hormone levels cause varying but transient elevations in IOP.

What You NEED TO KNOW

Clinical Manifestations

The signs and symptoms of glaucoma include slow, progressive visual loss. Individuals are usually unaware of the visual loss until late in the disease because central visual acuity generally remains intact until late in

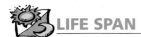

LIFE SPAN

Glaucoma is most common in African Americans between the ages of 45 and 65. The prevalence is 5 times that of Caucasians in the same age group.

the disease. IOP, indentation of the optic disc, and defects in the visual field are noted. The manifestations are the same, regardless of the type of glaucoma. The difference in manifestations is in the speed of onset and the severity of pressure elevations.

No early signs and symptoms are present to alert the patient with open-angle glaucoma that vision is deteriorating. IOP readings are in the normal range, the angle is normal, and the optic nerves are normal. Subtle peripheral vision deficits may occur. A small crescent shape (scotoma) appears in the visual field early in the disease. The signs and symptoms of closed-angle glaucoma appear suddenly, usually appearing in only one eye. Severe pain and blurred vision or vision loss is observed. Some patients see rainbow halos around lights, and some will experience nausea and vomiting. Larger areas of significant vision loss are noted with narrow-angle glaucoma. An eye exam may demonstrate a reddened conjunctiva and a cloudy cornea. The humor in the anterior chamber may appear cloudy and the pupil nonreactive. Pressures exceeding 23 mm Hg require further evaluation of the eye.

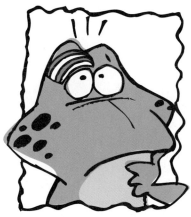

Symptom of glaucoma.

Prognosis

The Early Manifest Glaucoma Trial (EMGT) showed that early treatment of primary open-angle glaucoma significantly delays disease progression. The magnitude of initial IOP reduction was a major factor influencing disease progression. In most cases, blindness can be prevented if treatment is started early.

What You DO

Treatment

The treatment of glaucoma involves more than one drug, with different mechanisms of action. Patient adherence to therapy is decreased however when three or more drugs are required. Ocular miotics constrict the pupil and increase the outflow of humor (e.g., pilocarpine). Beta-blockers or alpha-adrenergics (e.g., timolol or epinephrine, respectively) are used to suppress the secretion of aqueous humor. Orally administered carbonic anhydrase inhibitors (e.g., acetazolamide) help reduce the production of aqueous humor. Mydriatic and cycloplegic drugs inhibit the parasympathetic nervous system by blocking acetylcholine (ACH) and paralyzing the ciliary and dilator muscle of the iris, thus causing both dilation of the pupil and paralysis of accommodation. All of these drug classes are contraindicated in patients who have narrow-angle glaucoma, primarily because dilation of the pupil further restricts outflow of aqueous humor.

Surgery may be required for patients in whom the progression of visual field loss and optic nerve damage cannot be halted. No single surgical procedure is available that is successful for all patients. The procedures that may be considered include the use of a laser to create an opening in the trabecular meshwork, thus enhancing drainage of aqueous humor. Channels can be surgically established to promote outflow of aqueous humor from the anterior chamber to the subconjunctival space. An iridectomy—the creation of a new route for the flow of aqueous humor to the trabecular meshwork—may also be performed. When other surgical procedures have failed, freezing of the ciliary body may be performed to decrease aqueous humor production.

Nursing Responsibilities

For the patient with glaucoma, the nurse should do the following:

- Review the signs and symptoms of IOP: unrelieved pain, nausea, and decreased vision.
- Encourage the patient to adhere to regular visits to the ophthalmologist. Vision and IOP testing should be done every 3 to 6 months. Visual field testing should be done every 6 to 18 months. The optic nerve should be evaluated every 3 to 18 months, depending on how well the pressure is controlled.
- Instruct patients to avoid alcohol and caffeine intake several hours before an eye examination.
- Teach patients to avoid activities that involve a Valsalva maneuver (e.g., straining at stool, bending over, lifting).
- Instruct the patient about what to expect at the time of surgery (e.g., popping sounds, flashing lights). A waiting period is required after surgery of approximately 1 to 2 hours to evaluate IOP.
- Position the postoperative patient on the nonoperative side to avoid pressure on the operative site.
- Review with the patient the signs and symptoms of postoperative infection: redness, swelling, drainage, blurred vision, and pain.
- Advise the patient that rubbing or applying pressure over the closed eye can damage healing tissue. Remind the patient of the importance of and rationale for eye protection after surgery, such as wearing an eye shield or eyeglasses at all times.

Do You UNDERSTAND?

DIRECTIONS: **Indicate which statements are *true* (T) and which are *false* (F). If false, correct the statement in the margin space to make it true.**

_____ 1. Glaucoma usually results from the overproduction of aqueous humor.

_____ 2. Prolonged exposure to sunlight and heavy smoking has been associated with an increased risk of glaucoma.

_____ 3. In the most common type of glaucoma, the abnormality involves obstruction of the trabecular meshwork and the anterior chamber.

What IS an Ocular Infection?

Pathogenesis

Infections of the eye can involve numerous eye structures. For example, blepharitis is a common bilateral inflammation of the eyelid margins. Dacryocystitis is an inflammation and blockage of the tear duct. A hordeolum (stye) is an infection of the glands of the eyelids. Conjunctivitis is an inflammation of the conjunctiva. Keratitis is an infection of the cornea. Vasodilation of the conjunctival, episcleral, and scleral vessels produces the red eye present in eye infections. Invasion of eye structures by microorganisms contributes to eye discomfort, a reduction of visual acuity, and, in some cases, photophobia.

Eye infections are usually the result of bacteria such as *Staphylococcus aureus, Pseudomonas aeruginosa,* and *Streptococcus pneumoniae.* Fungi such as *Candida* or *Aspergillus,* viruses such as adenovirus, herpes simplex, or herpes zoster, protozoa such as *Acanthamoeba,* or chlamydia can also cause eye infections.

At-Risk Populations

Patients who have systemic connective tissue disorders such as rheumatoid arthritis are particularly susceptible to corneal infections

Answers: 1. F—glaucoma usually results from degenerative changes of the trabecular meshwork; 2. F—prolonged exposure to sunlight and heavy smoking have been associated with cataracts; 3. T.

and ulceration. Dry eyes, trauma, or ineffective eyelid closure predispose the eye to infection.

What You NEED TO KNOW

Clinical Manifestations

The signs and symptoms of eye infections are summarized in the accompanying table. Occasionally, the patient may experience a headache or blurred vision.

Signs and Symptoms of Eye Infections

Infection	Eye Pain	Discharge	Visual acuity	Photophobia
Viral conjunctivitis	Mild, burning	Watery	Normal	No
Bacterial conjunctivitis	Mild to moderate, burning	Purulent	Normal	No
Keratitis	Moderate, aching	Clear	Decreased	Yes
Blepharitis	Mild	None	Normal	No
Hordeolum	Mild	Watery	Normal	Unusual
Dacryocystitis	Mild	Watery	Normal	Slight
Herpes infection	Mild to moderate	Watery	Decreased	Yes

Prognosis

The prognosis for the patient with an eye infection is generally good, providing that the infection is treated early. The patient usually remains at home but may need to be hospitalized if the infection progresses to the inside of the eye.

What You DO

Treatment

The goal of treatment for eye infections is to prevent progression of the infection and to promote healing. Infections are commonly treated with warm compresses applied to the eye several times daily. Topical antibiotic, antifungal, or antiviral therapy is prescribed, with the frequency of administration based on the severity of the infection. The infection usually disappears in 3 to 7 days.

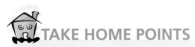

TAKE HOME POINTS

Recovery from most eye infections takes 3 to 7 days, providing the patient uses the eye drugs as ordered.

Nursing Responsibilities

For the patient with an eye infection, the nurse should do the following:

- Assess the patient's level of discomfort and possible lack of sleep. In some cases, eye drops may be given as often as every 15 minutes around the clock, thus the schedule is a challenge not only for the patient, but also for the nurse.
- Practice diligent hand washing, even when gloves are worn to apply the eye drops.
- Adhere to the drug administration schedule to reduce the risk of complications. Adhering to the schedule also builds patient's trust and reduces anxiety.
- Advise the patient that some drugs such as fortified bacitracin may cause stinging that lasts several minutes.
- Administer oral analgesics at regular intervals as indicated. Mild sleeping drugs may be helpful at bedtime.
- Cleanse the eye using warm tap water and a clean washcloth. Teach the patient to avoid using the same washcloth on the other eye.
- Provide patient and family teaching regarding drug administration and the signs and symptoms of increasing infection.
- Assess the home environment if the patient's vision is greatly reduced.

Do You UNDERSTAND?

DIRECTIONS: **Match the terms in Column A with the definitions in Column B.**

Column A	Column B
_____ 1. Dacryocystitis	a. Infection of the cornea
_____ 2. Hordeolum (stye)	b. Infection of the glands of the eyelids
_____ 3. Conjunctivitis	c. Inflammation of the lacrimal sac secondary to bacterial infection
_____ 4. Keratitis	d. Inflammation of the conjunctiva
_____ 5. Blepharitis	e. Bilateral inflammation of the eyelid margins

Answers: 1. c, 2. b, 3. d, 4. a, 5. e.

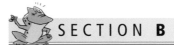

SECTION **B**

DISORDERS OF THE EAR

When sound strikes the ear, the eardrum (**tympanic membrane**) vibrates. The three small bones of the middle ear (hammer [malleus], anvil [incus], and stirrup [stapes]) function as levers, amplifying the motion of the eardrum and passing the vibrations on to the cochlea. The cochlea contains nerves that transmit sound. From this point, the eighth cranial nerve transmits the vibrations, translated into nerve impulses, to the hearing center in the brain. The inner ear also contains the semicircular canals that are essential to the sense of balance.

What IS Otosclerosis?

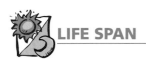

LIFE SPAN

Otosclerosis may worsen with pregnancy.

Pathogenesis

Otosclerosis is also known as "hardening of the ear" and is the leading cause of conductive hearing loss in adults. Approximately 10% of adults have otosclerosis. The cause is unknown. A formation of spongy bone occurs in the labyrinth of the ear. This formation of spongy bone causes the stapes to become immobile. Immobility of the stapes prevents the transmission of sound vibration to the inner ear. The loss of vibration results in a conductive hearing loss.

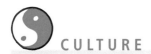

CULTURE

Otosclerosis is 10 times more common in Caucasians than it is in any other ethnic group.

At-Risk Populations

At one time, otosclerosis was thought to be a result of a vitamin deficiency or an infection of the middle ear (**otitis media**). Now, otosclerosis is known to be an autosomal dominant disorder, meaning transmission to children can occur when only one parent has the disorder. Of those affected, 60% have a positive family history of the disorder. This middle ear disorder usually begins during adolescence or the early 20s, affecting women approximately twice as frequently as it does men. The peak incidence is during the fourth and fifth decades of life.

What You NEED TO KNOW

Clinical Manifestations

The signs and symptoms of otosclerosis include a slow, progressive hearing loss. Changes can be noted as early as adolescence. An early symptom of otosclerosis is ringing in the ears; however, the most noticeable symptom is progressive loss of hearing. The hearing loss usually affects both ears. The patient commonly speaks in a soft voice and is aware of seemingly hearing better in noisy environments. Other symptoms include recurrent dizziness and postural imbalance.

The Rinne test compares air versus sensorineural conduction. A vibrating tuning fork is shifted between the mastoid bone (bone conduction) and the opening of the ear canal (air conduction). When the patient has otosclerosis, bone conduction is greater than air conduction. Normally air conduction exceeds bone conduction. The Weber test shows lateralization to the more affected ear when hearing loss is greater in one ear compared with the other. Audiometry testing confirms the hearing loss. A reddish blush from dilated blood vessels may be noted behind the eardrum (Schwartz's sign) on otoscopic exam.

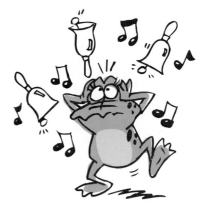

Ringing is an early symptom.

Prognosis

The conductive hearing loss that results from otosclerosis is one of the most common correctable middle ear disorders. It rarely progresses to deafness; however, progressive hearing loss is possible without treatment. Surgery improves hearing by at least 15 decibels in 90% of patients.

What You DO

Treatment

Because speech discrimination is usually unaffected, simple amplification of sound (with the use of hearing aids) is effective in treating otosclerosis. Although there is no known cure for otosclerosis, surgical techniques frequently restore conductive hearing loss by freeing the damaged ossicle or replacing it with other tissues. In this operation, the damaged ossicle is removed and replaced with stainless steel or a plastic prosthesis (**stapedectomy**). However, the procedure is performed less frequently today because of the risk of profound deafness and persistent postoperative vertigo.

People who are at risk for otosclerosis or who are not candidates for surgery can be given drugs to reduce the severity of bony fusion. Evidence suggests that sodium fluoride may help decrease the rate of hearing loss by replacing the hydroxyl ion in bone and decreasing resorption. Calcium gluconate and vitamin D can be used to retard bone resorption.

Nursing Responsibilities

For the patient with otosclerosis, the nurse should do the following:

- Speak directly to and clearly to (and face) the patient.
- Recognize that hearing-impaired patients pay increased attention to visual clues since they depend on them for understanding: therefore avoid showing annoyance with careless facial expressions.
- Use visual aids (e.g., pictures, diagrams, models) to help the patient understand medical terminology or procedures. An expert interpreter should be used when other attempts to communicate have failed or when speed and accuracy are important. The National Registry of Interpreters for the Deaf (NRID) has local chapters and can provide names of interpreters.
- Avoid the use of an intercom when caring for hospitalized patients. An intercom distorts sound and causes poor communication.
- Advise the patient to avoid aspirin or aspirin-containing products for 2 weeks before surgery to reduce the risk of bleeding.
- Have the patient lie on the nonoperative side, with the head of the bed elevated after surgery. This position reduces swelling and prevents dislodging of the prosthesis.
- Report any vertigo and nystagmus, and advise the patient not to disturb packing that may be placed in the ear canal.
- Advise the patient to avoid excessive exercise, straining, and activities that can lead to head trauma. Blow the nose gently, one nostril at a time. The nose should remain open when sneezing. Air travel should be avoided for up to 1 month after surgery.
- Encourage the patient to continue social involvement. Advocate the use of support groups for hearing-impaired persons.
- Teach the patient the proper way to use and care for a hearing aid, when prescribed, and the procedure to use should the aid malfunction.
- Encourage the patient to keep follow-up appointments to determine the degree of hearing regained.

Do You UNDERSTAND?

DIRECTIONS: **Indicate which statements are *true* (T) and which are *false* (F). If false, correct the statement in the margin space to make it true.**

_____ 1. Otosclerosis is caused by vitamin deficiency or ear infection.

_____ 2. Otosclerosis is an autosomal dominant disorder.

_____ 3. A spongy bone accumulates in the labyrinth of the ear with otosclerosis.

_____ 4. Surgery improves hearing by at least 15 decibels in 90% of patients.

_____ 5. Because speech discrimination is usually unaffected, simple amplification of sound (with the use of hearing aid) is effective in treating otosclerosis.

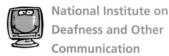

National Institute on Deafness and Other Communication Disorders

http://www.nidcd.nih.gov/health/balance/meniere.asp

What IS Ménière's Disease?

Pathogenesis

Ménière's disease is an inner ear (labyrinthine) disorder in which there is an increase in volume and pressure of the innermost fluid of the inner ear (endolymph). Endolymph is a clear, intracellular fluid found in the labyrinth of the inner ear. Normal balance is dependent on the stability of fluid pressure.

A change in the volume and fluid pressure contributes to recurrent attacks of hearing loss, tinnitus, vertigo, and a sensation of fullness. Vertigo is a perception that the patient or the environment is moving with the patient remaining seated or supine to prevent falling. Vertigo is not synonymous with dizziness. Patients who are dizzy have a feeling of confusion (**disorientation**) in space.

Most cases of Ménière's disease have no known cause. The idiopathic form of Ménière's is thought to be a result of a single viral injury to the transport system of the inner ear. Ménière's disease may develop after an injury to the head or a viral infection of the middle ear. A number of

Answers: 1. F—the cause of otosclerosis is unknown; 2. T; 3. T; 4. T; 5. T.

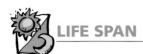

LIFE SPAN

Ménière's affects men and women equally between the ages of 20 and 60.

conditions are associated with Ménière's, including trauma, allergy, adrenal-pituitary insufficiency, and hypothyroidism. Anxiety appears to play an important role in triggering Ménière's attacks, as do abnormalities in the immune system. Over time the balance problem tends to resolve, but the hearing problem worsens.

At-Risk Populations

Patients who are at risk for Ménière's disease include those who have had a head injury or chronic infections of the middle ear. A relationship appears to exist between the number and severity of attacks of Ménière's disease and the degree of stress in a patient's life.

What You NEED TO KNOW

Clinical Manifestations

In approximately 90% of cases, only one ear is affected. Occasionally, Ménière's disease is referred to as a balance disorder, rather than a hearing disorder, because vertigo is frequently the most troublesome symptom in the early stages. Other clinical manifestations of Ménière's include ringing in the ears **(tinnitus)**, a feeling of fullness, sensitivity to loud noises, progressive hearing loss, and headache. In the acute stage, the patient have be pale, have severe nausea with vomiting, profuse sweating, and disabling vertigo; in addition, rapid, involuntary, rhythmic movement of the eyeball **(rotary nystagmus)** may occur. All symptoms are aggravated by motion. The accompanying sensorineural hearing loss is usually subtle, and the person may not realize that hearing has been lost because of the ringing in the ears. Between attacks the person may experience motion-related imbalance without vertigo.

Ménière's disease is an unpredictable chronic disorder. Those affected have symptoms that come in clusters. Some attacks last only minutes; other attacks may continue for hours, days, weeks, or months. Attacks may occur frequently or several weeks apart. Then, for some unknown reason, the episodes subside.

Prognosis

Control of Ménière's episodes is usually possible, although to date a cure is unavailable. The great majority of patients can be managed

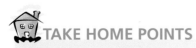

TAKE HOME POINTS

Few problems are more private than those involving the patient's balance. Balance problems, such as those found with Ménière's, may be debilitating and cause embarrassing gait problems. Patient safety can be jeopardized.

successfully with drugs. About 5% to 10% of patients require surgery for incapacitating vertigo.

What You DO

Treatment

A low-salt diet has been the mainstay of treatment for Ménière's disease. A variety of drugs have also been used in treatment. Although the scientific data supporting the use of diuretics in Ménière's is weak, many patients note an improvement in symptoms when taking them. Diuretics are thought to reduce the endolymphatic fluid volume within the cochlea. Drugs designed to suppress vertigo such as meclizine, diazepam, and dimenhydrinate may be useful in controlling the vertigo and alleviating acute symptoms. In severe cases, immunosuppressants such as prednisone may be used. Occasionally, sedatives are ordered to promote sleep and rest. When the ringing sensation becomes too disturbing to the patient, it may be masked (e.g., by music piped in through headphones) to make sleeping easier.

Fortunately, the majority of patients with Ménière's require no surgery. In a small number of persons, vertigo will be persistent and incapacitating, thus they may benefit from surgical treatment. Resection of the vestibular nerve remains the gold standard for eliminating vertigo while preserving hearing. This operation involves cutting the balance component of the eighth cranial nerve while leaving the hearing component intact. This operation offers a better than 95% chance of eliminating vertigo. Other surgical procedures may be directed toward relief of pressure by the bony structures surrounding the cochlea or diverting the flow of endolymphatic fluid by means of a shunt to the mastoid bone or to the subarachnoid space.

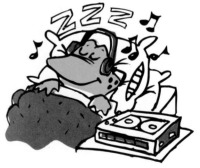

Mask the ringing.

Nursing Responsibilities

For the patient with Ménière's disease, the nurse should do the following:

- Advise the patient to rest quietly during an attack.
- Use non–drug therapies (e.g., meditation, imaging, deep breathing, quiet bedtime activities, among others) as much as possible to promote sleep and rest.

- Instruct patients to change position slowly to prevent injury.
- Teach the patient to reduce stress as much as possible and to avoid situations likely to trigger an attack.
- Assist the patient in identifying and avoiding food sources high in sodium and to avoid smoking.
- Teach the patient to avoid the use of ototoxic drugs when able (e.g., aspirin, quinine, aminoglycosides, furosemide) without first checking with the health care provider.

Do You UNDERSTAND?

DIRECTIONS: **Match the explanation in Column A with the appropriate term in Column B.**

Column A	Column B
_____ 1. Protects auditory apparatus from intense vibration	a. Tympanic membrane
_____ 2. Contains vestibule, cochlea, semi-circular canals; organ for hearing and balance	b. External auditory canal
	c. Inner ear
_____ 3. Organ of hearing	d. Malleus
_____ 4. Organs responsible for position sense and balance	e. Middle ear
	f. Annulus
_____ 5. Covers oval window of inner ear	g. Cochlea
_____ 6. Dense, fibrous rings surrounding the tympanic membrane	h. Footplate of stapes
	i. Semicircular canals

Answers: 1. a; 2. c; 3. g; 4. i; 5. h; 6. f.

What IS an Ear Infection?

Pathogenesis

The most common problems found in the ear are infections, primarily bacterial or fungal. Ear infections can be an acute or a chronic problem. The most frequent infection, otitis externa, involves the external ear canal and is the most common cause of ear pain in an adult. Otitis externa begins as a result of excessive dryness or wetness, which damages the protective waxy lining of the external ear canal. The most common form is known as "swimmer's ear" because it occurs as a result of water remaining in the ear canal. *Pseudomonas* is the usual offending organism. Occasionally, otitis externa can involve the cartilage of the pinna with resultant loss of the distinctive shape of the external ear.

Otitis media is the most common middle ear infection and is common in children, although it can occur in adults as well. Otitis media may also result from air pressure trauma to the middle ear and may occur after air travel or scuba diving. When symptoms occur suddenly and are of short duration, the diagnosis is acute otitis media. *Pseudomonas, Staphylococcus, Klebsiella,* or *Bacteroides* may be the contributing causes of otitis media.

Between bouts of otitis media, fluid may form in the middle ear, causing a serous otitis media. The fluid is formed when a blocked eustachian tube causes a vacuum to develop. When the swelling subsides, the fluid may be too thick to drain. Occasionally, serous otitis media is found in conjunction with upper respiratory infections or allergies.

Otitis media with effusion is the presence of middle ear fluid for 6 weeks or longer from the initial episode of acute otitis media. This occurs when the eustachian tube is not functioning to ventilate the ear and middle ear fluid develops without a prior ear infection.

Chronic otitis media develops with repeated episodes of acute otitis media. Chronic otitis media can lead to retraction of the eardrum, scarring and perforation of the eardrum, and death of the ossicles. The result of these disorders is a conductive hearing loss.

At-Risk Populations

The primary predisposing factor for all forms of otitis media appears to be poor eustachian tube function. Failure of the eustachian tube to allow air to enter the middle ear impairs normal function and creates an environment in which bacteria can grow. Infants who are bottle-fed in a supine position may develop repeated bouts of otitis media since the milk traverses the eustachian tube to the middle ear. Patients with debilitating systemic diseases such as diabetes mellitus are at risk for otitis externa.

What You NEED TO KNOW

Clinical Manifestations

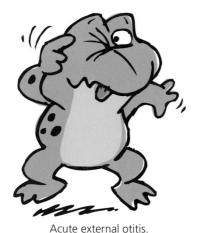

Acute external otitis.

Acute external otitis is characterized by the rapid onset of ear pain. The pain ranges from mild to severe and generally affects only one ear. The pain is more intense when the ear canal is edematous. An early symptom of otitis externa is itching in the ear canal. A tenderness that is present when the pinna is gently pulled is an early sign of external otitis. This finding is in contrast to otitis media, in which touching the external ear causes no pain.

Inflammation is easily identified using an otoscope. In early infectious disorders, the drainage may be clear and not discolored by pus.

A patient with acute otitis media may report bubbling, crackling, or popping sensations in the ear, especially during swallowing. A sense of fullness in the ear and a fluctuating conductive hearing loss may be reported. The eardrum is immobile and is dull or red, rather than the normal pearly gray color. The eardrum may be infected, perforated, retracted, or bulging, depending on the disease process involved.

Prognosis

Otitis is generally a self-limiting disorder. Although the problem may be recurrent in some people, when promptly treated, patients usually recover in less than 1 week.

TAKE HOME POINTS

Otitis media is generally easy to treat when promptly diagnosed. Without prompt diagnosis and treatment, otitis media can lead to sinusitis, meningitis, and brain abscess because of the general anatomy of the ear and surrounding tissues.

What You DO

Treatment

Acute otitis externa and otitis media are best treated with a 1-week course of antibiotic–steroid drops. This treatment usually results in resolution of the symptoms. Analgesics such as regular- or extra-strength acetaminophen are occasionally needed during the first 24 to 48 hours to control the pain. For some patients, decongestants may be used to help relieve the pressure within the ear.

Even though studies have shown that up to 80% of cases of acute otitis media will clear up on their own without medical treatment, the standard therapy for acute otitis media remains antibiotics. Even after effective antibiotic treatment, 40% of children may retain noninfected residual fluid in the middle ear that can cause some temporary hearing loss. This may last for 3 to 6 weeks after the initial antibiotic therapy.

Chronic otitis media is treated with a combination of eardrops and, occasionally, antibiotics by mouth. Ultimately, surgery (**myringotomy**) may be required to eradicate the infection and close the perforation of the eardrum resulting from the chronic infection. Systemic antibiotics may be needed for patients who have infection involving surrounding ear structures.

Nursing Responsibilities

For the patient with otitis externa and otitis media, the nurse should do the following:

- Advise the patient with otitis externa to use either earplugs or cotton coated with petroleum jelly to avoid getting water in the ear while bathing, showering, or swimming.
- Meticulously clean the external canal to allow the local antibiotic to reach the affected area. Suction, irrigation, or manual removal of earwax can be used. Ear irrigation should not be used when the patient is suspected of having a perforated eardrum.
- Administer eardrops as scheduled with the patient lying on the unaffected side for 3 to 5 minutes to allow gravity to promote movement of the drug into the ear canal. Wait 15 minutes between administrations when the drug is needed in both ears.
- When the external ear canal is swollen, insert a wick to allow the drops to penetrate the canal. Eardrops are placed directly on the wick.
- Instruct the patient to chew gum, suck on something sour, and swallow frequently. Yawning and blowing air out against closed nostrils may help open a swollen eustachian tube.

Do You UNDERSTAND?

DIRECTIONS: Compare the clinical manifestations of otitis externa with those of otitis media.

Disorder	Acute Otitis Externa	Acute Otitis Media
Onset		
Offending organism(s)		
Location of pain		
Discharge		
Swelling		
Complications		

References

Cataracts. Cecil textbook of medicine, URL http://textbook.cecilmedicine.com/content/.

Otitis. Cecil textbook of medicine, URL http://textbook.cecilmedicine.com/content/.

Glaucoma. Cecil textbook of medicine, URL http://textbook.cecilmedicine.com/content/.

Goldman L, Ausiello D: *Cecil textbook of medicine,* ed. 22, Philadelphia, 2004, Saunders.

Gutierrez K, Queener S: *Pharmacology for nursing practice,* Philadelphia, 2004, Mosby.

Huether S, McCance K: *Understanding pathophysiology,* ed 3, St Louis, 2005, Mosby.

Lewis S, Heitkemper M, Dirksen S: *Medical-surgical nursing: assessment and management of clinical problems,* ed 5, St Louis, 2004, Mosby.

Macular degeneration. Cecil textbook of medicine, URL http://textbook.cecilmedicine.com/content/.

Ménière's disease. Cecil textbook of medicine, URL http://textbook.cecilmedicine.com/content/.

Otosclerosis. Cecil textbook of medicine, URL http://textbook.cecilmedicine.com/content/.

Retinal detachment. Cecil textbook of medicine, URL http://textbook.cecilmedicine.com/content/.

Answers: **Acute otitis externa: rapid onset;** *Pseudomonas;* **external ear pain; discharge; swelling of external canal; loss of shape of pinna if external canal involved; acute otitis media: rapid onset;** *Pseudomonas, Staphylococcus, Klebsiella,* **or** *Bacteroides;* **no external ear pain; no obvious discharge; no obvious swelling of external canal; perforation, scarring, hearing loss, chronic otitis media.**

NCLEX® Review

Section A

1. Which statement about macular degeneration is true?
   1 Adequate intake of vitamin A can prevent macular degeneration.
   2 Peripheral vision remains intact.
   3 Laser therapy is used to successfully cure both the "wet" and "dry" types.
   4 Macular degeneration can be easily diagnosed using a slit-lamp.

2. Which of the following surgical procedures may be used to correct a retinal detachment?
   1 Iridectomy
   2 Keratoplasty
   3 Scleral buckling
   4 Trabeculectomy

3. Postoperative care of the patient with a detached retina includes
   1 Administering miotic eye drops.
   2 Allowing the patient to ambulate.
   3 Covering only the affected eye with a pressure dressing.
   4 Encouraging the patient to remain in a head-down, lateral position.

4. Your next-door neighbor is complaining of a sudden severe pain in the eye and a "curtain" closing in the field of vision. This person should be immediately referred to an
   1 Oculist.
   2 Ophthalmologist.
   3 Optician.
   4 Optometrist.

Section B

5. Conductive hearing loss is most commonly a result of
   1 A disease or trauma to the inner ear.
   2 Anything that blocks the external ear.
   3 Disease or trauma to the external ear.
   4 Nerve pathways leading to the brainstem.

6. The most common problem found in the external ear is(are)
   1 Invasion by insects and foreign bodies.
   2 Injury or trauma.
   3 Allergic reactions.
   4 Infection.

7. The organisms most often associated with acute otitis media include
   1 *Pseudomonas.*
   2 *Klebsiella.*
   3 *Staphylococcus.*
   4 *Bacteroides.*
   5 All of the above.

8. The technique used to administer eardrops to a child is to pull the pinna
   1 Up and back.
   2 Down and back.
   3 Forward and down.
   4 Forward and up.

NCLEX® Review Answers

Section A

1. **2** In macular degeneration, peripheral vision remains intact. Macular degeneration is neither prevented nor cured. The disorder is not easily diagnosed.

2. **3** Scleral buckling is used to correct retinal detachment. Iridectomy and trabeculectomy promote outflow of humor, thus reducing intraocular pressure. Keratoplasty redesigns the cornea.

3. **4** Remaining in a head-down, lateral position facilitates reattachment of the retina and prevents further problems. This postoperative care is appropriate for a patient treated for detached retina. Miotic eye drops will constrict only the pupil and may worsen the detachment. Allowing the patient to ambulate can cause further detachment. Covering only the affected eye does nothing to help but adds stress because the eyes work in tandem.

4. **2** Your neighbor should be referred to an ophthalmologist. An ophthalmologist is the only person qualified to treat a retinal detachment. An oculist, optician, or optometrist is not a physician and cannot treat retinal detachment.

Section B

5. **2** Anything that blocks the external ear canal can cause conductive hearing loss. Disease or trauma to the inner ear may cause balance problems, as well as hearing loss. Disease or trauma to the external ear may cause conductive hearing loss, depending on the situation. Damage to the nerve pathways causes a sensorineural hearing loss.

6. **4** The most common problem of the external ear is infection. The external ear may be invaded by insects and foreign bodies, be subject to injury or trauma, or suffer allergic reactions, but these situations are less common compared with infection.

7. The most common organisms associated with acute otitis media include *Pseudomonas, Staphylococcus, Klebsiella,* and *Bacteroides.*

8. **2** The pinna is pulled down and back in a child, and up and back in an adult. Pulling the pinna forward and down or forward and up will obstruct the canal.

Notes

Alterations in Integumentary Function

What You WILL LEARN

After reading this chapter, you will know how to do the following:

- ✔ List the various organisms that are associated with infections of the skin.
- ✔ Describe risk factors for skin infections.
- ✔ Summarize risk factors for skin cancer.
- ✔ Distinguish the differences between the symptoms associated with fungal, bacterial, and viral skin infections.
- ✔ Discuss nursing interventions used to care for patients with infectious skin diseases.
- ✔ Compare and contrast basal cell carcinoma, squamous cell carcinoma, and melanoma.
- ✔ Create a comprehensive list of interventions for patients with skin cancer.
- ✔ Explain the different types of burns.
- ✔ Describe potential complications of a severe burn.
- ✔ Identify a plan of care for a patient with a burn.

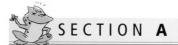

SECTION **A**

INFECTIOUS DISEASES OF THE SKIN

What IS Candidiasis?

Pathogenesis

Candida is a yeastlike fungus that is found in the vagina, in the gastrointestinal tract, and on the skin and mucous membranes. *Candida,* formerly known as *monilia,* is normally kept in check by resident bacteria that inhibits growth. Favorable growth factors include a warm, moist environment, a change in pH, an increase in blood glucose levels, or a decrease in immune system functioning. Other possible contributing factors include food allergies, diet, endocrine disorders, tightly fitting clothing, hypothyroidism, and douching. Candidiasis, also known as a yeast infection, can be a result of antibiotic therapy, which suppresses the protective flora of the mucous membranes and skin surfaces.

At-Risk Populations

Individuals at risk for candidiasis include those with endocrine diseases such as diabetes mellitus and Cushing's disease. Poor nutrition and debilitation can decrease resistance to infection. Patients with neoplastic diseases of the blood, those who are immunocompromised, and those who are receiving antineoplastic therapy are also at risk.

    Candida can reside in the skin folds of the abdomen, the inguinal area, or under the breasts of those who are obese. Uncircumcised males are at risk for candidiasis only when the foreskin is not retracted and washed on a daily basis. Individuals whose hands are frequently in water, such as dishwashers and bartenders, may also be susceptible to candidiasis. Poorly fitting and poorly cleaned dentures have also been found to be a source of the infection.

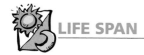

LIFE SPAN

Persons who are pregnant, on antibiotic therapy, or on birth control pills have an increased risk for candidiasis. Children and adults with incontinence are at risk for candidiasis from constant moisture and irritation.

What You NEED TO KNOW

Clinical Manifestations

Problems result when the *Candida* organism releases toxins that irritate the skin and mucous membranes. Physical appearance of a candida infection may vary depending upon the location of the infection.

Patients with oral candida often complain of taste changes. If the candida extends into their esophagus they may complain of a foreign body sensation every time they swallow.

Oral candidiasis (**thrush**) is characterized by the formation of a creamy white coating, white plaques, or flaking on a red, inflamed tongue or mucous membrane. The lesions may develop into shallow ulcers. The papillae on the tongue may appear large. The plaques on the tongue can be easily removed, but removal will cause bleeding. Denture wearers can also develop chronic candidiasis in areas under the dentures.

Candida infections of the skin are most likely to be found in any warm, dark, moist area such as the folds of the groin, under the breasts in women, and in the axillae. Skin lesions are typically moist, red, and pruritic with eroded scales. Candidiasis can also occur as a red, painful swelling around the nail beds.

Vaginal manifestations of *Candida* include vulvar pruritus and irritation, dysuria, erythema, dyspareunia, and a thick, cheesy vaginal discharge that may be odorless or foul-smelling. When severe, pustules may develop. A penile irritation (**balanitis**) that includes red lesions with defined borders and a white plaque with itching and burning may signal a *Candida* infection.

Prognosis

Candidiasis can be easily cleared with topical or oral antifungals that are available over-the-counter or by prescription. The infection is generally cleared in 3 to 7 days.

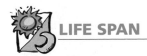

LIFE SPAN

Candidiasis has also been found on the lower back, the intergluteal folds, and the buttocks, particularly in children. Diaper rash from *Candida* may appear as mild redness and inflammation to an extremely erythematous area.

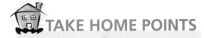

TAKE HOME POINTS

Candidiasis is generally cleared within 3 to 7 days with topical or oral antifungals available over-the-counter or by prescription.

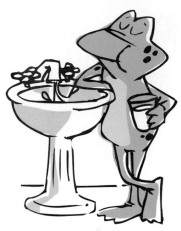

Swish and swallow!

What You DO

Treatment

The patient with candidiasis should begin treatment as soon as symptoms develop. Antifungal drugs such as topical clotrimazole or miconazole are effective against *Candida*. Oral candidiasis can be treated with oral suspensions of nystatin in the form of a "swish and swallow" treatment. Severe inflammation can also be treated with a combination drug that includes antifungal and topical steroids.

Nursing Responsibilities

For the patient with candidiasis the nurse should do the following:

* Advise the patient to wear loose-fitting clothing and to keep the skin clean and dry. Dry cotton cloths can be effective in separating areas that remain moist, such as skin folds and skin under the breasts.
* Encourage the patient with candidiasis infections of the hands to wear gloves during dishwashing and to dry the hands thoroughly afterward.
* Instruct the patient about the proper administration of prescribed drugs.

> ⚠ *Candida* infections should be treated immediately if the patient is severely immunocompromised. Otherwise the infection may become systemic, and can be life-threatening.

Do You UNDERSTAND?

DIRECTIONS: **Indicate which statements are *true* (T) and which are *false* (F). If false, correct the statement in the margin space to make it true.**

_____ 1. Candidiasis can occur as a red, painful swelling around the nail beds.

_____ 2. The candidal lesion is usually nodular and tan-colored, with the center depressed and the borders rolled.

_____ 3. Skin on the chest and legs is the most common site of candidiasis.

_____ 4. Candidiasis, also called yeast infection, *monilia,* and thrush, is caused by a yeastlike fungus.

Answers: 1. T; 2. F—lesions are usually red and edematous with well-defined borders; 3. F—areas under breasts, axillae, groin, perianal area, penis, and scrotum are the most common sites; 4. T.

What IS Folliculitis?

Pathogenesis

Folliculitis is a common skin infection of hair follicles caused by micro-organisms, injuries, or chemical irritation. Classification depends on the type of involvement. The disorder usually develops with an infection that proliferates from another site into the hair follicles. Folliculitis is caused primarily by *Staphylococcus aureus;* but other organisms such as *Klebsiella, Enterobacter, Pseudomonas,* or a dermatophyte such as a fungus can also cause an infection. The inflammation can be superficial or involve deep tissues.

At-Risk Populations

Predisposing factors to folliculitis include an abscess, a previous injury, an abrasion, or a wound located near the hair follicle. Enzymatic and chemotactic factors produced by the bacteria cause the inflammation. Pseudofolliculitis (also called razor bumps) occurs primarily on skin surfaces that are shaved.

Patients on long-term antibiotic therapy and those with existing injuries and infections are prone to folliculitis. An association also exists between folliculitis and persons who have poor hygiene. Patients with diabetes mellitus or who are taking corticosteroids are susceptible to the *Candida* form of folliculitis. *Pseudomonas aeruginosa* in swimming pools and whirlpool tubs with inadequate chloride levels can cause folliculitis.

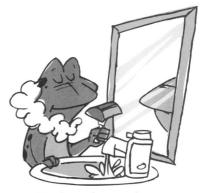

Watch out for razor bumps.

What You NEED TO KNOW

Clinical Manifestations

The hair follicle appears inflamed and tender. Some forms of folliculitis are painless. The patient may scratch the affected site. Small pustules, approximately 2 to 5 mm in size, form at the base of the hair follicle and may stay at the surface or go deeper, invading the entire follicle. The region becomes red, swollen, and tender, depending on the depth of infection. The hair shaft may not be visible in the center of the pustule. Lesions can appear singly or in masses. The most susceptible areas include the back, the scalp, the face, and the extremities. *Pseudomonas* folliculitis can be found on the buttocks, the hips, the axillae, or the external ear. *Candida* folliculitis can be found on the trunk, the upper extremities, and the face.

Prognosis

Recurrent infections may require more than one treatment period but usually resolve once the underlying factors contributing to the inflammation are resolved.

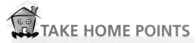

TAKE HOME POINTS

With adequate treatment, folliculitis should dissipate within 5 to 7 days.

What You DO

Treatment

Pustules can be cultured to determine the organism present. Oral antimicrobial therapy is useful, depending on the type of bacteria. Topical erythromycin, mupirocin, or antifungals such as clotrimazole are effective, depending on the type of infection. Saline compresses or Burow's compresses can be used to decrease swelling. Treatment also consists of keeping the area clean and dry.

Nursing Responsibilities

For the patient with folliculitis, the nurse should do the following:
- Advise the patient to keep the area as clean and dry as possible and to improve hygiene when this area is a source of infection.
- Encourage the patient to avoid shaving the affected area until the inflammation has resolved.
- Encourage patients to complete the prescribed course of antimicrobial therapy.

Do You UNDERSTAND?

DIRECTIONS: **Indicate which statements are *true* (T) and which are *false* (F). If false, correct the statement in the margin space to make it true.**

_____ 1. Folliculitis can occur as a red, painful swelling around the nail beds.

_____ 2. Folliculitis is most commonly caused by *S. aureus*.

Answers: 1. F—folliculitis does not occur around the nail beds; 2. T.

What IS a Furuncle or a Carbuncle?

Pathogenesis

Furuncles, also called boils, develop from folliculitis and are found primarily in skin areas containing infected hair follicles. The infection spreads from another site to invade hair follicles, which become swollen, red, and firm. The lesions will frequently fester, rupture, and drain. The anterior nares may be the source of initial infection by *S. aureus*.

Carbuncles are clusters of boils that begin in subcutaneous tissue, forming masses of painful, deep, swollen lesions. Carbuncles may drain through many different openings. *S. aureus* is the primary etiologic agent, but other aerobic and anaerobic organisms may also cause carbuncles. These lesions typically occur on the back of the neck, the lateral thighs, and the upper back.

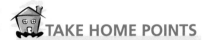

TAKE HOME POINTS

A carbuncle is a group of infected hair follicles that begins in subcutaneous tissue from masses of painful, deep, swollen lesions.

At-Risk Populations

People at risk for furuncles and carbuncles include those who are obese, debilitated, or who have diabetes mellitus, alcoholism, malnutrition, or acne. Patients who are immunocompromised or who have blood disorders such as anemia are also prone to these infections. A relationship to corticosteroid use has been noted.

What You NEED TO KNOW

Clinical Manifestations

Furuncles and carbuncles occur primarily on the upper back, thigh, or neck regions but may also appear in areas prone to friction or trauma. A carbuncle begins with a firm, tender, red nodule that is 1 to 5 cm in size. In a few days, the nodule becomes larger, painful, and cystlike. Cellulitis may also form before or in conjunction with the infection. The lesions will drain purulent material. Carbuncles can invade deep tissues, forming painful edematous masses with numerous open, draining sites. Systemic infection is possible and is evidenced by fever, chills, and malaise. Systemic infections can result in endocarditis or osteomyelitis.

Prognosis

Carbuncles and furuncles should heal with adequate treatment; some may resolve without any treatment. Numerous treatments may be required to eliminate the infection. Furunculosis is a chronic, recurrent form of the disease that may last from months to years.

What You DO

Treatment

Treatment includes moist heat and antibiotics. Moist heat provides some relief from discomfort and promotes drainage. Antibiotic ointments may be applied to the lesions. With larger lesions, an incision with drainage may be necessary. When cellulitis is evident or more than one lesion is present, a systemic cephalosporin or macrolide antibiotic is used. Treatment continues until the infection resolves but usually lasts 10 to 14 days.

Recurrent furunculosis is treated with longer episodes of antibiotics and general cleanliness. A culture should be obtained from patients with recurrent infection to determine the source of infection. Intranasal application of mupirocin calcium ointment for 5 days is also effective for patients who carry *S. aureus* in their nasal passages.

Nursing Responsibilities

For the patient with furuncles or carbuncles, the nurse should do the following:
- Advise the patient of the importance of keeping the area clean and dry to prevent further infection.
- Encourage the patient to use sterile dressings while lesions are draining, and emphasize that proper disposal of dressings is important.
- Isolate the hospitalized patient who has draining, methicillin-resistant *S. aureus* infections. Bed linens, towels, and clothing should be kept away from other individuals to prevent spread of the infection.
- Instruct the patient about the proper administration of nasal antibiotic creams.

Do You UNDERSTAND?

DIRECTIONS: **Indicate which statements are *true* (T) and which are *false* (F). If false, correct the statement in the margin space to make it true.**

_____ 1. Furuncles develop from carbuncles.

_____ 2. After a furuncle festers, it will rupture and drain, and the lesion will subside.

_____ 3. The staphylococcal organism frequently causes carbuncles.

_____ 4. Carbuncles are easily resolved in 3 to 4 days with local antibiotics.

What IS Impetigo?

Pathogenesis

Impetigo, a bacterial infection of the skin caused by group A streptococcus or *S. aureus,* or both, is spread by skin contact with contaminated surfaces such as other skin areas, fingernails, and objects of shared use. Impetigo can appear as a secondary infection from minor trauma, such as abrasions, eczema, insect bites, or poison ivy. Approximately 10 days after exposure to the bacteria, honey-colored crusts appear on the skin. Impetigo is more common in hot, humid weather. Scratching the lesions contributes to the spread of infection. After infection occurs, new lesions may develop on the skin even without any apparent break in the skin surface.

Common impetigo is the term used to describe an infection occurring in preexisting wounds. Bullous impetigo is characterized by small or large superficial bullae on the trunk or extremities.

At-Risk Populations

Impetigo is the most common skin infection in children. It is a highly communicable disease that spreads quickly among family members, in nurseries, in schools, and in crowded areas.

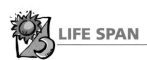

LIFE SPAN

Impetigo commonly occurs in infants and children, but adults who are in poor health, are malnourished, or have poor hygiene are also at risk.

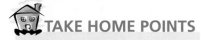

TAKE HOME POINTS

Impetigo is more common in hot, humid weather. Scratching the lesions contributes to spread of the infection.

Answers: 1. F—furuncles develop independently from carbuncles; 2. T; 3. T; 4. F—carbuncles may take 10 to 14 days to resolve.

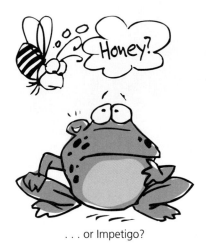

. . . or Impetigo?

What You NEED TO KNOW

Clinical Manifestations

Streptococcal impetigo appears as pustules, vesicles, or bullae on the skin. Inflammatory halos may appear around the lesion. As the lesions erupt, they leave a honey-colored serous liquid on the skin that forms a characteristic "stuck-on" crust. Clustered lesions create large crusts. Itching is common, although scratching excoriates the skin and spreads the infection. *S. aureus* also causes the bullous form of impetigo (**bullous impetigo**). These lesions begin as vesicles but enlarge to form bullae. The center may collapse, with fluid located in the periphery of the lesion. The center contains a varnishlike crust with reddened skin underneath.

Prognosis

With adequate treatment and good hygiene practices, impetigo can be resolved in 2 weeks without any further problems. A type of streptococcal impetigo, if not properly treated, may progress to cause poststreptococcal glomerulonephritis. Without adequate treatment, impetigo may cause other serious problems:
- Osteomyelitis
- Septic arthritis
- Lymphadenitis
- Meningitis or sepsis (in infants)
- Deep cellulitis
- Bacteremia
- Pneumonia

What You DO

Treatment

Interventions for impetigo include the application of topical mupirocin or triple antibiotic ointments. Systemic antibiotics such as penicillin or erythromycin are effective. For severe staphylococcal infections and bullous impetigo, intravenous (IV) therapy with a penicillinase-resistant penicillin is necessary. Topical applications of cool saline compresses are helpful in relieving the itching and discomfort.

Nursing Responsibilities

For the patient with impetigo, the nurse should do the following:

- Encourage the patient to keep the lesions clean and dry. The entire body can be cleaned with an antibacterial soap to prevent reoccurrence and spread to other areas. The crusts should be removed before the antibiotic cream is applied. To be effective, the cream is applied several times a day.
- Advise the caregiver to wear gloves to prevent spread of the infection. The patient's clothing and dishes should be washed separately to prevent the spread of infection.
- Advise the patient to avoid scratching.
- Encourage good hygienic measures to prevent spreading the infection to family members and others.

Do You UNDERSTAND?

DIRECTIONS: Fill in the blanks to complete the following statements.

1. Impetigo is highly _____.
2. Streptococcal impetigo appears as small pustules, vesicles, or bullae that erupt on the _____.
3. Impetigo lesions can be found anywhere on the body, especially in _____ areas such as the face, the hands, the neck, and the extremities.
4. _____ from impetigo is frequently a concern.

What IS Cellulitis?

Pathogenesis

Cellulitis is a bacterial infection of the dermis and subcutaneous tissue caused primarily by group A streptococcus or *S. aureus*, although many types of bacteria can cause cellulitis.

Answers: 1. contagious; 2. skin; 3. exposed; 4. scarring.

Erysipelas is an acute, inflammatory type of cellulitis that has lymphatic involvement. Paronychia is a cellulitis of the nail folds. Cellulitis can also develop around the eye. Group A streptococcus also causes perianal cellulitis. The erysipeloid form of cellulitis is found in individuals who handle saltwater fish, shellfish, meat products, and poultry. Cellulitis can also appear in normal, healthy skin.

At-Risk Populations

People who are at risk for cellulitis include those with diabetes mellitus, human immunodeficiency virus, or neoplasms; and IV–drug abusers, patients who are on antineoplastic therapy, and those with peripheral vascular disease. Patients who have had previous trauma to the skin or existing skin ulcers are also at risk.

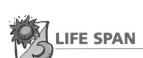

LIFE SPAN

Children under the age of 5 have a higher rate of facial cellulitis, particularly in the presence of an insect bite, laceration, or eczema.

What You NEED TO KNOW

Clinical Manifestations

Cellulitis is usually found on the lower legs, the ears, and the face, appearing a few days after the infectious organism invades the skin. Local swelling, tenderness, warmth, and pain may occur. Bright red patches or plaques with indefinite borders begin to appear. Edema may be present at the site. The skin may be tender and warm with toxic striations. Regional lymphadenopathy may be present. In later stages, pustules, abscesses, and necrosis may develop. With repeated bouts of infection, lymphatic drainage becomes impaired, which can result in repeated infections, lymphedema, and epidermal thickening known as elephantiasis nostras. Secondary infections of the site can also occur.

Prognosis

With adequate treatment, cellulitis should resolve. Some individuals continue to have recurrent episodes that are difficult to treat.

What You DO

Treatment

Treatment of cellulitis includes the use of systemic antibiotics such as cephalosporins or macrolides. Resistant strains are treated with penicillinase-resistant penicillin such as nafcillin or vancomycin. Analgesics and soaking in Burow's solution can be helpful in relieving discomfort. If a patient has cellulitis in the lower extremities, they should be elevated to reduce swelling.

Nursing Responsibilities

For the patient with cellulitis, the nurse should do the following:
- Advise the patient that most cellulitis is considered an infectious disorder.
- Encourage the patient to complete the course of antibiotic therapy.
- Remove any exudate and keep the area clean and dry. Dressings can be used when drainage is present.
- Elevate and immobilize the extremity when the involved area is edematous, and encourage the patient to wear support stockings.
- Encourage good hygiene to prevent further occurrences.
- Teach the patient how to prevent skin infections in the future.
- Instruct patients whose lesions have not resolved within 7 days to seek further medical care.

Do You UNDERSTAND?

DIRECTIONS: **Fill in the blanks to complete the following statements.**
1. When _____ first occurs, it appears as small _____, vesicles, or _____ on the skin.
2. Local _____, _____, warmth, and pain may occur.
3. _____ borders and edema may be present at the cellulitis site.

What IS Herpes Simplex?

Pathogenesis

Primary herpes simplex virus (HSV) infections affect 200,000 to 700,000 people every year, with as many as 2 million new cases occurring each year. Recurrent infections can affect up to 30 million Americans annually. Two serotypes cause HSV infections: type 1 (HSV-1) or type 2 (HSV-2). HSV-1 is usually responsible for nongenital infections found on the mouth, the face, and the cornea. Common names for the infection include cold sores, fever blister, and canker sores. HSV-1 is transmitted primarily by contact with infected saliva. Previous exposure to one type does not prevent infection from the other type. Genital herpes is the most common infectious genital disease in industrialized countries.

HSV infection occurs in two stages: primary infection and recurrent infection. Primary infection develops 3 to 12 days after initial exposure to the virus. The virus begins replicating in the dermis and epidermis and then travels down nerve roots to the dorsal root, where the virus lies dormant in the sensory ganglia until it is reactivated. During this latency period, the virus resides in the nuclei of host cells. After the virus is reactivated, it travels by way of the peripheral nerve root onto the skin or mucus membrane, creating lesions. Recurrent infections appear in the same manner as primary infections but may be less severe.

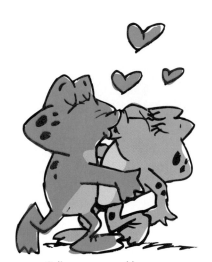

Saliva can spread herpes.

At-Risk Populations

Triggers for recurrent infections include stress, lack of sleep, sunburn, ultraviolet light, overexertion, menstruation, fever, trauma, and systemic infections. Eczema herpeticum is a form of atopic dermatitis that develops into herpes lesions.

The herpes virus is usually transmitted through intimate contact with another person who is shedding the virus from a mucosal surface or through body secretions. Seventy percent of transmission occurs when the individual has no symptoms. Oral transmission occurs through kissing, poor hand washing, and oral intercourse. Other patients at risk for HSV infection include those who are immunocompromised, those with cancer, or those receiving immunosuppressive drugs.

What You NEED TO KNOW

Clinical Manifestations

HSV can occur as a primary or recurrent infection. Patients with a primary HSV infection develop itching, burning, tingling, or pain in the affected area. A small cluster of vesicles appears on an erythematous base with vesicle rupture occurring in approximately 5 days. The vesicles may progress to pustules, ulcers, and crusts. The vesicles may be single or in groups on an erythematous base. A crust forms over the skin, with lesions taking 1 to 3 weeks to resolve. If the infection spreads to the oropharynx, patients may experience high fevers, headache, malaise, and sore throat.

Lesions can be found on the face, the lips, the mouth, the buttocks, or the genital region. Herpetic infection of the eye may manifest as pain, irritation, watery eyes, or photophobia and can lead to blindness.

Prognosis

Because no cure for the herpes virus is available, treatment measures are directed at the symptoms. Herpetic infections may lay dormant for long periods. After a primary infection, antibodies to the virus develop, creating recurrences that are usually more localized and less severe. Some patients have no further occurrence of the infection.

What You DO

Treatment

A diagnosis of herpes infection is made based on the appearance of the lesions, a Tzanck smear, a viral culture, or serologic testing. Acyclovir, famciclovir, and valacyclovir, when used early in an outbreak, have been found to be effective in most cases. A strain of acyclovir-resistant virus can develop in immunocompromised individuals. Penciclovir has also been found to be a possible treatment but must be applied every 2 hours while the patient is awake.

Therapy must be started early. When started within 48 hours of the beginning of prodromal symptoms, the effectiveness of treatment is increased. Therapy decreases viral shedding and promotes rapid healing. For individuals with frequent recurrences (e.g., six or more a year), oral acyclovir may be given for longer periods. Drying agents such as benzyl peroxide gel may be useful for facial lesions.

Nursing Responsibilities

For the patient with HSV infection, the nurse should do the following:

- Support the patient during any needed adjustments in lifestyle. Taking care of the overall health is important: including getting adequate rest, eating well, and reducing stress.
- Teach patients that transmission of the virus may occur even when they are asymptomatic.
- Prevent secondary infections. Good hand washing and hygiene must be performed during times of outbreak.

Do You UNDERSTAND?

DIRECTIONS: **Indicate which statements are *true* (T) and which are *false* (F). If false, correct the statement in the margin space to make it true.**

_____ 1. Acyclovir, famciclovir, and valacyclovir have been found to be effective in most cases of herpes infections.

_____ 2. Getting adequate rest, eating well, and reducing stress has little effect on the development or recurrence of herpes simplex.

Answers: 1. T; 2. F—these activities have a significant influence on the development or recurrence of HSV infections

What IS Herpes Zoster?

Pathogenesis

Herpes zoster is caused by the same virus—varicella-zoster—that produces chickenpox (varicella; shingles) and is characterized by acute inflammation along a dermatome of the skin. A decline in immunity, stress, or aging may cause reactivation of latent varicella-zoster virus. With initial exposure to chickenpox, the virus travels down the nerve fibers to the dorsal ganglion cells, where it resides in a dormant state. Once the varicella-zoster virus is reactivated, it replicates in the affected sensory ganglion. The virus moves through the sensory nerve pathways to the skin, where it creates pain, vesicles, and crusting. The inflammatory response along the nerve pathways and neuronal necrosis causes the intense pain. Reactivation is not completely understood, but it is believed to be a result of a decline in immunity.

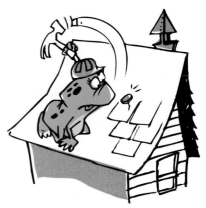

Shingles are painful.

At-Risk Populations

Individuals at risk for herpes zoster include patients who are immunocompromised, who have leukemia, or who have conditions that require an organ transplant. The incidence of shingles also increases with age.

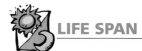

LIFE SPAN

Adults over age 50 have an increased incidence of shingles. Older adults are particularly susceptible to this herpes virus because of a loss of large nerve fibers and a shift to smaller nerve fibers.

What You NEED TO KNOW

Clinical Manifestations

Before the eruption of the lesions, the patient with herpes zoster may experience itching, pain, or tenderness at the site. In 3 to 5 days, vesicles begin to erupt on the skin. The lesions may appear "bubbly" or like cobblestones in clusters. The underlying skin is red and swollen.

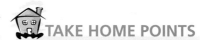

TAKE HOME POINTS

A direct relationship exists among postherpetic neuralgia is described as the presence of pain at least 1 month or more after the lesions have disappeared.

Vesicles usually develop on the posterior surface of the body and move peripherally along unilateral dermatomes to the anterior body surface. In 1 to 2 weeks, the crusts dry up.

Primary eruption sites are the facial, the thoracic, or the cervical nerve roots. A few lesions may be observed outside the primary area, particularly in children and immunocompromised individuals. Associated pain and paresthesia accompany this illness.

Permanent blindness can result when the herpes virus develops in the ophthalmic division of the trigeminal nerve. Rashes that resemble herpes zoster have been noted after the varicella vaccine has been given. The vaccine itself can cause an outbreak of herpes in a few individuals. A second and third reoccurrence of herpes zoster may occur but usually involves dermatomes other than those involved in the original attack.

Prognosis

No cure for herpes zoster is available. The pain of herpes zoster is intense and may last long after the vesicles have subsided. Postherpetic neuralgia may develop in 10% to 70% of the individuals who have this condition.

Treatment is directed at alleviating symptoms. The virus may lay dormant for long periods and arise during periods of stress, immunosuppression, or during aging. After an initial episode, most patients never experience another. The varicella vaccine has been found to be effective in preventing chickenpox. The hope is that the vaccine may also prevent the occurrence of herpes zoster.

What You DO

Treatment

The drug of choice in the treatment of herpes zoster is acyclovir although other antiviral drugs such as famciclovir, valacyclovir, vidarabine, and sorivudine have been used. Corticosteroid use is controversial but may be helpful for some patients to reduce the risk of postherpetic neuralgia.

Treatment begins as soon as possible after appearance of symptoms. When given before or during the vesicular phase, lesion development and pain is lessened. Burow's solution can be used to speed the drying of the lesions and remove crusts. Antibacterial sulfonamide cream can be applied to prevent secondary infections. Baking soda, aqueous alcohol lotions, or calamine lotion may be used for itching at the affected site.

Topical anesthetics may reduce pain at the site. Analgesics are frequently needed to relieve the pain. Opioid analgesics may be necessary when the pain is intense. Amitriptyline, an antidepressant, and a number of other drugs have been found useful because of their sedative effects.

Nursing Responsibilities

For the patient with herpes zoster, the nurse should do the following:

- Prevent secondary infection of the lesions. The area should be kept free of contaminants. Covering the lesions is not recommended during treatment.
- Manage pain. When pain becomes too severe, the patient may need to be referred to a pain clinic.
- Advise the patient to notify the health care provider if the eye becomes involved, so that a referral to an ophthalmologist can be made.
- Advise the patient with herpes zoster to avoid anyone who has not had chickenpox, women who are pregnant, and those who are immunocompromised. Herpes zoster can cause chicken pox in individuals who are susceptible.

Do You UNDERSTAND?

DIRECTIONS: **Indicate which statements are *true* (T) and which are *false* (F). If false, correct the statement in the margin space to make it true.**

_____ 1. Herpes zoster is an acute inflammation along the dermatomes of the skin.

_____ 2. The incidence of herpes zoster is not influenced by age.

_____ 3. Pain always disappears when lesions disappear.

_____ 4. Herpes zoster is easily cured with antibiotics.

What IS Tinea?

Pathogenesis

Tinea is a disease that results from invasion of the skin, the hair, or the nails by fungal organisms called **dermatophytes.** Tinea infections are described according to their location. Tinea capitis is a fungal invasion of the scalp, tinea pedis is of the feet, and tinea cruris is of the groin. Tinea corporis refers to all the other skin areas (excluding the scalp, the face, the hands, the feet, and the groin).

Various types of fungus may cause this disease. After the skin is inoculated by the fungus, the fungal hyphae grow into the stratum corneum layer of the skin. When the fungus invades a body area with hair, the fungus grows downward into the hair, disrupting and invading the keratin layer as it is formed within the follicle. By the third week of infection, broken, brittle hair may be seen.

At-Risk Populations

Patients with impaired cell-mediated immunity may acquire atypical and more aggressive forms of this disease. Other high-risk conditions include continual exposure to moist conditions, use of communal baths, and Cushing's syndrome.

What You NEED TO KNOW

Clinical Manifestations

Symptoms of the disease depend to some extent upon the area of the body where the infection is located. Tinea capitis is usually manifested as hair loss. Tinea corporis causes ring-shaped (annular) scaly patches with raised edges, vesicles, and pustules. Scaling, fissures, and maceration may occur on the feet, particularly between the toes. Tinea cruris is characterized by red, lesions with raised borders. Infections of the nail may cause separation from the nail bed. The nail itself will become thickened and discolored.

Prognosis

All forms of tinea will heal in a short time with appropriate treatment.

Treatment

Antifungal drugs are the mainstay of therapy for this disease. Some patients will require treatment for 2 months or more if the infection is severe or the nail bed is affected.

Nursing Responsibilities

For the patient with a tinea infection, the nurse should do the following:
- Teach the patient to avoid sharing combs, brushes, towels, or washcloths.
- Instruct the patient to dry intertriginous areas and the feet completely after bathing.
- Teach the patient how to take or apply topical drugs correctly.
- Instruct the patient to avoid touching newly appearing lesions while on treatment, and advise him or her to seek information from the health care provider if necessary.

Do You UNDERSTAND?

DIRECTIONS: **Circle the correct answer.**
1. Tinea corporis refers to a fungal infection of the
   a. Scalp.
   b. Groin.
   c. Torso.
   d. Feet.
2. Tinea infections are caused by
   a. Dermatophytes.
   b. Viruses.
   c. Bacteria.
   d. None of the above.

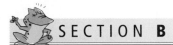

SECTION **B**

INFLAMMATORY SKIN DISORDERS

What IS Acne Vulgaris?

Pathogenesis

Acne vulgaris occurs when hormones called androgens overstimulate the skin's oil glands. The oil glands (**sebaceous glands**) secrete a substance called sebum, which normally travels up tiny hair follicles to the skin's pores, where it lubricates and protects the skin. However, excessive sebum can get trapped within the follicle. Simultaneously, overworked oil glands enlarge, accelerating the normal shedding of skin cells inside the follicle. These skin cells mix with trapped sebum and clog the skin's pores. Clogged pores promote overgrowth of the bacterium that causes acne *(Propionibacterium acnes)*. The bacteria in turn causes further inflammation of hair follicles and surrounding skin, resulting in acne.

Milder cases of acne will cause the development of noninflammatory papules. More severe forms cause inflamed papules, pustules, and nodules to develop. Acne is usually seen in areas of the skin that have the greatest concentration of pilosebaceous follicles, including the face and the upper part of the chest and back.

At-Risk Populations

A genetic predisposition to acne may be present. Acne affects men and women equally, but because males produce more androgen, they are prone to develop more severe cases of acne than females. Approximately 85% of the population is affected by this disorder at some time in their lives. Research studies failed to find a relationship between diet and acne, although stress is thought to play an important part in the longer prevalence of the condition among women. Although the exact link between stress and acne is unknown, theories suggest that stress increases the secretion of androgen.

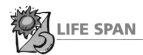

LIFE SPAN

Acne usually occurs between the ages of 10 and 13 and lasts 5 to 10 years. The hormonal fluctuations of the menstrual cycle can make young women more sensitive to androgens that are already present, causing flare-ups immediately before menses.

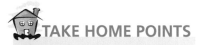

TAKE HOME POINTS

Overactivity of the skin's oil glands, not poor hygiene, poor character, or poor diet, is the cause of acne.

What You NEED TO KNOW

Clinical Manifestations

Acne typically occurs in areas where there are a large number of oil glands. The most common areas include the face, the scalp, the neck, the chest, the back, the upper arms, and the shoulders. Blackheads and whiteheads **(open and closed comedones)**, occasionally filled with pus **(pustules)**, and cysts may be present.

Prognosis

Whiteheads and blackheads drain and heal over time. Pustules and deeper cysts can cause scarring; however, the scarring tends to lessen with time. The tendency to scar varies from person to person. A severe inflammatory type of acne **(acne fulminans)** can cause arthritis and fever.

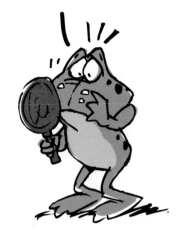

What You DO

Treatment

Many treatments for acne are available, including nonprescription and prescription drugs, and surgery. Topical treatments include benzyl peroxide, salicylic acid, and topical antibiotics. Benzyl peroxide is an antimicrobial agent effective against the bacteria associated with acne. Salicylic acid reduces abnormal shedding of skin cells along the hair follicle. Topical (as well as orally administered) antibiotics such as clindamycin and erythromycin kill acne bacteria on the skin's surface and reduce inflammation, but these antibiotics do not affect abnormal skin cell shedding or sebum production. For this reason, topical drugs are frequently used together with other acne preparations such as vitamin A derivatives **(retinoids)**. Retinoid and retinoid-like skin creams and lotions normalize skin cell shedding and growth and reduce inflammation, which combine to unclog pores. Retinoids are prescription drugs. All of these drugs have adverse effects that limit their use.

Acne treatment also includes the use of intralesional steroids and comedo extractions. In selected patients, cryosurgery is used. Dermabrasion is used for patients with severe scarring. A newer procedure, laser

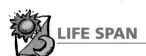

LIFE SPAN

During the teenage years, appearance is important to the patient. Acne may damage the adolescent's self-esteem. The nurse must counsel the patient in this regard.

resurfacing (also called laser peel), removes the top layers of skin without bleeding, the use of chemical peels, or dermabrasion. Laser resurfacing is typically performed under local or general anesthesia.

Nursing Responsibilities

For the patient with acne, the nurse should do the following:

- Identify persons at risk for acne. Provide patient and family teaching about the disorder and its treatment; this is important because many common misconceptions exist about the cause.
- Keep hands and face clean. Even resting the chin, forehead, or cheek on the hand can exacerbate the lesions. Hats, sweatbands, and shirt collars contribute to acne.
- Advise the patient to avoid mechanical trauma to the lesions, such as squeezing, rubbing, or picking at the comedones.
- Encourage the patient to use drug therapy as prescribed.

Do You UNDERSTAND?

DIRECTIONS: **Fill in the blanks to complete the following statements.**

1. Acne vulgaris is an inflammation within the area of the _____ _____.

2. _____ hormones do not contribute to the production of sebum.

3. Acne usually develops between the ages of _____ and _____.

4. The topical treatment of first choice for acne is _____ _____.

5. Two nursing responsibilities in reference to acne include _____ _____ and _____.

What IS Rosacea?

Pathogenesis

Rosacea, previously known as acne rosacea, is a chronic inflammatory process easily confused with acne vulgaris. In fact, rosacea may be present with acne. The cause of rosacea is unknown, although the pathogenesis is similar to that of acne vulgaris. Rosacea is a progressive, chronic dermatologic disorder that is characterized by papules, pustules, and tissue hyperplasia that typically appears in the central part of the face.

At-Risk Populations

Rosacea is more common in fair-skinned persons with an onset in middle-aged and older persons. The predisposing causes are unknown, but a family history and ruddy complexion are common findings.

What You NEED TO KNOW

Clinical Manifestations

In the early stages of development (before the age of 20), repeated episodes of flushing occur. The flushing eventually becomes a permanent, redness (**erythema**) on the nose and cheeks that occasionally extends to the forehead and chin. The flushing is common in women. Erythema persists as the person ages, with the sebaceous follicles enlarging and the skin changing to a purple-red color. The skin becomes coarse in texture. Eventually, vascular lesions form a group of small blood vessels (**telangiectasia**), and an irregular, bulbous thickening of the nose (**rhinophyma**) develops. Rhinophyma is present more frequently in men than it is in women.

Up to 58% of patients with this disorder may have visual symptoms. Conjunctivitis and keratitis, which are rare, may accompany rosacea. The patient may also have blepharitis, tearing, burning, iritis, episcleritis, and corneal vascularization with scarring. Severe forms of rosacea may threaten the patient's vision and require aggressive treatment.

Prognosis

Rosacea is characterized by periods of exacerbation and remission. The disorder requires prolonged treatment.

What You DO

Treatment

The treatment for rosacea is similar to those used for acne vulgaris. The antibiotic of choice is oral tetracycline. Topical metronidazole is an effective treatment, although it will make the affected area dry and red for a period. Metronidazole may have to be used for a prolonged period to suppress flare-up of symptoms. Telangiectases may be treated with electrodesiccation. Rhinophyma requires surgical removal of excess tissue through laser therapy.

Nursing Responsibilities

For the patient with rosacea, the nurse should do the following:
- Identify patients who are at risk for rosacea.
- Advise patients that although alcohol intake is not related to the development of rosacea, persons with rosacea are heat-sensitive. Patients should be taught to avoid vascular-stimulating agents, such as heat, cold, sunlight, hot liquids, highly seasoned foods, and alcohol.
- Provide patient and family teaching regarding the adverse effects of drugs and risks associated with surgical intervention.
- Provide emotional support. The disorder frequently alters the patient's self-image.

Do You UNDERSTAND?

DIRECTIONS: **Fill in the blanks to complete the following statements.**
1. Rosacea is characterized by periods of _____ and _____.
2. Telangiectasia is defined as _____.
3. The drugs commonly used in the treatment of rosacea include ___ _____ and _____.
4. Rosacea is more common in _____, with an onset occurring in _____ and _____ persons.

What IS Eczema?

Pathogenesis

The terms eczema and dermatitis are synonymous for the most common disorders (**dermatoses**) of the skin. Eczema is an inflammatory skin response to any injurious agent. Both endogenous and exogenous agents can cause an inflammatory response. Several types of dermatoses have been identified, including allergic contact dermatitis, irritant contact dermatitis, and atopic dermatitis.

More than 2000 allergens produce the inflammatory skin response, including clothing, cosmetics, cleaning products, occupational exposure, plants and woods, metal alloys found in jewelry, additives such as perfumes and dyes, and soap ingredients. An example of allergic contact dermatitis is that caused by contact with latex products, specifically examination gloves and condoms. Allergic contact dermatitis is a cell-mediated response brought about by sensitization to an allergen and is a type IV hypersensitivity reaction.

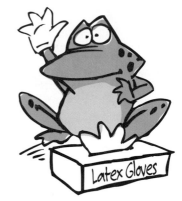

Latex can cause allergic contact dermatitis.

Irritant contact dermatitis can occur in persons who are in sufficient contact with the irritant to cause a reaction. For example, a reaction can occur from mechanical means (e.g., rubbing), chemical irritants (e.g., household cleaning products), or environmental irritants (e.g., wool, fiberglass, urine, plants). Another example is the reaction caused from contact with cement products.

Atopic dermatitis (also known as atopic eczema) occurs in two clinical forms: infantile and adult. Atopic dermatitis is a subtype of a type I hypersensitivity reaction. A family history of asthma, hay fever, or atopic dermatitis is usually present.

At-Risk Populations

Eczema has no age boundaries. This group of skin conditions can affect all ages and cultural groups.

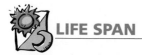

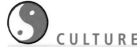
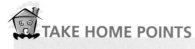

What You NEED TO KNOW

Clinical Manifestations

Vesicle formation, oozing, crusting, itching, erythema, and scaling characterize eczema, regardless of the specific form. The clinical manifestations can range from mild forms (e.g., itchy, hot, dry skin) to severe forms with raw, bleeding, and broken skin. The locations of the lesions are of great benefit in diagnosing the causative agent.

The infantile form usually becomes milder as the child ages, frequently disappearing by the age of 15. Adolescents and adults have dry, leathery, hyperpigmented or hypopigmented lesions located in the antecubital and popliteal areas. The lesions may spread to the neck, the hands, the feet, the eyelids, and behind the ears. Itching may be severe in both forms, and secondary infections are common.

Prognosis

Eczema is a life-long problem characterized by periods of exacerbation and remission.

What You DO

Treatment

The treatment of the various types of eczema is aimed at removing the source of the irritant or allergen, which may require the patient to modify behavior or even change employment to avoid the irritant or allergen. Modification measures may include wearing protective clothing such as goggles or gloves. Another modification measure may be alerting persons who have irritant contact dermatitis and who work in heavy industrial areas to avoid strong hand cleansers. Grease and grime can be removed with inert oil, such as salad oil or mineral oil, before washing with soap and water.

Washing the affected areas to remove further contamination by the irritant or allergen can treat minor cases of eczematous dermatitis. Avoidance of temperature changes and stress helps to minimize abnormal and cutaneous vascular and sweat responses.

Apply antipruritic creams or lotions, and bandage exposed areas. Topical steroids may be helpful in some cases. Chronic dry lesions are usually treated with ointments and creams that contain lubricating, keratolytic, or antipruritic drugs. Systemic interventions differ according to the type of irritant or allergen and the severity of the reaction. Extreme cases can be treated with oral antihistamines, systemic corticosteroids, and wet dressings.

Nursing Responsibilities

Care responsibilities for the person with eczematous dermatitis include primarily patient and family teaching about possible irritants, allergens, and avoidance behaviors.

Do You UNDERSTAND?

DIRECTIONS: **Provide answers to the following questions.**
1. What is the synonymous term for eczema? _____
2. What is a severe form of eczema? _____
3. What is a treatment for eczema? _____
4. With chronic eczema, how does the skin appear? _____
_____

What IS Psoriasis?

Pathogenesis

Psoriasis is a common, but chronic, inflammatory skin disease. It is characterized by inflamed, swollen skin lesions that have a typical silvery white scaling. The most common type of this disease is called *discoid* or *plaque psoriasis.*

Although the cause of psoriasis is uncertain, the most accepted theory attributes the cause to a T cell dermal immune response to an antigen. The activated T cells (primarily CD4-positive helper T cells) produce chemical messengers called **cytokines,** which stimulate keratinocyte

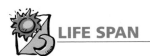

LIFE SPAN

All ages are affected; however, the onset of psoriasis usually occurs in the third decade of life. Childhood onset of psoriasis is associated with a familial history. Psoriasis can persist throughout life and flare up at unpredictable times.

Answers: 1. dermatitis; 2. allergic contact dermatitis; 3. removal of the source of the irritant or allergen; 4. dry and leathery, with hyperpigmented or hypopigmented lesions.

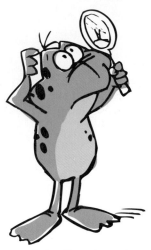

Psoriasis affects the scalp.

proliferation from the basal layer of the epidermis. The migration time of the keratinocyte from the basal cell skin layer decreases from the normal 26 to 30 days to 4 to 7 days. Cell turnover and metabolism increase. Capillary blood flow increases to support the metabolic demands. Infiltration of neutrophils and monocytes causes the accompanying inflammatory changes. Skin trauma is a common precipitating factor in individuals predisposed to the disorder.

At-Risk Populations

In the United States, psoriasis affects approximately 1% of the population. The incidence is decreased in warmer, sunny climates. An association appears to exist between psoriasis and arthritis. Psoriatic arthritis occurs in 5% to 7% of persons with psoriasis.

What You NEED TO KNOW

Clinical Manifestations

The body areas usually affected by this disorder include the scalp, the hairline, the elbows, the knees, and sites of trauma. The severity of psoriasis ranges from a life-threatening emergency to a minimal cosmetic problem. There is a characteristic circular, patchy appearance to the lesions of all sizes which are covered with heavy, dry, silvery scales. The increased rate of cell proliferation, capillary dilation, and cell metabolism creates the red appearance of erythema. The extent of inflammation determines the size and distribution of the lesions.

Prognosis

Wide variations exist in the severity and extent of the condition, as well as with the development of arthritis. There is no known cure at this time.

⚠ The pustular form of psoriasis may be fatal in individuals with suppressed immunity because of loss of fluid and electrolytes through the skin.

What You DO

Treatment

The goal of treatment is to suppress the clinical manifestations of the disorder. Treatment for psoriasis focuses on reducing epidermal cell proliferation and is used when less than 20% of the body surface is involved. Keratolytics, corticosteroids, and emollients are used in mild cases of psoriasis. Lesions of the genitalia, the scalp, and the nails are treated with shampoos and various lotions. Tar preparations and ultraviolet light or a combination of the two, as well as antimetabolites such as methotrexate and etretinate (vitamin A derivative), are used to treat moderate lesions. A combination of systemic corticosteroids, cyclosporin, topical agents, antimetabolites, and hospitalization may be used in severe cases.

Nursing Responsibilities

For the patient with psoriasis, the nurse should do the following:

- Instruct the patient to wear goggles to protect the eyes when ultraviolet light treatments are used.
- Teach the importance of hand washing before and after the application of topical drugs
- Teach the patient and family about the adverse effects of steroids and other drugs used in treatment of psoriasis.
- Allow patients to verbalize their feelings about the disorder. Encourage membership in a support group.

TAKE HOME POINTS

Support the body image of the patient with psoriasis. The disorder can be devastating to a patient's self-concept.

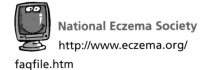

National Eczema Society
http://www.eczema.org/
faqfile.htm

Do You UNDERSTAND?

DIRECTIONS: **Indicate which statements are *true* (T) and which are *false* (F). If false, correct the statement in the margin space to make it true.**

_____   1. Psoriasis can be life-threatening.
_____   2. A person diagnosed with psoriasis can develop arthritis.

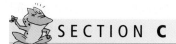

SECTION C

MALIGNANCIES OF THE SKIN

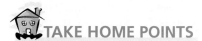
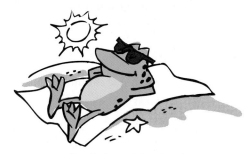

Don't stay out *too* long!

What IS Basal Cell Carcinoma?

Pathogenesis

Basal cell carcinoma (BCC) is a malignant lesion arising from epithelial cells. The most common sites of basal cell carcinoma are areas of the skin most exposed to the sun, such as the face and the neck. Ultraviolet (UV) light exposure, particularly UVB rays, creates DNA mutations. The p53 gene normally halts uncontrolled cell growth. However, mutations in the p53 gene allow cancer cells to grow and to become more aggressive. The *ras* oncogene (a tumor suppressor gene) has been implicated as a causative factor of BCC, squamous cell carcinoma, and melanomas.

At-Risk Populations

Melanin in the skin has a protecting effect. The populations at risk for basal cell carcinoma are older adults and light-skinned individuals. Patients with preexisting skin conditions or who have extensive time in the sun are at risk for basal cell carcinoma.

What You NEED TO KNOW

Clinical Manifestations

The clinical manifestations of basal cell carcinoma begin with a slightly elevated, pearl-colored nodule. Skin cells are not shed in the normal keratinization process, thus the tumor arises. The growth rate is slow. As the lesion grows, it frequently ulcerates. Usually the center of the lesion is depressed, and the borders are rolled and translucent.

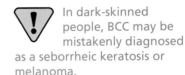 In dark-skinned people, BCC may be mistakenly diagnosed as a seborrheic keratosis or melanoma.

Prognosis

The prognosis of basal cell carcinoma is good, and with early diagnosis and treatment, a cure is expected. Metastatic spread is rare. Without treatment over months or years, basal cell carcinoma can destroy an ear lobe, eyelid, or other area by invading surrounding tissue. Large, deep, or infiltrating BCCs may show aggressive growth, but rarely metastasize to other areas of the body. Patients have an increased risk for tumor recurrence if the primary tumor is located in the midface or the ear, is of long duration, and is greater than 2 cm across at its largest dimension.

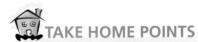
TAKE HOME POINTS

The early warning signs of skin cancer include changes in the size, color, borders, or texture of a mole and changes in the size or skin color of any spot or darkly pigmented growth. Early detection of unusual lesions is important.

What You DO

Treatment

Eradication of the tumor is the goal of therapy. The treatment for basal cell carcinoma includes surgery, radiation therapy, cryosurgery, photodynamic therapy, and electrodestruction.

Nursing Responsibilities

The nursing responsibilities for the patient with BCC are primarily preventative. Patients who have risk factors for skin cancer should have a thorough examination of all skin surfaces including genitals and scalp at least once year. The nurse should also do the following:

- Advise the patient to wear appropriate protective clothing and head covering when outdoors. Sunscreens with para-aminobenzoic acid (PABA) and a rating of at least 15 for UV protection should be used. Those who have a prior history of skin cancer should use sunscreen with a rating of 30.

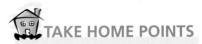
TAKE HOME POINTS

Teach the patient to avoid excessive exposure to UV light and to avoid the sun, particularly between the hours of 10:00 AM and 3:00 PM, when the ultraviolet light is strongest.

- Increase the patient's awareness of the potential harm to the skin from increasingly popular tanning booths.
- Teach the patient and family about the risk factors of skin cancer. The risk factors include a fair complexion, immunosuppression, and excessive UV exposure. The warning signs of skin cancer should also be included in the teaching.

Do You UNDERSTAND?

DIRECTIONS: **Indicate which statements are *true* (T) and which are *false* (F). If false, correct the statement in the margin space to make it true.**

_____ 1. No treatment is needed for basal cell carcinoma.

_____ 2. Change in size or color of any skin spot or dark pigmented growth is a warning sign of skin malignancy.

_____ 3. As the basal cell lesion grows, it frequently ulcerates. The center of the lesion is usually depressed, and the borders are rolled.

_____ 4. Skin on the chest and the legs is the most common site for basal cell carcinoma.

What IS Squamous Cell Carcinoma?

Pathogenesis

Squamous cell carcinoma (SCC) is a malignant tumor of the epidermis. These tumors grow more rapidly than basal cell tumors and can metastasize. Tumors can be limited to a localized area (**in situ**) or invasive and spread through to lymph. Squamous cell carcinoma tumors are firm. Unlike BCC, this cancer may originate in mucosal surfaces. The surface is elevated with a granular quality that easily bleeds. Most squamous cell carcinomas arise from skin lesions, including chronic ulcerated areas, sun-damaged skin, or areas of horny growth such as a wart, a callus, or scars.

At-Risk Populations

The cause of squamous cell carcinoma is unknown, although sun exposure and aging are the most common risk factors. Similar to basal cell carcinoma, UV exposure, particularly UVB rays, creates DNA mutations. Mutation of the p53 gene is considered part of the mechanism. The p53 gene normally halts uncontrolled cell growth. However, mutations in the gene allow cancer cells to become more aggressive.

Populations at risk for squamous cell carcinoma include older adults and light-skinned individuals. Environmental risk factors include exposure to insecticides and herbicides, chronic thermal injury and scars, and prolonged immunosuppression. Tumors that originated in the dorsal aspect of the hand, the lips, the ears and the penis have higher rates of recurrence.

What IS Malignant Melanoma?

Pathogenesis

Malignant melanoma is a cancerous lesion arising from epidermal melanocyte cells. Melanoma is the deadliest form of skin cancer. The cause of malignant melanoma is unknown. Melanocytes synthesize the pigment melanin. Malignant melanomas most commonly arise from an existing mole (**nevus**) but may also originate from normal skin surfaces. A nevus is a benign aggregation of melanocytes. When a nevus has a diameter of 6 mm or greater (about the size of the eraser on a pencil), it is considered highly suggestive for developing malignant melanoma.

Malignant melanoma is grouped into three varieties. Most malignant melanomas are the superficial spreading variety and occur in young and middle-aged adults. The lentigo malignant melanoma occurs during adolescence and middle age, and in older adults. The pattern of tumor growth for both lentigo and superficial spreading is horizontally along the skin surface. Their potential for metastasis is less than for the nodular variety of malignant melanoma. Nodular melanoma has a high potential of becoming metastatic because it grows vertically into deeper tissues. However, local invasion, regional lymph node metastasis, and distant metastasis are possible with all types of melanoma.

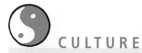

CULTURE

The populations that are most at risk for malignant melanoma are fair-skinned people and young to middle-aged adults who live in the sunbelt states.

At-Risk Populations

Sun exposure is the most common risk factor for malignant melanoma. Genetic predisposition, immunosuppression, and exposure to radiation or sunlight also increase the risk.

What You NEED TO KNOW

Clinical Manifestations of Squamous Cell Carcinoma

Skin exposed to the sun such as on the face and neck is most commonly affected. Squamous cell carcinoma is observed less frequently on the hands or other parts of the body. The lesions are scaly or keratotic, are slightly elevated with an irregular border, and usually have a shallow chronic ulcer. Later lesions grow outward, show large ulcerations, and have persistent crusts with raised, erythematous borders. SCC may grow under the nail bed and cause pain and swelling.

Prognosis for Squamous Cell Carcinoma

Squamous cell carcinoma remains confined at the epidermis for a long time. However, at some unpredictable time, the lesion may penetrate the basement membrane to the dermis and metastasize to regional lymph nodes. Invasive squamous cell carcinoma can be slow- or fast-growing with metastasis. Despite the unpredictable nature of the carcinoma, the prognosis of squamous cell carcinoma is good. A cure is expected with early diagnosis and treatment.

Clinical Manifestations of Malignant Melanoma

The manifestations of malignant melanoma vary. Most melanoma lesions are slightly raised and black or brown. The borders are irregular and the surfaces uneven. Periodically, melanomas ulcerate and bleed. Surrounding erythema, inflammation, and tenderness may occur. Dark melanomas are frequently mottled with red, blue, and white shades. The different colors represent three different concurrent processes: melanoma growth (blue), inflammation (red), and scar tissue formation (white).

Prognosis for Malignant Melanoma

The prognosis of malignant melanoma depends on several factors: the extent of metastasis, the initial lesion site and depth, lesion thickness, stage of the disease process, anatomic site, the patient's age, and the type

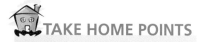

TAKE HOME POINTS

Nevi with a diameter of 6 mm or greater that bleed, itch, are deep brown, are asymmetrical, or that have irregular borders are considered suspicious for malignant melanoma.

of lesion. Initial lesions located on the extremities have the most favorable prognosis, and those located on the trunk, the head, or the neck have the poorest prognosis.

Lesions over 4 mm thick carry the poorest prognosis. Ten-year survival rates have increased steadily over the past 30 years, but the mortality rate continues to increase. Five-year survival rates are best for nonmetastatic lesions that are diagnosed and treated early.

What You DO

Treatment for Squamous Cell Carcinoma

Treatment for squamous cell carcinoma is similar to that for basal cell carcinoma. These measures include surgery, radiation therapy, cryosurgery, and electrodestruction. Reconstructive surgery may be required for extensive tumors. For metastatic squamous cell carcinoma, a combination of radiation and antineoplastic therapy may be required.

Treatment for Premalignant Melanoma Lesions

Most nevi never become malignant; however, suspicious pigmented nevi should be removed. Indications for biopsy and removal of the lesion are changes in size or color of a mole, irregular notched margins, nodularity, and ulceration, scab formation, itching, oozing, or bleeding. Treatment includes surgical excision, cryosurgery, and electrodestruction.

Treatment for Malignant Melanoma Lesions

The treatment of choice for known malignant melanoma is surgical excision. Dissection of regional lymph nodes may be required. After surgical excision, antineoplastic therapy is used for deep or extensive disease because there is a high risk for either recurrent or metastatic disease. Dacarbazine is the drug of choice. Combination regimens using dacarbazine, carmustine, cisplatin, and tamoxifen offer promising results, with response rates as high as 62%. Immunotherapy, such as the drug interferon, is also used to treat metastatic disease. Unfortunately, antineoplastic therapy does not appear to be helpful for patients with metastatic disease. Regional perfusion with antineoplastic drugs has been used for melanomas located on the extremities with varying degrees of success.

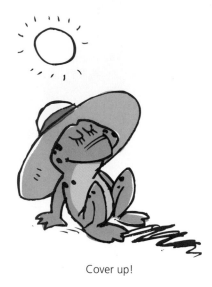

Cover up!

Nursing Responsibilities

For patients with squamous cell carcinoma and malignant melanoma, the nurse should do the following:

- Advise the patient to wear appropriate protective clothing and head covering when outdoors. Sunscreens with PABA and a rating of at least 30 for UV protection should be used.
- Increase the patient's awareness of the potential harm to the skin caused by increasingly popular tanning booths.
- Teach the patient and family the risk factors of skin cancer. The risk factors include a fair complexion, immunosuppression, and excessive UV exposure. The warning signs of skin cancer should also be included in the teaching.
- Allow the patient to express fears related to the diagnosis of malignant melanoma. The disfiguring surgical procedures that are necessary with large tumors and reconstruction efforts can cause problems with self-esteem and body image. Be certain to include counseling or refer the patient to support groups to allow the patient to heal emotionally, as well as physically.
- Patients with a prior history of skin cancer should see their health care provider at least every 4 to 6 months for a comprehensive examination of their skin. Early detection of recurrences offers the best chance for successful treatment.

Do You UNDERSTAND?

DIRECTIONS: **Indicate which statements are *true* (T) and which are *false* (F). If false, correct the statement in the margin space to make it true.**

_____ 1. Treatment for squamous cell carcinoma includes surgery, radiation therapy, cryosurgery, and electrodestruction.

_____ 2. Prevention includes using appropriate protective clothing and head coverings when outdoors.

_____ 3. Warning signs of skin cancer include changes in the size or color of a mole.

_____ 4. As the squamous cell carcinoma grows, it frequently ulcerates.

DIRECTIONS: **Fill in the blanks to complete the sentences using the words listed below. Words are only used once, and not all words are used.**

excision   malignant   expulsion   nonmalignant

prognosis   extremities   herbal therapy   warning

5. _____ is the preferred initial treatment for malignant melanoma.

6. An initial lesion located on the trunk, the head, or the neck has the poorest _____.

7. Metastatic spread is common with _____ melanoma.

8. Change in size or color of any skin spot or dark pigmented growth are _____ signs of malignancy.

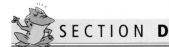

SECTION **D**

BURNS

WHAT IS A BURN?

Burns are injuries caused by application of heat, chemicals, electricity, or irradiation to the tissues. They are classified and described according to the source of injury. They are also described according to the depth and amount of injury to tissue.

Potential causes of thermal burns include flames, hot liquids, steam, semisolids, and hot objects. These types of burns are commonly seen in residential fires, explosions, and scald injuries. Electrical burns may occur after contact with exposed or faulty electrical wiring or high-voltage power lines. Lightning strikes are also a form of electrical injury.

Radiation burns are due to exposure to a radioactive source. This type of burn is rare and is associated with nuclear accidents and therapeutic radiation. Chemical burns are due to contact with strong acid, alkaline, or organic compounds. Certain household cleaning agents and chemicals used in industry and the military may cause chemical burns.

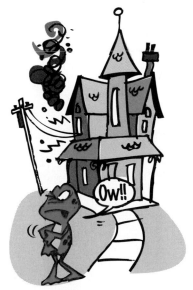

Don't get burned by faulty wiring.

Pathogenesis

Injury and damage occurs when energy from a heat source is transferred to the tissues. The chemical mediators associated with inflammation cause vasoconstriction. Arterial and venous blood flow decreases or may cease completely. Thrombosis may occur in peripheral vessels, with subsequent decrease in tissue perfusion that may lead to necrosis, which will then extend the area of injury.

After the initial period of vasoconstriction, vessels near the injured area dilate. This causes increased hydrostatic pressure within the capillaries and increased permeability within the capillary walls. Consequently, plasma moves from the circulation into the tissues. This process is called capillary leak syndrome. During this phase, the patient may experience severe generalized edema. Loss of intravascular fluid, electrolytes, and serum protein causes decreased osmotic pressure within the intravascular spaces. As a result of this fluid shift, severe hypovolemia, hyperkalemia, and hyponatremia may occur. Because of the lack of fluid within the vascular spaces, hemoconcentration occurs, which increases blood viscosity and worsens tissue hypoxia.

As the inflammatory response diminishes, capillary leak syndrome subsides and fluid returns to the intravascular spaces. Blood flow to the kidneys improves, which causes diuresis and loss of sodium in the urine. With the return of potassium to the cells, hypokalemia may occur. Tissue edema begins to resolve.

When capillary leaking is most severe, there is a decline in cardiac output because of hypovolemia. Cardiac output may remain decreased for up to 36 hours after the injury. Patients who have suffered electrical injury may also experience arrhythmias including ventricular fibrillation and asystole.

Burns of the head, neck and chest are more likely to result in pulmonary complications. Circumferential burns of the chest may compromise blood flow and limit respiratory expansion. If the patient inhaled superheated air, smoke, or steam, the respiratory tract may be compromised. Heated air and irritants within the upper airways cause the vocal cords to swell and close, leading to airway obstruction. Because of damage to the epithelial cells lining the airway, the lining of the trachea and bronchi may slough off 48 to 72 hours after the initial injury, resulting in further airway compromise. Intraalveolar edema may shift fluid into the interstitial spaces of the lungs. This causes fibrinous membranes to form within the lungs, leading to progressive respiratory failure.

The gastrointestinal system is also affected by decreased circulation during the period of hypovolemia. Because of decreased circulation, the mucosa of the gastrointestinal tract is damaged and decreased motility occurs. Peristalsis may decrease so much that a paralytic ileus results. Disruption in the gastric mucosa may lead to the development of Carling's ulcers, also known as acute gastroduodenal disease.

Catecholamines activated by the stress response will place the patient in a hypermetabolic state. This causes increased consumption of glucose and calories. The body temperature rises. The patient loses heat through burned skin surfaces, which then causes body temperature to rise even further in an attempt to compensate. For this reason, many patients develop a low-grade fever that is not always indicative of infection.

Burns larger than 12 to 16 cm^2 will develop a hard, leather-like crust (eschar) over the injured area, which is composed of dead dermal tissue. Because the eschar can limit circulation to underlying tissue, it must be removed and grafting done for healing to take place.

At-Risk Populations

There are many risk factors for burns; examples include hot water heaters set too high; workplace exposure to chemicals, electricity, or irradiation; and carelessness with burning cigarettes. Older houses and structures may have faulty wiring, which increases the risk for electrical fires. Young children and infants are at high risk for burns and scalds.

What You NEED TO KNOW

Clinical Manifestations

The severity of the injury is a function of the extent (depth of the burn) and the duration of exposure. Tissue damage is variable, depending upon the etiology of the burn. Different parts of the body are more susceptible to severe burn injuries. For example, the skin of the eyelids is much thinner than skin on the soles of the feet. Older adults have thinner skin overall, which puts them at risk for more severe burns, even by exposure at lower temperatures and of short duration.

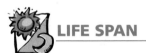 **LIFE SPAN**

Consider the possibility of child abuse when dealing with hot water burns in children. Observe the distribution of burns, paying attention to any straight lines, especially if bilateral.

 If a patient has singed nasal hairs or soot within the mouth and lips, he or she should be evaluated for respiratory injury. Signs and symptoms of respiratory damage may not occur until several hours after the original injury.

Burn Classification	Description
Superficial thickness	Devitalization of superficial layers of epidermis
	Basal epithelial cells and basement membranes remain intact
	Congestion of intradermal blood vessels
	Skin may be tender
Superficial partial-thickness	Involves varying degrees of epidermis and some of dermal layer with blister formation
Deep partial-thickness	Skin is red and very tender
Full-thickness	Involves epidermis and dermal layers with coagulation of subdermal plexis
	Skin is tough and leathery and nontender
Deep full-thickness	Involves skin, underlying muscle, fascia, tendons, and bones

Prognosis

The outcome of a burn is a function of the magnitude and the severity of the injury, the patient's age, and access to timely, appropriate care. Patients under the age of 4 or over the age of 65 are more likely to die from burns. Fifty percent survival can be expected from a 62% total body surface area burn in persons ages 0 to 14 years; from a 63% burn in persons ages 15 to 40 years; a 38% burn in those aged 40 to 65 years, and a 25% burn in persons over 65 years of age.

What You DO

Treatment

Therapy during the acute and emergent phases of injury is directed toward keeping the patient hemodynamically stable, supporting healing, relieving pain, and preventing infection. Minor burns may be successfully treated on an outpatient basis.

Burns must first be examined and classified according to their depth and size, as therapy for burns varies depending upon the extent of the injury and the patient's overall status. General treatment measures are determined based on an accurate assessment of total body surface area involved. The "Rule of Nines" is used for this purpose:

Affected Area*	Adult or Child	Percentage Involvement (TBSA)
Each upper extremity	Adult and child	9% BSA
Each lower extremity	Adult	18%
	Child	14%
Anterior trunk	Adult and child	18%
Posterior trunk	Adult and child	18%
Head and neck	Adult	10%
	Child	18%

*Quick estimate method for smaller burns: the surface area of the patient's hand is approximately 1% of TBSA.
TBSA; Total body surface area.

Transfer to a burn unit is required for all serious burns; partial thickness burns over 10% of total body surface area; any full-thickness burn; burns of the hands, the feet, the face, or the perineum; inhalation burns; electrical/or lightning burns; chemical burns; and circumferential burns.

Other patients requiring transfer to a burn center are those with a partial- or full-thickness burn involving over 10% of total body surface area in patients under 10 years and those over age 50, and any of the burns mentioned in the previous paragraph.

Patients with severe burns may require a surgical procedure called an escharotomy. This procedure involves making an incision in eschar tissue, which relieves pressure exerted by circumferential burns and indirectly improves blood flow to the area. If an escharotomy is unsuccessful, the patient may require a fasciotomy, which means that a deeper incision is made into the subcutaneous tissue and fascia.

Nursing Responsibilities

The first 48 hours after a burn injury is called the emergent phase. In the emergency setting, the nurse should do the following:

- Evaluate patency of the airway.
- Provide oxygen as needed.
- Obtain patient's age, baseline vital signs, and height and weight (where possible).
- Remove all smoldering or burning objects and clothing from the patient's skin.

- Keep the patient warm.
- Place the patient on NPO status (nothing by mouth).
- Elevate the extremities if there are no obvious fractures.
- Begin a large-bore IV (at least an 18-gauge), and initiate fluid resuscitation.
- Anticipate the need for a urinary catheter.
- Obtain a baseline electrocardiogram (ECG).
- Assess and document the severity of the burns according to percentage of total body surface area affected.

The acute phase of burn injury begins 48 hours after the burn occurred and continues until the wound is healed. During this time, on-going careful physical assessment is essential, along with measures designed to prevent or mitigate complications whenever possible. The nurse should do the following:

- When performing the physical assessment, remember to evaluate for possible complications associated with the injury. Symptoms of respiratory injury include a loud cough, drooling and difficulty swallowing, progressive hoarseness, and expiratory wheezes or stridor. Volume overload may cause progressive dyspnea and crackles upon auscultation.
- Since the protective barrier of the skin is no longer intact, scrupulous asepsis must be maintained when caring for these patients. Wear sterile gloves when caring for open wounds. Avoid sharing equipment between patients. Most patients with severe burns or widespread burns will require protective isolation. Monitor carefully for changes in vital signs, breath sounds, patterns of eliminations, and behavior. Review complete blood count (CBC) results daily, since a rising white blood cell (WBC) may also indicate infection.
- Listen to the abdomen for the presence or absence of bowel sounds. Patients with severe burns may have nausea, vomiting, and distention of the abdomen, or a developing paralytic ileus. Because these patients are at high risk for the development of gastrointestinal ulcers, check their stool and blood routinely for the presence of frank or occult blood.

In caring for all patients with burns, the nurse should address the following points:

- Patients who are immobilized by their burns are at risk for respiratory infections and require aggressive respiratory therapy and prompt treatment with the appropriate antibiotics(s). Turn these patients frequently and help them out of bed to a chair as soon as it is permitted.

- Burns can be extremely painful if nerve endings are spared. Assess patients for pain at least every 4 hours, and medicate accordingly. Premedicate with analgesics before painful procedures or dressing changes. Pain medications should be given intravenously to burn patients, because they are likely to have decreased absorption from muscle tissue and the gastric mucosa.

- For patients who do not require skin grafting, intensive nonsurgical management of the wound is required. In order for healing to take place, eschar and other cellular debris must be removed. This process is called **debridement**. Burns are usually debrided and cleaned two to three times daily during hydrotherapy. Nurses and technicians with special training use forceps and scissors to remove dead, loose tissue during hydrotherapy. After the wound has been cleaned, it is then covered with a sterile dressing.

- Make sure the patient is receiving adequate calories and nutrients. Some patients with large burns may require up to 5000 calories per day.

- Take steps to maintain range of motion and prevent joint contractures. Keep the patient in a neutral position with minimal flexion. Splints may be helpful on the hands, the elbows, the knees, the neck and the axillae. Assist the patient with range of motion exercises. Involve physical and occupational therapy in the patient's care early in treatment.

- Prevent scarring as much as possible. Patients with wounds that do not heal within 2 to 3 weeks are likely to have hypertrophied, contracted scar tissue. Pressure dressings and pressure garments, which are usually customized to the patient's size and stature, are extremely helpful in minimizing scarring.

- Offer emotional support, and encourage the participation of family and loved ones in the patient's care. These individuals are traumatized and isolated and may be facing permanent, severe disfigurement and incapacity.

- Once the patient's wounds have closed, rehabilitation begins. Emphasis during this phase is placed upon helping the patient achieve a positive psychosocial adjustment to his or her injury, optimal physical mobility, and the resumption of normal activities of daily living to the greatest extent possible.

Do You UNDERSTAND?

DIRECTIONS: **Circle the correct answer to the following questions.**

1. Which type of burn is most likely to cause cardiac dysrhythmias?
   a. Chemical
   b. Flame
   c. Electrical
   d. Radiation
2. A firefighter has just arrived in the emergency room seeking care after extinguishing a fire. The nurse notes he has a loud, brassy cough. The nurse should first
   a. Take his vital signs.
   b. Evaluate him for smoke inhalation.
   c. Inspect him for any smoldering ashes.
   d. Provide him with oxygen.
3. Escharotomies and fasciotomies are done to
   a. Relieve pressure.
   b. Restore circulation.
   c. Promote healing.
   d. All of the above.

References

American College of Preventive Medicine, Clinical Practice Guideline Committee: *Screening for skin cancer,* Washington, DC, 1998, Author.

American College of Preventive Medicine, Clinical Practice Guideline Committee: *Skin protection from ultraviolet light exposure,* Washington, DC, 1998, Author.

Barnhill RL: *Textbook of dermatopathology,* New York, 1998, McGraw-Hill.

Black J, Matassarin-Jacobs E: *Medical-surgical nursing: clinical management for continuity of care,* ed 5, Philadelphia, 1998, WB Saunders.

Braverman IM: *Skin signs of systemic disease,* ed 3, Philadelphia, 1998, WB Saunders.

Canadian Task Force on Preventive Health Care, Clinical Practice Guideline Committee: *Prevention of skin cancer,* Ottawa, 1999, Health Canada.

CancerNet: *Retinoblastoma,* 2000, URL http://cancernet.nci.nih.gov/ young_people/ yngconts.html.

Emmert DH: Treatment of common cutaneous herpes simplex virus infections, *Am Fam Physician* 61(6):1697, 2000.

Fultz J, Wells S, Welsh D: Acute burn injury. In Kidd PS, Wagner KD, editors: *High acuity nursing*, ed 4, Upper Saddle River, NJ, 2001, Prentice Hall.

Gutierrez K: *Pharmacotherapy: clinical decision-making in nursing,* Philadelphia, 1999, WB Saunders.

Hansen M: *Pathophysiology: foundations of disease & clinical interventions,* Philadelphia, 1998, WB Saunders.

Hay RJ: The management of superficial candidiasis, *J Am Acad Dermatol* 40(6):35, 1999.

McCance KL, Huether SE: *Pathophysiology: the biologic basis for disease in adults and children,* ed 4, St Louis, 2002, Mosby.

McCrary ML, Severson J, Tyring SK: Varicella zoster virus, *J Am Acad Dermatol* 41(1):1, 1999.

Morgan ED, Miser WF: *Treatment of minor thermal burns,* 2005, URL www.UpToDate.com.

Pinto DS, Clardy P: *Environmental electrical injuries,* 2005, URL www.UpToDate.com.

Porth C: *Pathophysiology: concepts of altered health states,* ed 7, Philadelphia, 2005, Lippincott.

Rhody C: Bacterial infections of the skin, *Prim Care Clin Office Pract* 27(2):459, 2000.

Rubin E, Farber JL: *Pathology,* ed 3, Philadelphia, 1999, Lippincott–Rubin.

Singleton JK et al: *Primary care,* Philadelphia, 1999, Lippincott–Williams & Wilkins.

Sorbel JD et al: Vulvovaginal candidiasis: epidemiologic, diagnostic, and therapeutic considerations, *Am J Obstet Gynecol* 178(2):203, 1998.

Wise RP et al: Post-licensure safety surveillance for varicella vaccine, *JAMA* 284(10):1271, 2000.

NCLEX® Review

Section A

1. The usual transmission mode for type 2 herpes simplex is through
   1 Kissing and touching.
   2 Sexual encounters.
   3 Contaminated food or water.
   4 Coughing.

Section B

2. The skin lesions of psoriasis are
   1 Nonscaling, violet-colored, pruritic papules.
   2 Black comedones.
   3 Pruritic vesicles.
   4 Thick, scaly, erythematous plaques.

3. Acne vulgaris is associated with
   1 Oily skin.
   2 Poor diet.
   3 Poor hygiene.
   4 Excessive melanocytes.

4. The health care provider instructs patients with rosacea to use caution with alcohol and hot drinks because they can cause
   1 Vasoconstriction.
   2 Vasodilation.
   3 Hypothermia.
   4 Hyperthermia.

Section C

5. What are the characteristic findings of the lesion of malignant melanoma?

   _____

6. Squamous cell carcinoma of the skin is manifested as
   1 Irregular pigmentation.
   2 An ulcerated, hyperkeratotic nodule with dermal invasion.
   3 A slightly elevated, pearl-colored nodule.
   4 Multifocal brown macules.

7. Which malignant skin lesion metastasizes the earliest?
   1 Basal cell carcinoma
   2 Kaposi's sarcoma
   3 Malignant melanoma
   4 Squamous cell carcinoma

8. An untreated basal cell carcinoma
   1 Metastasizes frequently.
   2 Frequently involves regional lymphatic tissues.
   3 Ulcerates and involves local tissues.
   4 Grows rapidly.

Section D

9. The capillary leak syndrome experienced by patients with severe burns may lead to
   1 Hypervolemia.
   2 Hypovolemia.
   3 Hypokalemia.
   4 Hypernatremia.

10. Patients who have suffered electrical injuries are at risk for
    1 Acute respiratory distress syndrome (ARDS).
    2 Secondary infections.
    3 Cardiac arrhythmias.
    4 Postural hypotension.

11. A patient has a full-thickness burn that encircles his entire right calf. After eschar begins to form, the nurse should be concerned about
    1 Infection.
    2 Circulatory compromise to the burned limb.
    3 Possible amputation.
    4 All of the above.

12. In the recovery phase of burn care, pressure garments are used to
    1 Protect delicate tissue.
    2 Minimize scarring.
    3 Cover unsightly scars.
    4 Help the patient maintain normal body temperature.

NCLEX® Review Answers

Section A

1. **2** The usual transmission route for type 2 herpes is by sexual encounter, not kissing and touching. Contaminated food and water and coughing do not spread the herpes virus.

Section B

2. **4** Thick, scaly, erythematous plaque lesions indicate psoriasis. Nonscaling, violet-colored, pruritic papules are associated with a number of disorders, the most common of which is Kaposi's sarcoma. Black comedones are associated with acne. Pruritic vesicles are associated with itching and allergic response.

3. **1** Oily skin contributes to acne vulgaris. That poor diet and hygiene causes acne vulgaris is a misconception. Excessive melanocytes cause a darkening of the skin.

4. **2** Alcohol and hot drinks cause vasodilation of the skin, thus making the face appear red. Body temperature (hypothermia and hyperthermia) and vasoconstriction are not associated with rosacea.

Section C

5. Most melanoma lesions are slightly raised and black or brown. The borders are irregular and the surfaces uneven. Periodically, melanomas ulcerate and bleed. Surrounding erythema, inflammation, and tenderness may be present. Dark melanomas are frequently mottled with red, blue, and white shades.

6. **2** An ulcerated, hyperkeratotic nodule with dermal invasion is characteristic of squamous cell carcinoma. Irregular pigmentation of the skin is associated with vitiligo. A slightly elevated, pearl-colored nodule may reflect basal cell carcinoma. Multifocal brown macules are known as nevi or freckles.

7. **3** Malignant melanoma metastasizes the earliest. Basal cell carcinoma rarely metastasizes. Kaposi's sarcoma is often found in patients with AIDS is confined to the skin and subcutaneous tissues, although it may become widespread to include the viscera.

8. **3** Untreated basal cell carcinoma ulcerates and involves local tissues. Untreated basal cell carcinoma grows slowly and does not involve regional lymph tissues or metastasize.

Section D

9. **2** Plasma moves from the vascular spaces into the tissues and causes severe intravascular volume depletion. Because the plasma is concentrated, hyperkalemia and hyponatremia may result. (Inadequate renal perfusion causes sodium to be lost in the urine.)

10. **3** Electrical shocks may disrupt the normal rhythm of the heart.

11. **4** All are possible complications of a severe burn.

12. **2** Pressure garments help to minimize the formation of hypertrophied scar tissue.

Notes

Alterations in Neuropsychiatric Function

What You WILL LEARN

After reading this chapter, you will know how to do the following:

- ✔ Discuss the 5 different types of schizophrenia and the various types of delusions seen in the disorder.
- ✔ Discuss the effects of depression in terms of behavior, emotion, and cognition.
- ✔ Correlate the clinical manifestations of bipolar disorder with the appropriate treatment modalities.
- ✔ Compare and contrast the various anxiety disorders with their clinical manifestations.
- ✔ Compare and contrast anorexia nervosa with bulimia in terms of clinical manifestations and treatment interventions.

A neuropsychiatric illness affects numerous aspects of a person's life, including the ability to work, succeed in school, live independently, socialize, and maintain family relationships. The stigma held by society often makes the illness all the more difficult for patients and their families.

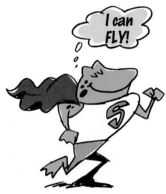

Superhero or Schizophrenic?

SECTION A

SCHIZOPHRENIA

What IS Schizophrenia?

Pathogenesis

Schizophrenia is a chronic psychotic disorder characterized by an altered perception of reality; affective, behavioral, and intellectual disturbances are often accompanied by hallucinations, delusions, and disturbed thought processes. Schizophrenia causes a withdrawal from real life and interferes with the ability to interpret reality. Inappropriate responses and altered mood are evident, hampering the ability to communicate with others, form meaningful relationships, and properly attend to activities of daily living.

There are five subtypes of schizophrenia:

1. *Paranoid type*—frequent auditory hallucinations or one or more delusions
2. *Disorganized type*—disorganized speech and behavior, and flat or inappropriate affect
3. *Catatonic type*—extreme motor immobility; purposeless, excessive motor activity; inappropriate physical postures; and repeating words or behaviors
4. *Undifferentiated type*—meets criteria for the general category of schizophrenia but does not fall into any of the other types
5. *Residual type*—one or more episodes of schizophrenia have occurred in the past but the current illness is essentially one of negative symptoms and mild positive symptoms

The cause of schizophrenia is unknown; however, stressful life events often precede the onset of schizophrenic symptoms. There is some evidence to support both genetic and neurochemical causes. Evidence for the neurochemical theory is found in the supportive data that the metabolites of neurotransmitters that control emotions and feelings are found at significantly higher levels in the urine of schizophrenic patients.

At-Risk Populations

A family history of schizophrenia occurs at a higher rate in those diagnosed with the disorder, reaching 40% for an identical twin. Schizophrenia typically first occurs during adolescence and young adulthood; however, onset can be in childhood or later adulthood.

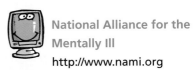

National Alliance for the Mentally Ill
http://www.nami.org
National Mental Health Association
http://www.nmha.org

What You NEED TO KNOW

Clinical Manifestations

Symptoms of schizophrenia include hallucinations, delusions, and disturbed thought processes and are categorized as positive or negative. The positive symptoms are the attention-getting symptoms and include hallucinations, delusions, bizarre behavior, paranoia, and social isolation. The negative symptoms are actually often more problematic for patients and include apathy, the inability to enjoy activities, poverty of speech (alogia), difficulty initiating activities, low energy, lack of motivation, poor thought processes, and an inability to make or keep friendships. Hallucinations in order of frequency of occurrence may be auditory, visual, tactile, olfactory or gustatory. Delusions are real to the schizophrenic patient and can be of various types:

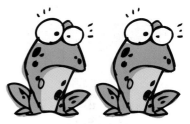

Schizophrenia can come in pairs.

- A *paranoid delusion,* also called a persecution delusion, is experienced when sufferers believes people are trying to harm them when evidence contradicts this belief.
- *Delusions of reference* occur when patients believe people are talking about them or information is communicated to them through media sources such as TV and radio.
- *Delusions of grandeur* cause patients to believe they have special abilities or powers.
- *Somatic delusions* occur when there is the belief that a serious physical illness or disorder exists when physical illness has been ruled out.
- *Delusions of jealousy* occur when patients have the false belief that a significant other is unfaithful.
- *Delusions of thought broadcasting* cause patients to believe their thoughts can be heard by others.

- *Thought insertion delusion* occurs when there is the belief that the thoughts of others are being inserted into the patient's mind.
- *Thought withdrawal delusion* causes patients to believe their thoughts have been removed from their mind by another person or agency.
- *Delusions of being controlled* are experienced when sufferers believe their body or mind is controlled by another person or agency.

Additional manifestations of schizophrenia include extremes of emotions ranging from extreme happiness to extreme depression; altered movement, to the extreme of no movement for long periods of time (catatonia); and inappropriate sexual or aggressive or violent behavior. Sufferers may lack the ability to enjoy or initiate activities (physical anhedonia); experience low energy and motivation; display flat affect; lack the ability to make or keep friends (social anhedonia); show poor memory, concentration, and problem solving. and display disorganized speech or behavior.

The American Psychiatric Association's *Diagnostic and Statistical Manual of Mental Disorders,* fourth edition (DSM-IV) criteria for the diagnosis of schizophrenia include two or more of the following during a 1-month period: delusions; hallucinations; disorganized speech (incoherence or looseness of association); grossly disorganized or catatonic behavior; negative symptoms (apathy), avolition (lack of motivation), or alogia (poverty of speech). If the delusions are bizarre or auditory hallucinations are present consisting of voices keeping a running commentary about the person's behavior or thoughts, or two or more voices conversing with each other, then only one criterion is needed.

The criteria also look at social and occupational dysfunction. One or more major areas of the person's life must be markedly below premorbid functioning (work, interpersonal relationships, or self-care); or, if the onset is in childhood or adolescence, there must be a failure to achieve expected level of interpersonal, academic, or occupational achievement.

The signs of schizophrenia must persist continuously for at least 6 months, with at least 1 month where all other mental diseases (schizoaffective disorder or mood disorder) and all other medical conditions (substance or drug use or general medical conditions) have been ruled out. If there is a history of a pervasive developmental disorder, including autistic disorder, then prominent hallucinations or delusions for 1 month are needed to make the diagnosis of schizophrenia.

Prognosis

The outcome of schizophrenia is poor in approximately 50% of cases; however, it is much improved with early diagnosis and adherence to a lifetime treatment plan. Lower rates of health-promoting behavior and higher mortality rates, partially explained by the high suicide risk, are evident in the affected population.

What You DO

Treatment

In general, there is no cure for schizophrenia, with the exception of a small percentage of patients experiencing a complete cure; however, the illness is treatable, with recovery typically taking at least several months. Ongoing and regular visits with a psychiatrist and therapist will be needed because the disorder is chronic and typically life-long.

Antipsychotic drugs combined with psychotherapy and social skills training is most often the treatment of choice. Additionally, regular sleep and exercise, along with eating well, managing daily stress, and avoiding alcohol and nicotine, helps in managing the disorder.

Nursing Responsibilities

For the patient suffering from schizophrenia, the nurse should do the following:

- Promote early detection with thorough patient assessment. Prodromal (warning) symptoms, which include reduced concentration and attention, withdrawal from friends and family, loneliness, reduced energy level, depressed mood, and anxiety, are experienced by a large percentage of patients months before the first psychotic break.
- Assess patients for positive and negative symptoms and thoughts of self-harm and suicide. For the hospitalized patient, institute suicide precautions, as needed, following hospital protocol. Continue to monitor symptoms and suicide risk throughout treatment.
- Establish a therapeutic nurse-patient relationship, listening to patient's views, maintaining eye contact, and showing empathy and understanding.

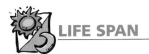

LIFE SPAN

Older women who suffer from schizophrenia have an increased risk of suicide and obesity. More than 10% of people diagnosed with schizophrenia die from suicide.

TAKE HOME POINTS

Sufferers of schizophrenia have a high self-harm and suicide risk. Feelings of confusion and isolation, combined with lack of supportive relationships, increase these risk factors.

TAKE HOME POINTS

- Approximately 50% of people suffering from schizophrenia abuse alcohol and drugs, requiring concurrent treatment.
- Do not use physical contact with the patient, asking for permission to do so if touch is necessary. Do not argue with the content of hallucinations or delusions.

• Empathize with the patient's feelings and focus on reality while taking care not to get drawn into talking about delusional material; however, it is important not to argue with the patient about the content of the delusion.

• Maintain a low level of stimuli, providing a structured environment (milieu) and quiet setting for hospitalized patients, with frequent patient observation (every 15 minutes).

• Manage violent behavior by setting firm limits.

• Assist the patient to sustain positive self-esteem during treatment because the level of self-esteem is significantly related to treatment outcome.

• Provide assistance and total care, when necessary, for self-care deficits of withdrawn or catatonic patients.

• Provide patient and family teaching (face-to-face, or with printed or video material works best) regarding the illness and required treatment. Research shows patients' and families' understanding of the illness and therapeutic effects of antipsychotic mediations significantly improves patient outcomes; less than 50% of patients in long-term treatment take their drugs as prescribed.

• Build collaborative relationships with patient caretakers and family members, supporting family interventions. Comprehensive family interventions postpone psychotic relapse and rehospitalization of patients.

• Monitor for any side effects from prescribed drugs, reporting findings to the primary care provider. Common side effects include weight gain, restlessness, tiredness, drooling, and muscle stiffness.

• Teach the patient ways to reduce stress and anxiety to avoid exacerbation of schizophrenic symptoms.

• Monitor for drug or alcohol use or abuse. Recommend drug and alcohol treatment and involvement in support programs such as Alcoholics Anonymous and Narcotics Anonymous for patients suffering from drug or alcohol dependency.

Tardive dyskinesia is a serious and irreversible side effect of antipsychotic drugs. It consists of involuntary tonic muscular spasms of the tongue, the fingers, the toes, the neck, the trunk, or the pelvis. Counsel the patient to avoid exposure to the sun and to wear sunblock to reduce the risk of tardive dyskinesia.

• It is important the patient and family be counseled to understand that antipsychotic drugs must not be stopped, even when symptoms subside, because the drug continues to prevent psychotic symptoms from returning.

Do You UNDERSTAND?

DIRECTIONS: **Fill in the blanks by unscrambling the italicized words.**

1. Delusions of _____ occur when patients believe people are talking about them. *(fneecrree)*

2. A negative symptom of schizophrenia is _____. *(yahpta)*

3. A positive symptom of schizophrenia is _____. *(stalliinunocha)*

4. Sufferers of schizophrenia have a high risk of _____. *(usedcii)*

5. _____ drugs must not be stopped, even when symptoms subside. *(canpihcistyto)*

SECTION B

MOOD DISORDERS

What IS Depression?

Pathogenesis

A depressive disorder is a severe mood disorder characterized by impaired functioning in behavior, emotion, and cognition. There is a decline in social activity and a decrease in the quality of social relationships. Occupational functioning is often affected, and psychotic features such as hallucinations and delusions may be present. Depression is the most common mental disorder and the second leading cause of disability after heart disease.

Various theories propose genetic, environmental, and biochemical factors for the cause of depression. Nearly 50% of identical twins are also found to have depression when one twin is affected. In support of the environmental theory, those with depression often report negative

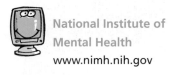

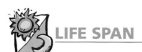

TAKE HOME POINTS

- Depression is often chronic and is frequently comorbid with anxiety disorder.
- Most patients diagnosed with depression will have multiple episodes, with those who experience early-onset depression being at highest risk for relapse.

LIFE SPAN

- Onset of depression typically does not occur before adolescence; however, it may occasionally be seen in children and is manifested by school phobias, underachievement, and antisocial behavior.
- In adolescents, depression may present as underachievement in school, truancy, hostility, drug use, and sexual promiscuity.
- The prevalence of depression declines in late middle age; however, medical illness, loneliness, and lack of social support correlate with higher rates of depressive symptoms in older adults.
- Although rates of depression are lower in the elderly population, suicide rates for elderly patients with a diagnosis of depression are the highest of all age groups.

experiences and distant relationships with parents during childhood; self-esteem is typically low with unreasonable self-expectations of perfectionism and overconcern about making mistakes. The neurotransmitters serotonin and norepinephrine are related to altered mood states. Antidepressant drugs inhibit the reuptake of these neurotransmitters, increasing availability and thus providing support for the biochemical theory.

At-Risk Populations

Depression is most prevalent in the 18- to 44-year-old age group, with an average age of onset of 27 years. Women are more likely to suffer from depression than men, with one in five women and one in eight men experiencing at least one episode of depression during their lifetime. Young married women with children are at higher risk and unmarried women with children at an even greater risk. Further, lower socioeconomic status, divorce, and social deprivation increase the risk for depression, and childhood physical and sexual abuse is associated with depression in adulthood. At 6% to 8%, the prevalence rate of depression in patients with a chronic medical diagnosis is double that of the general population.

What You NEED TO KNOW

Clinical Manifestations

The key symptoms of depression include a depressed mood, an inability to experience pleasure in events that normally give pleasure (**anhedonia**), lack of motivation, and pessimistic thinking. Additional manifestations often include a decline in the ability to concentrate, poor memory, reduced energy, low self-esteem, and changes in sleep and eating patterns. Patients are often observed to have poor posture, a sad facial expression, fixed gaze, and neglected personal hygiene. Complaints of headaches or backaches (somatic complaints) and decreased interest in sex (loss of libido) are common. Slowed movements (**psychomotor retardation**) are typical; however, constant pacing, hand wringing, and nail biting may instead be present (**psychomotor agitation**). Patients may report suicidal thoughts (**suicidal ideation**) or attempts and acts of self-harm. Some patients experience hallucinations and/or delusions.

The DSM-IV criteria for the diagnosis of depressive disorder includes a change in previous functioning and symptoms that cause clinically significant distress or impair social, occupational, or other important areas of functioning. In addition, five or more of the following occur nearly every day for most waking hours over the same 2-week period: depressed mood, an inability to enjoy life (anhedonia), significant weight loss or gain (more than 5% of body weight in 1 month), insomnia or hypersomnia, increased or decreased motor activity, fatigue or loss of energy (anergia), feelings of worthlessness or inappropriate guilt (may be delusional), decreased concentration or indecisiveness, and recurrent thoughts of death or suicidal ideation (with or without a plan).

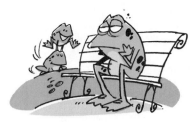

Don't let depression get you down.

The diagnosis may be further defined when other specific features are also present. The specific features include delusions and hallucinations; seasonal affective disorder (SAD)—related to either winter or summer; or catatonia, melancholy, or depression that occurs during the postpartum period.

Prognosis

It is estimated that nearly 50% of the cases of depression remain undiagnosed. Without diagnosis and treatment, prognosis is poor, with a high morbidity and mortality rate from lack of self-care, comorbid medical illness, and suicide. For many, depression becomes chronic with a high recurrence of symptoms. Long-term treatment and follow-up with the health care provider significantly improves outcome; however, the prognosis is poor without continued treatment. Because depression both occurs at a greater prevalence rate for those with medical illnesses, and increases the probability of a poorer outcome when a medical illness is comorbid, there is an overall decrease in the quality of life and life expectancy, with an increase in disability for these patients.

 Of those persons diagnosed with depression, 11% to 17% commit suicide.

What You DO

Treatment

The use of antidepressants alone or in combination with psychotherapy is most often the prescribed treatment for depression. In some instances, lithium, a mood-stabilizing drug used in the treatment of bipolar disorder, is used to treat recurring depression. When other therapy is not effective, electroconvulsive therapy may be indicated. For many, depression

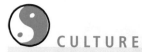

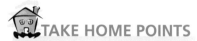

TAKE HOME POINTS

While research shows that nurses are good at identifying depression, the disorder is underrecognized by other health professionals and undertreated in general. Research shows that up to 50% of the cases of depression remain unidentified.

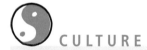

CULTURE

• Provide culturally sensitive care identifying the patient's beliefs about depression. Counsel the patient that the illness is treatable and help the patient to understand that the disorder is not his or her fault, nor under his or her direct control.
• Be sure to include the patient's favorite foods and drinks, providing preferred ethnic foods when available. Weekly weight readings will assist in evaluation of interventions and determining if goals have been met.

becomes chronic with a high recurrence of symptoms. In these cases long-term pharmacotherapy, mental health counseling, and regular follow-up with a mental health care provider is necessary.

Nursing Responsibilities

For the patient diagnosed with depressive disorder, the nurse should do the following:

• Promote early detection of depression with thorough patient assessment by identifying clinical manifestations and directly asking the patient, "Are you depressed?"
• Assess the patient for suicidal thoughts and attempts. Ask the patient, "Have you thought of killing yourself?" Institute suicide precautions as needed for the hospitalized patient, following hospital protocol.
• Establish a therapeutic nurse-patient relationship, conveying acceptance and caring while offering hope. The quality of the relationship between the nurse and the patient with depression is important for successful treatment.
• Provide patient and family education regarding the disorder, prescribed treatment plan, and drug side effects. Noncompliance with drug therapy is a major obstacle in effective treatment of depression. The nurse should use compliance-enhancing strategies. It may be necessary to specifically address the unsubstantiated, but common, belief that antidepressant drugs are addictive, while concurrently teaching the safety and effectiveness of antidepressant drug therapy.
• Schedule short, frequent visits with the hospitalized patient, informing the patient when you will visit, and establishing reliability by being on time for these sessions and staying the full scheduled time, even when the patient does not respond. Use active listening, maintaining a calm, caring, accepting approach, allowing time for the patient to respond. When the patient has periods of silence or is mute, quietly sit with the patient and occasionally make verbal observations such as, "I see you have a new picture on your wall."
• Involve the patient in activities that require minimal concentration skills. Begin with one-on-one activities, moving to group activities as tolerated.
• Maintain the hospitalized patient's nutritional status by offering frequent, small, high-calorie, high-protein snacks and drinks.

- Encourage self-care, allowing the patient to complete as much self-care as he or she is able, cueing and reminding as needed. Perform personal care and range of motion exercises, as needed, for the catatonic patient.
- Promote adequate sleep for the hospitalized patient by providing a relaxing routine in the evening and reducing stimulation. The patient should be encouraged to wake at a regular time, dress, and stay out of bed during the day to increase the likelihood of regular nighttime sleep. Teach the nonhospitalized patient the importance of maintaining this routine at home.
- Identify if drugs or alcohol are used or abused. Recommend drug and alcohol treatment and involvement in support programs such as Alcoholics Anonymous and Narcotics Anonymous for patients suffering from drug or alcohol dependency.

Do You UNDERSTAND?

DIRECTIONS: **Using the following illustrations, color the box on the graph provided that most accurately describes depressive disorder.**

1. The age group in which depression is most prevalent

8-12 years	13-18 years	18-44 years	44-69 years	70 years and older

2. The percentage of women likely to suffer from depression

4-5 %	6-8 %	11-17 %	20 %	50 %

3. The prevalence of depression in patients with a chronic medial diagnosis

4-5 %	6-8 %	11-17 %	20 %	50 %

4. The percentage of depression that goes undiagnosed

4-5 %	6-8 %	11-17 %	20 %	50 %

5. The percentage of people with depression who successfully commit suicide

4-5 %	6-8 %	11-17 %	20 %	50 %

Answers: 1. 18 to 44 years; 2. 20 %; 3. 6% to 8%; 4. 50%; 5. 11% to 17%.

What IS Bipolar Disorder?

Pathogenesis

Bipolar disorder, also known as manic-depressive illness, is a mood disorder consisting of two types of episodes, one in which the mood is either depressed **(hypomania)** and the other in which it is predominantly elated or irritable **(mania)**; and the periods of depression are long-lasting and frequent. Emotional, cognitive, and behavioral problems result from the long periods of depression alternating with periods of euphoria and psychosis. This cyclical pattern of depression and mania or hypomania causes significant disruption of daily life and future plans, and long-lasting negative psychologic and psychosocial effects. When in the depressed state, there is an overdependency upon others and feelings of hopelessness about the future. Manic episodes are typically characterized by grandiosity and excessive risk-taking. When in a manic phase, patients usually describe it as inescapable. The energy and elation of a manic episode is not easily resisted. Extreme goal-striving is common; however, occupational disability is high.

The genetic theory of the cause of bipolar disorder is supported by strong evidence. Bipolar disorder is clearly more prevalent within particular families, with the risk increasing by 10 times that of the general population when a first-degree relative is diagnosed with a mood disorder. Supportive data for the neurochemical theory exists in the evidence that norepinephrine and epinephrine are found at significantly higher levels in the blood of bipolar patients during a manic episode.

At-Risk Populations

Bipolar disorder affects 0.8% to 1.6% of the general population, with men and women affected equally. Typical onset is in late adolescence or early adulthood with recurrent episodes, leading to a chronic disorder.

What You NEED TO KNOW

Clinical Manifestations

Early warning signs **(prodromes)** vary between individuals with bipolar disorder; however, they are highly indicative of onset of a manic episode.

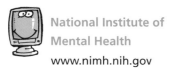

TAKE HOME POINTS

Alcohol and drug abuse and anxiety disorder occur commonly with bipolar disorder.

National Institute of Mental Health

www.nimh.nih.gov

In most cases, patients have learned to identify their own personal warning signs and report these accurately. There is constant physical and verbal activity, lack of ability to concentrate, poor judgment, decreased sleep, and possibly psychotic features (hallucinations and delusions) when in the manic phase. Dress and make-up is often bizarre and inappropriate. Continuous speech with abrupt changes in topic (**flight of ideas**) is typical, and the content of the conversation is often inappropriate, sexually explicit, or vulgar.

The DSM-IV criteria for the diagnosis of bipolar disorder include a distinct period of abnormality and persistently elevated, expansive, or irritable mood for at least 4 days of hypomania or 1 week of mania. During the period of mood disturbance the patient has at least three or more of the following symptoms, which have persisted (four if the mood is only irritable) and have been present to a significant degree: inflated self-esteem or grandiosity; decreased need for sleep (e.g., the person feels rested after only 3 hours of sleep); increased talkativeness or pressure to keep talking; flight of ideas or subjective experience that thoughts are racing; distractibility (i.e., the person's attention is too easily drawn to unimportant or irrelevant external stimuli); and increase in goal-directed activity (either socially, at work or school, or sexually) or psychomotor agitation; or excessive involvement in pleasurable activities that have a high potential for painful consequences (e.g., the person engages in unrestrained buying sprees, sexual indiscretions, or foolish business investments).

Further, bipolar disorder of the hypomanic type is diagnosed when the episode is associated with an unequivocal change in functioning that is uncharacteristic of the person when not symptomatic. There may be an absence of marked impairment in social or occupational functioning; delusions are never present; and hospitalization was not indicated.

Alternatively, bipolar disorder of the manic type is diagnosed when one the episode is severe enough to cause marked impairment in occupational activities, usual social activities, or relationships; or hospitalization is needed to protect client and others from irresponsible or aggressive behavior, or when there are psychotic features (e.g., grandiose and/or paranoid delusions).

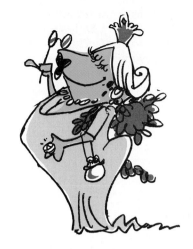

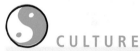

CULTURE

Bipolar disorder is more prevalent in the upper socioeconomic classes.

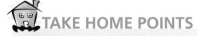

TAKE HOME POINTS

Patients with bipolar disorder report uncontrollable, racing thoughts and an altered interpretation of reality. In the hypomanic state, the symptoms are less severe and reality perception is not altered. The depressed phase typically manifests with increased sleep (hypersomnia) and decreased motor activity.

Monitor for lithium toxicity. Early signs of toxicity include nausea, vomiting, diarrhea, slurred speech, and thirst. Advanced signs of toxicity include hand tremor, mental confusion, nausea, and vomiting. Severe toxicity can lead to cardiac arrhythmia, coma, and death.

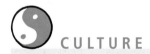

CULTURE

Provide culturally sensitive care. Counsel the patient that bipolar disorder is an illness that is treatable, and help the patient to understand the disorder is not his or her fault nor under the patient's direct control.

Prognosis

Research reveals that, on the average, individuals are not diagnosed as having bipolar disorder for 8 years after the emergence of symptoms, increasing morbidity and mortality. Occupational disability is high, and negative psychologic and psychosocial effects are long-lasting. The suicide risk in diagnosed cases is 15%. Additionally, the risk of suicide increases dramatically in undiagnosed bipolar disorder, contributing to a frequently poor outcome.

What You DO

Treatment

Long-term treatment with mood stabilizers is the cornerstone of treatment for bipolar disorder. Psychotherapy and social skills training often complement drug therapy. Treatment is difficult because of the altering states of depression, mania, and mixed states, with each state requiring different drug therapy, psychotherapy, and social interventions. Manic phases typically present the most difficult treatment challenge. Through psychotherapy, patients learn to identify warning signs (prodromal symptoms), enabling them to use coping skills and seek early treatment with the primary care provider and thus avoiding an actual manic episode.

Nursing Responsibilities

For the patient suffering with bipolar disorder, the nurse should do the following:

- Promote early detection of bipolar disorder with thorough patient assessment. Diagnosis is, on average, delayed by 8 years.
- Assess the patient for suicidal thoughts and attempts. Ask the patient, "Have you thought of killing yourself?" Institute suicide precautions as needed for the hospitalized patient, following hospital protocol.
- Establish a therapeutic, collaborative nurse-patient relationship, conveying acceptance and caring while offering hope; the quality of the relationship between the nurse and the patient is important for successful treatment.

- Provide patient and family education regarding the disorder, prescribed treatment plan, and drug side effects. Noncompliance with drug therapy is a major obstacle in the treatment of bipolar disorder. The nurse should encourage compliance-enhancing strategies.
- Monitor the patient for drug side effects and toxicity.
- Maintain a quiet, calm atmosphere during the manic phase for the hospitalized patient, redirecting the patient's energy into appropriate activities such as writing, painting, walking, and ping-pong and encouraging frequent rest periods.
- Set appropriate limits on patient's behavior and establish expectations to manage risk for self-injury and aggression toward other patients.
- Offer frequent high-calorie foods and drinks, avoiding caffeine. The patient may need cueing from the nurse to eat and drink.
- Teach the patient that manic episodes can be avoided by learning the early warning signs particular to each patient. Assist the patient to understand that although manic episodes are difficult to resist, negative consequences of previous episodes are a reminder of why it is so important to treat a manic episode before it becomes full-blown.
- Assist the patient to identify and avoid social events and activities that have a significant impact on mood, in particular, alcohol use and extreme sports. Counsel the patient to maintain a regular sleep schedule and regular daily routine to help protect against relapse.
- Encourage the patient to use his or her social support network.
- Identify if drugs or alcohol are used or abused. Recommend drug and alcohol treatment and involvement in support programs such as Alcoholics Anonymous and Narcotics Anonymous for patients suffering from drug or alcohol addiction.

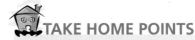

TAKE HOME POINTS

Ensure consistency among staff when implementing limit-setting interventions to avoid the often-used tactic by the patient suffering from bipolar disorder to divide staff, causing staff to become angry at each other, and decreasing the effectiveness of the nursing intervention.

Do You UNDERSTAND?

DIRECTIONS: **Indicate which statements are *true* (T) and which are *false* (F). If false, correct the statement in the margin space to make it true.**

_____   1. When in the manic state of bipolar disorder, the patient is overly dependent upon others and often has feelings of hopelessness about the future.

_____   2. The onset of bipolar disorder is typically in late adolescence or early adulthood.

_____   3. One of the manifestations of the depressed phase is insomnia.

_____   4. Antidepressant drugs are the mainstay of treatment for bipolar disorder.

_____   5. The energy expended during the acute manic phase should be controlled by allowing only rest and relaxation.

What IS Anxiety Disorder?

Pathogenesis

Experiences associated with danger trigger brain activity that serves functions of both reacting and remembering, protecting against current and future danger. In anxiety disorder this mechanism is faulty, triggering a response to stimuli that are neither unfamiliar nor actual threats and treating this information as dangerous: in essence, false alarms of danger. Often just the anticipation of the experience, or the thought of the experience, causes anxiety.

Anxiety disorder results in a decline in the ability to think. In some instances, anxiety disorder may include panic attacks, where normal functioning is drastically altered with subsequent risk for serious self-injury or suicide. When specific phobias are present in anxiety disorder,

Answers: 1. F—overdependence upon others and feelings of hopelessness typically occur when in the depressed state of bipolar disorder; 2. T; 3. F—increased sleep is common during the depressed phase of bipolar disorder. Insomnia is a manifestation of depressive disorders; 4. F—mood-stabilizers are the drug treatment of choice for bipolar disorder; antidepressant drugs are the treatment of choice for depressive disorders; 5. F—the energy expended during an acute manic phase should be redirected into appropriate activities such as writing, painting, walking, and playing ping-pong.

the persistent desire for, or actual avoidance of, an object or activity exists. Recurring thoughts or images (obsessions) and ritualistic behaviors (compulsions) may be the predominant characteristic of anxiety disorder; typically they occur together, but they can occur independently. Flashbacks and nightmares of a traumatic event may persist and are often accompanied by a lack of emotional responsiveness, a sense of detachment, and a lack of ability to trust. Occupational and social functioning and interpersonal relationships are affected, in many instances dramatically affected, by anxiety disorder.

Anxiety disorders are sub-divided into the following six types:

Panic Disorder. There are recurrent episodes of panic attacks AND at least one of the attacks has been followed by 1 month (or more) of the following: persistent concern about having additional attacks; worry about consequences ("going crazy," having a heart attack, losing control); or significant changes in behavior.

Panic disorder with **agoraphobia,** sometimes referred to as "adult separation anxiety," is intense anxiety or fear about being alone in places or situations where it might be difficult to escape, although a person can have a panic disorder without agoraphobia.

Phobias. The person has an irrational fear of an object or situation that persists even though the person may recognize it as unreasonable. There are three different types: (1) with **agoraphobia,** the fear of being alone in open or public places where escape might be difficult, the person may not leave home; (2) **social phobia** involves the fear of situations where one might be seen and embarrassed or criticized; typically, speaking to authority figures, public speaking, or performing; and (3) **specific phobias** refer to the fear of a single object, activity, or situation (e.g., snakes, closed spaces, flying). The anxiety is severe if the object, situation, or activity cannot be avoided.

Obsessive-Compulsive Disorder. The patient has either obsessions or compulsions; there is either preoccupation with persistent intrusive thoughts, impulses, or images **(obsession),** or repetitive behaviors or mental acts that the person feels driven to perform to reduce distress or prevent a dreaded event or situation **(compulsion).** The person knows the obsessions or compulsions are excessive and unreasonable, and the obsession or compulsion causes increased distress and is time-consuming.

Posttraumatic Stress Disorder. With posttraumatic stress disorder (PTSD) the person experienced, witnessed, or was confronted with an event that involved actual or threatened death to self or others, and responded in fear, helplessness, or horror. The event is persistently

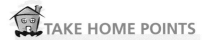

TAKE HOME POINTS

Anxiety disorder is frequently comorbid with depression.

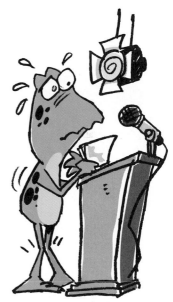

Social phobia includes the fear of public speaking.

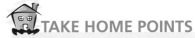

TAKE HOME POINTS

Fear of public speaking is the most common social phobia.

reexperienced by distressing dreams or images and reliving the event through flashbacks, illusions, and hallucinations. There is persistent avoidance of stimuli associated with the trauma such as avoidance of thoughts, feelings, conversations; avoidance of people, places, activities; inability to recall aspects of trauma; decreased interest in usual activities; feelings of detachment and estrangement from others; and restriction in feelings (love, enthusiasm, joy).

The symptoms are persistent, increased arousal and include two or more of the following: difficulty falling or staying asleep; irritability or outbursts of anger, and difficulty concentrating.

The symptoms may be acute—lasting less than 3 months; chronic—lasting 3 months or more; or delayed—with the onset of symptoms occurring at least 6 months after the stressful event.

Acute Stress Response. With an acute stress response the person experienced, witnessed, or was confronted with an event that involved actual or threatened death to self or others, and responded in fear, helplessness, or horror. Three or more of the following dissociative symptoms appear: a sense of numbing, detachment, or absence of emotional response; and reduced awareness of surroundings; derealization, depersonalization, and amnesia for an important aspect of the trauma. The event is persistently reexperienced through distressing dreams or images and reliving the events through flashbacks, illusions, or hallucinations. There is a marked avoidance of stimuli that arouse memory of trauma (thoughts, feelings, people, places, activities, conversations) and marked symptoms of anxiety such as difficulty falling or staying asleep; irritability or outbursts of anger; and difficulty concentrating. The symptoms cause impairment in social, occupational, and other functioning, or impair the patient's ability to complete some memory tasks. Symptoms last from 2 days to 4 weeks, which ordinarily occur within 4 weeks from the traumatic event.

Generalized Anxiety Disorder. With generalized anxiety disorder (GAD) there is excessive anxiety or worry more days than not over a 6-month period, and the person is unable to control the worrying. The anxiety and worry are associated with three or more of the following symptoms: restlessness, being keyed-up; being easily fatigued; having difficulty concentrating, mind goes blank; irritability; muscle tension; or sleep disturbance. In addition the anxiety or worry or physical symptoms cause significant impairment in social, occupational, or other areas of important functioning.

Strong evidence exists for the genetic theory. Of people diagnosed with anxiety disorder, 40% to 45% have a family member with the disorder.

Another theory proposes that damage to the hippocampus causes an overgeneralization of sensory inputs, recognizing what should be familiar input as unfamiliar and therefore dangerous. In support of the environmental theory, animal studies show a clear association between parenting in the formative years and later development of anxiety disorder.

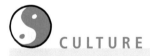

Anxiety Disorders
Association of America
www.adaa.org

At-Risk Populations

Panic disorder is twice as common in men as in women, with an onset typically between late adolescence and early adulthood. Obsessive-compulsive disorder and phobias affect men and women equally, typically manifesting during childhood, adolescence, or early adulthood. Women are more likely than men to have an anxiety disorder of the post-traumatic stress type, with the disorder affecting all age groups. General anxiety disorder can begin at any age and as early as during childhood, with women twice as likely as men to be affected.

What You NEED TO KNOW

Clinical Manifestations

The patient may present with heart palpitations, chest pain, difficulty breathing, restlessness, an inability to concentrate, dizziness, irritability, and sleep disturbance. During a panic attack the patient has feelings of impending doom, is unable to function appropriately, and may in extreme cases do him- or herself great physical harm or commit suicide. Depending upon the type of anxiety disorder, the fear of a specified situation or object **(phobia)**, intrusive thoughts or impulses (obsessions), repetitive, ritualistic behavior (compulsions), reexperiencing of a previous trauma (flashbacks), nightmares, feelings of detachment, and hallucinations are reported.

CULTURE

African Americans may report a "nervous breakdown" with feelings of tension and a deficit in self-care or activities of daily living.

Prognosis

There is significant occupational and social disability for patients suffering from an anxiety disorder as well as risk for suicide. Lack of a strong support network typically makes for a poor prognosis. Treatment does not provide a cure; however, ongoing treatment and a solid support system allows the patient with anxiety disorder to manage symptoms and minimize occupational, personal, and social disability.

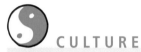
What You DO

Treatment

Treatment does not typically eliminate all problems caused by anxiety. The goal rather is to restore the occupational, social, and personal functioning that the anxiety disorder disrupts, and to relieve most of the suffering of physical and psychologic symptoms. Current treatment for anxiety disorder combines numerous therapies. Antianxiety drug therapy, usually with an antidepressant or benzodiazepine, combined with either psychotherapy, relaxation training, and systematic desensitization (gradual introduction to phobic object or situation) has been proven effective for treatment of anxiety disorders. Most patients benefits from some combination of these different forms of treatment.

Anxiety disorder is frequently comorbid with depressive disorder. Additionally, approximately 20% of patients diagnosed with social anxiety disorder, the most common type of anxiety disorder, suffer from alcoholism and require concurrent treatment for these comorbid disorders.

Nursing Responsibilities

For the patient diagnosed with anxiety disorder, the nurse should do the following:

- Assess the patient for suicidal thoughts and attempts. Ask the patient, "Have you thought of killing yourself?" Institute suicide precautions as needed for the hospitalized patient, following hospital protocol.
- Provide patient and family education regarding the disorder, prescribed treatment plan, and drug side effects. Noncompliance with drug therapy is a major obstacle in the treatment of anxiety disorder. The nurse should use compliance-enhancing strategies.
- Maintain a quiet, calm atmosphere with a structured daily routine for the hospitalized patient; stay with the patient; listen to the patient; engage the patient in activities he or she enjoys; acknowledge the patient's anxiety; and provide therapeutic interactions.
- Teach relaxation techniques and combine with deep breathing. The nurse should read the following relaxation exercise slowly and calmly, pausing for 5 to 30 seconds at each step:

  "Begin to relax by finding a comfortable position. Settle yourself, finding relaxing places for your arms, your hands, and your feet. Close your eyes gently. Now that you are settled, take three calming, deep breaths. Feel your stomach expand with each breath. Feel the tension leave your body each time you exhale. Think the word *calm* each time you exhale. Continue to breathe deeply and slowly as you relax by focusing on letting tension drift out of your body. Do not fight tension; instead, let it slide away."

- Encourage regular aerobic exercise for a minimum of 30 minutes four times per week; it is beneficial to add yoga or tai chi to this schedule. Caffeine should be avoided.
- Provide many opportunities for the patient to rehearse appropriate behavior for management of stressful situations.
- Encourage patients to use their social support network.

Do You UNDERSTAND?

DIRECTIONS: **Match the types of anxiety identified in Column B with their description in Column A.**

Column A

_____ 1. Extreme anxiety when in specific situations, such as in closed places, in high places, or flying, or about specific things, such as animals, birds, or insects.

_____ 2. Excessive anxiety or worry causing difficulty with concentration, sleep disturbance, and irritability.

_____ 3. Persistent, intrusive, unwanted thoughts and ritualistic behaviors.

_____ 4. Nightmares and flashbacks occur following a traumatic event and last more than 1 month.

_____ 5. Three or more dissociative symptoms (e.g., detachment, reduced awareness of surroundings, derealization, depersonalization, amnesia of a portion of the trauma); lasting from 2 days to 4 weeks.

Column B

a. General anxiety disorder

b. Acute stress response

c. Posttraumatic stress disorder

d. Obsessive-compulsive disorder

e. Phobias

Answers: 1. e; 2. a; 3. d; 4. c; 5. b.

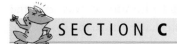

SECTION C

EATING DISORDERS

What IS Anorexia Nervosa?

Pathogenesis

Anorexia nervosa is a psychiatric disorder frequently misdiagnosed as a physical illness. The term anorexia means a loss of appetite. In anorexia nervosa, actual loss of appetite does not exist. Rather, a refusal to eat or an aberration in eating patterns and a loss of at least 15% to 25% of ideal body weight are present. Appetite is psychologic and is dependent on memory and associations, compared with hunger, which is physiologically aroused by the body's need for food. Low self-esteem is nearly always present, and the person suffering from anorexia nervosa carries on a self-dialogue of worthlessness and being unfit for love. Two types of anorexia nervosa have been defined: the food-restricting type and the binge-eating–purging type. Most patients with anorexia nervosa are women; men comprise 5% to 10% of patients with the disorder.

The cause of anorexia nervosa is unknown, but it is associated with emotional states such as anxiety, irritation, anger, and fear. One theory proposes that patients believe they have minimal control in other aspects of life, and the only part of life they can control is weight. Research reveals approximately 30% of people suffering from an eating disorder have been sexually abused. Bereavement, loss of a friend, physical abuse, and bullying are also triggers, as evidenced by the high frequency of these complaints by anorexic patients. The focus on food may be the way the anorexic patient regains control of her or his life. The societal ideal of "beautiful" or having the "right look" is also believed to be a factor in developing anorexia nervosa. Another theory proposes that because a patient with anorexia may not develop adult physical characteristics, excessive dieting may be a way of delaying maturity, thereby delaying sexual demands. Anorexia also appears to have a genetic basis, as evidenced by the high incidence of anorexia found in identical twins. Additionally, some evidence suggests that anorexia nervosa is, in part, a disorder of the hypothalamus.

Although a person with anorexia has a normal appetite, the feeling of hunger is ignored. During the course of the disease, gonadotropins are

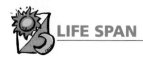

LIFE SPAN

Anorexia nervosa occurs primarily in girls after puberty. The prevalence of the disorder may be as high as 1 in 20.

not released from the anterior pituitary gland. The ovarian production of estrogens declines, and ovulation fails to occur. These conditions frequently persist long after nutritional status has improved. In some cases, menses cease before the actual weight loss becomes apparent. These factors indicate that the endocrine disturbance is not simply a consequence of malnutrition. In males who have anorexia nervosa, the level of gonadotropins and testosterone in the blood declines.

At-Risk Populations

The population at most risk for anorexia nervosa is young women, ages 12 to 18 years, who live in middle- to upper-class families. The risk for anorexia nervosa is also increased in members of professions that require low body weight, such as modeling, ballet, gymnastics, and wrestling.

What You NEED TO KNOW

Clinical Manifestations

The signs and symptoms of anorexia nervosa are usually found in a young person who is obsessed with the idea of being thin and an abnormal fear of becoming obese. Frequently, a prolonged refusal to eat occurs, to the point of danger. Patients with anorexia nervosa can also have bulimia. For patients to be diagnosed with anorexia nervosa, five criteria identified by the American Psychiatric Association must be met. These criteria include

- An intense fear of becoming obese that does not diminish as weight loss progresses.
- Disturbance of body image, such as claiming to feel fat even when emaciated.
- Refusal to maintain body weight over a minimal normal weight for age and height.
- No known physical illnesses that would account for the weight loss.
- Amenorrhea in postmenarchal women

Self-induced vomiting, use of laxatives or diuretics or both, and compulsive vigorous exercise typically accompanies these criteria. Additionally, the patient may experience weakness or exhaustion, hypotension, slow heart rate (**bradycardia**), edema, dry skin, cold hands and feet, low body temperature, and endocrine disturbances. Laboratory examination will

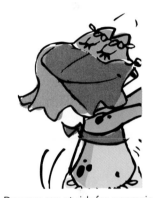

Dancers are at risk for anorexia.

CULTURE

Anorexia nervosa has been rapidly increasing throughout the world in developed countries as diverse as Russia, Japan, Australia, and the United States.

CULTURE

The population most at risk for anorexia nervosa is young women, ages 12 to 18 years, who live in middle- to upper-class families.

American Anorexia Bulimia Association, Inc.
http://www.aabainc

Eating Disorders Association
http://www.edauk.com

reveal low serum albumin and transferrin levels. A chronic state of anorexia causes decreased liver and renal function, anemia, osteoporosis from mineral loss, atrophy of the heart muscle, and cardiac arrest.

Prognosis

A cure is rare, with the goal focusing instead toward recovery by the formation of a healthy identity. Outcome is greatly improved when anorexia is diagnosed and treated early. The longer the gap between recognition of eating problems and appropriate intervention, the greater the likelihood the disorder will become chronic or result in early death. Lower weight and dysfunctional family relationships increase the likelihood of a poor outcome.

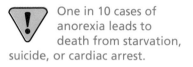

One in 10 cases of anorexia leads to death from starvation, suicide, or cardiac arrest.

What You DO

Treatment

Treatment of anorexia nervosa is difficult and lengthy, with an average duration of 5 to 7 years and including many setbacks. The primary goals are to restore normal nutrition and resolve the underlying psychologic problems. Intervention begins with hospitalization and efforts to treat the patient for starvation. Vitamins and minerals and a diet of 1200 to 1600 kcal/day is typically prescribed and given in three meals and two snacks to prevent abdominal distention. The calorie count is gradually increased. The goal of weight gain is 2 to 4 pounds per week. Milk products and fats are slowly added to the diet to avoid cramping. When a patient refuses to eat, intravenous (IV) fluid administration is necessary. Fluids are slowly introduced and gradually increased to improve fluid volume deficit. Enteral or parenteral nutrition may be required.

Various therapies help resolve the underlying psychologic problems, starting by assisting the patient to recognize and accept that at least one aspect of their behavior could be causing a serious problem. The sufferer must then be motivated to change, otherwise successful treatment is all but impossible. The patient's own strong willpower to continue maladaptive behavior throughout the course of the illness is redirected and harnessed to fight the illness instead. Treatment includes behavioral therapy, psychoanalysis, group therapy, insight-oriented therapy, and family therapy.

Nursing Responsibilities

The nurse is responsible for supporting the anorexic patient throughout therapy and helping the patient to eat. Therefore, the nurse should do the following:

- Promote early detection with thorough patient assessment. Probe in a nonjudgmental way by asking simple questions such as the following: Are you unhappy about the way you look? Would you like to be thinner than what you are? Are you dieting? Do you feel you have lost control of your eating? Do you think you have an eating problem? Do you think you might be suffering from a problem like anorexia or bulimia? (In approximately 50% of cases, the general practitioner will fail to diagnose the disorder, even in instances when the family has tried over a period of several months to alert the provider of concerns related to dysfunctional eating.)
- Assess the patient for suicidal thoughts and attempts. Ask the patient, "Have you thought of killing yourself?" Institute suicide precautions as needed for the hospitalized patient, following hospital protocol.
- Establish a therapeutic nurse-patient relationship. While this is typically challenging because anorexic patients often mistrust health professionals, research shows a therapeutic nurse-patient relationship is a pivotal factor in the treatment and recovery of patients diagnosed with anorexia nervosa.
- For the hospitalized patient, maintain a highly structured setting that includes precise meal times.
- Set firm limits regarding the selection of items from each category on the menu.
- Observe the patient during and after meals, and ensure that all food is eaten; purging is not practiced.
- Obtain daily weights each morning on the same scale and in the same type of clothing.
- Assess blood pressure, urinary output, skin turgor, and mucous membranes to monitor fluid volume status.
- Expect and manage setbacks in both the hospital and home settings.
- With management in the home setting for the patient not in need of hospitalization, teach the family to help the patient to build on the positive parts of the eating patterns rather than changing all bad habits at once. Encourage the family to reassure the anorexic patient

that she or he will be supported but that unacceptable behavior will not be ignored.

- Assist the patient in understanding that eating a healthy diet is a positive means for regaining control over behavior and activities.
- Provide patient and family education regarding the disorder and the prescribed treatment plan. Research shows training and supporting families significantly improves patient outcomes, reducing death rates and relapses.
- Provide emotional support and encouragement while allowing the patient opportunities to discuss feelings. The patient's strengths and positive coping skills are used as important parts of the care plan.
- Assist the patient to sustain positive self-esteem during treatment, because the level of self-esteem is significantly related to treatment outcome.
- Help the patient learn new methods of coping and achieve a sense of self-worth that is not exclusively based on appearance.
- Include the patient's family in therapy with the goal of enlisting the family to support the interventions of the health care providers.

Do You UNDERSTAND?

DIRECTIONS: **Indicate which statements are *true* (T) and which are *false* (F). If false, correct the statement in the margin space to make it true.**

_____   1. A clinical manifestation of anorexia nervosa is tachycardia.

_____   2. Anorexia nervosa can result in death from suicide.

_____   3. Females comprise an at-risk population for anorexia nervosa.

_____   4. Amenorrhea is a criterion used in the diagnosis of anorexia nervosa.

_____   5. Foods high in fat are immediately added to the diet plan for the anorexic patient to provide increased calories.

What IS Bulimia?

Pathogenesis

Bulimia is a compulsive eating disorder consisting of two types. Binge-purge disorder (**bulimia nervosa**) is characterized by recurrent episodes of binge eating (rapid consumption of a large quantity of food in 2 hours or less) and a sense of lack of control over eating. Purging in the form of self-induced vomiting or the use of laxatives or diuretics follows the episode of binge eating.

Binge-nonpurge disorder (**binge eating disorder**) involves uncontrolled eating that is usually kept secret. Patients engage in frequent binges but, unlike the patient with bulimia nervosa, they do not purge afterward. Up to 40% of people who are obese may be binge eaters.

The cause of bulimia or binge-eating disorder is unknown. A number of researchers believe that the eating disorder is a learned behavior that is associated with stress, anxiety, depression, loneliness, helplessness, and fear of becoming fat. The illness frequently occurs after a loss or the development of family problems. Another theory suggests that a disturbance in the appetite center of the hypothalamus contributes to bulimia or binge-eating disorder. In some cases, the onset can be traced to the patient being physically or sexually abused. A strict weight-loss diet has also been associated with the onset of bulimia.

In bulimia or binge-eating disorder, compulsive eating binges may occur as frequently as several times a day. The patient may consume thousands of calories at one sitting without hunger as a trigger. In other words, the amount of food consumed is out of proportion to the hunger that is felt. The patient is usually aware that the eating pattern is abnormal but has a preoccupying pathologic fear of becoming overweight. An unusually strong connection exists between feelings of self-worth and body shape and size. Poor impulse control results in overindulgence in other aspects of their life, such as substance abuse or sexual promiscuity.

Patients suffering from bulimia often have a history of being overweight and weight gain on low-calorie diets. When intake is restricted, patients have difficulty losing weight. These young women soon come to learn that a large intake of food, followed by purging, controls the weight.

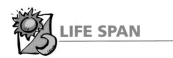

LIFE SPAN

Up to 5% of college-age women in the United States are bulimic.

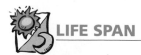

LIFE SPAN

Young women between the ages of 15 and 30 are at risk for bulimia and binge-eating disorder.

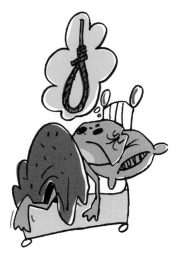

Depression is a symptom of bulimia.

TAKE HOME POINTS

Bulimia is frequently a hidden disorder that remains unnoticed by family, friends, and other acquaintances. Recognition and treatment of the disorder may not occur until the patient reaches age 40.

At-Risk Populations

The most common behavior that leads to anorexia, bulimia, or binge eating is dieting. Women with a history of poor family relationships, low self-esteem, and poor impulse control are most at risk.

What You NEED TO KNOW

Clinical Manifestations

Similar to the patient with anorexia nervosa, the patient with bulimia or binge-eating disorder uses self-destructive eating behaviors to deal with psychologic problems that may go much deeper than the obsession with food and weight.

Psychologic manifestations of bulimia include impaired impulse control, fear of obesity, and low self-esteem. Depression marked by feelings of gloom, suicidal ideation, irritability, and impaired concentration is common. Patients with long-term bulimia also report loneliness, boredom, and anger.

Other manifestations that frequently follow binge eating include abdominal pain and excessive sleeping. Frequent weight fluctuations of 10 pounds or more may be noted, although body weight is usually at or slightly below ideal. In patients suffering from the binge-purge type of bulimia, repeated vomiting can lead to bloodshot eyes, erosion of tooth enamel, swelling of the salivary glands that results from acid reflux and constant stimulation, and sore throat. The patient may complain of indigestion and heartburn from the vomiting, bloody emesis (**hematemesis**), constipation, hair loss, and irregular menses. Fistulas of the upper gastrointestinal (GI) tract may form. Additionally, because sufferers of bulimia nervosa are at high risk for self-injurious behavior, most often cutting, the patient may present with both new and old self-inflicted injuries. The patient can experience an irregular heartbeat that may lead to cardiac arrest. Fluid and electrolyte imbalances also develop. Elevated blood urea nitrogen (BUN) and serum amylase levels are found on laboratory analysis.

Prognosis

The prognosis is poor because many people with bulimia do not seek help until they reach their 40s. By this time, eating behaviors are deeply ingrained and difficult to change. The longer the gap between recognition of eating problems and appropriate intervention, the greater the likelihood the disorder will become chronic or result in early death. Drugs that are used to stimulate vomiting, bowel movements, or urination increase the risk of heart failure.

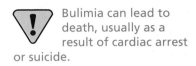 Bulimia can lead to death, usually as a result of cardiac arrest or suicide.

What You DO

Treatment

The treatment for bulimia has two goals: (1) to interrupt the binge-purge cycle by helping the patient gain control of eating habits and (2) to change attitudes toward food, eating, body size, and self. To accomplish these goals, a combination of diet management, drug therapy, psychotherapy, and exercise is used. When the patient also suffers from alcohol or drug dependency, the substance abuse is treated first.

Treatment begins with the patient being admitted to an inpatient eating disorders unit. A balanced diet is ordered that contains sufficient calories to meet the patient's basal metabolic needs. Drug therapy includes the use of an antidepressant, and potassium supplements are ordered as needed.

Psychotherapy is started while the patient is hospitalized, focusing on helping the patient develop positive coping skills for dealing with stress, anxiety, and feelings of powerlessness. Events and emotions preceding bulimic binges are identified, and the dysfunctional beliefs are modified. The patient is also educated in the importance of avoiding dieting and restricting caloric intake, which sets up the urge to binge-eat and then to compensate by purging. Lengthy outpatient treatment is usually required.

Physical exercise promotes self-regulation, possibly by reducing tension and improving ability to manage daily stress. It is important, however, that exercise activity be monitored because of the risk of using exercise as a form of purging method.

Nursing Responsibilities

The nurse is responsible for assisting the patient in breaking the binge-purge cycle and avoiding the complications associated with psychologic and metabolic upset. Therefore, the nurse should do the following:

- Promote early detection with thorough patient assessment. Probe in a nonjudgmental way by asking simple questions such as: Are you unhappy about the way you look? Would you like to be thinner than what you are? Are you dieting? Do you feel you have lost control of your eating? Do you think you have an eating problem? Do you think you might be suffering from a problem like anorexia or bulimia?
- Assist the patient in selecting the right portions of foods from all four food groups. The patient is usually allowed to refuse a specific number of foods (e.g., two or three), thus some sense of control is felt.
- Help the hospitalized patient understand that only the foods provided by the dietary department must be eaten and that all of the meal must be consumed. Remain with the patient for at least 1 hour after eating to provide support and reduce the likelihood the patient will induce vomiting.
- Encourage the patient to eat slowly and recognize feelings of satiety.
- Provide supervision and emotional support for the patient during stressful periods.
- Expect and manage setbacks in both the hospital and home settings.
- For the patient not in need of hospitalization, teach the family to help the patient to build on the positive parts of the eating patterns rather than changing all bad habits at once.
- Assist the patient in understanding that eating a healthy diet is a positive means for regaining control over behavior and activities.
- Allow the patient to express feelings and assist in developing positive coping skills to deal with anxiety and stress.
- Assist the patient and family in identifying other areas of self-regard that are unrelated to food.
- Provide age-appropriate and culturally appropriate patient and family teaching regarding the disorder and treatment to help prevent the development of anorexia nervosa.

- Monitor potassium levels at regular intervals, administering potassium supplements as prescribed. In some cases, IV potassium replacement may be needed.
- Encourage regular aerobic exercise for a minimum of 30 minutes four times per week; it is beneficial to add yoga or tai chi to this schedule.
- Determine whether drugs or alcohol are abused. Recommend drug and alcohol treatment and involvement in support programs such as Alcoholics Anonymous and Narcotics Anonymous for patients suffering from drug or alcohol addiction.

Do You UNDERSTAND?

DIRECTIONS: **Provide answers to each of the following questions.**

1. Name at least three methods that bulimic patients use to prevent weight gain _____ _____ _____.

2. In what age decade do most people with bulimia usually seek help _____?

3. What are the two most common causes of death related to bulimia _____, _____?

4. What are the three interventions used in the treatment of bulimia _____, _____, _____?

5. List six nursing responsibilities in caring for the bulimic patient.

_____

_____

_____

_____

_____

_____

Answers: 1. vomiting, laxatives, diuretics, fasting, excessive exercise 2. 40s 3. cardiac arrest, suicide; 4. diet management, drug therapy, psychotherapy; 5. assisting the patient in breaking the binge-purge cycle, helping the patient select the right portions of foods from all four food groups, observation of the patient during and after meals, allowing the patient to express feelings, providing emotional support to the patient during stressful periods, assisting the patient in developing positive coping skills, educating the patient regarding the long-term goal of improving self-esteem, monitoring potassium levels, and administering potassium as ordered.

References

American Psychiatric Association: *Diagnostic and statistical manual of mental disorders,* ed 4, Washington, DC, 1994, Author.

Anxiety Disorders Association of America: *Anxiety disorders,* 2005, URL http://www/adaa.org/AnxietyDisorderInfor/gad.cfm.

Badger F, Nolan P: Caring for people with depression, *Nurs Stand* 16(26):33, 2002.

Baethge C et al: Effectiveness and outcome predictors of long-term lithium prophylaxis in unipolar major depressive disorder, *J Psychiatry Neurosci* 28(5):355, 2003.

Charbonneau A et al: Measuring the quality of depression care in a large integrated health system, *Med Care* 41(5):669, 2003.

Chien W et al: Educational needs of families caring for patients with schizophrenia, *J Clin Nurs* 11(5):695, 2002.

Cooper LA et al: The acceptability of treatment for depression among African-American, Hispanic, and White primary care patients, *Med Care* 41(4):479, 2003.

Dickerson FB, Pater A, Origoni AE: Health behaviors and health status of older women with schizophrenia, *Psychiatr Serv* 53(7):882, 2002.

DuPont RL, Spencer ED, DuPont CM: *The anxiety cure,* Hoboken, NJ, 2003, John Wiley & Sons.

Embling S: The effectiveness of cognitive behavioural therapy in depression, *Nurs Stand* 17(14-15):33, 2002.

Gall SH et al: Supporting careers of people diagnosed with schizophrenia: evaluating change in nursing practice following training, *J Adv Nurs* 41(3):295, 2003.

Holzinger A et al: Subjective illness theory and antipsychotic medication compliance by patients with schizophrenia, *J Nerv Ment Dis* 190(9):597, 2002.

Huprich SK: Depressive personality and its relationship to depressed mood, interpersonal loss, negative parental perceptions, and perfectionism, *J Nerv Ment Dis* 191(2):73, 2003.

Internet Mental Health: *Eating disorders,* 2005, URL http://www.mentalhealth.com/dis/p20-et01.html.

Lloyd-Williams M et al: Is asking patients in palliative care, "Are you depressed?" appropriate? Prospective study, *BMJ* 327(10):372, 2003.

Maj M, Sartorius N: *Schizophrenia,* Hoboken, NJ, 2003, John Wiley & Sons.

Miller R, Mason SE: *Diagnosis schizophrenia: a comprehensive resource,* New York, 2002, Columbia University Press.

Minardi HA, Blanchard M: Older people with depression: pilot study, *J Adv Nurs* 46(1):23, 2004.

Ohayon MM, Schatzberg AF: Prevalence of depressive episodes with psychotic features in the general population, *Am J Psychiatry* 159(11):1855, 2002.

Paul T, Schroeter K, Dahme B, Nutzinger DO: Self-injurious behavior in women with eating disorders, *Am J Psychiatry* 159(3):408, 2002.

Power M: *Mood disorders,* Hoboken, NJ, 2004, John Wiley & Sons.

Ramjan LM: Nurses and the 'therapeutic relationship': caring for adolescents with anorexia nervosa, *J Adv Nurs* 45(5):495, 2004.

Roe D: A prospective study on the relationship between self-esteem and functioning during the first year after being hospitalized for psychosis, *J Nerv Ment Dis* 191(1):45, 2003.

Smith CE, Leenerts MH, Gajewski BJ: A systematically tested intervention for managing reactive depression, *Nurs Res* 52(6):401, 2003.

Smith G: *Anorexia and bulimia in the family: one parent's practical guide to recovery,* Hoboken, NJ, 2004, John Wiley & Sons.

Striegel-Moore RH et al: Abuse, bullying, and discrimination as risk factors for binge eating disorder, *Am J Psychiatry* 159(11):1902, 2002.

Sundgot-Borgen J et al: The effect of exercise, cognitive therapy, and nutritional counseling in treating bulimia nervosa, *Med Sci Sports Exerc* 34(3):190, 2002.

Thomas J et al: A descriptive and comparative study of the prevalence of depressive and anxiety disorders in low-income adults with type 2 diabetes and other chronic illnesses, *Diabetes Care* 26(8):2311, 2003.

Thomas SE, Randall CL, Carrigan MH: Drinking to cope in socially anxious individuals: a controlled study, *Alcohol Clin Exp Res* 27(12):1937, 2003.

Tryssenaar J, Gray H: Providing meaningful continuing education in a changing long-term care environment, *J Nurses Staff Dev* 20(1):1, 2004.

Willetts L, Leff J: Improving the knowledge and skills of psychiatric nurses: efficacy of a staff training programme, *J Adv Nurs* 42(3):237, 2003.

NCLEX® Review

1. The nurse is having a therapeutic conversation with a 47-year-old female patient diagnosed with schizophrenia. The patient perseverates on delusions of reference, becoming agitated and pointing to two other patients in the room who are quietly watching TV, saying "Those two are saying mean things about me!" The nurse knows the best course of action is to
   1 Allow the patient to spend some time alone, telling her you will return when she is calmer.
   2 Take a hold of the patient's hand to show empathy and support.
   3 Tell the two patients who are watching TV that they must leave the room, explaining that their presence is clearly upsetting for your patient.
   4 Maintain eye contact with the patient, focusing on discussing the patient's feelings and not arguing about the content of the delusion.

2. The pediatrician diagnoses a 9-year-old boy with depressive disorder. Which of the following complaints do you, as the nurse, expect to hear from the mother as a clinical manifestation of the boy's depressive disorder?
   1 Hostility
   2 Underachievement in school
   3 Drug use
   4 Backache

3. The nurse is caring for a 24-year-old patient with a diagnosis of bipolar disorder. The patient frequently confides in the nurse that she is sad to see the nurse's shift nearly ending because the evening shift nurses are uncaring and rarely talk to her. You recognize this as
   1 A serious issue of inappropriate behavior of the evening shift nursing staff to be handled by writing a formal complaint to the director of nursing.
   2 An indication that the patient has a comorbid alcoholism disorder.

3 An attempt by the patient to divide the staff and cause the staff to become angry at one another.
   4 Atypical behavior for the patient diagnosed with bipolar disorder.

4. Which of the following is NOT a manifestation of an anxiety disorder?
   1 Hypersomnia
   2 Irritability
   3 Chest pain
   4 Intrusive thoughts

5. A 17-year-old patient diagnosed with anorexia nervosa was a member of a predischarge support group. When she verbalized her financial inability to buy new clothes, other group members offer to provide her with some of their used clothes. The patient accepted the clothes but believed that they were too tight and she reduced her caloric intake. The nurse recognized this behavior as
   1 Normal behavior.
   2 Evidence of the patient's altered or distorted body image.
   3 Regression because the patient is approaching discharge.
   4 Indicative of the patient's ambivalence about moving towards outpatient treatment.

6. The nurse is evaluating the progress of a 28-year-old woman admitted to the psychiatric unit with a diagnosis of bulimia nervosa. Which of the following behaviors would indicate that the patient had progressed?
   1 Her conversations focus on food.
   2 She identifies healthy ways of coping with anxiety.
   3 She spends time alone in her room after each meal.
   4 She engages in rigorous exercise.

NCLEX® Review Answers

1. **4** The patient is experiencing strong feelings. Time should be spent in a therapeutic conversation allowing the patient the opportunity to express her feelings. The nurse should avoid physical contact with the patient because the patient may feel threatened by touch. There is no need to ask the uninvolved patients to leave the room.

2. **2** Depressive disorder in childhood is frequently manifested as underachievement in school. Hostility and drug use are commonly found in the adolescent population when afflicted with depressive disorder. Backache is often a complaint made by the adult suffering from depressive disorder.

3. **3** Splitting the staff is a common behavior of the patient who suffers from bipolar disorder, requiring consistency among staff of implementation of limit-setting interventions. There is no evidence provided in this scenario that indicates the patient has a comorbid alcoholism disorder or that the evening shift staff is providing inappropriate nursing care.

4. **1** The patient with anxiety disorder has difficulty sleeping, not hypersomnia. Hypersomnia is seen in the patient suffering from bipolar disorder during a depressive episode. Irritability, chest pain, and intrusive thoughts are all manifestations of anxiety disorder.

5. **4** The nurse realizes that this behavior indicates the patient is ambivalent about hospital discharge. This behavior is not normal. The patient already has an altered or distorted body image by virtue of her diagnosis. Her behaviors do not reflect regression to previous symptoms of her disorder.

6. **2** The patient who is identifying healthy ways to handle anxiety indicates that she has progressed. Conversations focusing on food, spending time alone after eating, and vigorously exercising are all signs that she will continue to practice bulimia.

Notes

Index